LUNG SURFACTANT
FUNCTION AND DISORDER

LUNG BIOLOGY IN HEALTH AND DISEASE

Executive Editor

Claude Lenfant

Former Director, National Heart, Lung, and Blood Institute
National Institutes of Health
Bethesda, Maryland

The opinions expressed in these volumes do not necessarily represent the views of the National Institutes of Health.

LUNG SURFACTANT FUNCTION AND DISORDER

Edited by

Kaushik Nag
Memorial University of Newfoundland
St. John's, Newfoundland and Labrador, Canada

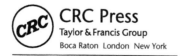

CRC Press
Taylor & Francis Group
Boca Raton London New York

CRC Press is an imprint of the
Taylor & Francis Group, an **informa** business

CRC Press
Taylor & Francis Group
6000 Broken Sound Parkway NW, Suite 300
Boca Raton, FL 33487-2742

First issued in paperback 2019

© 2011 by Taylor & Francis Group, LLC
CRC Press is an imprint of Taylor & Francis Group, an Informa business

No claim to original U.S. Government works

ISBN-13: 978-0-8247-5792-2 (hbk)
ISBN-13: 978-0-367-39289-5 (pbk)

A CIP record for this book is available from the British Library.

Library of Congress Cataloging-in-Publication Data available on application

Visit the Informa Web site at
www.informa.com

and the Informa Healthcare Web site at
www.informahealthcare.com

Introduction

Our odyssey of discovery and understanding with regard to lung surfactant has been long and fascinating. And indeed, the monographs found in the Lung Biology in Health and Disease series has given recognition to this journey through chapters in several monographs and through entire volumes devoted to lung surfactant and its function in health and disease. Some may ask the question "Why is there such an interest in this subject?"

Two reasons can be found in two remarkable books. In *Retrospectroscope—Insight into Medical Discovery* by Julius Comroe (1), the last three chapters titled "Premature Science and Immature Lungs, Part I to III" retrace the journey of surfactant from Laplace's Traite de Mecanique Celeste (2) to a life-saving treatment for prematurely born infants. This journey spanned almost two centuries. The second book, *The Restless Tide—The Persistent Challenge of the Microbial World*, by Richard M. Krause (3) can be summed up in a quotation from Thomas Babington (1830): "A single breaker may recede; but the tide is evidently coming in."

The essential message of these two books—that, often, we think we know what to do, but we really do not!—is actually the rationale for this new monograph *Lung Surfactant Function and Disorder*, edited by Dr. Kaushik Nag. The reader is introduced to many disciplines applicable to the study of lung surfactant, including chemistry, biochemistry, physics, genetics, computer science, physiology, and medicine. All are presented by well-known investigators from many countries and several continents.

Overall, this book illustrates the complexity, and expectations, of research on surfactant. In his Preface, Dr. Nag acknowledges Pierre De Gennes, who stated in his Nobel Lecture (1991) that "it is perhaps amazing to note that there is some overlap in thought between people who study high brow string theories, and description of soaps." This is reminiscent of a statement by C. V. Bogs in one of his lectures on "Soap Bubbles": "I hope that none of you are yet tired of playing with bubbles because, as I hope we shall see, there is more in a common bubble than those who have only played with them generally imagine" (4).

The series Lung Biology in Health and Disease is very pleased to present this latest volume on surfactant. It gives a new, and different perspective, reminding us that research and knowledge—like the tides—are a dynamic and an ever-renewed process.

Claude Lenfant, MD
Gaithersburg, Maryland

References

1. Comroe J. Retrospectroscope—Insight into Medical Discovery. Menlo Park, California: Von Gehr Press, 1977.
2. Laplace PS. Traite de Mecanique Celeste. Vol. 5. Crufelet and Courcier Paris, 1798–1827.
3. Krause RM. The Restless Tide—The Persistent Challenge of the Microbial World. The National Foundation for Infectious Diseases, 1981.
4. Bogs CV. Soap Bubbles: Their Colours and the Forces that Mold Them. London: Society for Promoting Christian Knowledge, 1890.

Preface

There have been major breakthroughs in lung surfactant (LS) research over the last two decades that have changed our concept of how and why the material works well at the lung air–water interface. From the initial ideas of a surface active material lining the alveoli to the seminal concepts of how low surface tension is reached, the classical ideas about Comroe's "extraordinary juice" requires revision and re-thinking. From the early concepts developed by Von Neergard, Pattle, Clements, Avery, and Bangham—to current status and future directions developed by others—LS research has come a long way.

The concept of this volume was developed about two years ago, at a Biophysical meeting and later at the American Thoracic Society meeting where I had the pleasure of meeting a number of upcoming researchers in the field. I was humbled to know how less a biophysicist like myself knew about the clinical and molecular biology aspects of LS. Our physicochemical way of looking at LS as a membranous or colloidal system was difficult to describe to the clinical scientists. This volume is a small contribution in explaining basic and clinical laboratory knowledge to the larger audience and surfactant researchers, at an advanced basic–clinical interface.

Although in recent years there have been a number of excellent reviews on various aspects of LS, like most reviews these tend to encompass a large volume of data and multiple interpretations and do not allow for easily bringing in new concepts from researchers. There are a number of other volumes included in the *Lung Biology in Health and Disease* series, such as volumes 1, 12, 24, 35, 55, 84, 121, 143 that have chapters devoted to LS related research, and have contributed to our understanding of LS over the last three decades. There is also a single authored volume (vol. 149), that focuses on biophysics as well as clinical aspects of LS at a basic level. There are also a few review books, almost a decade old, written by experts in the field. Normally, review books are written and edited by such experts. However, breaking this norm for this volume was due to my personal situation at the time of conception of this book as a post-doctoral fellow in an obscure university in Canada. At that time I was struggling with the toils and troubles of stable bubbles, and of securing a more permanent position (possibly in another obscure university in Canada). I have enthusiastically pursued respiratory research from my honors student days in India, leading to a masters in Physiology (Biophysics) and Biochemistry, and finally doctoral and postdoctoral training in lung biology. Over the past two decades I have had the opportunity to observe the LS system from a biophysical as well as a clinical viewpoint. During this period what fascinated me about surfactant was that the molecular mechanisms of its action could be interpreted from fields as diverse as neonatal physiology, genetic knockout mice, soft condensed matter, and nanobiology.

I had initially approached some new and upcoming researchers in this field who were at this stage of transition—from postdoctoral to the higher echelons of academia—to either create their own chapter or do so with co-contributors. This volume is thus designed to focus on laboratory research areas of some new and exciting semi-classical concepts of LS that try to encompass biophysics, molecular biology, clinical physiology, developmental and microbiology as well as surface and interfacial chemistry, physics, membranes, soft matter, and molecular imaging. The word "lung" is utilized throughout (and in the title) to replace "pulmonary," considering the presence of LS beyond the alveoli in the upper airways, and its role in asthma and upper respiratory tract disease. Also the parenthesis to the word (dys)function is used since some of the functional aspects of LS are not clear to date, and molecular mechanisms of disease and dysfunction of the material are only emerging.

This book is structured in a format where we attempt to broadly discuss the diversity of molecular composition (Chapters 1–5) and some current methodology in rapid analysis of LS lipids (Chapter 2) in various species and in health and disease (Chapter 1). The current status of surfactant proteins are presented in Chapters 3, 4, and 5. A few surprises have emerged along the way, as we now know that lung surfactant contain different disaturated lipids, other than DPPC (Chapter 1), and that some species breathe fine without this lipid being present in "large" amounts in their surfactant (Chapter 2). Others have recently compressed a fluid phospholipid film to reach near zero surface tensions in captive bubbles (Chapter 6) and observed similar properties of liquid crystalline membranes and LS (Chapter 7). The structure–function property of LS is too vast and detailed, thus I have taken the liberty to select a set of discussions on the function of lipids and lipid–protein systems, from a molecular mechanism and biophysics viewpoint (Chapters 6–13). Some of these (Chapters 9–13) discuss the classical concepts of the "laboratory assigned" roles of the surfactant proteins from SP-A to SP-D, while we wait for SP-Es and Fs to emerge. The book, however, includes other discussions especially for the possible new and emerging role of hydrophobic proteins in processes such as channel activity (Chapters 8 and 14) and in another section as antimicrobials (Chapter 17).

Although the final section of the book deals with (dys)function and disease aspects of surfactant from the clinical (Chapters 16 and 17), physiology (Chapter 15), replacement therapy aspects (Chapter 19), only a few contributions are assembled to provide a sample of such studies (Chapters 15–19). This is due to various aspects of lung disease related to LS discussed in previous books and volumes of this series. Thus I have only chosen a sample few, in order to provide researchers the necessary laboratory experience. I make no naive claims to either comprehend this vast area of respiratory distress, nor have I tried to attempt to provide a comprehensive and all inclusive glimpse at the complexity of LS dysfunction. My sincerest apologies to numerous upcoming and excellent researchers in this area for not being able include their work, due to shortage of textual space. This will possibly also allow one to avoid extreme physical discomfort and consumption of muscle (brain) relaxants which may be required while handling this volume. A future volume in editorial collaborations with experts in the clinical areas may be forthcoming, depending on the reception of this volume by the LS community.

I must confess my personal heavy-handedness in dealing with the Biophysics section (Chapters 6–14) since this is one area I feel comfortable with compared to my naivety in most others. (After all how do we study a floating membrane in the lung?) This section deals with the concept of low surface tension in the lung that may be induced by a fluid lipid defying some classical concepts (Chapter 7), to applying cell membrane "lipid rafts" or structural concept to surfactant (Chapter 6). Such methods rely heavily on new and powerful physicochemical techniques utilized to pin down single molecules, molecular motions, and aggressively define LS as soft matter—either inside an atomic force microscope (Chapters 11 and 12) or a computer (Chapter 9). Some of this methodology also requires a certain level of mathematical sophistication to be defined by experts (some of these colleagues are clinical scientists with doctorates in physical chemistry and physics). Someday these technologies may be helpful to new and emerging researchers who venture into the intricate world of nuclear spins of surfactant proteins (Chapter 11), knock-out genes (Chapter 13), and to smash DPPC under ion-beams (Chapter 10).

It would be a fallacy in even trying to acknowledge all the colleagues, co-authors, and experts that I have met and discussed LS research with for over two decades, having thus directly/indirectly contributed to this volume. However, I wish to thank a few, such as Dr. Claude Lenfant (Executive Editor of this series) for inviting me to edit this book, Prof. Fereidoon Shahidi (Biochemistry, Memorial University), and Anita Lekhwani (Acquisitions Editor, Taylor & Francis Group), for help in providing the necessary enthusiasm, editorial, and publication guidelines, without which this volume would never have seen publication. I would be remiss not to acknowledge the help and support of my mentor Dr. Kevin Keough (President, Alberta Heritage Foundation for Medical Research, Canada), who has continuously and enthusiastically encouraged as well as criticized my continuous adventure into the world of LS and membranes. A belated gratitude goes to the late Prof. Haripada Chattopadhayay of Presidency College, Kolkata (West Bengal, India) who had first showed me how breathing patterns of humans change due to circadian rhythms, in a dark room in India. Incidentally this room was above a floor of the Physics department, where C.V. Raman and S. Bose extrapolated their ideas on molecular vibration patterns and Bose–Einstein condensates, more than half a century ago. Funding for my studies in North America is gratefully acknowledged from the Medical Research Council of Canada, Ontario Thoracic Society, Canadian Lung Association, National Scientific and Educational Research Council, and recently from Canadian Institute of Health Research, Canada Foundation for Innovation, and Memorial University of Newfoundland.

Having actually watched the whales spray their lung surfactant in the bays of Newfoundland, to seeing and touching the terminal methyl chains of DPPC—or observing neonatal recovery after LS administration—I feel there are many fascinating discoveries yet to be made on Comroe's "extraordinary juice." As the master of analogy Pierre De Gennes stated in his Nobel Lecture "it is perhaps amusing to note that there is some overlap in thought between people who study high brow string theories and description of soaps" (see Chapter 6 for details). I sincerely hope this volume provides such overlap in lung surfactant researchers from biology, chemistry, physics, computer science, and medicine.

Kaushik Nag

Contributors

Mathias Amrein *Faculty of Medicine, University of Calgary, Alberta, Calgary, Canada*

Rinti Banerjee *School of Biosciences and Bioengineering, Indian Institute of Technology, Mumbai, India*

Timothy C. Bailey *Department of Physiology and Pharmacology and Department of Medicine, University of Western Ontario, London, Ontario, Canada*

Wolfgang Bernhard *Division of Neonatology, University of Tübingen, Tübingen, Germany*

Nikolaus Bourdos* *Institut für Biochemie, Westfälische Wilhelms-Universität Münster, Münster, Germany*

Current affiliation: Lehrstuhl für Biophysik, Ruhr Universität Bochum, Universitäts-strasse, Bochum, Germany.

Cristina Casals *Department of Biochemistry and Molecular Biology I, Complutense University of Madrid, Madrid, Spain*

Antonio Cruz *Department of Bioquímica, Universidad Complutense, Madrid, Spain*

Christopher B. Daniels *Department of Environmental Biology, University of Adelaide, Adelaide, Australia*

Haim Diamant *Department of Chemistry, Tel Aviv University, Tel Aviv, Israel*

Jonathan R. Faulkner *Departments of Ob/Gyn and Biochemistry, University of Western Ontario, London, Ontario, Canada*

Hans-Joachim Galla *Institut für Biochemie, Westfälische Wilhelms-Universität Münster, Münster, Germany*

Ignacio García-Verdugo *Department of Biochemistry and Molecular Biology I, Complutense University of Madrid, Madrid, Spain*

Donald P. Gaver III *Department of Biomedical Engineering, Tulane University, New Orleans, Louisiana, USA*

Stephan W. Glasser *Division of Pulmonary Biology, Cincinnati Children's Hospital Medical Center, Cincinnati, Ohio, USA*

Stephen B. Hall *Molecular Medicine, Oregon Health & Science University, Portland, Oregon, USA*

David Halpern *Department of Mathematics, University of Alabama, Tuscaloosa, USA*

Egbert Herting *Professor of Pediatrics, University of Lübeck, Lübeck, Germany*

Robert R. Harbottle *Department of Chemistry, University of Western Ontario, London, Ontario, Canada*

Jens M. Hohlfeld *Department of Respiratory Medicine, Hannover Medical School and Fraunhofer Institute of Toxicology and Experimental Medicine, Hannover, Germany*

M. G. Haufs *BGFA, Ruhr-Universität Bochum, Bochum, Germany*

Oliver E. Jensen *School of Mathematical Sciences, University of Nottingham, Nottingham, UK*

Chutima Jiarpinitnun *Department of Chemistry, The University of Chicago, Chicago, Illinois, USA*

Yiannis N. Kaznessis *Department of Chemical Engineering and Materials Science, and Digital Technology Center, University of Minnesota, Minneapolis/St. Paul, Minnesota, USA*

D. Knebel *JPK-Instruments AG, Berlin, Germany*

Thomas R. Korfhagen *Division of Pulmonary Biology, Cincinnati Children's Hospital Medical Center, Cincinnati, Ohio, USA*

Josh W. Kurutz *Department of Chemistry, The University of Chicago, Chicago, Illinois, USA*

Carol J. Lang *Department of Environmental Biology, University of Adelaide, Adelaide, Australia*

Ronald G. Larson *Department of Chemical Engineering, University of Michigan, Ann Arbor, Michigan, USA*

Stefan Malcharek *Institut für Biochemie, Westfälische Wilhelms-Universität Münster, Münster, Germany*

Jeya Nadesalingam *Department of Biochemistry, Oxford University, Oxford, UK*

Kaushik Nag *Department of Biochemistry, Memorial University of Newfoundland, St. John's, Newfoundland and Labrador, Canada*

David G. Oelberg *Center for Pediatric Research, Eastern Virginia Medical School and Children's Hospital of The King's Daughters, Norfolk, Virginia, USA*

Sandra Orgeig *Department of Environmental Biology, University of Adelaide, Adelaide, Australia*

Nades Palaniyar* *Department of Biochemistry, Oxford University, Oxford, UK*

Amiya K. Panda *Department of Chemistry, Behala College, Kolkata, West Bengal, India*

Jesús Pérez-Gil *Department of Bioquímica, Universidad Complutense, Madrid, Spain*

Inés Plasencia *Department of Bioquímica, Universidad Complutense, Madrid, Spain*

Fred Possmayer *Departments of Ob/Gyn and Biochemistry, University of Western Ontario, London, Ontario, Canada*

**Current affiliation*: Lung Biology Research Program, Hospital for Sick Children Research Institute, Toronto, Ontario, Canada.

Tony Postle *Division of Infection, Inflammation and Repair, School of Medicine and Southampton General Hospital, Southampton, UK*

Kenneth B. M. Reid *Department of Biochemistry, Oxford University, Oxford, UK*

Bengt Robertson *Laboratory for Surfactant Research, Department of Surgical Sciences, Karolinska University Hospital, Stockholm, Sweden*

Karina Rodriguez-Capote *Departments of Ob/Gyn and Biochemistry, University of Western Ontario, London, Ontario, Canada*

Sandra Rugonyi *Molecular Medicine, Oregon Health & Science University, Portland, Oregon, USA*

Ruud A. W. Veldhuizen *Department of Physiology and Pharmacology and Department of Medicine, University of Western Ontario, London, Ontario, Canada*

Sangeetha Vidyashankar *Department of Biochemistry, Memorial University of Newfoundland, St. John's, Newfoundland and Labrador, Canada*

Alan J. Waring *Department of Pediatrics, University of California, Los Angeles, California, USA*

Tom Witten *The James Franck Institute and Department of Physics, The University of Chicago, Chicago, Illinois, USA*

Ka Yee C. Lee *The Institute for Biophysical Dynamics, The University of Chicago, Chicago, Illinois, USA*

Contents

COMPOSITION, STRUCTURE, AND FUNCTION

Composition, Structure, and Function

1

Lung Surfactant Phospholipid Molecular Species in Health and Disease

TONY POSTLE

School of Medicine and Southampton
    General Hospital,
Southampton, UK

WOLFGANG BERNHARD

University of Tübingen,
Tübingen, Germany

I. Introduction

The importance of the phospholipid component for the physiological function of lung surfactant has been recognized for many years. However, the effects of development and disease on the detailed phospholipid composition of surfactant have received relatively little attention until recently, largely because of lack of sensitivity and specificity of the analytical methods available. Phospholipids are characterized either as glycerophospholipids, with fatty acids esterified at the *sn*-1 and *sn*-2 positions of the glycerophosphate backbone of the molecule, or as sphingolipids, with a fatty acid esterified to a sphingosine phosphate moiety (Fig. 1.1). The head group attached to the phosphate of glycerophospholipids can be choline, ethanolamine, serine, glycerol, or inositol to give, respectively, phosphatidylcholine (PtdCho), phosphatidylethanolamine (PtdEtn), phosphatidylserine (PtdSer), phosphatidylglycerol (PtdGly), or phosphatidylinositol (PtdIns). The vast majority of sphingolipids have choline esterified to the phosphate to generate sphingomyelin. Within each of these phospholipid classes, there is a spectrum of individual molecular species, defined by the combination of esterified fatty acids attached to the glycerol. Generally, membrane glycerophospholipids tend to have palmitoyl $(16:0)^1$ or stearoyl (18:0) at their *sn*-1 position and unsaturated fatty acids esterified at *sn*-2. The esterified fatty acid in sphingolipids is generally saturated, but can often contain as many as 22 or 24 carbon atoms.

Historically, techniques to measure individual molecular species of phospholipids have been very time consuming and either insensitive or technically demanding. An indication of the molecular species composition of surfactant phospholipid from newborn infants was provided by using thin-layer chromatography on silver nitrate-impregnated silica plates (1), which resolves phospholipids on the basis of their total number of unsaturated double bonds. More direct information about individual species can be provided by high-performance liquid chromatography (HPLC), with either precolumn (2–4) or postcolumn (5,6) derivative formation, but these techniques have proved too specialized and laborious to be adopted for widespread use. More recently, advances in instrument design have established electrospray ionization-mass spectrometry (ESI-MS) as a technique for analyzing phospholipid molecular species in great detail and with exquisite sensitivity (7). ESI-MS is a soft ionization technique that generates molecular ions with minimal fragmentation and is ideally suited to characterizing surfactant phospholipid molecular species (8,9).

Perhaps ironically, one additional reason for the relative lack of interest in individual surfactant phospholipid molecular species was the early identification of the importance of PC16:0/16:0 for surfactant function. Demonstrations

---

[1]The abbreviation for fatty acids is given by the number of carbon atoms and carbon:carbon double bonds in the molecule. Thus, the saturated 16 carbon atom palmitate molecule is 16:0, the monounsaturated palmitoleate and oleate molecules are, respectively, 16:1 and 18:1, and the more unsaturated linoleate and arachidonate molecules are, respectively, 18:2 and 20:4. Individual molecular species of glycerophospholipids are designated first by the identity of the polar headgroup and then by the combination of fatty acids. Consequently, dipalmitoyl phosphatidylcholine is PC16:0/16:0, whereas 1-stearoyl-2arachidonoyl phosphatidylinositol is PI18:0/20:4.

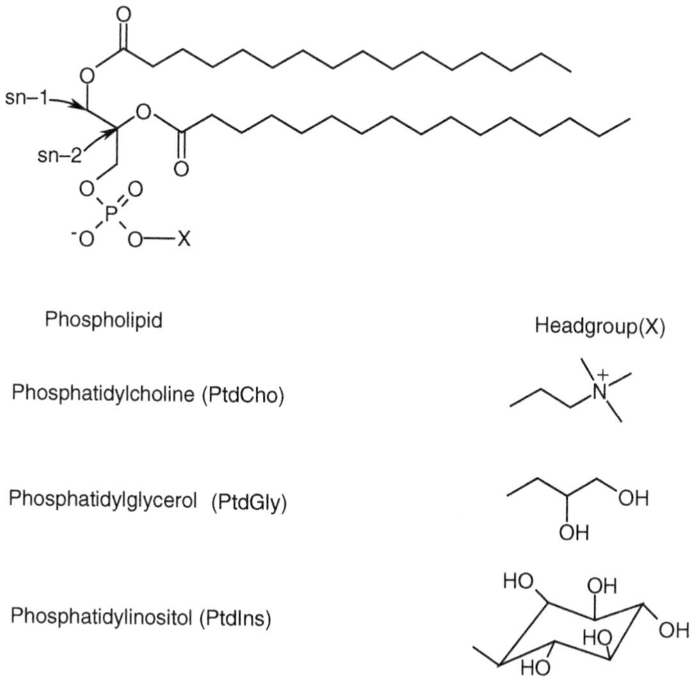

Figure 1.1 Molecular structures of phospholipids.

in vitro that PC16:0/16:0 could mimic many of the surface properties of surfactant meant that little attention was paid in clinical studies to the precise identities of the other phospholipid species. In addition, development of simple robust techniques to quantify disaturated PtdCho (DSPC) as the residue after the oxidative destruction of unsaturated species (10) led to the general identification of DSPC as PC16:0/16:0. This concentration on the central importance of PC16:0/16:0 in surfactant function has been reinforced by more recent observations that an effective exogenous surfactant can be constructed from this single PtdCho species together with acidic phospholipids and hydrophilic surfactant peptides (11). However, considerable evidence now suggests that surfactant phospholipid composition varies in response to the physiological demands of breathing (12) and that PtdCho species other than PC16:0/16:0 may contribute to surfactant function. This is especially relevant in the light of experiments showing that monounsaturated PtdCho species can display surface properties generally attributed to PC16:0/16:0 (13). Moreover, recent studies have demonstrated that under dynamic conditions surface tension lowering function of surfactants is inferior for preparations which are highly enriched in PC16:0/16:0 but are deprived in other characteristic PtdCho molecular species (discussed subsequently), irrespective of the presence of the hydrophobic surfactant protein SP-B (12).

II. Composition of Surfactant Phospholipid Molecular Species in the Adult Lungs

Estimates that PC16:0/16:0 contributes 70–80% of surfactant PtdCho, based on the OsO_4 oxidation technique, are now generally recognized as too high (14) both because of the presence of other disaturated species including PC16:0/14:0 and PC16:0/18:0 and because of the oxidation of monounsaturated species is often incomplete. In contrast, analysis by either HPLC or ESI-MS provides a good agreement about the molecular species of PtdCho in lung surfactant, but this composition can vary considerably between different animal species and will alter to adapt to pulmonary structure and the physiological demands put on the lungs. Values for the PC16:0/16:0 content in native mammalian surfactants vary between 35.6% for rabbit and 54% for humans (15) and in therapeutic surfactants from 39.4% in bovine Alveofact to 50.2% in porcine Curosurf (16). Examples of ESI-MS analysis of lung surfactant PtdCho are shown in Fig. 1.2, which details mass spectra of material isolated from adult mouse, rabbit, and human lungs. Apart from the variation in PC16:0/16:0, it is clear that surfactant PtdCho from all these animals contains the same overall range of molecular

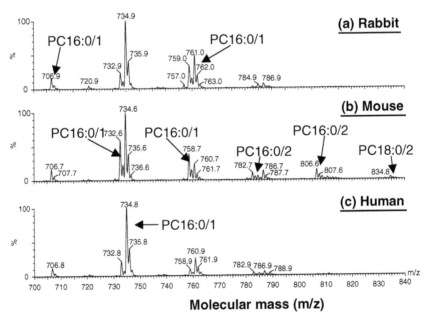

Figure 1.2 ESI-MS of PtdCho molecular species from adult (a) rabbit, (b) mouse, and (c) human surfactant. PtdCho species were determined as precursor scans of the phosphorylcholine fragment ($m/z = 184$).

species, but with different distributions. Strikingly, all surfactants analyzed contained predominantly 16:0 at their *sn*-1 position, with *sn*-1 stearoyl and *sn*-1 oleoyl together accounting for <10%. These surfactants contained essentially only four major PtdCho molecular species other than PC16:0/16:0 and small amounts of polyunsaturated species. As will be discussed later, PC16:0/18:2 and PC16:0/18:1 are major components of plasma lipoprotein and inflammatory cell membrane PtdCho, respectively, in addition to being minor components of surfactant. In contrast, PC16:0/14:0 and PC16:0/16:1 are minor components of cell membrane PtdCho and can be regarded as diagnostic for surfactant. This conclusion is supported by metabolic labeling experiments showing identical kinetics for the incorporation of [³H]choline into alveolar PC16:0/14:0, PC16:0/16:1, and PC16:0/16:0 for mouse and perfused rat lungs (17). The combined synthesis and synthetic rates of these three species were all greater than those of longer chain monounsaturated species such as PC16:0/18:1.

In most mammalian surfactants, with the exception of the rhesus monkey (18) and newborn piglet (unpublished data) where PtdIns predominate, the anionic phospholipids PtdGly, generally, is the most abundant surfactant glycerophospholipid after PtdCho. When compared with PtdCho, PtdGly has a much greater variation between different animal species. Schlame et al. (19) found rat surfactant PtdGly to contain 26.7% PG16:0/18:1, 16.9% PG16:0/16:0, 11.2% PG16:0/20:4, and 10.6% PG16:0/22:6. Using similar HPLC techniques, Akino and coworkers (2) reported rabbit surfactant PtdGly to contain 34.7% PG16:0/16:0, 32% PG16:0/18:1, and 10.5% PG16:0/18:2 with negligible polyunsaturated species. In contrast, human lung surfactant PtdGly has a very different composition to either rat or rabbit, being dominated by three monounsaturated species with low amounts of PG16:0/16:0 (15). This variation of PtdGly composition between animal species is shown clearly by the spectra detailed in Fig. 1.3.

The variation in PtdIns composition between different animal species is even more striking (Fig. 1.4). PI16:0/16:0 was a minor component of surfactant PtdIns from all animals, whereas human and rabbit surfactant PtdIns were essentially monounsaturated (15). However, although human surfactant PtdIns comprised largely three species in approximately equal proportions (PI16:0/18:1, PI18:1/18:1, PI18:0/18:1), rabbit surfactant PtdIn was dominated by PI16:0/18:1 as a single species. In complete contrast, the dominant species of rat PtdIns was PI18:0/20:4, and this difference was even more marked in the mouse. Although the anionic phospholipids PtdGly and PtdIns apparently can replace each other in their contribution to the dynamic properties of alveolar surfactants (18), their relation to respiratory physiology is even less clear than for PtdCho composition, which correlates with respiratory rate (20). In addition, it is not clear how differences in surfactant phospholipids composition related to the significant differences in both the macroscopic and microscopic structures of lungs from varied mammalian species (21).

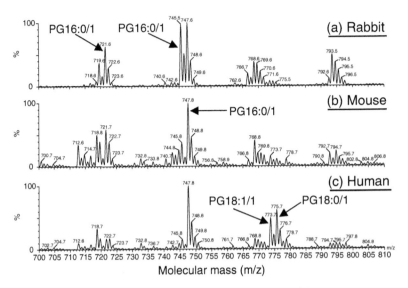

Figure 1.3 ESI-MS of PtdGly molecular species from adult (a) rabbit, (b) mouse, and (c) human surfactant. All samples were analyzed under negative ion conditions over the mass range $m/z = 700$–810. The ion peaks at $m/z = 718$, 766, and 768 are derived from PtdCho.

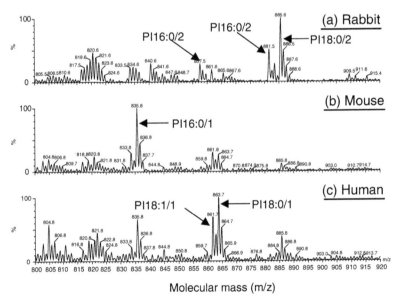

Figure 1.4 ESI-MS of PtdIns molecular species from adult (a) rabbit, (b) mouse, and (c) human surfactant. All samples were analyzed under negative ion conditions over the mass range $m/z = 800$–920.

III. Molecular Species of Surfactant Phospholipid During Fetal Development

The development of the surfactant system during late fetal growth is extremely well documented. For many years, the ratio of PtdCho to sphingomyelin (lecithin:sphingomylein or L:S) or the appearance of PtdGly in amniotic fluid has been used as indicators of fetal lung maturity (22–24). However, at least for PtdCho, this development is also accompanied by significant alterations to the molecular species of surfactant. No information is available for the molecular specificity of surfactant PtdGly or PtdIns during fetal development.

PtdCho from immature human fetal lung and liver at 15 weeks of gestation, before the expression of the surfactant system, is largely monounsaturated comprising almost 50% PC16:0/18:1 (25). It is significant, however, that the same analysis showed immature fetal lung PtdCho to contain 25% PC16:0/16:0. Subsequent tissue differentiation until term was then characterized by increasing unsaturation of liver PtdCho and increasing saturation of lung PtdCho, both at the expense of temporal decreases in PC16:0/18:1 content (25,26). However, the greatest fractional increases in PtdCho molecular species during fetal lung development are not only restricted to PC16:0/16:0, but also involve in PC16:0/16:1 and, particularly, PC16:0/14:0. Importantly, turnover rates of both PC16:0/16:0 and PC16:0/14:0 are 3-fold decreased at end gestation, leading to an accumulation of these components not only in guinea pigs (27) but also in human fetuses (20).

IV. Molecular Species of Phospholipid During Postnatal Development

In surfactants, PtdCho molecular species comprise 80% of total phospholipids. Both across mammalian and even avian species, and independent from postnatal age, the sum of PC16:0/16:0, PC16:0/14:0, and PC16:0/16:1 comprise 75–80% of total PtdCho (12,28). In general, there is a negative correlation between the fraction of PC16:0/16:0 and respiratory rate, whereas PC16:0/14:0 and/or PC16:0/16:1 positively correlate with respiratory rate. Consequently, PC16:0/16:0 concentration is lower in neonatal when compared with adult mammals, whereas PC16:0/14:0 and/or PC16:0/16:1 are increased. Strikingly, during alveolarization of rat and mouse lungs between days 4 and 14 after birth when respiratory rate increased to $300-400\ \mathrm{min}^{-1}$, the concentration of PC16:0/16:0 was low at 33% of total PtdCho. In contrast, at the same postnatal age, PC16:0/14:0 comprised some 25–27% of total PtdCho when compared with $<10\%$ in adult animals (20).

The physiological meaning of such compositional changes, however, is still unclear. High respiratory rates may cause a positive end-expiratory pressure that stimulates branching and organ development, precludes collapse of the pulmonary air spaces and consequently reduces the need for large amounts of PC16:0/16:0. The relatively high concentrations of PC 16:0/14:0 and PC16:0/16:1, species with lower gel to fluid phase transition temperatures, may promote surfactant spreading but, if so, it remains unclear why this is not achieved with a surfactant enriched, for instance, in PC16:0/18:1. Intriguingly, the adult cow and the rabbit both have low concentrations of PC16:0/16:0, together with low respiratory rates of $\sim$60 min^{-1}. Surfactant from these adult animals, however, is enriched in PC16:0/18:1 rather than in PC16:0/16:1 supporting a specific contribution of PC16:0/16:1 and PC16:0/14:0 enrichment to the lung physiology of fast breathing mammals. The precise functions of PC16:0/14:0 and PC16:0/16:1 and their potential contribution to therapeutic surfactants in the clinical management of patients ventilated at different frequencies remain to be investigated.

V. Modification of Surfactant Phospholipid Molecular Species in Disease States

A. Respiratory Syncytial Virus Bronchiolitis

Infants respiratory syncytial virus (RSV) bronchiolitis are deficient in surfactant, both in quantity and ability to reduce surface tension. Ventilated RSV positive infants treated with exogenous surfactant (Survanta) showed a more rapid improvement in oxygenation and ventilation indices over the first 60 h when compared with infants in an air placebo group (29). ESI-MS of BALF phospholipid generated an index of surfactant status from the concentration ratio of PC16:0/16:0 to PC16:0/18:1. This ratio correlated with both lung compliance and resistance, and over time increased in the treated group and declined in the placebo group. These data suggest that functional surfactant has a role in maintaining small airway patency in RSV infected infants and supplementation has the potential to reduce length of ventilation and barotrauma.

B. Respiratory Diseases in Children

Surfactant phospholipid composition in children changes both with postnatal development and with disease. Total phospholipid concentration in bronchoalveolar lavage fluid decreased exponentially with age in children without respiratory disease (16), but were higher in children with cystic fibrosis. Surfactant from this disease group was dysfunctional, could not generate low minimal surface tension values, and was characterized by accumulation of inactive large aggregates. For these children, surfactant PC16:0/16:0 decreased proportionately with disease progression and correlated directly with airway resistance (FEV$_1$). Molecular species analysis by ESI-MS showed that decreased PC16:0/16:0 was accompanied by increased PC16:0/18:1, suggesting accumulation in the airways of inflammatory cell membranes which are enriched in this PtdCho species.

C. Asthma

Considerable evidence suggests that impaired surfactant function in conducting airways leads to liquid filling and formation of mucus plugs, and therefore contributes to the severity of the asthmatic response (30). Surfactant can be recovered from all levels of the bronchial tree, but most evidence suggests that the phospholipid component at least is almost exclusively alveolar in origin. In healthy lungs, PtdCho species from airway surfactant are almost identical to those from the alveolar compartment (31) and, for individual people, PtdCho species compositions of sputum surfactant correlated directly with BALF surfactant compositions measured some weeks earlier (9). Studies in isolated rat trachea show clearly that airway epithelia makes little if any contribution to airway surfactant (32).

Impaired surfactant function after local allergen challenge to mild asthmatic subjects was associated with decreased PC16:0/16:0 but, in contrast to cystic fibrosis, the concentration of PC16:0/18:2 rather than PC16:0/18:1 was increased in the asthmatic group (8). As PC16:0/18:2 is the major PtdCho of human plasma lipoprotein (33), this was interpreted as influx of plasma phospholipid components during the allergic response, in contrast to the appearance of inflammatory cell membrane components in respiratory infections. Although it is not yet clear to what extent interactions between surfactant and the lipoprotein component of plasma contribute to surfactant dysfunction, in addition to inhibition by protein components such as fibrin monomers, ESI-MS analysis of phospholipids in bronchoalveolar lavage and sputum samples provides a sensitive means to monitor the airway infiltration of large plasma proteins during the asthmatic response.

D. Acute Respiratory Distress Syndrome

Similarities between neonatal RDS and acute respiratory distress syndrome (ARDS) led many research groups to investigate the potential of exogenous surfactant replacement as a therapy (34–36) with varying results. Analysis of surfactant phospholipid fatty acid composition showed decreased palmitate and increased monounsaturated fatty acids (37), changes consistent with accumulation of membrane material derived from inflammatory cells. In addition, increased activity of phospholipase A_2 in ARDS (38,39) may contribute to the hydrolysis of surfactant phospholipid, generating chaotropic lysophospholipid species. Secretory phospholipase A_2 binds preferentially to anionic phospholipids, which might help to explain the preferential loss of both PtdGly and PtdIns in ARDS. It does not, however, exhibit any substrate specificity for individual PtdCho species (40) and consequently its action would not be expected to contribute to selective loss of PC16:0/16:0 when compared with other PtdCho species. Despite extensive studies on surfactant replacement therapy in ARDS, very little is published regarding disease-related changes to the molecular species compositions of surfactant phospholipids. One preliminary study in children with acute lung injury/ARDS (Dr. Todd, personal communication) has shown a progressive loss of surfactant PC16:0/16:0 with increasing disease severity, accompanied by increased PC16:0/18:1. There was a general loss of PtdGly species accompanied by a fractional increased concentration of the poly-unsaturated PI18:0/20:4 species that is the predominant PtdIns species of inflammatory cells but only a minor component of human lung surfactant. These changes are all consistent with the well-documented increased activity and numbers of lung inflammatory cells, especially neutrophils, in ARDS contributing both membrane material to lung secretions and releasing hydrolytic phospholipase A_2 enzymes.

VI. Conclusion

It has now become clear that, far from being a rigidly defined composition, surfactant phospholipids exhibit a wide range of variation, both between different animal species and between different stages of development. The molecular species composition of surfactant PtdCho both responds dynamically to physiological constraints, such as patterns of respiration, and is dramatically altered in a variety of disease states. Moreover, the precise details of the alterations of surfactant phospholipid molecular species can provide direct information about the mechanisms of surfactant inactivation in these various diseases. Challenges for the future include definition of the precise roles of the surfactant specific phospholipids other than PC16:0/16:0 (PC16:0/14:0, PC16:0/16:1, and PtdGly) and establishing the relative roles that altered specificities of surfactant phospholipid synthesis and hydrolysis contribute to disease-mediated changes. In this context, the ability to quantify rates of synthesis of individual surfactant phospholipid molecular species *in vivo* using ESI-MS combined with deuteriated substrates is a very exciting possibility.

References

1. Hill CM, Brown BD, Morley CJ, Barson AJ. Pulmonary surfactant. 1. In immature and mature babies. Early Hum Dev 1988; 6:143–151.
2. Hayashi H, Adachi H, Kataoka K, Sato H, Akino T. Molecular species profiles of acidic phospholipids in lung fractions of adult and perinatal rabbits. Biochim Biophys Acta 1990; 1042:126–131.
3. Kahn MC, Anderson GJ, Anyan WR, Hall SB. Phosphatidylcholine molecular species of calf lung surfactant. Am J Physiol Lung Cell Mol Physiol 1995; 269:L567–L573.
4. Schlame M, Casals C, Rustow B, Rabe H, Kunze D. Molecular species of phosphatidylcholine and phosphatidylglycerol in rat lung surfactant and different pools of pneumocytes type II. Biochem J 1998; 253:209–215.

5. Ashton MR, Postle AD, Hall MA, Smith SL, Kelly FJ, Normand ICS. Phosphatidylcholine composition of endotracheal tube aspirates of neonates and subsequent respiratory disease. Arch Dis Child Fetal Neonatal 1992; 67:378–382.

6. Poets CF, Arning A, Bernhard W, Acevedo C, von der Hardt H. Active surfactant in pharyngeal aspirates of term neonates: lipid biochemistry and surface tension function. Eur J Clin Invest 1997; 27:293–298.

7. Han XL, Gross RW. Structural determination of picomole amounts of phospholipids via electrospray ionization tandem mass spectrometry. J Am Soc Mass Spectrom 1995; 6:1202–1210.

8. Heeley EL, Hohlfeld JM, Krug N, Postle AD. Phospholipid molecular species of bronchoalveolar lavage fluid after local allergen challenge in asthma. Am J Physiol Lung Cell Mol Physiol 2000; 278:L305–L311.

9. Wright SM, Hockey PM, Enhorning G, Strong P, Reid KBM, Holgate ST, Djukanovic R, Postle AD. Altered airway surfactant phospholipid composition and reduced lung function in asthma. J Appl Physiol 2000; 89:1283–1292.

10. Mason RJ, Nellenbogen J, Clements JA. Isolation of disaturated phosphatidylcholine with osmium tetroxide. J Lipid Res 1976; 17:281–284.

11. Hall SB, Venkitaraman AR, Whitsett JA, Holm BA, Notter RH. Importance of hydrophobic apoproteins as constituents of clinical exogenous surfactants. Am Rev Respir Dis 1992; 145:24–30.

12. Bernhard W, Gebert A, Vieten G, Rau GA, Hohlfeld JM, Postle AD, Freihorst J. Pulmonary surfactant in birds: coping with surface tension in a tubular lung. Am J Physiol Regul Integr Comp Physiol 2001; 281:R327–R337.

13. Crane JM, Hall SB. Rapid compression transforms interfacial monolayers of pulmonary surfactant. Biophys J 2001; 80:1863–1872.

14. Holm BA, Wang ZD, Egan EA, Notter RH. Content of dipalmitoyl phosphatidylcholine in lung surfactant: ramifications for surface activity. Pediatr Res 1996; 39:805–811.

15. Postle AD, Heeley EL, Wilton DC. A comparison of the molecular species compositions of mammalian lung surfactant phospholipids. Comp Biochem Physiol A Mol Integr Physiol 2001; 129:65–73.

16. Mander A, Langton-Hewer S, Bernhard W, Warner JO, Postle AD. Altered phospholipid composition and aggregate structure of lung surfactant is associated with impaired lung function in young children with respiratory infections. Am J Respir Cell Mol Biol 2002; 27:714–721.

17. Bernhard W, Bertling A, Dombrowsky H, Vieten G, Rau G, von der Hardt H, Freihorst J. Metabolism of surfactant phosphatidylcholine molecular species in cftr (tm1HGU/tm1HGU) mice compared to MF-1 mice. Exp Lung Res 2001; 27:349–366.

18. Egberts J, Beintema-Dubbledam A, de-Boers A. Phosphatidylinositol and not phosphatidylglycerol is the important minor phospholipid in rhesus-monkey surfactant. Biochim Biophys Acta 1981; 919:90–92.

19. Schlame M, Rustow B, Krunze D, Rabe H, Reichmann G. Phosphatidylglycerol of rat lung. Intracellular sites of formation de novo and acyl species pattern in mitochondria, microsomes and surfactant. Biochem J 1986; 240:247–252.

20. Bernhard W, Hoffmann S, Dombrowsky H, Rau GA, Kamlage A, Kappler M, Haitsma JJ, Freihorst J, von der Hardt H, Poets CF. Phosphatidylcholine molecular species in lung surfactant: composition in relation to respiratory rate and lung development. Am J Respir Cell Mol Biol 2001; 25:725–731.

21. Mercer RR, Russell ML, Crapo JD. Alveolar septal structure in different species. J Appl Physiol 1994; 77:1060–1066.

22. Hallman M, Arjomaa P, Mizumoto M, Akino T. Surfactant proteins in the diagnosis of fetal lung maturity. 1. Predictive accuracy of the 35 kDa protein, the L/S ratio and PG. Am J Obstet Gynecol 1988; 158:531–535.

23. Tsai MY, Shultz EK, Williams PP, Bendel R, Butler J, Farb H, Wager G, Knox EG, Julian T, Thompson TR. Assay of disaturated phosphatidylcholine in amniotic fluid as a test of fetal lung maturity: experience with 2000 analyses. Clin Chem 1987; 33:1648–1651.

24. Ishizuka T, Ishikawa K, Maseki M, Tomodo Y, Tsnda T. Determination of phosphatidylglycerol in amniotic fluid for prediction of fetal lung maturity by microbore column liquid chromatography. J Chromatogr 1986; 380:43–54.

25. Caesar PA, Wilson SJ, Normand ICS, Postle AD. A comparison of the specificity of phosphatidylcholine synthesis by human fetal lung maintained in either organ or organotypic culture. Biochem J 1988; 253:451–457.

26. Hunt AN, Kelly FJ, Postle AD. Developmental variation in whole human lung phosphatidylcholine molecular species: a comparison with guinea pig and rat. Early Hum Dev 1991; 25:157–171.

27. Burdge GC, Kelly FJ, Postle AD. Synthesis of phosphatidylcholine in guinea-pig fetal lung involves acyl remodelling and differential turnover of individual molecular species. Biochim Biophys Acta 1993; 1166:251–257.

28. Bernhard W, Postle AD, Rau GA, Freihorst J. Pulmonary and gastric surfactants. A comparison of the effect of surface requirements on function and phospholipid composition. Comp Biochem Physiol A Mol Integr Physiol 2001; 129:173–182.

29. Tibby SM, Hatherill SM, Wright SM, Wilson P, Postle AD, Murdoch IA. Exogenous surfactant supplementation in infants with respiratory syncytial virus bronchiolitis. Am J Respir Crit Care Med 2000; 162:1251–1256.

30. Enhorning G, Holm BA. Disruption of pulmonary surfactant's ability to maintain openness of a narrow tube. J Appl Physiol 1993; 74:2922–2927.

31. Bernhard W, Haagsman HP, Tschernig T, Poets CF, Postle AD, van Eijk ME, von der Hardt H. Conductive airway surfactant: surface-tension function, biochemical composition, and possible alveolar origin. Am J Respir Cell Mol Biol 1997; 17:41–50.

32. Rau GA, Dombrowsky H, Gebert A, Thole HH, von der Hardt H, Freihorst J, Bernhard W. Phosphatidylcholine metabolism of rat trachea in relation to lung parenchyma and surfactant. J Appl Physiol 2003; 95:1145–1152.

33. Postle AD, Al MD, Burdge GC, Hornstra G. The composition of individual molecular species of plasma phosphatidylcholine in human pregnancy. Early Hum Dev 1995; 43:47–58.

34. Seeger W, Günther A, Walmrath HD, Grimminger F, Lasch HG. Alveolar surfactant and adult respiratory distress syndrome. Pathogenetic role and therapeutic prospects. Clin Invest 1993; 71:177–190.

35. Hartog A, Gommers D, Lachmann B. Role of surfactant in the pathophysiology of the acute respiratory distress syndrome (ARDS). Monaldi Arch Chest Dis 1995; 50:372–377.

36. Gregory TJ, Steinberg KP, Spragg R, Gadek JE, Hyers TM, Longmore WJ, Moxley MA, Cai GZ, Hite RD, Smith RM et al. Bovine surfactant therapy for patients with acute respiratory distress syndrome. Am J Respir Crit Care Med 1997; 155:1309–1315.

37. Schmidt R, Meier U, Yabut-Perez M, Walmrath D, Grimminger F, Seeger W, Gunther A. Alteration of fatty acid profiles in different pulmonary surfactant phospholipids in acute respiratory distress syndrome and severe pneumonia. Am J Respir Crit Care Med 2001; 163:95–100.

38. Kim DK, Fukuda T, Thompson BT, Cockrill B, Hales C, Bonventre JV. Bronchoalveolar lavage fluid phospholipase A_2 activities are increased in human adult respiratory distress syndrome. Am J Physiol Lung Cell Mol Physiol 1995; 269:L109–L118.

39. Furue S, Kuwabara K, Mikawa K, Nishina K, Shiga M, Maekawa N, Ueno M, Chikazawa Y, Ono T, Hori Y et al. Crucial role of group IIA phospholipase A(2) in oleic acid-induced acute lung injury in rabbits. Am J Respir Crit Care Med 1999; 160:1292–1302.

40. Burdge GC, Creaney A, Postle AD, Wilton DC. Mammalian secreted and cytosolic phospholipase A_2 show different specificities for phospholipid molecular species. Int J Biochem Cell Biol 1995; 27:1027–1032.

2

New Insights into the Thermal Dynamics of the Surfactant System from Warm and Cold Animals

CAROL J. LANG, CHRISTOPHER B. DANIELS, and SANDRA ORGEIG

University of Adelaide,
Adelaide, Australia

I. Introduction

A. Pulmonary Surfactant

A surface tension is created at any air–liquid interface because the forces of attraction between water molecules are stronger than the forces between water and air. In the lungs, such a surface tension would promote lung collapse and increase the work required to inflate the lung (1). Surface tension is usually defined as the force required to stretch a rectangular surface fluid by a known length (usually 1 cm) and is expressed either as dyn/cm or mN/m (where 1 dyn/cm = 10^{-5} N/cm or 1 mN/m). Pure water has a surface tension of 70 dyn/cm (or 70 mN/m) at 37°C. Pulmonary surfactant interferes with the interaction of the surface water molecules and varies the surface tension at the air–liquid interface. This behavior is termed "surface activity" (2). Pulmonary surfactant can reduce surface tension in the lung to <5 mN/m in mammals (3).

B. Surfactant Composition

Pulmonary surfactant is a complex mixture of lipids (90% by weight) and proteins (10% by weight). Phospholipids (PL) comprise 80–90% of the surfactant lipids and are present in different molecular species (forms) that differ from each other in the fatty acid moiety and degree of saturation. Phosphatidylcholine (PC) is the most abundant PL (70–85%) (4) and the disaturated form; dipalmitoylphosphatidylcholine (DPPC) containing two molecules of the fatty acid, palmitate, is the major contributor to surfactant surface activity (1,5). The two other major PL, phosphatidylinositol (PI), and phosphatidylglycerol (PG) have negatively charged acidic headgroups and vary in their ratio to each other throughout development and between different mammalian and nonmammalian species (2,6). Surfactant also contains minor PL, including sphingomyelin (S), phosphatidylserine (PS), and phosphatidylethanolamine (PE), which make up 1–7% of the surfactant lipids (7–9). The remainder of the surfactant lipids include the neutral lipids, primarily cholesterol, but also lesser amounts of mono-, di-, and triglycerides and free fatty acids (9). Cholesterol (CHOL) is the second most abundant lipid in surfactant (6) comprising 10% by weight (4) and 20 mol% of the total lipid (10). CHOL and unsaturated phospholipids (USP) increase the fluidity of the surfactant monolayer and are particularly important in maintaining the spreadability of surfactant over the alveolar surface (11,12). In addition, four surfactant proteins have been identified. Surfactant protein A (SP-A) and surfactant protein D (SP-D) are hydrophilic, calcium-dependent, carbohydrate-binding proteins (13,14). Surfactant protein B (SP-B) and surfactant protein C (SP-C) are hydrophobic proteins (15,16). SP-A is the most abundant surfactant protein and is highly conserved within the vertebrates (17). In addition to their roles in the surfactant system (discussed subsequently), SP-A and SP-D are involved in lung defense against bacteria (18), and SP-B and SP-C are important in surfactant biosynthesis (19). SP-A in its delipidated form also regulates surfactant secretion from alveolar type II cells (ATII cells) (20).

C. Alveolar Type II Cells

The alveolar epithelium is composed of two main cell types, alveolar type I cells and ATII cells. Type I cells cover 97% of the alveolar surface area (21), and in mammals, ATII cells are located in crevices between the alveoli (7). ATII cells are cuboidal in shape and contain microvilli and specialized secretory organelles known as lamellar bodies (9). A photograph of an ATII cell isolated from the Australian marsupial mammal, *Sminthopsis crassicaudata*, is given in Fig. 2.1. ATII cells are the main site for the synthesis, storage, and release of surfactant (9). ATII cells are capable of *de novo* synthesis of all the major PL of the surfactant system (22) and the major surfactant proteins. In addition to their crucial function in the surfactant system, ATII cells are involved in the repair of the alveolar epithelium after lung injury (by differentiation into type I cells) and the regulation of the amount and composition of the fluid lining the alveoli (aqueous hypophase) (20). Lamellar bodies are stabilized by the surfactant protein SP-B (19) and consist of a proteinaceous core, around which are stacked bilayers of lipids within a limiting membrane. The limiting membrane of the lamellar bodies fuses with the plasma membrane of ATII cells to release the surfactant components into the hypophase (23).

D. The Surfactant Cycle

In mammals, lamellar bodies are secreted in response to local biochemical factors (7), signals from the autonomic nervous system (24), and deep breathing (25) or stretch (26) (Fig. 2.2). In the aqueous hypophase, the lamellar body contents

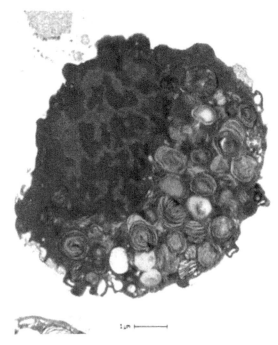

Figure 2.1   Electronmicrograph of an ATII cell isolated from the lungs of *Sminthopsis crassicaudata*. Scale bar = 1 μm.

hydrate and unravel to form tubular myelin, a characteristic crosshatched structure (27). Surfactant components are released from the tubular myelin and form a "surface-active" layer at the air–liquid interface (27). The surfactant layer at the air–liquid interface has long been considered a simple monolayer. However, recent electron microscopic and surface activity studies suggest that several lipid layers are closely associated with the surface film at the air–liquid interface (23,28). When the alveoli are compressed during expiration, USP and neutral lipids are thought to be excluded from the surface film, and may be recycled or degraded under the control of SP-A, and possibly SP-D (5,29). The remaining surface film is rich in DSP (disaturated phospholipids), particularly DPPC, and by the end of expiration, the surface tension is almost zero (22). At this point, the surface film exists in a gel state because DPPC has a phase transition temperature of 41°C (temperature at which it changes from a solid, tightly packed gel to a liquid-crystalline state). During compression at 37°C, the DPPC-rich surface film is packed tightly together, excluding water molecules and lowering surface tension (1). A low surface tension makes it easier to inflate the lungs during inspiration and as the alveoli expand, the DPPC-rich surface film probably pulls apart into rafts (11). As the alveoli

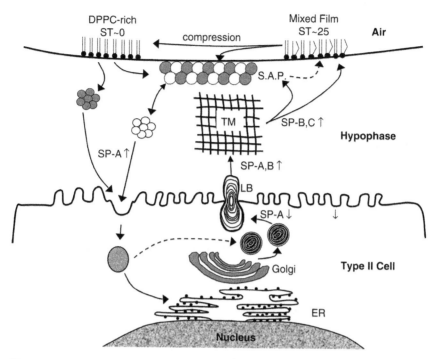

Figure 2.2 Schematic diagram of the life cycle of pulmonary surfactant. Pulmonary surfactant components are synthesized in the endoplasmic reticulum (ER), transported to the golgi apparatus (Golgi), and packaged into lamellar bodies (LB). Lamellar bodies are secreted into the liquid lining the alveoli (hypophase) via exocytosis across the type II cell plasma membrane. Here the lamellar bodies swell and unravel, forming a cross-hatched structure, termed tubular myelin, which consists of lipids and proteins. This structure supplies lipids to the surface film as well as the surface-associated phase (S.A.P.). As the mixed molecular film is compressed, lipids are squeezed out of the film into the S.A.P. to produce a DPPC-enriched film, which is capable of reducing surface tension (ST) to near 0 mN/m. It is possible that some lipids from the S.A.P. re-enter the surface film (dashed line arrow). Lipids from the surface film and the S.A.P. are eventually recycled and taken back up by the type II cell via endocytosis. The role of some of the surfactant proteins (SP-A, -B, and -C) in regulating these processes is indicated with ↑ (stimulation) or ↓ (inhibition). Figure reproduced from Fig. 1 in Ref. (31).

expand, CHOL and USP are retrieved from the secondary lipid layers or released from tubular myelin and adsorbed into the surface layer between the DPPC rafts (7). SP-B and SP-C promote this rapid adsorption of lipids to the air–liquid interface (30). Neutral lipids and USP lower the phase transition temperature of the surface layer mixture and therefore, increase the fluidity of surfactant (1) so that it can re-spread over the expanding alveolar surface (7).

E. Temperature

Given the biophysical properties (e.g., phase transition temperature) of the lipid constituents, temperature is of profound importance to the behavior and function of pulmonary surfactant. Homeothermic mammals, such as humans and rats, experience respiratory distress and surfactant dysfunction with relatively small fluctuations in body temperature (31–33). However, ectothermic animals, including fish, reptiles, and amphibians, experience fluctuations in body temperature on a daily and/or seasonal basis (2). In addition, many small mammals and birds allow their body temperature to decrease during periods of inactivity when they enter a reduced metabolic state, known as torpor. The depth, frequency, and length of torpor bouts vary from mild hypothermia in bears and small birds to daily torpor in bats, stress-induced torpor in small marsupials, and prolonged hibernation in rodents such as the ground squirrel (34). However, despite experiencing very large and often very rapid changes in body temperature, both ectotherms and heterothermic mammals do not suffer from any apparent respiratory distress or surfactant dysfunction. Understanding how the surfactant system can remain functional over a range of body temperatures in ectotherms and heterothermic mammals has the potential to be extremely useful in helping us to understand biochemical, biophysical, and regulatory mechanisms involved in surfactant function (35). The determination of those aspects of the surfactant system that are modified during temperature changes may also enable us to manipulate or exploit these same regulatory and biochemical mechanisms in humans to improve surfactant function. In addition to improving recovery after lung transplantation (36–38), this may lead to new and innovative treatments for asthma (39,40), cystic fibrosis (41), acute respiratory distress syndromes (35,37–42), and both medically and environmentally-induced hypothermia (43). Hence, this chapter summarizes our current knowledge of the thermal dynamics of the surfactant system and in particular, the compositional and biophysical aspects of surfactant that are important to surfactant function (Sections II, III). We also review the mechanisms controlling surfactant secretion at the cellular level and the effects of temperature on these regulatory factors (Section IV).

II. Temperature and the Biophysical Properties of Surfactant

A. Comparative Biology of Surfactant Function

The primary role of surfactant in mammals is to reduce and vary surface tension at the air–liquid interface and thus, reduce lung compliance (work of breathing), provide alveolar stability, and prevent alveolar edema (2). However, in reptiles and amphibians, removal of surfactant has little effect on lung compliance because respiratory units are large and extremely compliant (2). In addition, avian lungs are rigid and nondistensible (2). The different function of surfactant in the lungs of mammals and nonmammals is reflected in differences in surface activity (Table 2.1). In mammals, highly surface-active material is crucial to prevent atelectasis (collapse) of the alveoli and to increase static compliance. However, the mode of breathing and ventilatory mechanics observed in reptiles, amphibians, and fish seems to require a less surface-active surfactant. In these animals, surfactant acts as an "antiadhesive" to prevent alveolar surfaces from adhering to each other (44) (Section II.B). An antiadhesive function may also be important in heterothermic mammals during torpor when they experience extended nonventilatory periods (45). Furthermore, diving mammals, amphibians, and reptiles collapse their alveoli at depth when external compression forces are elevated (2). Thus, the antiadhesive function of surfactant, in preventing alveolar surfaces from sticking together, may be essential in cold and diving animals regardless of phylogenetic grouping or lung structure. In all the vertebrate groups, or more accurately, in all lung types, controlling lung fluid balance and thereby, preventing pulmonary edema is another important function of surfactant (2). Filtration, or the movement of fluid from capillaries into the lung tissue, is highest in amphibians and reptiles (44,46–50). Therefore, the tendency for fluid to enter the lungs in amphibians and reptiles is much greater than in mammals. In addition, birds have minute air capillaries and the "antiedema" function may in fact be the major physical function of avian surfactant (2,51). Hence, the functions of pulmonary surfactant differ slightly between mammalian and nonmammalian animals and these functional differences are reflected in the surface activity of the surfactant in their lungs (Table 2.1).

B. Function of Surfactant as an Antiadhesive in Ectothermic Animals

In ectothermic animals, the surface activity of surfactant is significantly lower than that observed in mammalian lungs (Table 2.1) and this corresponds to differences in surfactant composition (Section III.B). Moreover, most lungs of ectothermic vertebrates are 100–200 times more compliant than mammalian lungs and this alleviates the need to drastically reduce surface tension at the air–liquid interface during inspiration (2). Thus, the main function of surfactant in ectotherms may be in preventing alveolar surfaces from adhering together at low lung volumes (52). Using scanning electron microscopy to demonstrate the breathing dynamics of the lizard *Ctenophorus nuchalis*, Daniels et al. (53) showed that during lung deflation, the epithelial tissues fold in on each other like a concertina. This results in large portions of epithelial tissue coming into contact during low lung volumes. The work required to initially separate these surfaces is dependent upon the distance originally separating the surfaces, the areas of surfaces in contact, and the surface tension lining the surfaces (54). A fluid lining of low surface tension between the surfaces would prevent the adhesion of alveolar surfaces in contact and reduce the work of separating the surfaces (54). Hence, the pressure initially required to open a completely

Table 2.1 Summary of Surface Activity Parameters of Surfactants from a Range of Vertebrates

Species	T_A (°C)	Device	ST_{eq} (mN/m)	ST_{min} (mN/m)	%SAcomp	Surface activity
I. Osteichthys						
1. Teleostei						
Carassius auratus[a]	22	BS	—	26	—	Very low
Hoplias malobaricus[b]	37	WLB	—	22	70*	Very low
Hoplerythrinus unitaeniatus[b]	37	WLB	—	22	80*	Very low
Arapaima gigas[b]	37	WLB	—	22	75*	Very low
2. Ginglymodi						
Lepisosteus osseus[c]	24	WLB	25 ± 1.3	17.0 ± 1.0	70	Very low
3. Dipnoi						
Lepidosiren paradoxa[c]	37	WLB	—	22	70	Very low
II. Amphibia						
1. Caudata						
Amphiuma tridactylum[c]	24	WLB	27.7 ± 0.4	17.6 ± 1.1	62	Low
2. Anura						
Bufo marinus[c]	24	WLB	26.7 ± 1.1	18.6 ± 0.5	55	Low
III. Reptilia						
1. Ophidia						
Eunectes murinus[d]	37	WLB	—	22	70*	Very low
2. Crocodilia						
Alligator mississippiensis[c]	24	WLB	32.9 ± 1.1	19.6 ± 0.5	70	Very low

		T_A	ST_{eq}	ST_{min}	%SAcomp	
3. Testudinata						
Trachemys scripta[c]	WLB	24	26.7 ± 1.7	18.0 ± 0.4	60	Low
Testudo hermanni[e]	WLB	24	40 ± 6	4.0 ± 1.7	65*	Intermediate
4. Lacertilia						
Pogona vitticeps[c]	WLB	24	24.6 ± 1.9	14.4 ± 0.8	30	High
Trachydosaurus rugosus[c]	WLB	24	24.4 ± 0.6	13.2 ± 1.5	30	High
IV. Aves						
Gallus gallus domesticus[c]	WLB	24	28.6 ± 4.9	18.8 ± 0.2	75	Very low
Meleagris gallapavo[f]	WLB	22	—	5.6 ± 2.1	57*	Intermediate
V. Mammalia						
Mus musculus[c]	WLB	24	25.8 ± 1.5	5.1 ± 1.1	46	Very high
Sminthopsis crassicaudata[c]	WLB	24	26.3 ± 0.5	5.4 ± 0.3	43	Very high
Rattus norvegicus[g]	CBS	37	25	<1	15–30	Very high
Chalinolobus gouldii	CBS	37	25	<1	11.8	Very high

Note: Data are mean ± SEM. T_A, ambient temperature; ST_{eq}, equilibrium surface tension; ST_{min}, minimum surface tension; %SAcomp, %surface area compression; WLB, Wilhelmy–Langmuir surface balance; BS, Enhorning bubble surfactometer; CBS, captive bubble surfactometer.
*Values for %SAcomp were recalculated from data in the literature as the compression required to achieve ST_{min} from 100% Area.
[a](47).
[b](48).
[c](2).
[d](49).
[e](50).
[f](51).
[g](3).

Source: Table modified from Table 1 in Ref. (2).

collapsed lung (opening pressure) can provide an indication of the antiadhesive function of surfactant (47,52,55). Removing surfactant from lungs isolated from lizards (52), actinopterygiian fishes (47,55), garter snakes (56), and tiger salamanders (57) significantly increases opening pressure of the lungs. However, in all cases, filling pressure (i.e., after initial lung opening) was extremely low (1–4 cm H_2O) and remained unchanged before and after lavage (2). This indicates that surfactant is important in these lungs only during the initial phase of inflating a collapsed lung and not during further inflation or deflation, as is the case in mammals.

The antiadhesive function of surfactant may be particularly important when ectotherms are cold because the normal respiratory cycle of many reptiles and amphibians is characterized by low lung volumes and long nonventilatory periods (58,59). Two studies have investigated the effect of changes in body temperature on the antiadhesive function of surfactant in ectothermic animals. Daniels et al. (52) demonstrated that increasing body temperature from 27°C to 37°C in central netted dragons, *Ctenophorus nuchalis*, decreases the opening pressure of the lungs without affecting lung compliance. This may reflect an increase in fluidity due to the increase in temperature and thus, an increase in the spreadability of surfactant over alveolar surfaces at 37°C (52). In bearded dragons, *Pogona vitticeps*, increasing body temperature from 18°C to 37°C had no effect on opening pressure or filling pressure (60). Hence, a decrease in body temperature does not affect the antiadhesive properties of surfactant in bearded dragons. Furthermore, the increase in amount of PL observed in bearded dragons at 37°C does not appear to affect opening pressure and thus, surfactant antiadhesive function. Hence, the observed increases in surfactant PL at 37°C in bearded dragons may be due to increases in metabolic rate and thus, increased secretion of lamellar bodies from ATII cells. Although a critical amount of surfactant may be necessary to serve an antiadhesive function, increases above this amount do not appear to further promote the nonadherence of epithelial surfaces (60). The antiadhesive properties of surfactant appear to be dependent on its ability to reduce surface tension to some extent and to remain fluid and readily adsorbed to the air–liquid interface (2). Hence, the more detergent-like surfactant of ectothermic animals is capable of lowering, but not necessarily varying surface tension to any great extent. However, ectothermic surfactant can spread easily over lung epithelial surfaces to prevent adhesion, even when animals are cold.

C. Surface Activity Measurements

The surface activity of surfactant has been measured using a variety of procedures (12,60–68), but more recently using a primed Wilhelmy–Langmuir surface balance (WLB) and a captive bubble surfactometer (CBS). The WLB consists of a half-filled deep Teflon trough fitted with a tight barrier on top (11,12). Before application of surfactant material, the Teflon trough and leading side of the barrier are primed with DPPC to prevent surfactant material from adhering to the walls of the trough and thereby leaking from the surface (31). Surface-active materials are placed on the surface of the liquid, where they spread. The mechanically driven barrier compresses the film and a dipping plate attached to a force transducer is then used to calculate surface tension (12). In the CBS, a liquid bubble floats (is buoyant) against a hydrophilic roof of 1% agarose gel and bubble volume can be controlled by varying the pressure in the chamber (69,70). As volume is reduced, the surface area is reduced and the surface tension of the surfactant film at the bubble surface falls. The bubble shape changes from spherical to oval depending on the surface tension. Surface tension measurements are made through shape analysis of the bubble using digital image processing techniques (3). A temperature-controlled jacket surrounds the chamber containing the bubble so that experiments can be conducted at different temperatures (3). In the CBS, the surface film is not interrupted by barriers such as plastic walls or outlets and therefore, provides a leak proof system, unlike the WLB (70).

When measuring surface activity, a number of biophysical properties are usually examined (Fig. 2.3). Adsorption is a measure of the rate at which surface-active material accumulates at the air–liquid interface from the aqueous subphase and reduces surface tension (2). Both the rate of adsorption and the resulting equilibrium surface tension (ST_{eq}) indicate the ability of surfactant to form a surface-active film; they are strongly dependent on the concentration of PL in the measured sample. A "good" surfactant usually has an ST_{eq} of 25 mN/m (3). When the surfactant film is cyclically compressed under dynamic conditions *in vitro*, surface tension decreases below ST_{eq} to the ST minimum (ST_{min}). A measure of how efficiently surfactant reduces surface tension under compression can be obtained from the change in surface area (%SAcomp) required to achieve ST_{min}. The ST_{min} and %SAcomp are therefore the best indicators of the ability of surfactant to lower surface tension under dynamic compression. Generally, a "good" surfactant is able to reach an ST_{min} of <5 mN/m, and an excellent surfactant <1 mN/m (3).

Homeothermic Mammals

The effect of temperature on the surface activity of surfactant isolated from homeothermic mammals appears to be controversial and is largely dependent on the procedures employed to measure surface tension (71–76). The apparent increases in ST_{min} with increasing temperature, seen in some of the earlier studies, are most probably due to surface film leakage in the apparatus used (72). Recent techniques such as the primed WLB, CBS, and the *in situ* microdroplet technique generally demonstrate that in vitro, temperature does not greatly affect the surface properties of isolated pulmonary surfactant (72). Miles et al. (73) reported that ventilating isolated rat lungs at 37°C and 22°C had no effect on the ST_{min} of the surfactants measured using a primed WLB at 22°C and

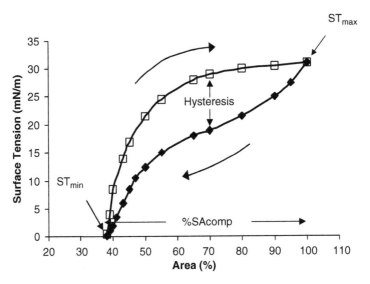

Figure 2.3 Schematic diagram of a typical surface tension-area isotherm during dynamic compression of a surfactant film *in vitro*. Arrows indicate the expansion and compression limbs of the curve. The difference in surface tension at the same area% between the compression and expansion limbs is termed hysteresis and represents the irreversible heat loss in the cycle. Upon repeated cycling, the hysteresis rapidly diminishes as the curve is shifted to the right. This has the effect that the %SAcomp required to achieve minimum surface tension (ST_{min}) is reduced; that is, the film is capable of generating low surface tensions more rapidly and efficiently. Furthermore, the maximum surface tension (ST_{max}) frequently decreases with repeated dynamic cycling. Figure reproduced from Ref. (31).

37°C, respectively. However, ST_{min} did increase significantly when measured on the WLB at 42°C (19 mN/m) (73). Using an improved microdroplet technique to measure surface tension over the entire pressure volume curve at 22°C and 37°C, Schürch et al. (74) also determined that the alveolar surface tension and the surface tension to volume relationship are both essentially identical at the two temperatures. Thus, within this temperature range, temperature seems to have little effect on the surface activity of homeothermic surfactant and this may have profound implications *in vivo*.

Breathing requires the contraction of muscles and is, therefore, an energy-requiring process. The amount of energy required to breathe (work of breathing W_t) is dependent on the type of breathing pattern [frequency (f) and tidal volume (V_t)], airways resistance (W_{raw}), and lung compliance (ease of inflation) (C), where $W_t = W_{raw} + (f \times V_t^2/2C)$ (75). Lung compliance (C), or the ease of inflation, is determined by the elasticity of lung tissue and by the surface tension of the fluid lining the alveoli (76). Lung connective tissue is composed of collagen fibers, which are highly sensitive to temperature (77). Decreasing temperature significantly increases the elasticity of lung tissue and therefore, decreases lung tissue compliance (77). A decrease in lung compliance makes it harder to inflate the lungs and thus, increases the work of breathing (75). An increase in the work of breathing leads to an increase in the amount of oxygen required to ventilate the lungs and thus decreases the efficiency of oxygen extraction with each breath (75). However, overall lung compliance could be maintained despite decreases in tissue compliance if the surface tension of the fluid lining the alveoli was further decreased by increases in surfactant surface activity, which are induced by changes in surfactant composition (45). Unfortunately, no studies have examined the behavior or composition (Section III.A) of surfactant from homeotherms at temperatures lower than the relatively mild 20–25°C. At temperatures >20°C, there are also some discrepancies between the studies using cats (78), dogs (79,80), rabbits (35,77,80,81), and rats (82). The discrepancies may be due, in part, to the different species, methods, temperature regimes, and data analysis used (35). However, although the details and mechanisms remain unclear, it is generally agreed that cooling of lungs from homeothermic mammals is associated with decreases in overall lung compliance (35). This suggests that the surface-active properties of homeothermic surfactant and thus, its composition are not altered by a decrease in temperature. Hence, although homeothermic mammals can modify their surfactant composition under certain physiological conditions (Section III.A), they do not appear to do so under temperature stress. This may explain the respiratory distress experienced during hypothermia by homeothermic animals.

Heterothermic Mammals

In heterothermic mammals, the surfactant system is very dynamic and responds rapidly to changes in physiological conditions experienced throughout torpor and activity (83). Most research on the effects of temperature on the surfactant of heterothermic mammals has involved two species: fat-tailed dunnarts, *Sminthopsis crassicaudata* and Gould's wattled bats, *Chalinolobus gouldii*. Dunnarts are small marsupial mammals that live in the semi-arid regions of Australia. Dunnarts enter torpor in response to food deprivation and low ambient temperatures. During torpor, body temperature decreases from ~35°C in active (warm) dunnarts to a few degrees above ambient temperature (often between 10°C and 20°C) in torpid (cold) dunnarts (84). Torpor in dunnarts is also accompanied by changes in ventilatory pattern and torpor can last for >8 h (84). Dunnarts can be maintained in breeding colonies in the laboratory and thus, like rats and mice, are an ideal research model. Gould's wattled bats are small insectivorous bats that are widespread and common throughout Australia. During daily torpor in bats, body temperature can drop as low as 5°C (85,86). In torpor, bat ventilation undergoes marked changes, with episodic breathing bouts alternating with long nonventilatory periods (87).

As in homeothermic mammals, decreases in body temperature in heterothermic mammals are associated with increases in tissue elasticity and thus,
decreases in lung tissue compliance, at least in the early stages of torpor (45).
However, in heterothermic mammals, torpor is accompanied by marked
decreases in metabolic rate (88) and thus, oxygen extraction. Consequently,
the work of breathing, as a percentage of metabolic rate, may be expected to
rise dramatically (Section on *Homeothermic Mammals*) as body temperature
falls (89). Hence, reducing the work of breathing is likely to be of greater importance in ectothermic and heterothermic animals than in homeothermic mammals.
However, although tissue compliance decreased at 1 and 4 h of torpor in
dunnarts, overall lung compliance measured in the presence of surfactant was
unaffected by torpor. If tissue compliance decreases, then the surface tension
of the alveolar fluid must also decrease in order for overall lung compliance to
remain unchanged. Therefore, surfactant appears to counteract the decrease in
tissue compliance during torpor in heterothermic mammals and thus, maintain
the work of breathing at a minimum. Furthermore, ventilatory periods are
much more infrequent during torpor (88) and as a result, the work of breathing
(as a percentage of metabolic rate) may over time, actually decrease even
further (89). Therefore, both dunnarts and bats must optimize their surfactants
at low temperatures to decrease surface tension in the lung and thus, reduce
the work of breathing. The fluidity of surfactant must also be maintained at
cold body temperatures and this may be achieved by lowering the phase transition temperature of the lipid mixture, and thus, changing the composition of
the surfactant mixture (Section III.A). Consequently, mechanisms that alter
and maintain surfactant amount and composition in the lung must function
adequately at both warm and cold body temperatures (Section IV).

The surface activity properties of surfactant collected from active, torpid,
and arousing dunnarts and bats are provided in Tables 2.2 and 2.3, respectively.
Surfactant collected from active and torpid dunnarts appears to function optimally at the body temperature of the animal from which it was isolated. A
surface tension of 9.12 ± 0.3 mN/m at $37°C$ was found for surfactant obtained
from torpid dunnarts killed after being in torpor for 8 h with a body temperature
of $15°C$. However, a surface tension of 6.41 ± 0.3 mN/m at $37°C$ was found for
surfactant obtained from active dunnarts. Furthermore, adsorption (movement to
the air–liquid interface) of surfactant collected from torpid dunnarts is significantly slower than surfactant collected from active dunnarts when measured at
an ambient temperature of $37°C$. Conversely, surfactant from torpid dunnarts
adsorbs much faster at $15°C$ than surfactant from active dunnarts (72). Surfactant
from torpid dunnarts also requires a smaller change in compressibility
(%SAcomp) to attain ST_{min} compared with surfactant from active dunnarts
measured at either $20°C$ or $37°C$ (72). Similar changes in surface activity have
been observed during torpor in Gould's wattled bats. When surfactant from
active and torpid Gould's wattled bats were analyzed on a CBS at a temperature
matching the body temperature of the bat, equilibrium surface tensions of

Table 2.2 Effect of Temperature on Surface Activity of Pulmonary Surfactant from Mice and the Fat-Tailed Dunnart, *Sminthopsis crassicaudata*

Animal/activity state	ST_{min}	%SAcomp
Properties measured at 20°C in WLB		
Mice	5.3 ± 0.3	46.0 ± 3.0
Active dunnart	5.4 ± 0.2	48.3 ± 0.5
4 h Torpor dunnart	4.0 ± 0.3	36.0 ± 3.2*
8 h Torpor dunnart	4.43 ± 0.19	26.5 ± 2.2**
Properties measured at 37°C in CBS		
Active dunnart	6.4 ± 0.3	89.1 ± 0.8
8 h Torpor dunnart	9.1 ± 0.3*	84.9 ± 1.8*

Note: Data expressed as mean ± SE; $n = 4–6$ animals. Values for surface tension parameters are in mN/m. ST_{min}, minimum surface tension; %SAcomp required to achieve ST_{min} from 25 mN/m; WLB, Wilhelmy–Langmuir surface balance; CBS, captive bubble surfactometer.
*Significantly different from active dunnarts.
**Significantly different from active and 4 h torpid dunnarts. Data from Lopatka et al. (72).

25 mN/m and minimum surface tensions of 1 mN/m were achieved. These values are similar to the literature values for other mammals (11,90). Adsorption was significantly slower when surfactant from active bats was analyzed at 24°C compared with 37°C. Conversely, surfactant from torpid bats demonstrated much faster adsorption at 24°C compared with 37°C. Quasistatic and dynamic cycling of surfactant from active bats at 37°C yielded lower ST_{min} and %SAcomp than

Table 2.3 The Effect of Temperature on the Surface Activity of Pulmonary Surfactant from Gould's Wattle Bat, *Chalinolobus gouldii*

Activity status	Temp (°C)	N	ST_{min} (mN/m) (mean ± SE)	ST_{max} (mN/n) (mean ± SE)	%SAcomp
Active	37	6	1.2 ± 0.01*	27.7 ± 0.17*	11.8 ± 0.1*
bat	24	6	2.5 ± 0.09*	31.9 ± 0.15*	17.2 ± 0.5*
Torpid	37	6	3.8 ± 0.04#	23.4 ± 0.26#	10.1 ± 0.2#
bat	24	6	1.2 ± 0.2#	23.0 ± 0.13	8.8 ± 0.2#
Arousing	37	6	1.8 ± 0.51^	28.6 ± 0.3^	11.9 ± 0.1
bat	24	6	2.2 ± 0.1^	26.5 + 1.21^	11.3 + 0.3

Note: Data expressed as mean ± SE for ST_{min}, ST_{max}, and %SAcomp for surfactant isolated from active, torpid, and arousing bats dynamically cycled at 25 cycles/min and examined at 24°C and 37°C using a CBS. Pairs of symbols denote values that are significantly different. Bat data from Codd et al. (90).

when measured at 24°C. Conversely, surfactant from torpid bats reached a lower ST_{min} and required less %SAcomp to reach low ST_{min} at 24°C than at 37°C (90). Hence, in heterothermic mammals, surfactant from active (warm) animals appears to be more suited to function at higher temperatures (37°C) and surfactant from torpid (cold) animals appears to function better at lower temperatures.

Rapid Arousals from Torpor

Arousal from torpor by heterothermic mammals can be very rapid. During arousal in dunnarts, body temperature increases from 10–15°C to 32–35°C at a rate of 0.7–1°C per min (91). Bats also arouse very rapidly from torpor with warming rates of 0.81°C per min having been recorded (83). Surfactant isolated from bats arousing from torpor ($T_b = 28$–32°C) adsorbs much faster at 37°C than at 24°C and functions optimally at 37°C (as indicated by a decrease in ST_{min} and %SAcomp) (90). Surfactant isolated from dunnarts killed immediately after arousal from torpor, adsorbs slowly at 37°C at a rate similar to that of surfactant from torpid animals. When assayed at 15°C, surfactant from aroused dunnarts adsorbs faster than that of active dunnarts but more slowly than that of torpid dunnarts. However, as in bats, ST_{min} and %SAcomp decrease rapidly in dunnart surfactant immediately after arousal, which results in a pronounced improvement in surface tension-lowering ability at 37°C. Thus, surfactant from heterothermic mammals undergoes rapid changes in surface activity and lipid composition (Section III.A), which enables the mixture to function effectively at rapidly increasing body temperatures. At least in dunnarts, but probably also in bats, the surface activity of surfactant undergoes virtually simultaneous changes with increasing body temperature as they rapidly arouse from torpor. Rapid improvements in surface activity occur immediately after arousal and may be necessary to optimize the alveolar surface area for gas exchange when rapid increases in breathing frequency and lung tidal volume occur. Slower changes in surface activity to warm-active levels may reflect a post-arousal stabilization of the respiratory system at the higher body temperature (92).

III. Temperature and Surfactant Composition

A. Lipid Composition

The composition of surfactants from a wide range of animal species and their preferred body temperatures are given in Table 2.4. The amount of surfactant lipids, when normalized to wet lung mass, is lowest in fish, intermediate in amphibians, and highest in reptiles and mammals (57). However, when normalized to the surface area of the lungs, fish and reptiles contain greater amounts of lipid than occurs in the lungs of mammals (57). When expressed as a percentage of PL, fish contain much greater levels of CHOL and USP than members of the other vertebrate groups, and the percentage of CHOL relative to disaturated phospholipids (DSP) decreases 10- to 15-fold in the tetrapods (57). The lowest CHOL

Table 2.4 Summary of Surfactant Lipid Composition from a Range of Vertebrates

Species	N	$T_{A/B}$ (°C)	PL (mg/ gWL)	PC	PG	PE	SM	PI	PS	LPC/ Unk	CHOL (mg/ gWL)	CHOL/ PL	DSP (mg/ gWL)	%DSP/ PL
							%PL							
Mammalia														
Eutheria														
Rattus norvegicus[a]	6	37	1.70[b]	75.5	11.0	4.6	0.2	3.0	1.9	ND	0.130[b]	0.071[b]	0.78[b]	45.7[b]
Rattus norvegicus[c,#]	6	37	ND	83.6	8.3	0.7	4.0	4.0	4.0	4.0	ND	ND	ND	61[§]
Mus musculus[d]	6	37	16.9*	72.3	18.1	1.9	3.3	4.5	4.5	0	1.49*	0.097	7.46*	44.5
Nyctophilus geoffryi[y]	36	32	14.6*	ND	ND	ND	ND	ND	ND	ND	0.1*	0.008	6.2*	42.27
Chalinolobus gouldii[z]	37	32	17.3*	ND	ND	ND	ND	ND	ND	ND	0.268*	0.019	7.7*	44.1
Homo sapiens[e]	14	37	ND	72.8	9.5	5.3	1.3	11.1	11.1	ND	1.54[f,#,*]	0.071[b]	ND	48.5[b]
Homo sapiens[c,#]	6	37	ND	80.5	9.1	2.3	8.1	8.1	8.1	8.1	ND	ND	ND	68[§]
Metatheria														
Macropus eugenii[g,#]	3	37	ND	55.0	9.0	13.0	0.0	22.0	22.0	0	ND	ND	ND	
Sminthopsis crassicaudata[w]	6	~35	21.8*	70.7	6.0	2.1	7.7	13.5	13.5	0	1.48*	0.068	9.0*	40.2
Sminthopsis crassicaudata[d]	6	~15	38.4*	58.7	6.4	3.9	9.2	21.8	21.8	0	4.14*	0.107	18.9*	49.3
Aves														
Meleagris gallopavo[h]	6	~37	0.17	86.4	ND	5.6	0.3	ND	ND	ND	ND		ND	
Gallus gallus[i]	1	~37	ND	79.2	0	5.2	2.9	8.9	3.0	ND	ND		ND	
Domestica	5	~37												
Domestica[f,#]	6	RT	15.7*	43.5	ND	21.9	10.1	17.7		2.4	18.8*	0.065[j]	ND	30.6[j]
Reptilia														
Ophidia														
Eunectes alv.lung[k]	1	~37	ND	54.0	0	12.0	20.0	7.0	8.0	ND	ND	ND	ND	ND
Murinus sac.lung	1	~37	ND	46.0	0	14.0	25.0	5.0	100	ND	ND	ND	ND	ND
Thamnophis ordinoides[l]	3	23	0.69	64.0	4.1	0	1.0	16.9		14.2	0.023	0.035	0.21	33.9
Crotalus atrox[l]	3	23	2.42	68.6	0	0	11.7	1.4		17.7	0.17	0.079	1.14	43.6

(continued)

Table 2.4 Continued

Species	N	$T_{A/B}$ (°C)	PL (mg/gWL)	PC %PL	PG	PE	SM	PI	PS	LPC/Unk	CHOL (mg/gWL)	CHOL/PL	DSP (mg/gWL)	%DSP/PL
Lacertilia														
Ctenophorus nuchalis[m]	8	37	2.16[b]	72.5	0	0	3.1	24.5		ND	0.24[b]	0.080[b]	1.06[b]	46.4[b]
Pogona vitticeps[n]	6–7	37	27.8*	80.1	0	0	3.6	16.2		0	NS	0.086	ND	ND
	4–7	18	20.2*	76.6	0	0	5.4	18.0		0	NS	0.083	ND	ND
Testudinata														
Malaclemys geographica	4	14	0.19	70.7	0	8.4	3.9	7.6	2.7	ND	ND	ND	ND	ND
Malaclemys geographica[o]	4	32	0.47	77.1	0	6.7	3.5	10.0	2.8	ND	ND	ND	ND	ND
Natator depressus[n]	5	RT	1.47	70.7	0	0	9.9	19.4		0	NS	0.061	NS	27.9
Caretta caretta[n]	5	RT	2.7	66.7	0	0	10.4	22.8		0	NS	0.099	NS	26.7
Pseudemys scriptas[f,#]	8	RT	14.2*	47.5	ND	24.8	8.7	13.2		3.4	11.5*	ND	ND	ND
Crocodilia														
Crocodylus porosus[n]	3	RT	0.96	67.6	0	2.5	4.7	2.5		0	NS	0.067	NS	27.7
Amphibia														
Anura														
Rana catesbiana[i]	1	?	ND	76.3	9.1	6.4	0.8	4.5	1.5	ND	ND	ND	ND	ND
Rana pipiens[f,#]	7	RT	11.7*	49.9	ND	21.5	6.3	14.4		2.4	17.7*	ND	ND	ND
Rana pipiens[p]	10	14	1.07	73	11.7	2.8	3.5	1.0	ND	ND	ND	ND	ND	ND
Bufo marinus[q]	3	23	0.33	62.6	13.1	9.0	6.7	8.6		0	0.02	0.035	ND	13.2
Gymnophiona														
Typhlonectes natans[r]	8	23	0.44	66.1	0	0	9.1	13.1	1.2	Unk 10.4	0.043	0.107	0.181	43.4
Caudata														
Amphiuma tridactylum[q]	3	23	0.27	77.5	0	1.2	3.9	17.5	0	0	0.023	0.076	0.075	25.8

Osteichthys

Dipnoi

Neoceratodus forsteri[s]	3	23	0.084	59.6	0.5	14.4	15.3	10.2	0	0	0.022	0.242	0.006	8.9
Lepidosiren paradoxa[t]	1–3	RT	ND	46.0	8.0	19.0	11.0	0		0	ND	ND	ND	ND
Lepidosiren paradoxa[s]	3	23	0.22	73.9	1.8	6.9	7.3	9.3		0.8	0.010	0.044	0.059	27.8
Protopterus annectens[s]	4	23	0.61	80.2	3.0	3.0	5.6	7.9		0.4	0.028	0.052	0.126	20.4

Teleostei

Hoplias malabaricus[t]	1–3	RT	ND	70	0	7	5	0	12	5	ND	ND	ND	ND
Hoplerythrinus unitaeniatus[t]	1–3	RT	ND	69	0	25	2	0	2	0	ND	ND	ND	ND
Erythrinus erythrinus[t]	1–3	RT	ND	93	0	3	2	2	0	0	ND	ND	ND	ND
Arapaima gigas[t]	1–3	RT	ND	39	6	7	24	8	8	8	ND	ND	ND	ND
Carassius (posterior[u] Auratus swimbladder)	9	23	0.14	75	1.2	4.7	15.9	5.1		0	0.051	0.328	0.036	20.8

Ginglymodi

Lepisosteus osseus[v]	5–8	23	0.50	76.4	1.4	4.6	5.9	7.9		3.0	0.09	0.175	0.069	14.1

Arthropoda

Mollusca

Helix aspersa[x]	1	RT	ND	45.3	2.9	32.4	0	4.3	8.6	Unk 6.5	ND	0.041	ND	8.6

Note: $T_{A/B}$, ambient or body temperature; PL, phospholipid; CHOL, cholesterol; DSP, Disaturated PL, gWL (gram wet lung mass); *dry lung mass; RT, room temperature (22–25°C); PC, phosphatidylcholine; PG, phosphatidylglycerol; PE, phosphatidylethanolamine; SM, sphingomyelin; PI, phosphatidylinositol; PS, phosphatidylserine (a single value for PI and PS indicates that bands could not be resolved); LPC, lysophosphatidylcholine; unkwn, unknown PL; ND, not determined. #Whole lung extracts. §%Disaturated PC. [a](99). [b](57). [c](100). [d](45). [e](101). [f](102). [g](103). [h](51). [i](104). [j](105). [k](48). [l](106). [m](107). [n](108). [o](109). [p](110). [q](53). [r](111,112). [s](48). [t](47). [u](55). [v](72). [w](113). [x](93). [z](90). Table has been modified from Ref. (95).

levels are found in the highly specialized lungs of microchiropteran bats. Choco-
late wattled bats, *Nyctophilus geoffroyi* and Gould's wattled bats, *Chalinolobus
gouldii* have 15 and 6 times less cholesterol, respectively, than has been reported
in the surfactant of any other mammal (83). The complexity of the bat lung and
the tiny size of the alveoli may explain the low levels of CHOL observed in bat
surfactant. In bats, the air spaces are finely subdivided such that the alveolar
diameter is smaller than that of most other similar sized mammals (93). The
small alveolar surface area may reduce or alleviate the need for a "spreading"
agent in the surfactant of bats. Alternatively, bats may exhibit a decreased
CHOL as an adaptive strategy to maximize the surface activity. High surface
activity may be necessary to counteract the higher collapse pressures associated
with the rapid cycling in volume of small alveoli and the increased ventilation
necessary for the high metabolic cost of flight (94). Therefore, a high CHOL/
low DSP mixture could be a primitive surfactant that was modified through the
evolution of the vertebrates by a range of selection pressures, including terrestri-
ality, habitat, lung structure, lung function, and temperature (2).

It is clear from Table 2.4 that temperature has been a powerful evolutionary
force on the lipid composition of the surfactant system (1). Animals with lower
preferred body temperatures have much higher ratios of CHOL/DSP in their
surfactants (e.g., fish and amphibians, generally $T_b < 25°C$) than animals with
"warm" body temperatures (some reptiles, birds, and mammals, $T_b \sim 37°C$)
(95). This pattern is consistent across the vertebrates, despite differences in lung
structure and phylogeny and is undoubtedly a result of the thermal and biophysical
properties of the surfactant lipids. CHOL-rich surfactant can function at low body
temperatures because cholesterol lowers the phase transition temperature of the
lipid mixture over a broad range of temperatures and acts as a fluidizer at the
air–liquid interface (45,72,92). CHOL acts as a fluidizer at low temperatures
(96), disrupting the Van der Waals forces between adjacent PL fatty acid chains
and forcing the mechanical separation of PL headgroups to enhance adsorption
and promote surfactant respreading upon inspiration (97). USP also have much
lower phase transition temperatures and can increase surfactant fluidity at low
temperatures (2). There is, however, an evolutionary trade-off between temperature and the relative amount of saturated PL. At low body temperatures, increasing
surfactant fluidity can occur by diluting DSP content with CHOL (usually a short-
term response) or USP (a long-term response), but these changes will also decrease
the surface tension-lowering ability (2,72,92,98). In nonmammalian vertebrates, a
decrease in surface tension-lowering ability is a feasible evolutionary trade-off,
given the primary antiadhesive function of their surfactants. However, surfactant
in heterothermic mammals must be fluid at cold body temperatures, yet still remain
surface-active. Heterothermic mammals also maintain fluidity and surface
activity, at least in part, by varying the relative proportions of CHOL and USP
to DSP during activity and torpor. Thus, CHOL appears to be very important to
the thermal dynamics of surfactant, both in a long-term evolutionary sense and
during daily or seasonal changes in body temperature.

Ectothermic Animals

Keough and colleagues (109,114) were the first to demonstrate that surfactant lipid composition could alter in response to relatively short-term changes in body temperature. Lau and Keough (109) observed that surfactant collected from cold-acclimated map turtles, *Malaclemys geographica*, after 2–3 months of hibernation was less lavageable and higher in unsaturated fatty acids than surfactant from warm-acclimated turtles (109). Since then, Daniels et al. (113) have demonstrated that the central netted dragon, *Ctenophorus nuchalis*, doubles the CHOL/PL ratio in its surfactant after a 4 h decrease in body temperature from 37°C to 14°C (Fig. 2.4). The overall amount of alveolar surfactant collected from central netted dragons did not change with a 4 h decrease in body temperature (113). In another agamid lizard (the bearded dragon), *Pogona vitticeps*, both CHOL and total PL increased after acclimation for 4 h at 37°C compared with 18°C (60). However, the relative proportions of CHOL/PL did not change in these lizards and this may indicate that bearded dragons need longer than 4 h, given their larger sizes (120.7 $\pm$ 5.2 g; mean $\pm$ SE) to bring about the changes in CHOL/PL ratio that was observed in the smaller central netted dragons (30.2 $\pm$ 4.7 g; mean $\pm$ SD) (60). Alternatively, CHOL/PL may not be as critical to surfactant fluidity in bearded dragons (60) and they may use other methods such as increasing USP, fatty acids, and proteins to increase fluidity when cold. Clearly, more research is needed to determine the full complement of compositional changes and the importance of these changes on surfactant function in ectothermic animals. The consequence of changing surfactant composition on the antiadhesive function of ectothermic surfactant has also not been studied.

Heterothermic Mammals

Surfactant collected from torpid dunnarts (45) and cold-acclimated ground squirrels (114) is higher in total PL than surfactant collected from active dunnarts and warm-acclimated squirrels. During torpor in dunnarts, there are increases in total PL, the relative amounts of DSP, CHOL, and PI, and a decrease in the predominant phospholipid, PC (45). These changes correlate with changes in surface activity (Section II.C) and thus enable dunnart surfactant to function effectively at low body temperatures experienced during torpor (72,92). In contrast, during torpor in the microchiropteran bats, measures of total surfactant PL and DSP did not change in *C. gouldii* (90) and decreased in *N. geoffroyi* (93). In both these bats, the DSP/PL ratio also did not change between torpor and activity. The different response of bats and dunnarts may reflect the different physiological states of the animals during torpor (90). Unlike bats, torpor in dunnarts is a stress response to low ambient temperatures and food shortages and may be associated with elevated levels of cortisol, which are known stimuli for surfactant PL synthesis (22). In addition, in the laboratory studies, torpor in bats ($T_b = 24–25°C$) was likely to be more shallow than that experienced by dunnarts ($T_b = 13–15°C$). There is also evidence that the lung of bats may not completely

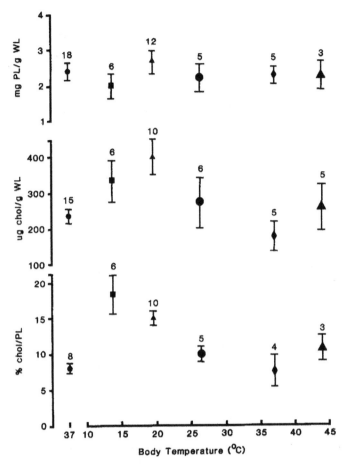

Figure 2.4 Changes in the amount of PL and CHOL harvested by lavage and expressed per gram wet lung, together with cholesterol expressed as percentage of PL, in *C. nuchalis* maintained at different body temperatures for 4 h. Results are expressed as means ± SEM. Numbers of lizards are above each data point. Reproduced from Ref. (113).

deflate during torpor, even at very low ambient temperatures (115,116) and this may lead to differences in surfactant composition and function during torpor. Despite differences in the response of their surfactant PL to decreasing body temperature, both *C. gouldii* and dunnarts increase their CHOL during torpor (Fig. 2.5). This suggests a fundamental role for CHOL in cold heterothermic mammals. However, CHOL did not increase during torpor in *N. geoffroyi*. Furthermore, the relatively low levels of CHOL in bat surfactant, compared with other animals (Table 2.4), suggest that other components must be acting to aid in the spreading and fluidity of bat surfactant at low body temperatures.

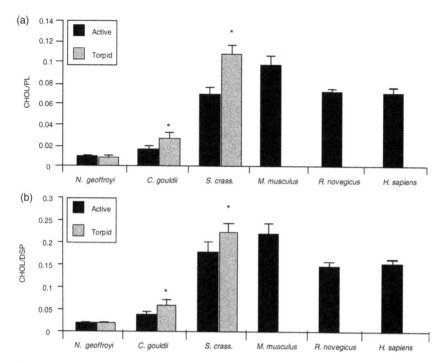

Figure 2.5 (a) Relative amounts of total CHOL as a fraction of total PL ($\mu g/\mu g$) for active bats, dunnarts, mice, rats, and humans as well as torpid bats and dunnarts. (b) Cholesterol as a fraction of DSP ($\mu g/\mu g$) for active bats, dunnarts, mice, rats, and humans and torpid bats and dunnarts. Data are from Refs. (45,90,93).

Veldhuizen et al. (8) have demonstrated that the addition of acidic PL, mono-, di-, and triglycerides, and the hydrophobic surfactant proteins, SP-B and SP-C enhance adsorption rate of surfactant to the air–liquid interface (8). Surfactant proteins are ideal for increasing fluidity because unlike CHOL and other fatty acids, they do not influence surface activity *per se*, but they do enhance the adsorption rate by interacting with the PL (8). Therefore in bats, and possibly in other animals, the surfactant proteins and other fatty acids may be important in maintaining surfactant function at cold temperatures, in preference, or in addition, to increasing CHOL, which also lowers surface activity.

Homeothermic Mammals

Homeothermic mammals rarely experience significant body temperature fluctuations and when they do, as in hypothermia, they can suffer respiratory distress (32,33,77). Consequently, experimental manipulations in homeothermic mammals are not ethical or feasible and little is known about the effects of altering body temperature on surfactant composition in these animals. Using isolated perfused rat lungs, King and Martin (117) observed that lowering the incubation temperature to 13°C virtually abolished surfactant PL secretion. However, an increase in total surfactant PL has been observed in isolated perfused rat lungs incubated at 22°C (73). Similar increases in the amount of alveolar PL, despite decreases in surfactant secretion occur during torpor in dunnarts (118) and may act to improve surfactant spreadability and function at cold body temperatures (45). Thus, decreases in phospholipid turnover may be a regulatory mechanism that is exploited in hypothermic homeotherms and heterothermic mammals to increase the amount of surfactant phospholipid and thus maintain surfactant function as body temperature begins to fall. Alterations in surfactant composition, and particularly in CHOL, occur in response to swimming exercise in rats (119) and cycling exercise in humans (120). In humans, the direction of change in the CHOL/DSP ratio is dependent on the fitness of the individuals and possibly their ventilatory capabilities (120). In perfused rat lungs, the direction of change in the CHOL/DSP ratio is dependent on the type of breathing pattern (high tidal volume or high frequency) (119). Thus, homeothermic mammals can modify their surfactant composition under certain physiological conditions. This would suggest that the surfactant systems of homeothermic mammals possess the mechanisms needed to alter surfactant composition under conditions of temperature stress. Whether or not these mechanisms occur in response to temperature changes *in vivo*, such as those experienced in hypothermia or in isolated lungs transplants, is not known. However, temperature-induced alterations in surfactant composition seem unlikely, given that decreases in temperature decrease lung compliance and have little effect on surfactant surface activity (Section II).

B. Protein Composition

There is no doubt that the four surfactant proteins play a very important role in the function of all mammalian lungs and consequently, they have become a hot topic of research in recent times (Section III.B). However, the effects of changes in body temperature on the amount, synthesis, behavior, and function of SP-A, SP-B, SP-C, and SP-D have yet to be examined. Other studies on other proteins demonstrate that during hibernation gene expression decreases while the half-life of mRNA increases (121). This preservation of mRNA is thought to aid the resumption of gene expression during inter-bout arousals and allows for the replenishment of protein pools. During hibernation, there are also changes in differential gene expression and the differential control of enzymatic activity through phosphorylation or sequestering of enzymes (121). Hence, it is possible that temperature also influences the rates of surfactant protein synthesis, secretion, and the activity of degradation pathways within ATII cells, Clara cells, and the alveolar compartment. In addition, temperature may alter interactions between the surfactant proteins and the surfactant phospholipids that are important in the adsorption of surfactant lipids to the air–liquid interface

(8). Furthermore, protein clearance in the lung is temperature-dependent and alveolar liquid and protein clearance decreases in isolated goat lungs as temperature is reduced from 30°C to 18°C (122). Therefore, as temperature decreases, total protein, and thus, probably the amount of the surfactant proteins, increases in the lung. Increases in the surfactant proteins may lead to disruption of the surfactant monolayer (39). Therefore, we hypothesize that at low temperatures, increases in alveolar protein may act to reduce the surface activity of surfactant. Changes to surface activity could increase surfactant fluidity and either improve or hamper the adsorption of lipids to the air–liquid interface. Whether or not the surfactant protein themselves increase (change in their relative proportions to each other) or alter their function at low temperatures still remains to be examined. However, there can be no doubt that the findings will be extremely important to our understanding of the thermal dynamics of the entire surfactant system.

IV. Temperature and Control of Surfactant Secretion

There are two pools of surfactant in the lungs: the intracellular pool in lamellar bodies of ATII cells and the extracellular pool in the alveolar hypophase (22). The turnover of surfactant is rapid, with 10–40% of the intracellular pool secreted and removed from the extracellular pool per hour (5). Therefore, in order to maintain the composition and amount of alveolar surfactant, these two pools must be tightly regulated by the processes of surfactant synthesis, secretion, and turnover (25). The effect of temperature on surfactant synthesis and turnover has yet to be examined in detail. In addition, the neutral lipid, cholesterol, appears to be titrated rapidly and independently of the PL components of surfactant (60) and studies using isolated lungs indicate that there may be an alternate (i.e., non-lamellar body) source of cholesterol, which is rapidly mobilized by hyperventilation (119). Adrenergic and cholinergic agonists control PL release but do not appear to influence CHOL release in isolated lungs of reptiles. Exercise and temperature can also influence CHOL/PL ratios in a variety of species (60,89,118,119,123). However, mechanisms controlling CHOL release into the lung have so far received only limited experimental attention. Hence, in the following paragraphs, we will focus on the effects of temperature on the control of PL secretion from ATII cells. A schematic representation of the factors controlling surfactant secretion and the intracellular signaling pathways they activate is given in Fig. 2.6.

A. Basal Secretion

Temperature undoubtedly affects the rate of basal secretion from ATII cells. The kinetic effects of temperature on the rate of metabolic processes, such as surfactant secretion, are defined by the Q_{10}. Q_{10} relates the rate of a stimulatory or secretory pathway to temperature. A Q_{10} of 2–3 means that the rate will decrease by one-half for every 10°C fall in body temperature (124). High temperatures

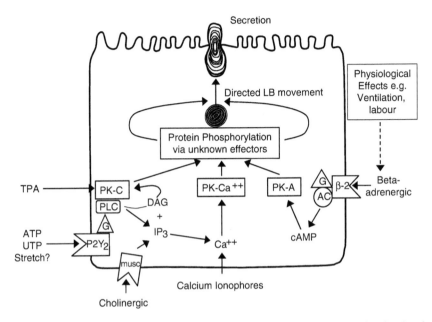

Figure 2.6 Regulation of surfactant secretion from ATII cells. Secretion is stimulated by at least three different signaling pathways. Several different receptors may be involved in signaling through the protein kinase C pathway. The interactions of second messengers have been simplified. For example, cAMP can also increase levels of intracellular calcium. Figure modified from Refs. (20) and (31).

increase the metabolic rate of ATII cells and may directly stimulate the rate of synthesis and/or secretion of lamellar bodies (26). Low temperatures decrease metabolic rate, and therefore, the rate of surfactant secretion. In ATII cells isolated from homeothermic rats, a decrease in incubation temperature to 5°C virtually abolishes surfactant secretion (125). However, lizard (ectothermic) and dunnart (heterothermic) ATII cells secrete surfactant at both low (18°C) and high (37°C) incubation temperatures (118,126). In ATII cells isolated from dunnarts, surfactant secretion was significantly lower at 18°C than at 37°C, but the Q_{10} for the process was 1.3. Hence, the secretory pathway in dunnart ATII cells is relatively insensitive to temperature change and is regulated or altered in some way to counteract the kinetic effects of a decrease in temperature (118,124). These temperature-resistance mechanisms remain unknown. Whether ATII cells isolated from ectothermic animals are also resistant to temperature change is not yet known. Moreover, Van Breukelen and Martin (121) suggest that the same biochemical mechanisms that act to counteract the kinetic effects of temperature during torpor and hibernation in heterothermic animals probably also exist in homeothermic mammals. Hence, homeothermic mammals may possess the biochemical mechanisms used by heterotherms to survive temperature stress, but do not utilize these regulatory mechanisms during thermal stress.

B. Ventilation (Mechanical Stimulation)

Homeothermic Mammals

Ventilation is the major stimulus for surfactant release in homeothermic mammals (127). Increasing the volume of air inhaled (ventilatory tidal volume) stimulates surfactant secretion in homeothermic mammals (25). A significant decrease in the number of lamellar bodies has been observed in rat lungs inflated by one deep breath in a 1 h period of otherwise normal tidal volume ventilation (128). Ventilation-induced increases in surfactant secretion occur via direct mechanical stimulation of ATII cells and subsequent increases in cytosolic calcium (129) (Fig. 2.6). A deep breath is associated with greater inflation of the alveoli and stretching of the alveolar walls. ATII cells are located in crevices between alveoli, where they are exposed to the maximum amount of movement (25). Physical stretch of isolated rat type II cells results in an increase in surfactant secretion equivalent to a combination of agonists, indicating that ventilation is an important stimulus for surfactant release in homeotherms (127,129). Recent technological advances have made it possible for researchers to mimic different ventilatory patterns *in vitro* by mechanically stretching ATII cells. Thus, in the near future, researchers should be able to define in detail the effects of different ventilatory regimes on mechanical stimulation on homeothermic ATII cells. A much better understanding of the involvement of intracellular calcium and other intracellular signaling pathways, that are activated by the mechanical distortion of ATII cells is also possible with this technology (129).

Ecothermic Animals

In lizard lungs, ventilatory pattern does not affect surfactant release or composition (60) and this is probably because the breathing cycle of reptiles is highly variable and consists of short ventilatory periods followed by nonventilatory periods (89). Such a respiratory pattern is discontinuous (60) and therefore, does not guarantee a regular mechanical stimulation of the ATII cells (60). In addition, the actual arrangement of ATII cells in the lizard lung may be such that they do not actually experience much mechanical deformation during ventilation (60). Thus, the increases in surfactant PL and changes in composition that are observed at warm body temperatures in lizard lungs cannot be attributed to changes in breathing pattern (60).

Heterothermic Mammals

Given its importance in homeothermic mammals, ventilation is also likely to be an important stimulus in heterothermic animals, at least, when they are active and warm. However, as body temperature decreases, metabolic rate, and thus the requirement for oxygen also decrease, which reduces the need to breathe. Consequently, both tidal volume and frequency decrease markedly as body temperature decreases during torpor or hibernation in heterothermic mammals (45). Therefore, mechanical distortion (stretch) of ATII cells also decreases in cold animals and thus, ventilation is unlikely to be an effective regulator of surfactant release during torpor or hibernation. Yet, surfactant levels remain elevated or even increase in cold animals (Section III.A) and this may reflect a decrease in alveolar fluid clearance or surfactant turnover in the lung (45). Alternatively, other regulatory mechanisms, such as the parasympathetic nervous system (PNS), may become more important in regulating surfactant secretion when ventilation decreases during torpor in heterothermic animals.

C. Adrenergic Agonists

Homeothermic Mammals

Adrenergic agonists are released from the sympathetic nervous system (SNS) *in vivo* and are a major stimulus of surfactant release in homeothermic mammals (89,130,131). In rats, rabbits, and humans, stimulation of surfactant secretion by β-adrenergic agonists has been observed in isolated ATII cells, isolated perfused lungs, and *in vivo* (26). β-adrenergic agonists bind to membrane-bound β_2-adrenergic receptors on ATII cells and activate the second messenger, cAMP (Fig. 2.6). Stereologic analyses demonstrate that this stimulatory response is rapid in mammals, with lamellar body volume density decreasing within 0.5 h after injection (31).

Ectothermic Animals

It is not known whether ectothermic animals possess β_2 adrenergic receptors. The SNS appears to be absent or poorly developed in lungfish (132) and consequently, adrenaline does not stimulate surfactant release in ATII cells isolated from the Australian lungfish, *Neoceratodus forsteri* (133). However, the SNS is more highly developed in reptiles and amphibians and adrenaline does stimulate surfactant release in ATII cells isolated from bearded dragons, *Pogona vitticeps* and the North American bullfrog, *Rana catesbeiana* (133). In addition, perfusing isolated lizard lungs of *P. vitticeps* with adrenaline also stimulates surfactant release (60), suggesting that surfactant release is under sympathetic control in these animals. Hence, it is possible that adrenaline acts in ectothermic animals through similar receptors and biochemical pathways to those reported in homeothermic mammals.

Temperature does not appear to affect the overall response of lizard ATII cells to stimulation by adrenergic agonists. Decreasing incubation temperature of isolated lizard ATII cells from 37°C to 18°C has no effect on the stimulatory response of adrenaline (126). Furthermore, increases in body temperature in *P. vitticeps* are accompanied by increases in the amount of surfactant PL (60) and plasma levels of the β agonists, adrenaline, and noradrenaline (89). Hence, the increase in PL found *in vivo* with increases in body temperature may be triggered by an increase in plasma catecholamines (89). However, the observed increases in circulating catecholamines may also reflect an overall increase in sympathetic activity and thus, the activity of sympathetic nerve terminals within the lizard lung. Therefore, PL secretion may be stimulated by direct sympathetic innervation of the ATII cells, or indirectly, by circulating catecholamines. The release of catecholamines by the SNS may result in an increase in local or physiological metabolic activity (89). Consequently, regulation by the SNS may be inefficient in cold lizards conserving metabolic energy. Thus, other regulatory mechanisms, with the exception of ventilation, may become more important at cold body temperatures in ectotherms.

Heterothermic Mammals

As in homeothermic mammals, adrenergic agonists appear to be central in controlling surfactant release in heterothermic mammals, at least when they are warm. Adrenergic agonists increase surfactant secretion in ATII cells isolated from fat-tailed dunnarts, *Sminthopsis crassicaudata* at both warm (37°C) and cold (18°C) incubation temperatures (Table 2.5). However, sympathetic activity

Table 2.5 Comparison of Agonist-Stimulated Secretion (Expressed as a Percentage of Basal Secretion) Between Different Animals Studied and Between Two Incubation Temperatures

Animal	Time (h)	Temp (°C)	Percentage of basal secretion	
			Adrenergic	Cholinergic
Dunnart[a]	4	37	141	121
Dunnart[a]	4	18	129	136
Dunnart[b]	3	37	132	124
Lizard[c]	3	37	106 Ad	100
Lizard[c]	3	18	113 Ad	108
Rat[d]	3	37	147 Tb (10 μM)	102
Rat[e]	3	37	290 (10 μM)	
Rat[f]	1.5	37	300 (10 μM)	97

Note: Agonist-stimulated secretion is presented as the percent of basal secretion, where basal secretion is given the value of 100%. [a](118). [b](134). [c](126). [d](135). [e](131). [f]Dobbs and Mason (130). Values from Dobbs and Mason (125) and Ormond et al. (124) are calculated from data collected as the percent of incorporated ³H-choline secreted. Values from Wood et al. (126,133) are calculated from a nonradiolabelled study, where data were presented as the percent increase in secretion of total phospholipid after a 3 h incubation in the presence of agonist relative to the secretion during a 3 h control period, without agonist. Isoproterenol was used as the adrenergic agonists unless otherwise stated as follows: Ad, Adrenaline HCL and Tb, Terbutaline (10 μM). Carbamylcholine chloride was used as the cholinergic agonist. Concentrations of agonists were at 100 μM, unless otherwise indicated in brackets. Reproduced from Ref. (118).

probably decreases *in vivo* during torpor in dunnarts. Wood et al. (133) postulated that sympathetic control of secretion in torpid animals is unlikely because the release of adrenergic factors would increase metabolic rate, causing them to arouse from torpor. However, despite decreases in ventilation and probably sympathetic activity, the amount of surfactant PL increases during torpor in dunnarts (45). As in lizards, temperature does not alter the stimulatory response of dunnart ATII cells to adrenergic agonists. Dunnart ATII cells incubated at both 37°C and 18°C respond equally well to adrenergic stimulation (118). Furthermore, recent research in our laboratory demonstrates that dunnart ATII cells maintain the number and function of β_2-adrenergic receptors and upregulate intracellular cAMP levels during torpor. These modifications may lead to an increased sensitivity of ATII cells to β-adrenergic agonists during torpor and enable adrenergic control despite a lower sympathetic output. Retaining the capacity to respond to sympathetic stimulation during torpor may allow dunnart ATII cells to respond rapidly to increases in sympathetic activity during the early stages of arousal from torpor, prior to increase in body temperature, metabolic rate, and ventilation. Alternatively, or in addition, regulation by the PNS and cholinergic agonists, which do not increase metabolic rate, may be important in controlling surfactant release during torpor.

D. Cholinergic Agonists

Homeothermic Mammals

There appears to be some controversy about the role of acetylcholine and the PNS in stimulating surfactant release. Acetylcholine has been found to act on muscarinic receptors to increase PL release in intact rabbit (136) and isolated rat (131) lungs. However, Nicholas and Barr (137) failed to find a similar increase in the isolated perfused rat lung. In addition, the cholinergic agonist, carbamylcholine chloride does not stimulate surfactant secretion from ATII cells isolated from humans and rats (125). Although, ATII cells do possess muscarinic receptors, cholinergic nerves have not been found in the alveolar regions of the mammalian lung. Therefore, in homeothermic mammals, cholinergic agonists may not act directly on muscarinic receptors on ATII cells. Wood et al. (137) postulated that cholinergic factors released by the PNS may influence surfactant secretion in reptiles by stimulating contraction of pulmonary smooth muscle cells and subsequently distorting the ATII cells (mechanical stimulation) (24). This mechanism may also occur in homeothermic mammals because distortion of ATII cells represents the major stimulus for surfactant release (127).

Ecothermic Animals

Reptiles, unlike mammals, have lungs richly innervated with both cholinergic and adrenergic nerves (138,139). However, regulation by the SNS (adrenergic) is likely to be inappropriate in cold ectotherms because catecholamines will increase metabolic rate locally, regionally, and globally within the animal (139). It is disadvantageous to increase the metabolic activity and hence oxygen consumption of tissues when torpor is clearly designed to reduce these processes. Therefore, in ectotherms at low body temperatures and during nonventilatory periods, the PNS may stimulate activity in pulmonary smooth muscle, thereby promoting gas exchange and ventilation of respiratory surfaces without increasing metabolic rate (139). In reptilian lungs, PNS nerve endings are located in the alveolar region (138). Therefore, the release of acetylcholine from parasympathetic nerves could stimulate surfactant secretion by direct interaction with muscarinic receptors on ATII cells. Carbamylcholine chloride increases PC secretion in ATII cells isolated from Australian lungfish, *Neoceratodus forsteri,* bearded dragons, *Pogona vitticeps,* and the North American bullfrog, *Rana catesbeiana* (133). Furthermore, in isolated perfused lungs of the bearded dragons, the stimulatory activity of acetycholine is inhibited by atropine, an antagonist (inhibitor) of muscarinic cholinergic receptors (139). In addition, the sympathetic ganglion blocker, hexamethonium does not inhibit cholinergically stimulated secretion in isolated lizard lungs (128). This suggests that the response to cholinergic agonists is not mediated indirectly through preganglionic stimulation of sympathetic nerve fibers (139). Therefore, cholinergic agonists can interact directly with muscarinic receptors, which are located in the smooth muscle and on ATII cells in the lizard lung (139).

However, regulation by the PNS is temperature dependent in bearded dragons, at least at the cellular level. Carbamylcholine chloride stimulated surfactant secretion from bearded dragon ATII cells incubated at 20°C, but not at 37°C (126). As the response of lizard ATII cells to adrenergic agonists is not sensitive to temperature, the switch in the response of ATII cells to cholinergic factors at cold temperatures may be due to temperature-sensitive muscarinic receptors or enzymes that are specifically part of the cholinergic signaling pathway. Alternatively, low temperatures may reduce the activity of enzymes, such as acetylcholinesterase, which break down acetylcholine and therefore, increase the amount of acetylcholine interacting with the cholinergic receptors on ATII cells at low temperatures (139). Consequently, in lizards, adrenergic stimulation is particularly important at warm body temperatures when the cholinergic pathway is not activated (126). In contrast, direct cholinergic stimulation may be more important in cold lizards with decreased metabolic rates.

Heterothermic Mammals

Cholinergic agonists also act directly on ATII cells isolated from heterothermic mammals to stimulate surfactant secretion. Carbamylcholine chloride increases PC secretion in ATII cells isolated from fat-tailed dunnarts, *Sminthopsis crassicaudata* (Table 2.5) and juvenile, unfurred, heterothermic tammar wallabies, *Macropus eugenii* (118,126,133,140). The cholinergic response may reflect thermoregulatory plasticity, a characteristic of these two marsupials. This finding is in direct contrast to observations made in homeothermic mammals. It is possible that mammals, which maintain a constant body temperature, need only the actions of the SNS (adrenergic) to efficiently regulate surfactant secretion. Heterothermic mammals may have a direct role for the PNS in regulating surfactant secretion at low body temperatures. Studies examining the innervation of the lungs of dunnarts or tammar wallabies have not yet been completed. Therefore, we do not know whether the alveolar regions of these marsupials are innervated with cholinergic nerves (like lizards) or if they lack cholinergic innervation (like homeothermic mammals). Studies examining the effects of cholinergic agonists on surfactant release *in vivo* or in isolated lungs of heterothermic mammals have also not been completed. However, it is possible, given the observations in both ectotherms and homeotherms, that the PNS of heterotherms also stimulates surfactant secretion indirectly via stimulation of receptors on pulmonary smooth muscle and thus, distortion of ATII cells.

As in cold lizards, the amount of surfactant PL increases in dunnarts during torpor. However, unlike in lizards, carbamylcholine chloride can stimulate surfactant secretion in isolated dunnart ATII cells at both cold (18°C) and warm (37°C) incubation temperatures (Table 2.5) (118). Therefore, both adrenergic and cholinergic control of surfactant secretion is insensitive to temperature in dunnart ATII cells and this further supports the hypothesis that dunnart ATII cells are highly insensitive to temperature changes (Section IV.A) (118). However, changes in the adrenergic and cholinergic regulation of surfactant secretion must occur at some physiological level in dunnarts, because the release of catecholamines by the SNS may increase metabolic rate and cause dunnarts to arouse from torpor. Hence, the SNS is probably suppressed during torpor and thus, the PNS may become an important stimulus of secretion in cold animals. Dunnart ATII cells may have lost or not evolved the temperature-sensitive cholinergic switch, that is found in lizard ATII cells, and this has a number of advantages (118). Firstly, dunnart ATII cells can respond quickly to a physiological change in autonomic stimulation during the rapid entry and arousal from torpor. Secondly, the retention of both parasympathetic and sympathetic stimulation at 37°C may enable the combined action of adrenergic and cholinergic factors on ATII cells, increasing surfactant secretion above that obtained with either factor alone (118).

E. Other Factors

A great number of other biochemical factors influence the secretion of surfactant. ATP, through purinergic receptors on ATII cells, is a powerful stimulator for surfactant release (141,142). Metabolites of arachidonic acid (20), calcium ionophores (143), endothelin-1 (144), vasopressin (145), lipoproteins (146), and phorbol esters (145) all stimulate surfactant secretion. Once secreted, the surfactant components themselves can also regulate further secretion. At low lung volumes, USP and surfactant proteins (especially SP-A) are squeezed out of the surfactant film and these components act to inhibit further secretion (20). If delipidated, purified SP-A can inhibit all forms of agonist-induced secretion *in vitro*, suggesting that SP-A acts to inhibit secretion at a stage shared by all the regulatory mechanisms (147). Below the phase transition temperatures, saturated PC also inhibits surfactant secretion *in vitro* (148). The effects of temperature on the responses of the secretory pathways to these biochemical factors still need to be examined.

V. Summary and Future Directions

Since the early 20th century, substantial research has been undertaken to understand the pulmonary surfactant system in humans and its function in healthy and diseased states. Research concerning the surfactant system of other animals has been largely ignored, except by a few dedicated researchers. Yet, ectotherms and heterothermic mammals are clearly excellent models for investigating how the surfactant system copes with physiological variables. Despite differences in lung structure, temperature has had a profound effect on the evolution of the surfactant system. Temperature also affects the physical properties of the surfactant components. Consequently, heterothermic animals alter the composition and surface activity of their surfactant in order to respond to changes in body temperature. The compositional change that occurs during torpor in heterothermic mammals, and particularly increases in the cholesterol to phospholipid ratio, appear to facilitate faster adsorption, low ST_{min}, and low compressibility at the reduced temperature. This suggests that *in vivo*, surfactant from torpid animals functions very similarly to surfactant in warm-active animals. However, not all of the observed changes in surface activity can be attributed to cholesterol. Bats have extremely low levels of cholesterol compared with other mammals, which may indicate that other surfactant components such as the surfactant proteins and acidic fatty acids may be involved in fluidizing the surfactant mixtures during torpor. Thus, the surfactant system appears to be highly sensitive to temperature changes and in heterothermic animals, responds rapidly with changes in surfactant amount, composition, and surface activity with entry and arousal from torpor. However, in order for the observed changes in lipid composition and increases in surfactant to occur during torpor, there are also changes in the regulatory and secretory pathways controlling surfactant release into the lung. Understanding how the surfactant system can remain functional over a range of temperatures may have important medical consequences in the treatment of hypothermia (35), hyperthermia (32), cystic fibrosis (41), and asthma (39). The consequences of temperature on the function of surfactant are also important in hypothermic surgery, lung transplantation (33,36,37), and in the development of artificial surfactants for the treatment of respiratory distress syndromes (36,37,149,150).

References

1. Possmayer F. Physicochemical aspects of pulmonary surfactant. In: Polin RA, Fox WW, eds. Fetal and Neonatal Physiology. WB Saunders Company, 1997:1259–1275.

2. Daniels CB, Lopatko, OV, Orgeig S. Evolution of surface activity related functions of vertebrate pulmonary surfactant. Clin Exp Pharmacol Physiol 1998; 25:716–721.
3. Schürch S, Bachofen H, Goerke J, Green F. Surface properties of rat pulmonary surfactant studied with the captive bubble method: adsorption, hysteresis, stability. Biochim Biophys Acta 1992; 1103:127–136.
4. King R. Pulmonary surfactant. J Appl Physiol 1982; 53:1–8.
5. Wright JR. Clearance and recycling of pulmonary surfactant. Am J Physiol 1990; 259:L1–L12.
6. Batenburg JJ. Surfactant phospholipids: synthesis and storage. Am J Physiol 1992; 262(6):L367–L385.
7. Goerke J. Pulmonary surfactant: functions and molecular composition. Biochim Biophys Acta 1998; 1408:79–89.
8. Veldhuizen RAW, Nag K, Orgeig S, Possmayer F. The role of lipids in pulmonary surfactant. Biochim Biophys Acta 1998; 1408:90–108.
9. Wright JR, Clements JA. Lung surfactant turnovers and factors that affect turnover. In: Massaro D, ed. Lung Cell Biology. New York: Marcel Dekker Inc, 1989:655–699.
10. King RJ, Clements JA. Lipid synthesis and surfactant turnover in the lungs. In: Fishman AP, Fisher AB, Geiger SR, eds. Handbook of Physiology. 1st ed. Bethesda: American Physiological Society, 1985:309–336.
11. Goerke J, Clements JA. Alveolar surface tension and lung surfactant. In: Macklem PT, Mead J, eds. Handbook of Physiology, Section 3: The Respiratory System. Vol 3: Mechanics of Breathing, Part I. Washington DC: American Physiological Society, 1985:247–260.
12. Possmayer F. Biophysical activities of pulmonary surfactant. In: Polin RA, Fox WW, eds. Fetal and Neonatal Physiology. 1st ed. Philadelphia: WB Saunders Co., 1991:459–962.
13. Haagsman HP, Hawgood S, Sargeant T, Buckley D, White RT, Drickamer K, Benson B. The major lung surfactant protein 28-36, is a calcium-dependent carbohydrate-binding protein. J Biol Chem 1987; 262:13877–13880.
14. Persson A, Chang D, Crouch E. Surfactant protein D is a divalent cation-dependent carbohydrate-binding protein. J Biol Chem 1990; 265(10):5755–5760.
15. Hawgood S, Derrick M, Poulain F. Structure and properties of surfactant protein B. Biochim Biophys Acta 1998; 1408:150–160.
16. Johansson J. Structure and properties of surfactant protein C. Biochim Biophys Acta 1998; 1408:161–172.
17. Sullivan LC, Daniels CB, Phillips ID, Orgeig S, Whitsett JA. Conservation of surfactant protein A: evidence for a single origin for vertebrate pulmonary surfactant. J Mol Evol 1998; 46:131–138.
18. McCormack FX. Structure, processing and properties of surfactant protein A. Biochim Biophys Acta 1998; 1408:109–131.
19. Weaver TE. Synthesis, processsing and secretion of surfactant proteins B and C. Biochim Biophys Acta 1998; 1408:173–179.
20. Mason RJ, Voelker DR. Regulatory mechanisms of surfactant secretion. Biochim Biophys Acta 1998; 1408:226–240.
21. Ward HE, Nicholas TE. Alveolar type I and type II cells. Aust NZ J Med 1984; 14:731–734.

22. Haagsman HP, Van Golde LMG. Synthesis and assembly of lung surfactant. Ann Rev Physiol 1991; 53:441–464.
23. Johansson J, Curstedt T. Molecular structures and interactions of pulmonary surfactant components. Eur J Biochem 1997; 244:675–693.
24. Massaro D, Clerch L, Massaro GD. Surfactant secretion: evidence that cholinergic stimulation of secretion is indirect. Am J Physiol 1982; 243:C39–C45.
25. Wirtz H, Schmidt M. Ventilation and secretion of pulmonary surfactant. Clin Invest 1992; 70:3–13.
26. Chander A, Fisher AB. Regulation of lung surfactant secretion. Am J Physiol 1990; 258:L241–L253.
27. Lumb RH. Phospholipid transfer proteins in mammalian lung. Am J Physiol 1989; 257:L190–L194.
28. Schürch S, Qanbar R, Bachofen H, Possmayer F. The surface-associated surfactant reservoir in the alveolar lining. Biol Neonate 1995; 67(suppl):61–76.
29. Kuroki Y, Voelker DR. Pulmonary surfactant proteins. J Biol Chem 1994; 269:25943–25946.
30. Eiijk MV, DeHaas CGM, Haagsman HP. Quantitative analysis of pulmonary surfactant proteins B and C. Anal Biochem 1995; 232:231–237.
31. Orgeig S, Daniels CB, Sullivan LC. The development of the pulmonary surfactant system. In: Harding R, Pinkerton K, Plopper C, eds. The Lung: Development, Aging and the Environment, London: Academic Press, 2004; Chapter 10, 150–167.
32. Peterson DR, Davis N. Sudden infant death syndrome and malignant hyperthermia diathesis. Aust Paediatr J 1986; (Suppl 1):33–35.
33. Meban C. Influence of pH and temperature on behaviour of surfactant from human neonatal lungs. Biol Neonate 1978; 33:106–111.
34. Geiser F, Ruf T. Hibernation versus daily torpor in mammals and birds—physiological variables and classification of torpor patterns. Physiol Zool 1995; 68(6):935–966.
35. Inoue H, Inoue C, Hildebrandt J. Temperature and surface forces in excised rabbit lungs. J Appl Physiol 1981; 51:823–829.
36. Erasmus ME, Petersen AH, Hofstedt G, Haagsman HP, Bambang Oetomo S, Prop J. Surfactant treatment before reperfusion improves the immediate fuction of lung transplants in rats. Am J Respir Crit Care Med 1996; 153:665–670.
37. Osanai K, Takahashi K, Sato S, Iwabuchi K, Ohtake K, Sata M, Yasui S. Changes of lung surfactant and pressure–volume curve in bleomycin-induced pulmonary fibrosis. J Appl Physiol 1991; 70:1300–1308.
38. Possmayer F, Novick RJ, Rudd AW, Veldhuizen JL, Bjarneson D, Lewis JF. Potential role for pulmonary surfactant in lung transplantation. In: Matalah S, Sznadger JI, eds. ARDS: Cellular and Molecular Mechanisms and Clinical Management, New York: Plenum Pub Corp, 1998:117–124.
39. Postle AD. The role of pulmonary surfactant in the asthmatic response. Clin Exp Allergy 2000; 30(9):1201–1204.
40. Penn RB, Panettieri RA Jr, Benovic JL. Mechanisms of acute desensitization of the beta2AR-adenylyl cyclase pathway in human airway smooth muscle. Am J Respir Cell Mol Biol 1998; 19(2):338–348.
41. Postle AD, Mander A, Reid KB, Wang JY, Wright SM, Moustaki M, Warner JO. Deficient hydrophilic lung surfactant proteins A and D with normal surfactant phospholipid molecular species in cystic fibrosis. Am J Respir Cell Mol Biol 1999; 20(1):90–98.

42. Bernard S. Induced hypothermia in intensive care. Anaesth Intensive Care 1996; 24:382–388.

43. Frappell PB, Daniels CB. Ventilation and oxygen consumption in agamid lizards. Physiol Zool 1991; 64:985–1001.

44. Daniels CB, Orgeig S, Wilsen J, Nicholas TE. Pulmonary-type surfactants in the lungs of terrestrial and aquatic amphibians. Respir Physiol 1994; 95:249–258.

45. Langman C, Orgeig S, Daniels CB. Alterations in composition and function of surfactant associated with torpor in *Sminthopsis crassicaudata*. Am J Physiol 1996; 271:R437–R445.

46. Burggren WW, West NH. Changing respiratory importance of gills, lungs and skin during metamorphosis in the bullfrog *Rana catesbeiana*. Respir Physiol 1982; 47:151–164.

47. Daniels CB, Skinner CH. The composition and function of surface active lipids in the goldfish swim bladder. Physiol Zool 1994; 67(5):1230–1256.

48. Phleger CF, Saunders BS. Swim-bladder surfactants of Amazonian air-breathing fishes. Can J Zool 1978; 56:946–952.

49. Phleger CF, Benson AA. Cholesterol and hyperbaric oxygen in swimbladders of deep sea fishes. Nature 1971; 230:122.

50. Meban C. Physical properties of surfactant from the lungs of the tortoise *Testudo hermanni*. Comp Biochem Physiol 1980; 67(2):253–257.

51. Fujiwara T, Adams FH, Nozaki M, Dermer GB. Pulmonary surfactant phospholipids from turkey lung: comparison with rabbit lung. Am J Physiol 1970; 218:218–225.

52. Daniels CB, Eskandari-Marandi BD, Nicholas TE. The role of surfactant in the static lung mechanics of the lizard *Ctenophorus nuchalis*. Respir Physiol 1993; 94:11–23.

53. Daniels CB, McGregor LK, Nicholas TE. The dragon's breath: a model for the dynamics of breathing and faveolar ventilation in agamid lizards. *Herpetologica* 1994; 50:251–261.

54. Sanderson RJ, Paul GW, Vatter AE, Filley GF. Morphological and physical basis for lung surfactant action. Respir Physiol 1976; 27(3):379–392.

55. Smits AW, Orgeig S, Daniels CB. Surfactant composition and function in lungs of air-breathing fishes. Am J Physiol 1994; 266:R1309–R1313.

56. Daniels CB, Smits AW, Orgeig S. Pulmonary surfactant lipids in the faveolar and saccular lung regions of snakes. Physiol Zool 1995; 68(5):812–830.

57. Daniels CB, Orgeig S, Smits AW. The composition and function of reptilian pulmonary surfactant. Respir Physiol 1995; 102:121–135.

58. Milsom WK. Intermittent breathing in vertebrates. Annu Rev Physiol 1991; 53:87–105.

59. Martin KM, Hutchison VH. Ventilatory activity in *Amphiuma tridactylum* and *Siren lacertina* (Amphibia, Caudata). J Herpetol 1979; 13:427–434.

60. Wood PG, Daniels CB, Orgeig S. Functional significance and control of release of pulmonary surfactant in the lizard lung. Am J Physiol 1995; 269:R838–R847.

61. Pattle RE. Properties, function, and origin of the alveolar lining layer. Proc R Soc Lond 1958; 148:217–240.

62. Pattle RE. The cause of the stability of bubbles derived from the lung. Phys Med Biol 1960; 5:11–26.

63. Porter AW. The calculation of surface tension from experiment—Part 1. Sessile drops. Philos Mag 1933; 15:163–170.

64. Putz G, Goerke J, Schurch S, Clements JA. Evaluation of a pressure-driven captive bubble surfactometer. J Appl Physiol 1994; 76:1417–1424.

65. Putz G, Goerke J, Taeusch HW, Clements JA. Comparison of captive and pulsating bubble surfactometers with use of lung surfactants. J Appl Physiol 1994; 76:1425–1431.

66. Enhorning G. Pulmonary surfactant function studied with the pulsating bubble surfactometer (PBS) and the capillary surfactometer (CS). Comp Biochem Physiol A Mol Integr Physiol 2001; 129(1):221–226.

67. Keough KMW, Parsons CS, Tweeddale MG. Interactions between plasma proteins and pulmonary surfactant; pulsating bubble studies. Can J Physiol Pharmacol 1989; 67:663–668.

68. Yu S, Harding PGR, Smith N, Possmayer F. Bovine pulmonary surfactant: chemical composition and physical properties. Lipids 1983; 18:522–529.

69. Schürch S, Bachofen H, Goerke J, Possmayer F. A captive bubble method reproduces the in situ behaviour of lung surfactant monolayers. J Appl Physiol 1989; 67:2389–2396.

70. Schürch S, Bachofen H, Possmayer F. Surface activity in situ, in vivo, and in the captive bubble surfactometer. Comp Biochem Physiol A 2001; 129:195–207.

71. Avery ME. Surfactant deficiency in hyaline membrane disease. The story of discovery. Am J Respir Crit Care Med 2000; 161:1074–1075.

72. Lopatko OV, Orgeig S, Daniels CB, Palmer D. Alterations in the surface properties of lung surfactant in the torpid marsupial *Sminthopsis crassicaudata*. J Appl Physiol 1998; 84(1):146–156.

73. Miles PR, Bowmen L, Frazer DG. Properties of lavage material from excised lungs ventilated at different temperatures. Respir Physiol 1995; 101:99–108.

74. Schürch S, Goerke J, Clements JA. Direct determination of surface tension in the lung. Proceedings of the National Academy of Science of the United States of America. 1976; 73:4698–4702.

75. Crosfill ML, Widdicombe JG. Physical characteristics of the chest and lungs and the work of breathing in different mammalian species. J Physiol 1961; 158:1–14.

76. von Neergaard KV. New notions on a fundamental principle of respiratory mechanics: the retractile force of the lung, dependent on the surface tension in the alveoli. Zeitschrift für Gesamte Experimentelle Medizin 1929; 66:373–394.

77. Inoue H, Inoue C, Hildebrandt J. Temperature effects on lung mechanics in air- and liquid-filled rabbit lungs. J Appl Physiol 1982; 53:567–575.

78. Horie T, Ardila R, Hildebrandt J. Static and dynamic properties of excised cat lung in relation to temperature. J Appl Physiol 1974; 36:317–322.

79. Diaz G, Gunther B. Shear viscosity of the surfactant from dog lungs. Arch Biol Med Exp 1984; 17:21–27.

80. Wildeboer-Venema F. The influences of temperature and humidity upon the isolated surfactant film of the dog. Respir Physiol 1980; 39:63–71.

81. Lempert J, Macklem PT. Effect of temperature on rabbit lung surfactant and pressure–volume hysteresis. J Appl Physiol 1971; 31:380–385.

82. Clements JA. Functions of the alveolar lining. Am Rev Respir Dis 1977; 115:67–71.

83. Codd JR, Daniels CB, Orgeig S. Thermal cycling of the pulmonary surfactant system in small heterothermic mammals. In: Heldmeier G, Klingenspor M, eds.

Life in the Cold. 11th International Hibernation Symposium. Berlin: Springer-Verlag, 2000:187–197.

84. Godfrey GK. Body-temperatures and torpor in *Sminthopsis crassicaudata* and *S. larapinta* (Marsupialia-Dasyuridae). J Zool 1968; 156:499–511.

85. Hosken DJ, Withers PC. Metabolic physiology of euthermic and torpid lesser long-eared bats, *Nyctophilus geoffroyi* (Chirpotera:Vespertilionidae). J Mammal 1999; 80(1):42–52.

86. Hosken DJ, Withers PC. Temperature regulation and metabolism of an Australian bat, *Chalinolobus gouldii* (Chiroptera:Vespertilionidae) when euthermic and torpid. J Comp Physiol B 1997; 167:71–80.

87. Morris S, Curtin AL, Thompson MB. Heterothermy, torpor, respiratory gas exchange, water balance and the effect of feeding in gould's long eared bat *Nyctophilus gouldi*. J Exp Biol 1994; 197:309–335.

88. Geiser F, Ruf T. Hibernation versus daily torpor in mammals and birds: physiological variables and classification of torpor patterns. Physiol Zool 1995; 68:935–966.

89. Wood PG, Daniels CB. Factors affecting opening and filling pressures in the lungs of the lizard *Pogona vitticeps*. Respir Physiol 1996; 103:203–210.

90. Codd JR, Schürch S, Daniels CB, Orgeig S. Torpor-associated fluctuations in surfactant activity in Gould's wattled bat. Biochim Biophys Acta 2002; 308:463–468.

91. Geiser F, Baudinette RV. The relationship between body mass and rate of rewarming from hibernation and daily torpor in mammals. J Exp Biol 1990; 151:349–359.

92. Lopatko OV, Orgeig S, Palmer D, Schurch S, Daniels CB. Alterations in pulmonary surfactant after rapid arousal from torpor in the marsupial *Sminthopsis crassicaudata*. J Appl Physiol 1999; 86(6):1959–1970.

93. Slocombe NC, Codd JR, Wood PG, Orgeig S, Daniels CB. The effect of alterations in activity and body temperature on the pulmonary surfactant system in the lesser long-eared bat *Nyctophilus geoffroyi*. J Exp Biol 2000; 203(16):2429–2435.

94. Codd JR, Slocombe NC, Daniels CB, Wood PG, Orgeig S. Periodic fluctuations in the pulmonary surfactant system in Gould's wattled bat (*Chalinolobus gouldii*). Physiol Biochem Zool 2000; 73(5):605–612.

95. Daniels CB, Orgeig S. The comparative biology of pulmonary surfactant: past, present and future. Comp Biochem Physiol A Mol Integr Physiol 2001; 129(1):9–36.

96. Notter RH, Tabak SA, Mavis RD. Surface properties of binary mixtures of some pulmonary surfactant components. J Lipid Res 1980; 21:10–22.

97. Presti FT, Pace RJ, Chan SI. Cholesterol phospholipid interaction in membranes. 2. Stoichiometry and molecular packing of cholesterol-rich domains. Biochemistry 1982; 21:3831–3835.

98. Daniels CB, Orgeig S, Wood PG, Sullivan LC, Lopatko OV, Smits AW. The changing state of surfactant lipids: new insights from ancient animals. Am Zool 1998; 38:305–320.

99. Hallman M, Gluck L. Phosphatidylglycerol in lung surfactant II. Subcellular distribution and mechanism of biosynthesis in vitro. Biochim Biophys Acta 1975; 409:172–191.

100. Shelley SA, Paciga JE, Balis JV. Lung surfactant phospholipids in different animal species. Lipids 1984; 19:857–862.

101. Neumann MA, McMurchie EJ, Gibson RA. A comparison of lung lamellar body phospholipids from premature and term infants: is sphingomyelin a contaminant of surfactant? Pediatr Pulmonol 1990; 9:162–165.

102. Harlan WR, Margraf JH, Said SI. Pulmonary lipid composition of species with and without surfactant. Am J Physiol 1966; 211:855–861.

103. Ribbons KA, Baudinette RV, McMurchie EJ. The development of pulmonary surfactant lipids in a neonatal marsupial and the rat. Respir Physiol 1989; 75:1–10.

104. Hallman M, Gluck L. Phosphatidylglycerol in lung surfactant. III. Possible modifier of surfactant function. J Lipid Res 1976; 17:257–262.

105. Johnston SD, Orgeig S, Lopatko OV, Daniels CB. Development of the pulmonary surfactant system in two oviparous vertebrates. Am J Physiol 2000; 278(2):R486–R493.

106. Daniels CB, Orgeig S, Smits AW. Invited perspective: the evolution of the vertebrate pulmonary surfactant system. Physiol Zool 1995; 68(4):539–566.

107. Daniels CB, Barr HA, Nicholas TE. A comparison of the surfactant associated lipids derived from reptilian and mammalian lungs. Respir Physiol 1989; 75:335–348.

108. Daniels CB, Orgeig S, Smits AW, Miller JD. The influence of temperature, phylogeny, and lung structure on the lipid composition of reptilian pulmonary surfactant. Exp Lung Res 1996; 22:267–281.

109. Lau K, Keough KMW. Lipid composition of lung and lung lavage fluid from map turtles (*Malaclemys geographica*) maintained at different environmental temperatures. Can J Biochem 1981; 59:208–219.

110. Vergara GA, Hughes GM. Phospholipids in the washings from the lungs of the frog (*Rana pipiens*). J Comp Physiol 1980; 139:117–120.

111. Orgeig S, Daniels CB, Smits AW. The composition and function of the pulmonary surfactant system during metamorphosis in the tiger salamander *Ambystoma tigrinum*. J Comp Physiol B 1994; 164:337–342.

112. Orgeig S, Daniels CB. The evolutionary significance of pulmonary surfactant in lungfish (*Dipnoi*). Am J Respir Cell and Mol Biol 1995; 13:161–166.

113. Daniels CB, Barr HA, Power JHT, Nicholas TE. Body temperature alters the lipid composition of pulmonary surfactant in the lizard *Ctenophorus nuchalis*. Exp Lung Res 1990; 16:435–449.

114. Melling J, Keough KMW. Major phospholipids from the lung and lung lavage fluid from warm and cold acclimated Richardson's ground squirrels (*Spermophilus richardsoni*). Comp Biochem Physiol B 1981; 69:797–802.

115. Hays GC, Webb PI, Speakman JR. Arrhythmic breathing in torpid pipistrelle bats, *Pipistrellus pipistrellus*. Respir Physiol 1991; 85:185–192.

116. Szewczak JM, Jackson DC. Apneic oxygen uptake in the torpid bat, *Eptesicus fuscus*. J Exp Biol 1992; 173:217–227.

117. King RJ, Martin HM. Effects of inhibiting protein synthesis on the secretion of surfactant by type II cells in primary culture. Biochim Biophys Acta 1981; 663:289–301.

118. Ormond CJ, Orgeig S, Daniels CB. Neurochemical and thermal control of surfactant secretion by alveolar type II isolated from the marsupial Sminthopsis crassicaudata. J Comp Physiol B 2001; 171:223–230.

119. Orgeig S, Barr HA, Nicholas TE. Effect of hyperpnea on the cholesterol to disaturated phospholipid ratio in alveolar surfactant of rats. Exp Lung Res 1995; 21:157–174.

120. Doyle IR, Jones ME, Barr HA, Orgeig S, Crockett AJ, McDonald CF, Nicholas TE. Composition of human pulmonary surfactant varies with exercise and level of fitness. Am J Respir Crit Care Med 1994; 149:1619–1627.

121. Van Breukelen F, Martin SL. Invited review: molecular adaptations in mammalian hibernators: unique adaptations or generalized responses? J Appl Physiol 2002; 92:2640–2647.

122. Serikov VB, Grady M, Matthay MA. Effect of temperature on alveolar liquid and protein clearance in an in situ perfused goat lung. J Appl Physiol 1993; 75:940–947.

123. Orgeig S, Daniels CB, Lopatko OV, Langman C. Effect of torpor on the composition and function of pulmonary surfactant in the heterothermic mammal (*Sminthopsis crassicaudata*). In: Geiser F, Hulbert AJ, Nicol SC, eds. Adaptations to the Cold: 10th International Hibernation Symposium. Armidale: University of New England Press, 1996:223–232.

124. Schmidt-Nielson, K. Animal Physiology: adaptation and environment. Animal Physiology: Adaptation and Environment, 5th ed. Cambridge: Cambridge University Press, 1997.

125. Dobbs LG, Mason RJ. Pulmonary alveolar type II cells isolated from rats. J Clin Invest 1979; 63:378–387.

126. Wood PG, Lopatko OV, Orgeig S, Codd JR, Daniels CB. Control of pulmonary surfactant secretion from type II pneumocytes isolated from the lizard, *Pogona vitticeps*. Am J Physiol 1999; 277(46):R1705–R1711.

127. Wirtz HRW, Dobbs LG. Calcium mobilization and exocytosis after one mechanical stretch of lung epithelial cells. Science 1990; 250:1266–1269.

128. Nicholas TE, Barr HA. The release of surfactant in the rat lung by brief periods of hyperventilation. Respir Physiol 1983; 52:69–83.

129. Edwards YS. Stretch stimulation: its effects on alveolar type II cell function in the lung. Comp Biochem and Physiol 2001; 129:245–260.

130. Dobbs LG, Mason RJ. Stimulation of secretion of disaturated phosphatidylcholine from isolated alveolar type II cells by 12-O-tetradecanoyl-13-phorbol acetate. Am Rev Respir Disease 1978; 113:705–713.

131. Brown LS, Longmore WJ. Adrenergic and cholinergic regulation of lung surfactant secretion in the isolated perfused rat lung and in the alveolar type II cell in culture. J Biol Chem 1981; 256:66–72.

132. Fritsche R, Axelsson M, Franklin CE, Grigg GG, Holmgren S, Nilsson S. Respiratory and cardiovascular responses to hypoxia in the Australian lungfish. Respir Physiol 1993; 94:173–187.

133. Wood PG, Lopatko OV, Orgeig S, Joss JM, Smits AW, Daniels CB. Control of pulmonary surfactant secretion: an evolutionary perspective. Am J Physiol Regul Integr Comp Physiol 2000; 278(3):R611–R619.

134. Wood PG, Lopatko OV, Orgeig S, Joss JM, Smits AW, Daniels CB. Control of pulmonary surfactant secretion: an evolutionary perspective. Am J Physiol 2000; 278(3):R611–R619.

135. Dobbs LG, Gonzalez R, Williams MC. An improved method for isolating type II cells in high yield and purity. Am Rev Respir Disease 1986; 134:141–145.

136. Oyarzun MJ, Clements JA. Ventilatory and cholinergic control of pulmonary surfactant in the rabbit. J Appl Physiol 1977; 43:39–45.

137. Nicholas TE, Barr HA. Control of release of surfactant phospholipids in the isolated perfused rat lung. J Appl Physiol 1981; 51:90–98J.

138. Campbell G, Duxson MJ. The sympathetic innervation of lung muscle in the toad *Bufo marinus*: a revision and an explanation. Comp Biochem Physiol 1978; 60(C):65–73.

139. Wood PG, Andrew LK, Daniels CB, Orgeig S, Roberts CT. Autonomic control of the pulmonary surfactant system and lung compliance in the lizard. Physiol Zool 1997; 70:444–455.

140. Miller NJ, Orgeig S, Daniels CB, Baudinette RV. Postnatal development and control of the pulmonary surfactant system in the tammar wallaby *Macropus eugenii*. J Exp Biol 2001; 204(Pt 23):4031–4042.

141. Rice WR, Dorn CC, Singleton FM. P2-purinoceptor regulation of surfactant phosphatidylcholine secretion. Relative roles of calcium and protein kinase C. Biochem J 1990; 266(2):407–413.

142. Griese M, Gobran LI, Rooney SA. A2 and P2 purine receptor interactions and surfactant secretion in primary cultures of type II cells. Am J Physiol 1991; 261:L140–L147.

143. Sano K, Voelker DR, Mason RJ. Effect of secretagogues on cytoplasmic free calcium in alveolar type II epithelial cells. Am J Physiol 1987; 253(5 Pt 1): C679–C686.

144. Sen N, Grunstein MM, Chander A. Regulation of lung surfactant secretion by endothelin-1 rat alveolar type II cells. Am J Physiol 1994; 266(10):L255–L262.

145. Wright JR, Dobbs LG. Regulation of pulmonary surfactant secretion and clearance. Annu Rev Physiol 1991; 53:395–414.

146. Pian MS, Dobbs LG. Lipoprotein-stimulated surfactant secretion in alveolar type II cells: mediation by heterotrimeric G proteins. Am J Physiol 1997; 273(3 Pt 1): L634–L639.

147. Dobbs LG, Wright JR, Hawgood S, Gonzalez R, Venstrom K, Nellenbogen J. Pulmonary surfactant and its components inhibit secretion of phosphatidylcholine from cultured rat alveolar type II cells. Proc Nat Acad Sci USA 1987; 84: 1010–1014.

148. Suwabe A, Mason RJ, Voelker DR. Calcium dependent association of surfactant protein A with pulmonary surfactant: application to simple surfactant protein A purification. Arch Biochem Biophys 1996; 2:285–291.

149. Postle AD, Heeley EL, Wilton DC. A comparison of the molecular species compositions of mammalian lung surfactant phospholipids. Comp Biochem Physiol A Mol Integr Physiol 2001; 129(1):65–73.

150. Taylor AE, Rehder K, Hyatt RE, Parker JC. Pulmonary fluid exchange. In: Wonsiewicz M, ed. Clinical Respiration Physiology. Philadelphia: Saunders, 1989:169–191.

3

Molecular and Functional Properties of Surfactant Protein A

CRISTINA CASALS and IGNACIO GARCÍA-VERDUGO

Complutense University of Madrid,
Madrid, Spain

I. Introduction

Surfactant protein A (SP-A) is a large oligomeric apolipoprotein primarily found in the alveolar fluid of mammalians. SP-A belongs to the "collectin" (collagen–lectin) family characterized by an N-terminal collagen-like domain and a globular C-terminal domain that includes a C-type carbohydrate recognition domain (CRD). Collectins bind to a wide range of sugar residues that are rich in microbial surfaces in a Ca^{2+}-dependent manner. The collectin family has five well-characterized members: lung surfactant protein A (SP-A) and D (SP-D), serum mannose binding protein (MBP), serum bovine conglutinin, and collectin-43 (1). Recently, another novel human collectin from liver (CL-L1) has been cloned (2). Together with the first component of the complement (C1q), these proteins are also called defense collagens, and play important roles in innate immunity (1).

Substantial evidence indicates that SP-A is involved in innate host-defense and inflammatory immunomodulator processes of the lung (3–5). Unlike other collectins, SP-A is a lipid binding protein, a property that allows this collectin to position and concentrate along with the extracellular membranes that line the alveolar epithelium. Thus, SP-A is tightly associated with surfactant membranes and enriched in lattice-like arrays of intersecting membranes, characteristic of the alveolar fluid, called tubular myelin. In fact, SP-A is necessary for the formation of tubular myelin. These structures do not disrupt surface activity but optimize the surface properties of lung surfactant. This ability of SP-A to bind lipids is of relevance in several aspects of pulmonary surfactant biology (5,6).

The primary structure of mature SP-A is highly conserved among different mammalians with some important differences. It consists of four structural domains (Fig. 3.1): (1) an N-terminal segment (7–10 amino acids) involved in intermolecular disulfide bond formation; (2) a 79 residue collagen-like domain characterized by 23 Gly-X-Y repeats with an interruption near the midpoint of the domain; (3) a 35 aminoacid segment with high α-helical propensity, which constitutes the neck region between the collagen and the globular domain; and (4) a 115 residue C-terminal globular domain involved in lipid binding and also in Ca^{2+}-dependent binding of oligosaccharides. This domain contains two conserved tryptophan residues (located at positions 191 and 213) and a glycosylation site (located at residue Asn^{187}). SP-A is modified after translation (cleavage of the signal peptide, proline hydroxylation, and N-linked glycosylation) and assembled into a complex oligomeric structure that resembles a flower bouquet. In one of the initial steps of the assembly of SP-A, trimers of SP-A are built up by the association of three polypeptide chains, the collagen regions of which intertwine to form a collagen triple-helix that is stabilized by interchain disulfide bonds. In the final stage of the assembly, the octadecamers appear to be formed by lateral association of the N-terminal half of six triple-helical stems (7,8) (Fig. 3.2). Like SP-A, MBP and C1q are assembled into hexamers of trimers whereas SP-D and conglutinin form cruciform-shaped oligomers of four trimers (1).

In humans, there are two functional genes (*SP-A1* and *SP-A2*) (9) corresponding to two different SP-A cDNA sequences (10); however, in other mammalian species studied, except baboons (11), there is only one. The nucleotide sequence differences between the two human genes that result in amino acid

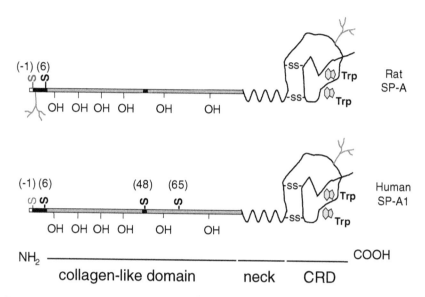

Figure 3.1 Domain structures of the polypeptide chain of human SP-A1 and rat SP-A. Branched structures represent N-linked carbohydrates. [-S] denotes cysteine residues at different positions of mature hSP-A1 and rat SP-A. The collagen regions below and above the triple-helix interruption are shown. [OH] represents hydroxylation of proline residues at the Y position of G-X-Y tripeptide units.

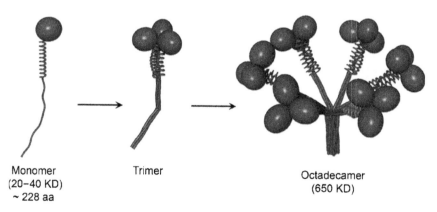

Figure 3.2 Three-dimensional model of SP-A monomer, trimer, and octadecamer. Oligomerization is an intracellular process that occurs in a zipper-like fashion along the C-terminal to N-terminal axis. Triple-helix formation from separated polypeptide chains requires previous trimerization of C-terminal globular domains, by a trimeric α-helical coiled-coil structure. Octadecamers appear to be formed by lateral association of the N-terminal half of six triple-helical stems, forming a microfibrillar end piece stabilized by disulfide bonds.

changes are located in the signal peptide, collagen-like, and globular domains of the resulting proteins (12,13). Interestingly, although both genes are expressed in lung alveolar type II cells, the *SP-A2* gene is expressed primarily (if not exclusively) in tracheal and bronchial submucosal gland cells (14–16). Octadecameric oligomers of human SP-A isolated from the bronchoalveolar lavage may be hetero-oligomers of both SP-A1 and SP-A2 homotrimers; alternatively, Voss et al. (17) have postulated that human SP-A may consist of homo-oligomers of heterotrimers composed of two SP-A1 molecules and one SP-A2 molecule. Whether the two gene products are expressed in a 2:1 (SP-A1/SP-A2) ratio and actually form heterotrimeric structures remains to be defined. The functional importance of having two distinct chain types in human SP-A is also unknown.

The present chapter will focus on the structural aspects of SP-A from human and experimental animals and the role of structural domains of SP-A in the binding of this protein to surfactant membranes, microbes, and alveolar and inflammatory cells present in the alveolar fluid. The binding capabilities of SP-A are involved in its putative biological functions: (a) improvement of surfactant biophysical function and integrity, (b) defense against alveolar pathogens, and (c) immunomodulation of the inflammatory response (Fig. 3.3).

II. Structure/Function Relationship

A. Domains Required for Oligomeric Assembly

The domains of SP-A that are essential for trimerization are the collagen-like region and the neck domain, which likely forms a rigid α-helical coiled-coil

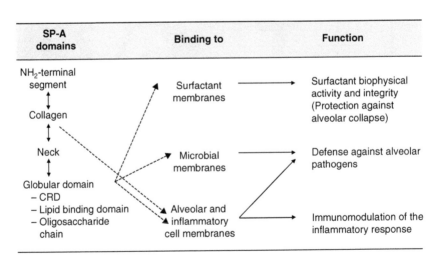

Figure 3.3 Relationships among structural domains, binding capabilities, and potential biological functions of SP-A.

(Figs. 3.1 and 3.2). Interchain disulfide cross-linkage at the N-terminal region stabilizes this structure. SP-A is assembled as multimers of trimeric subunits (Fig. 3.2). The N-terminal region is involved in covalent interactions between triple-helix stems to form higher oligomers. Researchers believe that SP-A oligomerization occurs in a zipper-like fashion along the C-terminal to N-terminal axis (18) as occurs with other collectins (SP-D and MBP-C) (19,20). Thus, the triple-helix formation from separate polypeptide chains requires previous trimerization of C-terminal globular domains, likely by a trimeric α-helical coiled-coil. In turn, triple-helix formation aligns the polypeptide chains for disulfide bond formation at the N-terminal segment, and, in the case of human SP-A, at the collagen interruption (Fig. 3.1).

Scientists assume but have not yet shown that the linking region between the collagen-like domain and the globular domain form a rigid coiled-coil structure. An α-helical coiled-coil can be predicted from the amino acid sequence by its characteristic heptad repeat pattern a-b-c-d-e-f-g-d, where residues "a" and "d" are hydrophobic aminoacids. Figure 3.4 shows alignment of the potential coiled-coil region of human SP-A from different species. For comparison, human SP-D is also shown. The X-ray crystallographic data for SP-D (21) demonstrated the existence of a coiled-coil organization in the neck domain as it was found for MBP (22). In the SP-A neck fragment, most of the residues in "a" and "d" of the four heptad repeat are hydrophobic (Leu, Val, Ile, Met, Ala, and Phe) or amphipathic (Gln, Tyr), although there are some departures from this role (i.e., hydrophilic residues such as Thr, Ser, and His) as occurs in MBP (22). There are two highly conserved positively charged residues (Lys/Arg^{95} and His^{96} at positions "e" and "f", respectively) and one negatively charged residue (Glu/Asp^{93} at position "c") in this otherwise very hydrophobic region. Hydrophobic amino acids at every turn of the helix form the interior of the coiled-coil and stabilize this rigid structure. Between the staggered

```
  ---                    ++
AHLDEE  LQSA LHE  IRHQ ILQ   SMGV LSF  QEFM LAV  G       Pig
ASLDEE  LQTT LHD  LRHQ ILQ   TMGV LSL  HESL LVV  G       Canine
AYLDEE  LQAT LHE  LRHH ALQ   SIGV  LSL  QGSM KAV  G       Rabbit
AYLDEE  LQTE LYE  IKHQ ILQ   TMGV LSL  QGSM LSV  G       Rat
AYLDEE  LQTA SYE  IKHQ ILQ   TMGV LSL  QGSM LSV  G       Mouse
81      87        94          101       108       115
AHLDEE  LQAT LHD  FRHQ ILQ   TRGA LSL  QGSI MTV  G       hSP-A
        d efg a bc  d efg a bc  d efg a bc  d efg  a bc
        204
        VASLRQQ    VEALQGQ    VQHLQAA   FSQYKKV   ELFP  hSP-D
        a    d     a    d     a    d    a    d
```

Figure 3.4 Sequences of the neck region of SP-A from different species. Human SP-D sequence is also shown. Most of the residues in "a" and "d" position of the heptad repeat are hydrophobic.

triple-helix of the collagen portion and the coiled-coil structure, in which the three polypeptide chains are in register, there is a highly conserved sequence with three contiguous negatively charged residues (Asp^{84}-Glu^{85}-Glu^{86}). This short region between the collagen and coiled-coil regions cannot be aligned in perfect register. The potential function of this very acidic region, besides serving as an adapter between the aligned and the nonaligned regions of SP-A trimer, has not been examined.

Oligomerization in SP-A and other collectins seems to be needed for many of their functions. Although most SP-A interactions with ligands occur in the globular domain, the binding affinity depends on the oligomeric status of SP-A. The binding affinity of a single SP-A lectin domain for carbohydrates is very low. However, the greater multiplicity of lectin domains found in higher-order oligomers and self-aggregated forms of SP-A is required to give high-affinity binding to carbohydrate-bearing surfaces (1,3,4). In addition, the degree of SP-A oligomerization and stability of the collagen domain is correlated with lipid-related functional capabilities of SP-A (23,24).

In relation to the functions of the collagen domain of SP-A, it is clear that its high tensile strength, stability, and relative resistance to proteolysis make this domain perfect as a cross-linker between globular domains and the N-terminal segment. However, the collagen-like domain not only functions as scaffolding that amplifies the ligand binding activities of globular domains. Table 3.1 shows structural and functional properties of SP-A related to a structurally intact collagen-like domain (23–36).

No mutation in SP-A associated with a respiratory pathology has yet been identified. Interestingly, an association has been found between a mutation in the collagen-like region of MBP and low levels of MBP in serum, which results in an infantile illness characterized by recurrent infections and failure to thrive (37,38). In the bronchoalveolar lavage from patients with birch pollen allergy, SP-A exists not only in fully assembled complexes of octadecamers as in healthy individuals, but also in smaller oligomeric forms (e.g., dodecameric, nonameric, or hexameric) (39).

B. The Globular Domain

The C-terminal globular domain is involved in the binding of SP-A to calcium, carbohydrates, and phospholipids, and is critical for host defense, immuno-modulation of the inflammatory response, and surfactant-related functions. This region contains ~115 amino acids, including four conserved cysteines that form two intramolecular disulfide loops (Cys^{204}-Cys^{218} and Cys^{135}-Cys^{226}), and 18 highly conserved amino acid residues common to the C-type lectines (40). The three-dimensional structure of SP-A is not known, but the X-ray crystallographic structures of rat and human MBP fragments (22) and human SP-D fragments (21), as well as those from four other C-type lectins, are useful models for SP-A [see Ref. (22,41,42) for reviews].

Table 3.1 Requirement of a Structurally Intact Collagen-Like Domain for Structural and Functional Properties of SP-A

Structure	In vitro activities of SP-A	Potential in vivo functions of SP-A
• Structural stability at physiological temperatures (human, dog, pig SP-A) (23–26) • Oligomerization (human and rat SP-A) (23,24,29) • Ca^{2+}-dependent self-aggregation (pig, human SP-A) (23–25)	• Tubular myelin formation (mouse SP-A) (27,28) • Prevention of surfactant inactivation by serum (mouse SP-A) (27,28)	→ Surfactant biophysical activity and integrity (protection against alveolar colapse)
	• High affinity for lipid and carbohydrate binding (rat SP-A) (29,30) • Aggregation of bacterial lipopolysaccharide (human SP-A) (23,24)	→ Host-defense: binding to pathogen surface membranes and endotoxins
	• Binding to the C1qRp (CD93) receptor in phagocytic cells (human SP-A) (31) • Phagocytosis of Mycobacterium through SPR210 (human SP-A) (32) • Upregulation of Mannose receptor in alveolar macrophages (human and rat SP-A) (33) • Stimulation of chemotaxis in alveolar macrophages and neutrophils (human SP-A) (34,35) • Inhibition of lymphocyte proliferation and IL-2 secretion through SPAR210 (human, bovine and rat SP-A) (36)	→ Host-defense: binding to receptors on cell membranes
	• Type II cell receptor binding (rat SP-A) (29,30) • Specific inhibition of lipid secretion by type II cells (rat SP-A) (29,30) • Lipid up-take by type II cells (rat SP-A) (29,30)	→ Regulation of type II cell function

The basic structure of the globular domain consists of a structural core made up of α-helical and β-strands. MBP and SP-D modeling predicts that one important structural domain is a hydrophobic cluster containing the conserved residues Phe-178, Tyr-188, Trp-191, Pro-196, Trp-213, and Val-205 (SP-A numbering). These amino acids hold together the carbohydrate/calcium binding region (CRD). MBP modeling predicts that one of the two Ca^{2+} binding sites (named site 2) is located in the center of the sugar binding site. The binding of sugar involves hydrogen bonding and Van der Waal's interactions, and it is stabilized by coordination bonds to the calcium ion. MBP modeling also predicts that the SP-A residues Glu195, Glu202, Asn214, and Asp215 are responsible for those interactions. The two tryptophans (Trp-191 and Trp-213) are located near the calcium binding site 2 and are sensitive markers of conformational changes in this region. Using the fluorescent apolar probe *bis*-ANS, we recently found that hydrophobic sites in SP-A increase upon addition of calcium, indicating that the binding of calcium to the protein leads to a conformational change in the protein, which makes it more hydrophobic (Casals and García-Verdugo, unpublished data). This conclusion is confirmed by intrinsic fluorescence studies of human SP-A, in which the tryptophan fluorescence emission maximum of SP-A is blue-shifted upon addition of calcium (23,24). This conformational shift enhances lipid binding and allows carbohydrate binding, protein self-association, and SP-A-mediated lipid aggregation.

Carbohydrate Binding and Specificity

The collectins show preference either for D-hexoses with an equatorial orientation of the 3- and 4-hydroxyl groups (such as mannose, glucose, N-acetylglucosamine, or mannosamide) or for L-fucose with a similar arrangement of hydroxyl groups at positions 2 and 3 (40,43). Sequence analysis of C-type CRDs in comparison with monosaccharide specificity indicates that C-type lectins can be divided into two groups according to a three-residue motif in the CRD (carbohydrate/calcium binding region): (1) mannose/glucose-binding C-type lectins that contain a highly conserved sequence (Glu-Pro-Asn) in their CRDs that bind mannose/glucose. All collectins, except for SP-A, contain the Glu-Pro-Asn motif. In SP-A this sequence is Glu[195]-Pro[196]-Ala/Arg[197], where Ala[197] is present in humans and Arg[197] in other mammalians. (2) Galactose-binding C-type lectins contain the sequence Gln-Pro-Asp in their CRDs (40).

SP-A binds preferentially to mannose and fucose (44). These sugars are commonly found on fungal and micrococcal surfaces. Discrepancy has been reported on the affinity of SP-A for the galactose residue. It has been demonstrated that SP-A binds to galactose by affinity chromatography (44), but not by inhibition of SP-A binding to solid-phase mannan by specific sugars (45). On the other hand, SP-A binds galactosylceramide coated on a solid support (46). Galactosylceramide is a common glycolipid asymmetrically located in the extracellular face of mammalian cell membranes. Site-directed mutagenesis of the CRD of rat SP-A indicated that substitution of Glu^{195}-Pro^{196}- Arg^{197} by Gln^{195}-Pro^{196}-Asp^{197} changed the specificity of SP-A from mannose to galactose. Curiously, the latter mutations inhibited the capability of SP-A to aggregate phospholipid vesicles in the presence of calcium but not the ability of SP-A to bind dipalmitoylphosphatidylcholine (DPPC) (47). Alanine mutations of residues within the calcium/carbohydrate coordination set blocked SP-A binding to phospholipids (48). Monoclonal antibodies against the CRD domain containing these residues also abrogated the binding of SP-A to phospholipids (49). These studies are consistent with the location of the major lipid binding site(s) of SP-A to the globular lectin C-terminal domain and indicate that the critical region for carbohydrate binding and the lipid binding domain might overlap. Recent studies using transmission electron microscopy confirm that the globular region of SP-A is responsible for interaction with lipid vesicles (50). Whether the carbohydrate binding region in SP-A interacts directly with the phosphocholine moiety of DPPC is still not known. However, the binding of SP-A to DPPC is Ca^{2+}-independent (51–53), and is not reversed or prevented by adding sugars (54) or galacotosylcermide (unpublished data) in the presence of calcium. In contrast, MBP and SP-D interact with phosphatidylinositol (PI) and glycosphingolipids through a lectin-mediated binding (55,56).

Lipid Ligands for SP-A and the Nature of SP-A/Lipid Interaction

SP-A interacts with a broad range of insoluble amphipathic lipids present in surfactant and cellular membranes or bacterial envelopes (6). Several studies indicated that SP-A preferentially binds to phospholipids whose headgroups are phosphocholine [phosphatidylcholine (PC) or sphingomyelin (SM)] and whose lipid moiety consists of long and saturated hydrocarbon chains. Both DPPC and SM fulfill these requirements (52,53,57). Several studies indicated that the binding of SP-A to DPPC vesicles is independent of Ca^{2+} but dependent on the physical state of the vesicle (52,53). SP-A interacts in a Ca^{2+}-independent manner with the interfacial region of saturated PC bilayers in the gel or ripple phase, which is characterized by a specific conformation of the phosphocholine moiety.

It remains questionable whether hydrophobic interactions occur between the amino acid side chains of the protein and the phospholipid acyl chains in the bilayer. Several lines of evidence indicate the involvement of hydrophobic binding forces in the interaction of SP-A with DPPC vesicles or DPPC monolayers (52,58–61). It is reasonable to think that hydrophobic interactions of SP-A with DPPC-rich bilayers can only be explained if SP-A partly penetrates into the membrane interface due to the existence of lipid packing defects. We recently found partial solubilization of surfactant membranes in Triton X-100, suggesting that liquid ordered (Lo) and liquid disordered (fluid) (Lα) domains coexist in these membranes. Lipid analysis of detergent resistant membranes (DRMs) or triton-insoluble floating fractions (TIFFs) indicated that they were enriched in cholesterol and DPPC (C. Casals, unpublished data).

DRMs (or TIFFs) seem to function as platforms for the attachment of SP-A to surfactant membranes because SP-A was absolutely segregated in DRMs or TIFFS (C. Casals, unpublished data). Fluid and liquid ordered phase coexistence in surfactant membranes could favor partition of SP-A into those membranes. Interestingly, SP-A also interacts with the gel-like regions in monolayers of pulmonary surfactant lipid extracts (62) and causes a reorganization or rearrangement of solid domains in the surfactant monolayer. It is noteworthy that SP-A in the subphase only associates with the DPPC monolayer when gel-like domains begin to appear upon compression and liquid expanded (fluid) and liquid condensed (gel) domains coexist (59). Under these conditions, SP-A interacts with the monolayer in packing defects at fluid–gel boundaries (59). These results are consistent with the concept that SP-A recognizes the lipid in the gel phase but can only penetrate into the membrane interface in lipid packing defects at liquid disordered-liquid ordered boundaries. At a surface pressure of 10 mN/m (plateau region, in which there is phase coexistence), SP-A in the subphase is able to perturb the lipid packing of DPPC monolayers at neutral pH in the absence of Ca^{2+} (59,60). Globular domains of SP-A (comprising lipid binding domains) must interact with acyl chains of phospholipid monolayers sufficiently to perturb the usual lipid packing. It was recently demonstrated that SP-A induces a decrease in the average acyl chain tilt angle of DPPC monolayers (at a surface pressure of 10 mN/m) from 35° to 28° (61). This indicates that SP-A increases lipid packing efficiency and that hydrophobic interactions must be involved.

In contrast, SP-A binds poorly to neutral or acidic phospholipid vesicles in the fluid phase, and detection of binding requires the presence of Ca^{2+} (53,63). The Ca^{2+}-dependent binding of immobilized SP-A to negatively charged phospholipid vesicles shows a preference for PI over phosphatidylglycerol (PG) (63). Similarly to SP-D or MBP, it is possible that the Ca^{2+}-dependent binding of SP-A to PI vesicles involves the CRD site. However, the inhibition of SP-A binding to PI by sugars has not been studied.

Lipomannan and mannosylated lipoarabidomannan, two major mycobacterial cell-wall lipoglycans, are also ligands for SP-A (64,65). The binding of SP-A to lipoglycans from the mycobacterial envelope seems to be dependent on Ca^{2+} (64). Both the terminal mannose residues and the fatty acids of lipoglycans are critical for binding. SP-A-lipoglycan interaction involves the CRD of SP-A. The carbohydrate binding site of SP-A seems to recognize the terminal mannosyl epitopes of lipoglycans from supramolecular assemblies of lipoglycan in solution. The lipid moiety of the lipoglycan seems to be necessary for the formation of those supramolecular assemblies. This supramolecular organization of these amphipathic molecules in solution might allow a repetitive and ordered presentation of terminal mannosyl epitopes, increasing recognition by the multiple CRDs of SP-A (65).

On the other hand, there are contradictory results about the Ca^{2+}-dependence of the binding of SP-A to rough lipopolysacchride (rough LPS) via lipid A (66–68) and to glycosphingolipids (46,69). It is also not clear whether

SP-A interacts with these lipids through a lectin-mediated binding. Our recent data indicated that SP-A is able to bind rough LPS in solution or rough LPS monolayers in a Ca^{2+}-independent manner (unpublished data).

III. SP-A Functions

A. Surfactant-Related Functions

Table 3.2 (51,53,54,58,70–82) summarizes *in vitro* lipid-related activities of SP-A and potential functions of SP-A in the integrity and biophysical activity of surfactant. The recent availability of SP-A knockout mice allows assessment of these functions. Evidence derived from SP-A knockout mice supports the concept that (1) SP-A does not directly contribute to surface properties of pulmonary surfactant, but the interaction of SP-A with surfactant membranes aids to maintain optimal surface activity in response to alterations in the alveolar microenviroment (83). *In vitro* experiments with surfactant isolated from transgenic mice that overexpress SP-A (78) or from SP-A knockout mice (27,83) corroborate that SP-A enhances the resistance of surfactant to protein inhibition. (2) SP-A is necessary for the formation of tubular myelin, a unique structure of surfactant in the alveolar spaces, whose presence has been correlated with high surface activity but is not absolutely required for breathing (27,83). (3) *In vivo* experiments from SP-A-deficient mice do not support a critical role of SP-A in surfactant homeostasis by controlling the secretion and uptake by alveolar cells (27,83). It is possible that some compensatory mechanism may function in the absence of SP-A.

Table 3.2 Surfactant-Related Functions of SP-A

"*In vitro*" surfactant-related activities of SP-A	Surfactant-related functions of SP-A
Induces Ca^{2+}-dependent aggregation of lipid vesicles with or without SP-B or SP-C (51,53,54,58,70,71)	Promotion of surfactant biophysical activity
Enhances adsorption of phospholipids along the air/liquid interface in a concerted action with SP-B (72,73)	
Mediates the formation of large ordered tubular myelin, when added to DPPC, PG, and SP-B mixtures in the presence of Ca^{2+} (74–76)	
Reduces inhibition of surfactant activity by foreign lipid binding proteins or serum lipoproteins (27,77,78)	Prevention of surfactant inactivation
Inhibits conversion of large (active) to small (inactive) surfactant aggregates (79)	
Enhances surfactant uptake into type II cells (80) and alveolar macrophages (81)	Surfactant homeostasis
Inhibits surfactant secretion by type II cells (82)	

The mechanism of stabilization and protection of surfactant mediated by SP-A is not known. One of the most interesting effects of SP-A on surfactant-like phospholipid vesicles is its ability to induce rapid aggregation of these vesicles with or without surfactant hydrophobic proteins SP-B and SP-C (51,53,54,58,70,71). This process is dependent on calcium, and predicts the surface active properties of the protein in concerted action with SP-B (72,73).

The mechanism involved in the vesicle aggregation phenomenon is poorly understood. It was suggested that the process of lipid aggregation mediated by SP-A could be correlated with that of self-association of the protein (84). Recent evidence indicates that vesicle aggregation and SP-A self-association might be related phenomena:

1. The calcium activation constant ($K_a^{Ca^{2+}}$) for both processes is similar. It is in the micromolar range in the presence of physiological saline (0.74 ± 0.2 and 2.4 ± 0.5 μM, for SP-A-induced lipid aggregation and protein self-association, respectively) (25,54).
2. The extent of SP-A-mediated lipid aggregation depends on proline hydroxylation in the collagen domain and the degree of SP-A oligomerization (23,24). Likewise, the ability of SP-A to self-associate depends on the stability of the collagen-like domain, which is correlated to proline hydroxylation and the degree of oligomerization (23,24). In addition, self-association activity of human or porcine SP-A is completely inhibited by unfolding of the collagen-like domain (24,25). SP-A self-association depends on calcium, and Ca^{2+} induces a conformational change on the globular domain of the protein identified by intrinsic fluorescence (23,24). Thus, it is possible that SP-A–SP-A association occurs among globular heads. A structurally intact collagen domain would ensure the grouping and orientation of globular heads in the oligomer.
3. Tubular myelin or multilamellar vesicles from native surfactant contain arrays of SP-A (76,85). Those structures seem to remain intact when the lipid is partially removed with acetone (76,85), and their spacing is comparable to the size of SP-A. These results suggest that interconnected SP-A molecules form the skeleton of these multilamellar structures or tubular myelin.

Figure 3.5 illustrates self-associated SP-A molecules connecting surfactant membranes by interaction of their globular heads with membrane surfaces of contiguous bilayers. The SP-A protein network interacting with DPPC monolayers is visible by transmission dectron microscopy (86) and fluorescence microscopy (59,60). This type of supraquaternary organization of SP-A and cooperative interaction with surfactant membranes could stabilize large surfactant aggregates, decrease surfactant inactivation in the presence of serum protein inhibitors, and, more importantly, prevent adherence of endotoxin or bacteria to the alveolar epithelium. Interestingly, Palaniyar et al. (87) showed that

AIR   BILAYER-MONOLAYER TRANSITION

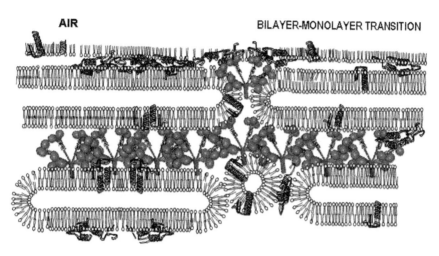

Figure 3.5   Model of the interaction of self-associated SP-A with surfactant membranes containing the hydrophobic surfactant proteins SP-B and SP-C.

recombinant rat SP-A with a deletion of the collagen-like domain failed to form protein networks and interacted with lipid monolayers in an unorganized manner. The collagen-like region and/or full oligomeric assembly of SP-A actually play an important role in the accommodation of SP-A in the alveolar fluid, because *in vivo* experiments demonstrate that the collagen-deficient mutant converts SP-A into an inhibitor of surfactant function (27). Deletion of the collagen-like domain also disrupts tubular myelin formation (27).

Figure 3.6 shows a schematic model of SP-A/SP-B-dependent tubular myelin structure. The mechanism involved in the formation of tubular myelin is poorly understood. However, it is likely that the formation of these complex structures requires (1) close contacts between opposing DPPC-rich membranes mediated by SP-A; (2) SP-A self-association mediated by calcium; and (3) fusion of membranes mediated by SP-B and facilitated by nonbilayer lipids such as unsaturated-PG-Ca^{2+} (these cone-shaped lipids are likely present in the corners of tubular myelin structures).

The functional significance of these complex structures is not known. Interestingly, tubular myelin-rich fraction is the most active fraction of all surfactant subfractions assayed *in vitro* (88), and morphological studies indicate that tubular myelin figures are in close proximity to the surface layer of the alveolar fluid. These structures seem to function as a membrane reservoir in the alveolar fluid in which SP-A is highly concentrated at the interface in a configuration that does not disrupt but optimizes the biophysical activity of surfactant lipids. Because of the high concentration of SP-A in these membrane traps close to the surface layer, McCormack and Whitsett (5) suggested that tubular myelin could have a primary antimicrobial function. Tubular myelin may function as

(a)   (b)

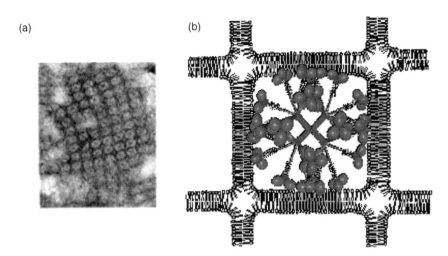

Figure 3.6 Tubular Myelin (TM). (a) Typical electron microscopy (EM) micrograph of tubular myelin. The EM image shows X-shaped structures (probably protein) in the square-lattice regions. [From Nag et al. (76) with permission]. (b) Scheme of TM: the globular heads of self-associated SP-A likely interact with DPPC-rich bilayers. Unsaturated PG-Ca^{2+} and SP-B (not shown) are likely present in the corners of TM. They probably make possible nonbilayer structures at the membrane intersection.

an extracellular surfactant reservoir that serves to collect inhaled microbes at the air–liquid interface due to the high concentration of SP-A in these structures. It seems possible that surfactant membranes and their apolipoproteins simultaneously function as the primary antimicrobial defense in the alveolar fluid and as a protective layer against alveolar collapse.

B. Host-Defense and Immunomodulation of the Inflammatory Response in the Alveolus

SP-A binds to a variety of nonself molecular structures including allergens, lipopolysaccharides, and other components of bacteria, viral, and fungi surfaces. This binding neutralizes, agglutinates, and/or enhances the uptake of pathogens by phagocytes of the innate immune system such as alveolar macrophages and neutrophils. Moreover, SP-A is capable of direct interaction with immune cells through binding to the cell membrane receptors resulting in modulation of immune cell functions such as phagocytosis, chemotaxis, proliferation, cytokine production, respiratory burst, and expression of surface receptors (Fig. 3.7).

Binding of SP-A to Pathogen Surfaces

SP-A recognizes complex arrays of polysaccharides and other glycoconjugates, including polysaccharide constituents of capsules, Gram-negative (GN)

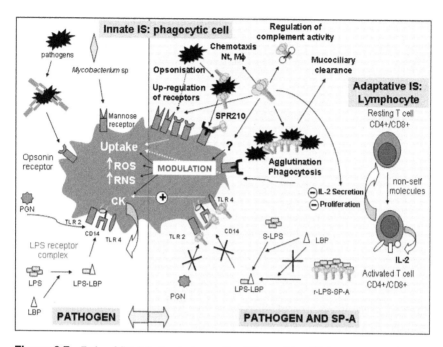

Figure 3.7 Role of SP-A in innate immunity. CK, cytokine; IS, immune system; LPS, smooth or rough lipopolysaccharide; LBP, LPS binding protein; Mφ, macrophage; Nt, neutrophil; PGN, peptidoglycan; r-LPS, rough LPS; s-LPS, smooth LPS; ROS, reactive oxygen species; RNS, reactive nitrogen species; SP-AR, SP-A receptor; TLR, Toll-like receptor.

lipopolysaccharides, lipoglycans, and glycoproteins that are present in pathogen surfaces (4). The C-terminal globular domain of SP-A seems to be responsible for these interactions. As we discussed earlier, this domain is involved in the binding of SP-A to lipids, Ca^{2+}, and carbohydrates. The globular domain also contains a conserved Asn187 which is posttranslational glycosylated (Fig. 3.1). Glycosylation in Asn187 is important in the binding of SP-A to certain viruses.

Table 3.3 shows different mechanisms of SP-A interaction with pathogen surfaces (65,66,89–99). The binding of SP-A to influenza virus A involves the sialic acid residues on Asn^{187}-linked oligosaccharide moiety of SP-A (90,91). Deglycosylation of SP-A or enzymatic digestion to remove only sialic acid residues inhibits the binding of SP-A to influenza virus A, whereas mannan, which binds to the CRD of SP-A, has no effect (91). In contrast, SP-A binds to cytomegalovirus (CMV) proteins in a Ca^{2+}-dependent manner. In addition, the binding of SP-A to CMV proteins is inhibited by mannan, suggesting that interaction between SP-A and CMV proteins involves the carbohydrate recognition activity of SP-A (92). Participation of the CRD–lectin activity of SP-A has also been

Table 3.3 Interaction of the C-Terminal Domain of SP-A with Pathogens

Structural motif in SP-A	Structural motif in the pathogen surface	Pathogen type
Asn[187]-linked carbohydrates	Lectin	Herpes Simplex virus 1 (89)
		Influenza A virus (90,91)
Lectin domain	Envelope glycoproteins	Cytomegalovirus (92)
	G,F-Glycoproteins	Respir. Syncytial Virus (93,94)
	Major surface glycoprotein	*Pneumocystis carinii* (95,96)
	Capsular polysaccharide	*Klebsiella pneumoniae* (97)
	Mannosylated lipoarabinomannan	*Mycobacterium sp.* (65)
	Lipomannan	
	Glycoproteins (gp45, 55)	*Aspergillus fumigatus* (98)
Lipid binding domain	Lipopolysaccharide (lipid A)	Gram-negative bacteria (66)

reported in the interaction of SP-A with lipoglycans of mycobacteria (65) and with the major surface glycoprotein of *Pneumocystis carinii* (95,96) (4).

The interaction of SP-A with GN and Gram-positive (GP) bacteria is not fully understood. Some authors have suggested that SP-A may recognize peptido-glycan or lipoteichoic acid from the GP cell wall but convincing results have not been published yet (99,100). SP-A has been described as binding to rough but not to smooth LPS from GN strains (66,67). Bacteria with rough LPS phenotypes are most common among species that colonize the surfaces of the respiratory tract (101). Binding studies in the presence of mannan or deglycosylated SP-A indicated that neither the carbohydrate binding region nor the carbohydrate moiety of SP-A are involved in its binding to rough LPS (66,68). It is likely that SP-A binds to the lipid A moiety of rough LPS by the lipid binding domain of SP-A instead of through a lectin-mediated binding (66). Interaction of SP-A with rough LPS seems to interfere with the subsequent binding of rough LPS to LPS binding protein (LBP) (102). LBP binds to the lipid A domain of LPS, catalyzes the binding of LPS to CD14, and enhances CD14-mediated cell activation. The complex CD14/TLR4/MD2 leads to stimulation of cells via induction of NF-κB (103). The presence of SP-A results in significant inhibition of NF-κB activation in alveolar macrophages stimulated with rough LPS (102) (Fig. 3.7).

Once SP-A has recognized the nonself structure in the pathogen surface, different mechanisms are involved in the neutralization and clearance of patho-gens. SP-A is able either to opsonize nonself structures for disposal by immune cells (104,97) or to agglutinate various microorganisms, including bac-teria, fungi, and viruses (104–106). Agglutination facilitates the mechanical removal of bacteria from the lungs by mucociliary clearance and also increases the phagocytosis of bacteria by alveolar macrophages (107) (Fig. 3.7).

Interaction of SP-A with Immune Cell Membranes

SP-A may have three modes of binding to immune cells: (a) through a lectin-mediated event to glycoproteins present in the surface of monocytes and macrophages (108,109); (b) through the N-linked carbohydrate on the C-terminal domain of SP-A, which binds to a lectin present in the plasma membrane of alveolar macrophages (110); and (c) through the collagen-like domain of SP-A, which binds to a protein receptor on the surface of alveolar macrophages (111,112) (Fig. 3.7).

Several cell surface proteins that bind SP-A have been identified (Table 3.4) (31,32,36,67,100,113–116). However, the specific contributions of these molecules to the biological activities of SP-A remain unclear.

SPR210

Chroneos et al. (114) described a specific receptor of 210 kDa, named SPR210, that binds to SP-A with high affinity in a Ca^{2+}-dependent manner but independent of the carbohydrate binding activity of SP-A. The collagen-like domain of SP-A

Table 3.4 Potential SP-A Receptors in Cells Present in the Alveolar Fluid

SP-A domain	Receptor	Expression in alveolar cells	SP-A function
Collagen-like	Calreticulin/ CD91	Macrophages[a]	Clearance of apoptotic cells (113), macropinocytosis (116)
Collagen-like	C1qRp (CD93)	Monocyte/ macrophages Type II cells (murine)	Phagocytosis (31)
Collagen-like	SPA receptor (SPR210)	Lymphocytes Macrophages (Mϕ) Type II neumocytes	Inhibition of T cell proliferation and IL-2 production (36) Enhanced uptake of BCG by Mϕ (32) Inhibition of phospholipid secretion (114)
Neck	CD14 m	Macrophages[a]	Modulation of LPS response (67)
nd	Toll-like 4	Macrophages[a]	Activation of macrophages (115)
nd	Toll-like 2	Macrophages[a]	Inhibition of cytokine-PGN induced response (100)
Globular domain	SIRP-α	Macrophages[a]	Inhibition of inflammatory mediator production (116)

[a]Expressed in more cell types; nd, not determinated; BCG, bacillus Calmette–Guerin; PGN, peptidoglycan; SIRP-α, signal-inhibitory regulatory protein-α.

has been suggested as the putative domain that interacts with SPR210 (36,114). This receptor mediates SP-A-induced inhibition of phospholipid secretion by type II cells (114), SP-A-induced inhibition of T-cell proliferation (36), and SP-A-enhanced uptake of bacillus Calmette–Guérin by macrophages (32).

C1qRp (CD93)

C1q receptors (C1qR) trigger effects on a wide range of immune cells. C1qRp has been identified as the leukocyte antigen CD93 and is expressed in human endothelial cells, monocytes, and immature dendritic cells. It has been suggested that SP-A, MBL, and C1q directly bind to C1qRp through their collagen-like domains and enhance phagocytosis (31). Recent studies suggest that C1qRp is involved primarily in adhesion events rather than C1q-mediated phagocytosis (117). The role of C1qRp in phagocytosis requires further studies.

CD14

CD14 is a 53 kDa GPI-anchored protein that also exists as a soluble form. Nowadays, CD14 stands as a major receptor for various bacterial components, and is considered as a pattern-recognition receptor (103). SP-A directly interacts with CD14 via its neck domain (118). The binding of SP-A to CD14 might prevent the binding of smooth LPS to CD14 (67). This would explain the inhibition mediated by SP-A of TNF-alpha release from rat alveolar macrophages stimulated with smooth LPS (119), because SP-A poorly binds to smooth LPS. SP-A also reduced the cytokine release from human alveolar macrophages (120) and human buffy coat cells (121) stimulated with smooth LPS. Consistent with these data, *in vivo* experiments showed that SP-A-deficient mice intratracheally challenged with smooth *Escherichia coli* 026:B6 LPS produce significantly more tumor necrosis factor than the wild-type mice (122). In contrast, Bufler et al. (123) recently reported that SP-A has no major effects on the response of a macrophage cell line to smooth and rough *Pseudomonas aeruginosa* strains.

Toll-Like Receptors

SP-A also interacts with toll-like receptors (TLR). TLR are pattern recognition receptors that participate in signaling a variety of microbial infections (103). The interaction of SP-A with the extracellular domain of TLR2 inhibits peptidoglycan-mediated response (100). On the other hand, SP-A from alveolar proteinosis patients seems to interact with TLR4 complex, inducing activation of the NF-kB pathway and up-regulation of cytokine synthesis (115). However, the detailed mechanism by which SP-A interacts with TLR4 receptor requires further studies. Phelps and co-workers also demonstrated that human SP-A from alveolar proteinosis patients and recombinant human SP-A stimulate TNF-alpha secretion by THP-1 cells (124,125). The precise mechanism of the interaction of SP-A with this monocytic cell line has not been described yet.

Beside cytokine modulation, SP-A itself can modulate other functions in monocytes/macropahges such as reactive oxygen (ROS) and nitrogen species

(RNS) production. Both ROS and RNS are involved in antibacterial and antiviral defense. However, these reactive species, as well as cytokines, have the potential to exacerbate an inflammatory response if their levels are not tightly regulated. Alveolar macrophages incubated with SP-A have a decrease in superoxide production, indicating a dampening of the respiratory burst and suggesting a protective role against the oxidant injury caused by alveolar macrophages in the lung (126,127). Others, however, have found SP-A to stimulate the respiratory burst (128). The reasons for these different findings are not completely understood but may be related to different methods used to purify SP-A (128). On the other hand, SP-A seems to enhance the production of nitric oxide by alveolar macrophages (129) although removal of endotoxin from SP-A preparation reverses this effect (130). In contrast, SP-A with low endotoxin level has been shown to enhance the production of nitric oxide metabolites by alveolar macrophages activated with IFN-gamma and challenged *in vitro* with *Mycoplasma pneumoniae* (131). *In vivo* studies using SP-A-deficient mice indicate that these mice produce more nitric oxide upon intratracheal challenge of *P. aeruginosa* or LPS (122,132). The response to SP-A seems to vary with the pathogen challenge, the state of cell activation (133), cell source (134), and SP-A nature (135). SP-A domains involved in the regulation of the cited inflammatory mediators are unknown and requires further studies.

Finally, there are different studies that support an activating ligand role of SP-A. SP-A enhances phagocytosis of IgG or complement-coated sheep erythrocytes, presumably due to up-regulation of Fc and CR1 receptors by SP-A (136). The treatment of human monocytic cell line THP-1 with SP-A leads to a significant increase of the expression of CD14, ICAM1, and CD11b (137). Pretreatment of macrophages with SP-A stimulates phagocytosis of *M. tuberculosis* probably by up-regulation of mannose receptor (108). More recently, it was shown that SP-A increases the surface expression of functional mannose receptor on macrophages, as demonstrated by both flow cytometry and confocal microscopy (33). Using recombinant mutants of rat SP-A, these authors demonstrate a critical role for both the CRD and the collagen-like region of SP-A in mediating up-regulation of mannose receptor.

IV. Concluding Remarks

Lung SP-A is part of the naturally occurring innate immune system which provides an immediate defense against a wide range of lung pathogens (viruses, bacteria, and fungi). The high affinity of SP-A to surfactant membranes allows the concentration of this protein in the alveolar fluid. Levels of SP-A have been reported to fall during infections and lung inflammation. Therefore, the use of recombinant forms of human SP-A together with surfactant lipids may alleviate the need for administration of antibiotics and/or anti-inflammatory drugs, especially in the very young and in the immunocompromised adults. One of the open questions in surfactant molecular biology is why there are two functional genes (SP-A1 and SP-A2) in humans, corresponding to two different SP-A cDNA sequences. A complete understanding of the structure and function of human SP-A will allow the production of recombinant SP-A to be used in human therapies.

Acknowledgment

We thank Dr. M. L. F. Ruano for drawing the three-dimensional model of SP-A monomer, trimer, and octadecamer. This work was supported by P103013 from F15 and QLK2-CT-2000-00325 from the European Community.

References

1. Lu J, Teh C, Kishore U, Reid KB. Collectins and ficolins: sugar pattern recognition molecules of the mammalian innate immune system. Biochim Biophys Acta 2002; 1572:387–400.

2. Ohtani K, Suzuki Y, Eda S, Kawai T, Kase T, Yamazaki H, Shimada T, Keshi H, Sakai Y, Fukuoh A, Sakamoto T, Wakamiya N. Molecular cloning of a novel human collectin from liver (CL-L1). J Biol Chem 1999; 274:13681–13689.

3. Lawson PR, Reid KB. The roles of surfactant proteins A and D in innate immunity. Immunol Rev 2000; 173:66–78.

4. Crouch E, Wright JR. Surfactant proteins A and D and pulmonary host defense. Annu Rev Physiol 2001; 63:521–554.

5. McCormack FX, Whitsett JA. The pulmonary collectins, SP-A and SP-D, orchestrate innate immunity in the lung. J Clin Invest 2002; 109:707–712.

6. Casals C. Role of surfactant protein A (SP-A)/lipid interactions for SP-A functions in the lung. Pediatr Pathol Mol Med 2001; 20:249–268.

7. Voss T, Eistetter H, Schafer KP, Engel J. Macromolecular organization of natural and recombinant lung surfactant protein SP 28–36. Structural homology with the complement factor C1q. J Mol Biol 1988; 201:219–227.

8. Haas C, Voss T, Engel J. Assembly and disulfide rearrangement of recombinant surfactant protein A *in vitro.* Eur J Biochem 1991; 197:799–803.

9. White RT, Damm D, Miller J, Spratt K, Schilling J, Hawgood S, Benson B, Cordell B. Isolation and characterization of the human pulmonary surfactant apoprotein gene. Nature 1985; 317:361–363.

10. Floros J, Steinbrink R, Jacobs K, Phelps D, Kriz R, Recny M, Sultzman L, Jones S, Taeusch HW, Frank HA, Fritsch EF. Isolation and characterization of cDNA clones for the 35-kDa pulmonary surfactant-associated protein. J Biol Chem 1986; 261:9029–9033.

11. Gao E, Wang Y, McCormick SM, Li J, Seidner SR, Mendelson CR. Characterization of two baboon surfactant protein A genes. Am J Physiol 1996; 271:L617–L630.

12. Floros J, Hoover RR. Genetics of the hydrophilic surfactant proteins A and D. Biochim Biophys Acta 1998; 1408:312–322.

13. DiAngelo S, Lin Z, Wang G, Phillips S, Ramet M, Luo J, Floros J. Novel, non-radioactive, simple and multiplex PCR-cRFLP methods for genotyping human SP-A and SP-D marker alleles. Dis Markers 1999; 15:269–281.

14. Saitoh H, Okayama H, Shimura S, Fushimi T, Masuda T, Shirato K. Surfactant protein A2 gene expression by human airway submucosal glands and cells. Am J Respir Cell Mol Biol 1998; 19:202–209.

15. Goss KL, Kumar AR, Snyder JM. SP-A2 gene expression in human fetal lung airways. Am J Respir Cell Mol Biol 1998; 19:613–621.

16. Khubchandani KR, Goss KL, Engelhardt JF, Snyder JM. *In situ* hybridization of SP-A mRNA in adult human conducting airways. Pediatr Pathol Mol Med 2001; 20:349–366.

17. Voss T, Melchers K, Scheirle G, Schafer KP. Structural comparison of recombinant pulmonary surfactant protein SP-A derived from two human coding sequences: implications for the chain composition of natural human SP-A. Am J Respir Cell Mol Biol 1991; 4:88–94.

18. Spissinger T, Schäfer KP, Voss T. Assembly of the surfactant protein SP-A. Deletions in the globular domain interfere with the correct folding of the molecule. Eur J Biochem 1991; 199:65–71.

19. Hoppe HJ, Barlow PN, Reid KB. A parallel three stranded alpha-helical bundle at the nucleation site of collagen triple-helix formation. FEBS Lett 1994; 344:191–195.

20. Wallis R, Drickamer K. Asymmetry adjacent to the collagen-like domain in rat liver mannose-binding protein. Biochem J 1997; 325:391–400.

21. Hakansson K, Lim NK, Hoppe HL, Reid KB. Crystal structure of the trimeric alpha-helical coiled-coil and the three lectin domains of human lung surfactant protein D. Structure Fold Des 1999; 7:255–264.

22. Weis WI, Drickamer K. Trimeric structure of a C-type mannose-binding protein. Structure 1994; 15:1227–1240.

23. García-Verdugo I, Guirong G, Floros J, Casals C. Structural analysis and lipid binding properties of recombinant human surfactant protein A (SP-A) derived from one (SP-A1 or SP-A2) or both genes. Biochemistry 2002; 41:14041–14053.

24. García-Verdugo I, Sánchez-Barbero F, Bosch FU, Steinhilber W, Casals C. Effect of hydroxylation, oligomerization, and glycosylation on structural and biochemical properties of recombinant human SP-A1. Biochemistry 2003; 42:9532–9542.

25. Ruano ML, Garcia-Verdugo I, Miguel E, Perez-Gil J, Casals C. Self-aggregation of surfactant protein A. Biochemistry 2000; 39:6529–6537.

26. Haagsman HP, White RT, Schilling J, Lau K, Benson BJ, Golden J, Hawgood S, Clements JA. Studies of the structure of lung surfactant protein SP-A. Am J Physiol 1989; 257:L421–L429.

27. Ikegami M, Elhalwagi BM, Palaniyar N, Dienger K, Korfhagen TR, Whitsett JA, McCormack FX. The collagen-like region of surfactant protein A (SP-A) is required for correction of surfactant structural and functional defects in the SP-A null mouse. J Biol Chem 2001; 276:38542–38548.

28. Palaniyar N, Zhang L, Kuzmenko A, Ikegami M, Wan S, Wu H, Korfhagen TR, Whitsett JA, McCormack FX. The role of pulmonary collectin N-terminal domains in surfactant structure, function, and homeostasis *in vivo*. J Biol Chem 2002; 277:26971–26979.

29. McCormack FX, Pattanajitvilai S, Stewart J, Possmayer F, Inchley K, Voelker DR. The Cys6 intermolecular disulfide bond and the collagen-like region of rat SP-A

play critical roles in interactions with alveolar type II cells and surfactant lipids. J Biol Chem 1997; 272:27971–27979.

30. McCormack FX, Damodarasamy M, Elhalwagi BM. Deletion mapping of N-terminal domains of surfactant protein A. The N-terminal segment is required for phospholipid aggregation and specific inhibition of surfactant secretion. J Biol Chem 1999; 274:3173–3181.

31. Nepomuceno RR, Ruiz S, Park M, Tenner AJ. C1qRp is a heavily O-glycosylated cell surface protein involved in the regulation of phagocytic activity. J Immunol 1999; 162:3583–3589.

32. Weikert LF, Edwards K, Chroneos ZC, Hager C, Hoffman L, Shepherd VL. SP-A enhances uptake of bacillus Calmette-Guerin by macrophages through a specific SP-A receptor. Am J Physiol 1997; 272:L989–L995.

33. Beharka AA, Gaynor CD, Kang BK, Voelker DR, McCormack FX, Schlesinger LS. Pulmonary surfactant protein A up-regulates activity of the mannose receptor, a pattern recognition receptor expressed on human macrophages. J Immunol 2002; 169:3565–3573.

34. Wright JR, Youmans DC. Pulmonary surfactant protein A stimulates chemotaxis of alveolar macrophage. Am J Physiol 1993; 264:L338–L344.

35. Schagat TL, Wofford JA, Greene KE, Wright JR. Surfactant protein A differentially regulates peripheral and inflammatory neutrophil chemotaxis. Am J Physiol Lung Cell Mol Physiol 2003; 284:L140–L147.

36. Borron P, McCormack FX, Elhalwagi BM, Chroneos ZC, Lewis JF, Zhu S, Wright JR, Shepherd VL, Possmayer F, Inchley K, Fraher LJ. Surfactant protein A inhibits T cell proliferation via its collagen-like tail and a 210-kDa receptor. Am J Physiol 1998; 275:L679–L686.

37. Super M, Thiel S, Lu J, Levinsky RJ, Turner MW. Association of low levels of mannan-binding protein with a common defect of opsonisation. Lancet 1989; 2:1236–1239.

38. Matsushita M, Ezekowitz RA, Fujita T. The Gly-54 → Asp allelic form of human mannose-binding protein (MBP) fails to bind MBP-associated serine protease. Biochem J 1995; 311:1021–1023.

39. Hickling TP, Malhotra R, Sim RB. Human lung surfactant protein A exists in several different oligomeric states: oligomer size distribution varies between patient groups. Mol Med 1998; 4:266–275.

40. Drickamer K. C-type lectin-like domains. Curr Opin Struct Biol 1999; 9:585–590.

41. Hakansson K, Reid KB. Collectin structure: a review. Protein Sci 2000; 9:1607–1617.

42. McCormack FX. Structure, processing and properties of surfactant protein A. Biochim Biophys Acta 1998; 1408:109–131.

43. Weis WI, Drickamer K. Structural basis of lectin-carbohydrate recognition. Annu Rev Biochem 1996; 65:441–473.

44. Haagsman HP, Hawgood S, Sargeant T, Buckley D, White RT, Drickamer K, Benson BJ. The major lung surfactant protein, SP 28–36, is a calcium-dependent, carbohydrate-binding protein. J Biol Chem 1987; 262:13877–13880.

45. Haurum JS, Thiel S, Haagsman HP, Laursen SB, Larsen B, Jensenius JC. Studies on the carbohydrate-binding characteristics of human pulmonary surfactant-associated protein A and comparison with two other collectins: mannan-binding protein and conglutinin. Biochem J 1993; 293:873–878.

46. Childs RA, Wright JR, Ross GF, Yuen CT, Lawson AM, Chai W, Drickamer K, Feizi T, Specificity of lung surfactant protein SP-A for both the carbohydrate and the lipid moieties of certain neutral glycolipids. J Biol Chem 1992; 267:9972–9979.

47. McCormack FX, Stewart J, Voelker DR, Damodarasamy M. Alanine mutagenesis of surfactant protein A reveals that lipid binding and pH-dependent liposome aggregation are mediated by the carbohydrate recognition domain. Biochemistry 1997; 36:13963–13971.

48. McCormack FX, Kuroki Y, Stewart JJ, Mason RJ, Voelker DR. Surfactant protein A amino acids Glu195 and Arg197 are essential for receptor binding, phospholipid aggregation, regulation of secretion, and the facilitated uptake of phospholipid by type II cells. J Biol Chem 1994; 269:29801–29807.

49. Kuroki Y, McCormack FX, Ogasawara Y, Mason RJ, Voelker DR. Epitope mapping for monoclonal antibodies identifies functional domains of pulmonary surfactant protein A that interact with lipids. J Biol Chem 1994; 269:29793–29800.

50. Palaniyar N, Ridsdale RA, Holterman CE, Inchley K, Possmayer F, Harauz G. Structural changes of surfactant protein A induced by cations reorient the protein on lipid bilayers. J Struct Biol 1998; 122:297–310.

51. King RJ, Carmichael MC, Horowitz PM. Reassembly of lipid-protein complexes of pulmonary surfactant. Proposed mechanism of interaction. J Biol Chem 1983; 258:10672–10680.

52. King RJ, Phillips MC, Horowitz PM, Dang SC. Interaction between the 35 kDa apolipoprotein of pulmonary surfactant and saturated phosphatidylcholines. Effects of temperatura. Biochim Biophys Acta 1986; 879:1–13.

53. Casals C, Miguel E, Perez-Gil J. Tryptophan fluorescence study on the interaction of pulmonary surfactant protein A with phospholipid vesicles. Biochem J 1983; 296:585–593.

54. Ruano ML, Miguel E, Perez-Gil J, Casals C. Comparison of lipid aggregation and self-aggregation activities of pulmonary surfactant-associated protein A. Biochem J 1996; 313:683–689.

55. Ogasawara Y, Kuroki Y, Akino T. Pulmonary surfactant protein D specifically binds to phosphatidylinositol. J Biol Chem 1992; 267:21244–21249.

56. Persson AV, Gibbons BJ, Shoemaker JD, Moxley MA, Longmore WJ. The major glycolipid recognized by SP-D in surfactant is phosphatidylinositol. Biochemistry 1992; 31:12183–12189.

57. Kuroki Y, Akino T. Pulmonary surfactant protein A (SP-A) specifically binds dipalmitoylphosphatidylcholine. J Biol Chem 1991; 266:3068–3073.

58. Ruano ML, Perez-Gil J, Casals C. Effect of acidic pH on the structure and lipid binding properties of porcine surfactant protein A. Potential role of acidification along its exocytic pathway. J Biol Chem 1998; 273:15183–15191.

59. Ruano ML, Nag K, Worthman LA, Casals C, Perez-Gil J, Keough KM. Differential partitioning of pulmonary surfactant protein SP-A into regions of monolayers of dipalmitoylphosphatidylcholine and dipalmitoylphosphatidylcholine/dipalmitoylphosphatidylglycerol. Biophys J 1998; 74:1101–1109.

60. Ruano ML, Nag K, Casals C, Perez-Gil J, Keough KM. Interactions of pulmonary surfactant protein A with phospholipid monolayers change with pH. Biophys J 1999; 77:1469–1476.

61. Bi X, Taneva S, Keough KM, Mendelsohn R, Flach CR. Thermal stability and DPPC/Ca^{2+} interactions of pulmonary surfactant SP-A from bulk-phase and mono-layer IR spectroscopy. Biochemistry 2001; 40:13659–13669.

62. Worthman LA, Nag K, Rich N, Ruano ML, Casals C, Perez-Gil J, Keough KM. Pulmonary surfactant protein A interacts with gel-like regions in monolayers of pulmonary surfactant lipid extract. Biophys J 2000; 79:2657–2666.

63. Meyboom A, Maretzki D, Stevens PA, Hofmann KP. Interaction of pulmonary sur-factant protein A with phospholipid liposomes: a kinetic study on head group and fatty acid specificity. Biochim Biophys Acta 1999; 1441:23–35.

64. Sidobre S, Puzo G, Riviere M. Lipid-restricted recognition of mycobacterial lipo-glycans by human pulmonary surfactant protein A: a surface-plasmon-resonance study. Biochem J 2002; 365:89–97.

65. Sidobre S, Nigou J, Puzo G, Riviere M. Lipoglycans are putative ligands for the human pulmonary surfactant protein A attachment to mycobacteria. Critical role of the lipids for lectin-carbohydrate recognition. J Biol Chem 2000; 275:2415–2422.

66. Van Iwaarden, JF, Pikaar JC, Storm J, Brouwer E, Verhoef J, Oosting RS, van Golde LM, van Strijp JA. Binding of surfactant protein A to the lipid A moiety of bacterial lipopolysaccharides. Biochem J 1994; 303:407–411.

67. Sano H, Sohma H, Muta T, Nomura S, Voelker DR, Kuroki Y. Pulmonary surfac-tant protein A modulates the cellular response to smooth & rough lipopolysacchar-ides by interaction with CD14. J Immunol 1999; 163:387–395.

68. Kalina M, Blau H, Riklis S, Kravtsov V. Interaction of surfactant protein A with bacterial lipopolysaccharide may affect some biological functions. Am J Physiol 1995; 268:L144–L151.

69. Kuroki Y, Gasa S, Ogasawara Y, Makita A, Akino T. Binding of pulmonary surfac-tant protein A to galactosylceramide and asialo-GM2. Arch Biochem Biophys 1992; 299:261–267.

70. Casals C, Ruano ML, Miguel E, Sanchez P, Perez-Gil J. Surfactant protein-C enhances lipid aggregation activity of surfactant protein-A. Biochem Soc Trans 1994; 22:370S.

71. Hawgood S, Benson BJ, Jr., Hamilton RL. Effects of a surfactant-associated protein and calcium ions on the structure and surface activity of lung surfactant lipids. Biochemistry 1985; 24:184–190.

72. Hawgood S, Benson BJ, Schilling J, Damm D, Clements JA, White RT. Nucleotide and amino acid sequences of pulmonary surfactant protein SP 18 and evidence for cooperation between SP 18 and SP 28–36 in surfactant lipid adsorption. Proc Natl Acad Sci USA 1987; 84:66–70.

73. Schürch S, Possmayer F, Cheng S, Cockshutt AM. Pulmonary SP-A enhances adsorption and appears to induce surface sorting of lipid extract surfactant. Am J Physiol 1992; 263:L210–L218.

74. Suzuki Y, Fujita Y, Kogishi K. Reconstitution of tubular myelin from synthetic lipids and proteins associated with pig pulmonary surfactant. Am Rev Respir Dis 1989; 140:75–81.

75. Williams MC, Hawgood S, Hamilton RL. Changes in lipid structure produced by surfactant proteins SP-A, SP-B, and SP-C. Am J Respir Cell Mol Biol 1991; 5:41–50.

76. Nag K, Munro JG, Hearn SA, Rasmusson J, Petersen NO, Possmayer F. Correlated atomic force and transmission electron microscopy of nanotubular structures in pulmonary surfactant. J Struct Biol 1999; 126:1–15.

77. Cockshutt AM, Weitz J, Possmayer F. Pulmonary surfactant-associated protein A enhances the surface activity of lipid extract surfactant and reverses inhibition by blood proteins *in vitro*. Biochemistry 1990; 29:8424–8429.

78. Elhalwagi BM, Zhang M, Ikegami M, Iwamoto HS, Morris RE, Miller ML, Dienger K, McCormack FX. Normal surfactant pool sizes and inhibition-resistant surfactant from mice that overexpress surfactant protein A. Am J Respir Cell Mol Biol 1999; 21:380–387.

79. Veldhuizen RAW, Yao LJ, Hearn SA, Possmayer F, Lewis JF. Surfactant-associated protein A is important for maintaining surfactant large-aggregate forms during surface-area cycling. Biochem J 1996; 313:835–840.

80. Stevens PA, Wissel H, Zastrow S, Sieger D, Zimmer KP. Surfactant protein A and lipid are internalized via the coated-pit pathway by type II pneumocytes. Am J Physiol Lung Cell Physiol 2001; 280:L141–L151.

81. Quintero OA, Wright JR. Clearance of surfactant lipids by neutrophils and macrophages isolated from the acutely inflamed lung. Am J Physiol Lung Cell Mol Physiol 2002; 282:L330–L339.

82. Dobbs LG, Wright JR, Hawgood S, Gonzalez R, Venstrom K, Nellenbogen J. Pulmonary surfactant and its components inhibit secretion of phosphatidylcholine from cultured rat alveolar type II cells. Proc Natl Acad Sci USA 1987; 84:1010–1014.

83. Korfhagen TR, Bruno MD, Ross GF, Huelsman KM, Ikegami M, Jobe AH, Wert SE, Stripp BR, Morris RE, Glasser SW, Bachurski CJ, Iwamoto HS, Whitsett JA. Altered surfactant function and structure in SP-A gene targeted mice. Proc Natl Acad Sci USA 1996; 93:9594–9599.

84. Haagsman HP, Sargeant T, Hauschka PV, Benson BJ, Hawgood S. Binding of calcium to SP-A, a surfactant-associated protein. Biochemistry 1990; 29:8894–8900.

85. Palaniyar N, Ridsdale RA, Hearn SA, Possmayer F, Harauz G. Formation of membrane lattice structures and their specific interactions with surfactant protein A. Am J Physiol 1999; 276:L642–L649.

86. Palaniyar N, Ridsdale RA, Possmayer F, Harauz G. Surfactant protein A (SP-A) forms a novel supraquaternary structure in the form of fibers. Biochem Biophys Res Commun 1998; 250:131–136.

87. Palaniyar N, McCormack FX, Possmayer F, Harauz G. Three-dimensional structure of rat surfactant protein A trimers in association with phospholipid monolayers. Biochemistry 2000; 39:6310–6316.

88. Magoon MW, Wright JR, Baritussio A, Williams MC, Goerke J, Benson BJ, Hamilton RL, Clements JA. Subfractionation of lung surfactant. Implications for metabolism and surface activity. Biochim Biophys Acta 1983; 750:18–31.

89. van Iwaarden JF, van Strijp JA, Visser H, Haagsman HP, Verhoef J, van Golde LM. Binding of surfactant protein A (SP-A) to herpes simplex virus type 1-infected cells is mediated by the carbohydrate moiety of SP-A. J Biol Chem 1992; 267:25039–25043.

90. Malhotra R, Haurum JS, Thiel S, Sim RB. Binding of human collectins (SP-A and MBP) to influenza virus. Biochem J 1994; 304:455–461.

91. Benne CA, Kraaijeveld CA, van Strijp JA, Brouwer E, Harmsen M, Verhoef J, van Golde LM, van Iwaarden JF. Interactions of surfactant protein A with influenza A viruses: binding and neutralization. J Infect Dis 1995; 171:335–341.

92. Weyer C, Sabat R, Wissel H, Kruger DH, Stevens PA, Prosch S. Surfactant protein A binding to cytomegalovirus proteins enhances virus entry into rat lung cells. Am J Respir Cell Mol Biol 2000; 23:71–78.

93. Barr FE, Pedigo H, Johnson TR, Shepherd VL. Surfactant protein-A enhances uptake of respiratory syncytial virus by monocytes and U937 macrophages. Am J Respir Cell Mol Biol 2000; 23:586–592.

94. Ghildyal R, Hartley C, Varrasso A, Meanger J, Voelker DR, Anders EM, Mills J. Surfactant protein A binds to the fusion glycoprotein of respiratory syncytial virus and neutralizes virion infectivity. J Infect Dis 1999; 180:2009–2013.

95. Zimmerman PE, Voelker DR, McCormack FX, Paulsrud JR, Martin WJD. 120-kDa surface glycoprotein of *Pneumocystis carinii* is a ligand for surfactant protein A. J Clin Invest 1992; 89:143–149.

96. McCormack FX, Festa AL, Andrews RP, Linke M, Walzer PD. The carbohydrate recognition domain of surfactant protein A mediates binding to the major surface glycoprotein of *Pneumocystis carinii*. Biochemistry 1997; 36:8092–8099.

97. Kabha K, Schmegner J, Keisari Y, Parolis H, Schlepper-Schaeffer J, Ofek I. SP-A enhances phagocytosis of *Klebsiella* by interaction with capsular polysaccharides and alveolar macrophages. Am J Physiol 1997; 272:L344–L352.

98. Madan T, Kishore U, Shah A, Eggleton P, Strong P, Wang JY, Aggrawal SS, Sarma PU, Reid KB. Lung surfactant proteins A and D can inhibit specific IgE binding to the allergens of *Aspergillus fumigatus* and block allergen-induced histamine release from human basophils. Clin Exp Immunol 1997; 110:241–249.

99. van de Wetering JK, van Eijk M, van Golde LM, Hartung T, van Strijp JA, Batenburg JJ. Characteristics of surfactant protein A and D binding to lipoteichoic acid and peptidoglycan, 2 major cell wall components of gram-positive bacteria. J Infect Dis 2001; 184:1143–1151.

100. Murakami S, Iwaki D, Mitsuzawa H, Sano H, Takahashi H, Voelker DR, Akino T, Kuroki Y. Surfactant protein A inhibits peptidoglycan-induced tumor necrosis factor-alpha secretion in U937 cells and alveolar macrophages by direct interaction with toll-like receptor 2. J Biol Chem 2002; 277:6830–6837.

101. Griffiss JM, Schneider H, Mandrell RE, Yamasaki R, Jarvis GA, Kim JJ, Gibson BW, Hamadeh R, Apicella MA. Lipooligosaccharides: the principal glycolipids of the neisserial outer membrane. Rev Infect Dis 1988; 10:S287–S1095.

102. Stamme C, Muller M, Hamann L, Gutsmann T, Seydel U. Surfactant protein A inhibits lipopolysaccharide-induced immune cell activation by preventing the interaction of lipopolysaccharide with lipopolysaccharide-binding protein. Am J Respir Cell Mol Biol 2002; 27:353–360.

103. Heumann D, Roger T. Initial responses to endotoxins and Gram-negative bacteria. Clin Chim Acta 2002; 323:59–72.

104. McNeely TB, Coonrod JD. Aggregation and opsonization of type A but not type B *Haemophilus influenzae* by surfactant protein A. Am J Respir Cell Mol Biol 1994; 11:114–122.

105. Tino MJ, Wright JR. Surfactant protein A stimulates phagocytosis of specific pulmonary pathogens by alveolar macrophages. Am J Physiol 1996; 270:L677–L688.

106. Madan T, Eggleton P, Kishore U, Strong P, Aggrawal SS, Sarma PU, Reid KB. Binding of pulmonary surfactant proteins A and D to *Aspergillus fumigatus* conidia enhances phagocytosis and killing by human neutrophils and alveolar macrophages. Infect Immun 1997; 65:3171–3179.

107. Pikaar JC, Voorhout WF, van Golde LM, Verhoef J, Van Strijp JA, van Iwaarden JF. Opsonic activities of surfactant proteins A and D in phagocytosis of Gram-negative bacteria by alveolar macrophages. J Infect Dis 1995; 172:481–489.

108. Manz-Keinke H, Egenhofer C, Plattner H, Schlepper-Schafer J. Specific interaction of lung surfactant protein A (SP-A) with rat alveolar macrophages. Exp Cell Res 1991; 192:597–603.

109. Wintergerst E, Manz-Keinke H, Plattner H, Schlepper-Schafer J. The interaction of a lung surfactant protein (SP-A) with macrophages is mannose dependent. Eur J Cell Biol 1989; 50:291–298.

110. Gaynor CD, McCormack FX, Voelker DR, McGowan SE, Schlesinger LS. Pulmonary surfactant protein A mediates enhanced phagocytosis of *Mycobacterium tuberculosis* by a direct interaction with human macrophages. J Immunol 1995; 155:5343–5351.

111. Pison U, Wright JR, Hawgood S. Specific binding of surfactant apoprotein SP-A to rat alveolar macrophages. Am J Physiol 1992; 262:L412–L417.

112. Malhotra R, Thiel S, Reid KB, Sim RB. Human leukocyte C1q receptor binds other soluble proteins with collagen domains. J Exp Med 1990; 172:955–959.

113. Vandivier RW, Ogden CA, Fadok VA, Hoffmann PR, Brown KK, Botto M, Walport MJ, Fishe JH, Henson PM, Greene KE. Role of surfactant proteins A, D, and C1q in the clearance of apoptotic cells in vivo and in vitro: calreticulin and CD91 as a common collectin receptor complex. J Immunol 2002; 169:3978–3986.

114. Chroneos ZC, Abdolrasulnia R, Whitsett JA, Rice WR, Shepherd VL. Purification of a cell-surface receptor for surfactant protein A. J Biol Chem 1996; 271:16375–16383.

115. Guillot L, Balloy V, McCormack FX, Golenbock DT, Chignard M, Si-Tahar M. Cutting edge: the immunostimulatory activity of the lung surfactant protein-A involves Toll-like receptor 4. Immunol J 2002; 168:5989–5992.

116. Gardai SJ, Xiao YQ, Dickinson M, Nick JA, Voelker DR, Greene KE, Henson PM. By binding SIRP-α or calreticulin/CD9I, lung collectins act as dual function surveillance molecules to suppress or enhance inflammation. Cell 2003; 115:13–23.

117. Reid KB, Colomb M, Petry F, Loos M. Complement component C1 and the collectins-first-line defense molecules in innate and acquired immunity. Trends Immunol 2002; 23:115–117.

118. Sano H, Chiba H, Iwaki D, Sohma H, Voelker DR, Kuroki Y. Surfactant proteins A and D bind CD14 by different mechanisms. J Biol Chem 2000; 275:22442–22451.

119. McIntosh JC, Mervin-Blake S, Conner E, Wright JR. Surfactant protein A protects growing cells and reduces TNF-alpha activity from LPS-stimulated macrophages. Am J Physiol 1996; 271:L310–L319.

120. Arias-Diaz J, Garcia-Verdugo I, Casals C, Sanchez-Rico N, Vara E, Balibrea L. Effect of surfactant protein A (SP-A) on the production of cytokines by human pulmonary macrophages. Shock 2000; 14:300–306.

121. Hickling TP, Sim RB, Malhotra R. Induction of TNF-alpha release from human buffy coat cells by *Pseudomonas aeruginosa* is reduced by lung surfactant protein A. FEBS Lett 1998; 437:65–69.

122. Borron P, McIntosh JC, Korfhagen TR, Whitsett JA, Taylor J, Wright JR. Surfactant-associated protein A inhibits LPS-induced cytokine and nitric oxide production *in vivo*. Am J Physiol Lung Cell Mol Physiol 2000; 278:L840–L847.

123. Bufler P, Schmidt B, Schikor D, Bauernfeind A, Crouch EC, Griese M. Surfactant Protein A and D differently regulate the immune response to nonmucoid *Pseudomonas aeruginosa* and its lipopolysaccharide. Am J Respir Cell Mol Biol 2003; 28:249–256.

124. Kremlev SG, Umstead TM, Phelps DS. Surfactant protein A regulates cytokine production in the monocytic cell line THP-1. Am J Physiol 1997; 272:L996–L1004.

125. Wang G, Phelps DS, Umstead TM, Floros J. Human SP-A protein variants derived from one or both genes stimulate TNF-alpha production in the THP-1 cell line. Am J Physiol Lung Cell Mol Physiol 2000; 278:L946–L1004.

126. Katsura H, Kawada H, Konno K. Rat surfactant apoprotein A (SP-A) exhibits antioxidant effects on alveolar macrophages. Am J Respir Cell Mol Biol 1993; 9:520–525.

127. Weber H, Heilmann P, Meyer B, Maier KL. Effect of canine surfactant protein (SP-A) on the respiratory burst of phagocytic cells. FEBS Lett 1990; 270:90–94.

128. van Iwaarden JF, Teding van Berkhout F, Whitsett JA, Oosting RS, van Golde LM. A novel procedure for the rapid isolation of surfactant protein A with retention of its alveolar-macrophage-stimulating properties. Biochem J 1995; 309:551–555.

129. Blau H, Riklis S, van Iwaarden JF, McCormack FX, Kalina M. Nitric oxide production by rat alveolar macrophages can be modulated *in vitro* by surfactant protein A. Am J Physiol 272:L1198–L1204.

130. Wright JR, Zlogar DF, Taylor JC, Zlogar TM, Restrepo CI. Effects of endotoxin on surfactant protein A and D stimulation of NO production by alveolar macrophages. Am J Physiol 1999; 276:L650–L658.

131. Hickman-Davis J, Gibbs-Erwin J, Lindsey JR, Matalon S. Surfactant protein A mediates mycoplasmacidal activity of alveolar macrophages by production of peroxynitrite. Proc Natl Acad Sci USA 1999; 96:4953–4958.

132. LeVine AM, Kurak KE, Bruno MD, Stark JM, Whitsett JA, Korfhagen TR. Surfactant protein-A deficient mice are susceptible to *Pseudomonas aeruginosa* infection. Am J Respir Cel Mol Biol 1998; 19:700–708.

133. Stamme C, Walsh E, Wright JR. Surfactant protein A differentially regulates IFN-gamma- and LPS-induced nitrite production by rat alveolar macrophages. Am J Respir Cell Mol Biol 2000; 23:772–779.

134. Hickman-Davis JM, O'Reilly P, Davis IC, Peti-Peterdi J, Davis G, Young KR, Devlin RB, Matalon S. Killing of *Klebsiella pneumoniae* by human alveolar macrophages. Am J Physiol Lung Cell Mol Physiol 2002; 282:L944–L956.

135. Allen MJ, Harbeck R, Smith B, Voelker DR, Mason RJ. Binding of rat and human surfactant proteins A and D to *Aspergillus fumigatus* conidia. Infect Immun 1999; 67:4563–4569.

136. Tenner AJ, Robinson SL, Borchelt J, Wright JR. Human pulmonary surfactant protein (SP-A), a protein structurally homologous to C1q, can enhance FcR- and CR1-mediated phagocytosis. J Biol Chem 1989; 264:13923–13928.

137. Kremlev SG, Phelps DS. Effect of SP-A surfactant lipids on expression of cell surface markers in the THP-1 monocytic cell line. Am J Physiol 1997; 272:L1070–L1077.

4

Receptors and Ligands for Collectins Surfactant Proteins A and D

NADES PALANIYAR, * **JEYA NADESALINGAM, and KENNETH B. M. REID**

Oxford University,
Oxford, UK

Current affiliation: Hospital for Sick Children Research Institute, Toronto, Ontario, Canada.

I. Introduction

Pulmonary surfactant is a mixture of lipids (90% w/w) and proteins ($\sim$10% w/w), and these proteolipid complexes are known to maintain low surface tension. However, recent studies show that surfactant also plays vital roles in immunity. The major proteins present in the bronchoalveolar lavage (BAL) fluid include antibodies, albumin, antimicrobial proteins, and surfactant proteins or surfactant-associated proteins (SPs). The SPs constitute $\sim$20% (w/w of the total protein) of the proteins present in the lung washings (1). The hydrophilic collectins SP-A ($\sim$90%, w/w of the SPs) and SP-D ($\sim$2–5%, w/w of the SPs) are the major proteins associated with surfactant lipids. Although most of the SP-A isolated from the BAL is associated with large aggregate form of the surfactant lipid, >70% of the SP-D is present in the nonsedimentable aqueous fraction. Interestingly, SP-A and SP-D do not affect the surface tension reducing property of surfactant, under normal conditions. Both *in vitro* and *in vivo* experiments clearly established that hydrophobic proteins SP-B and SP-C ($\sim$5%, w/w of the SPs) are the proteins that directly participate in this function. Gene-knockout mouse models suggest that SP-A and SP-D affect both innate immunity and lipid-related functions to varying degrees. In this chapter, we focus on the ligands and receptors for SP-A and SP-D. Our discussions highlight recent advances in the interactions of SP-A and SP-D with lipids, novel receptors, and microbial surfaces ligands. We also critically evaluate collectin-mediated surfactant dysfunction both in terms of lipid- and innate immune-related functions.

II. Collectins and Related Proteins

Collectins are a group of proteins that contain fibrillar collagen-like region and globular C-type lectin domains, which bind carbohydrate ligands in a calcium-ion dependent manner (Fig. 4.1) (2,3). This family of proteins is known to participate in innate immunity via recognizing the arrays of carbohydrates present

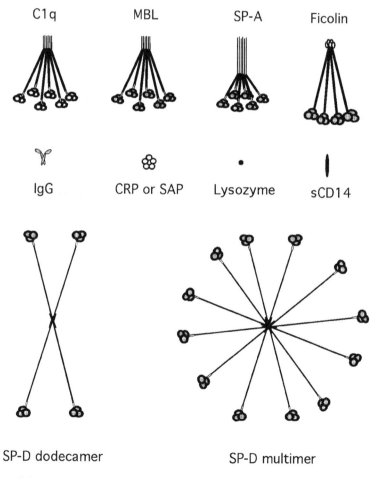

Figure 4.1 Oligomeric structures of collectins and related proteins. The molecules are drawn to show approximate relative dimensions.

on microbial surfaces (4). Although SP-A and SP-D are the two major collectins present in the lungs, they do not appear to activate the complement system. Mannose-binding lectin (MBL), a well-characterized collectin, is an acute phase serum protein, which binds several types of microbial cell wall carbohydrates and activates complement via the lectin pathway (5). Subcomponent C1q, of the first component of complement, is structurally similar to those of SP-A and MBL, but it is not a collectin. C1q binds Fc regions of antibody via protein–protein interactions and activates complement via the classical pathway (6,7). Other serum collectins include bovine conglutinin (8,9), bovine CL-43 (10,11), bovine CL-46 (12), human CL-P1 (placenta) (13) and human, and mouse CL-L1 (liver) (14). The recently reported collectin, CL-P1 is a 140 kDa type II transmembrane protein, and is present on the surface of endothelial cells but not on macrophages. This novel collectin acts as a scavenger receptor and mediates the phagocytosis of microbes and oxidized LDL (13). The 40 kDa CL-L1 is synthesized in many tissues with predominant expression in the liver, placenta, and adrenal glands. CL-L1 is present in the cytoplasm in contrast to the other secreted collectins and shows very weak affinity for carbohydrate ligands (14). Therefore, functions other than innate immunity have been envisaged for this collectin. The bovine CL-46 is highly expressed in thymus and liver and shows typical carbohydrate binding abilities (12).

Ficolins (H, L, M types) belongs to another class of collagen-like region-containing oligomeric carbohydrate binding proteins that contain nonclassical lectin domains (15–17). These proteins have fibrinogen-like globular domains instead of C-type lectin domains (17). Like MBL, H-ficolin and L-ficolin/P35 activate complement via the lectin pathway (5,9,17). Microfibril-associated protein 4 (MFAP-4) is another protein (250 kDa oligomer with 36 kDa subunits) found in the lung washings that has fibrinogen-like carbohydrate recognition domains (CRDs) but it lacks collagen-like regions (18). This protein has been suggested to play roles in leukocyte adhesion.

Other oligomeric globular carbohydrate binding proteins include pentraxins such as C-reactive protein (CRP), serum amyloid component P (SAP), and PTX-3 (7). These proteins bind pathogens and dying cells and directly interact with Fc receptors or activate complement by interacting with C1q (7). The CD14, a well-studied LPS receptor, is another example for soluble lectin (19). Many of these lectins are involved in opsonizing/clearing pathogens and various forms of lipids from the lung, serum, and other tissues. Some of the innate immune functions of these proteins overlap with those of SP-A and SP-D.

The group of membrane-anchored lectins or collagen-like proteins includes the IgE receptor FcεRII (CD23), mannose receptor (MR), complement receptor 3 (CR3), scavenger receptor (SR-CL1), LOX1, and MARCO (3). Glycosylphosphatidylinositol (GPI)-anchored form of CD14 is also present on the surface of many phagocytes. Dendritic cell-specific ICAM-grabbing nonintegrin (DC-SIGN) and liver-SIGN (L-SIGN) are two recently characterized receptors that contain extracellular lectin domains, and specifically binds ICAM-3 present on resting T-cells (20–22). As DC-SIGN is present on the surfaces of both DCs and alveolar macrophages, this lectin appears to play critical roles in effective clearance of pathogen and antigen presentation (23). Therefore, in contrast to soluble opsonic globular lectins and fibrillar collectins, these membrane-anchored lectins are likely to act as true receptors for carbohydrate ligands present on the microbial surfaces.

III. Tissue Distribution of SP-A and SP-D

Although both SP-A and SP-D were discovered in the pulmonary surfactant and named as surfactant proteins or SPs (24–27), recent reports that use sensitive detection methods indicate that they are also expressed in many other tissues (28–32). At the protein level, although SP-D is present in many tissues including epithelial cells, vasculature, gut, urogenital tract, and many secretory glands, SP-A is clearly detectable only in the lungs (31). In general, SP-D is detectable in many exocrine secretions, mucosal surfaces, and the tissues that come in contact with external environment. Although some of these tissues contain surfactant-like lipids (e.g., intestine and middle ear), many other regions contain mucus membranes. How SP-D is anchored to these surfaces is not clearly understood. Our data indicate that SP-D binds mucin which suggests that the collectin may be anchored to mucus membranes via this glycoprotein (Palaniyar et al., unpublished data). Distribution of collectins, particularly SP-D, in various mucosal surfaces implies that these molecules participate primarily in immunity.

IV. Potential Functions of SP-A and SP-D

As these collectins bind to a variety of ligands, they could potentially modulate several functions in addition to their roles in innate immunity (3,33). The functions attributed to these proteins include the alleviation of allergic response (34–38), maintenance of surfactant homeostasis (39,40) and surface activity of surfactant in the presence of inhibitors (41,42), prevention of lipid oxidation (43,44), opsonization of apoptotic cells (45,46) and their debris (47,48) for removal, enhancement of pathogen clearance, and maintenance of inflammation free lung and other tissues (49–51).

V. Structure of SP-A and SP-D

Collectins have a short interchain disulfide bond-forming N-terminal segment, a collagen-like region with Gly-X-Y repeats (where X is any amino acid and Y is often hydroxyproline or hydroxylysine), a hydrophobic neck region, and a C-terminal globular CRD (25,26,52,53). The globular domains of collectins also contain phospholipid-binding domain (PBD), and both of these regions appear to overlap with each other (54–56). Three CRDs are held together by protein–protein interactions at the hydrophobic neck region (57,58). The adjacent collagen-like region folds into a triple helix, and the three peptide chains are tethered at the N-terminal segment by disulfide bonds (Figs. 4.1 and 4.2).

Trimeric SP-A subunits (3 × ~26–32 kDa) further assemble as octadecamer (540 kDa) by forming a common collagenous stem up to the kink. These oligomers are further stabilized by covalent interchain disulfide bond formation at the short N-terminal segment (2,41). This ~20 nm long quaternary structural assembly orients all the CRDs to a similar plane (59,60). Further oligomerization of SP-A results in the formation of multi or unidirectional protein fibers, ranging up to a few micrometers in length (61,62). This supra-quaternary organization can provide a high affinity interaction between the SP-A and the ligands (62). Trimeric SP-D subunits (3 × 43 kDa), however, assemble as higher order oligomers via the interactions at N-terminal segments and only the proximal parts of the collagen-like regions (63,64). Dodecameric SP-D molecules appear as X-shaped ~100 nm long assemblies (516 kDa) whereas higher order multimers appear as "asterisks or fuzzy balls" (53,63).

Molecular information about the CRDs of SP-D has been elaborated in detail by X-ray crystallography (Fig. 4.2) (57). Three CRDs assemble to form a stable trimer subunits, and each CRD with a single carbohydrate binding site points to the same plane, and these three carbohydrate binding pockets are spaced in a triangle with ~51 Å to each side. These sites can bind hydroxyl groups of glucose and related saccharides (65) (Shrive et al., unpublished data). Although, this CRD organization does not favor the interaction of the collectins with mannosyl residues present on the host cells, they can effectively bind saccharide arrays present on the microbial surfaces with high avidity. The center of three CRDs has a positively charged surface suggesting that SP-D can interact effectively with negatively charged components such as LPS by electrostatic interaction (4,57).

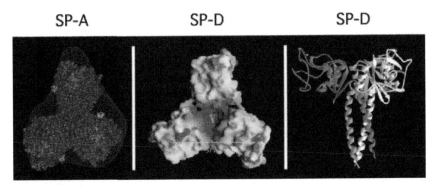

Figure 4.2 **(See color insert)** Molecular organization of CRDs of SP-A and SP-D. See Refs. (56,57) for further details.

Low-resolution molecular information obtained from the CRDs of SP-A by single particle electron crystallography and homology modeling suggests that CRDs of SP-A also form stable trimers and interact with ligands such as lipid monolayers (56). The amino acids that are known to alter the lipid-protein interactions (41,55,66) are present at the lipid–protein interface. The N-linked glycosylation site is present at the sides of the SP-A trimers. This structural organization is consistent with the idea that the N-linked sugars provide stability to the protein whereas the CRDs/PBDs interact directly with ligands. X-ray crystallographic information should provide clearer information about this CRD (67). SP-A selectively interacts with lipids that are present in surfactant and presumably in microbial membranes. Moreover, the ability of SP-A to bind to lipids and carbohydrates appears to have a physiological and immunological relevance in the lungs.

VI. Ligands for SP-A and SP-D

SP-A and SP-D bind to diverse classes of ligands, which belong to two main categories: lipids and saccharides. Experiments with fragments of native collectins (68,69), site directed mutagenesis (41), molecular modeling (56), and X-ray crystallography (67) and recent electron microscopic studies (56,60) suggest that the recognition of these ligands occurs via the CRD/PBD of these collectins.

A. Lipid Ligands for SP-A and SP-D

SP-A and SP-D bind to some of the lipid ligands present in the pulmonary surfactant. Binding of these ligands conveniently anchors these innate immune collectins in the air–liquid interface, where the air-borne microbes and external agents make the primary contact with lungs (2,3).

SP-A and Lipids

SP-A preferentially binds dipalmitoylphosphatidylcholine (DPPC), the major surface tension reducing lipid component (~40–50%, w/w) of the pulmonary surfactant (70,71). This lipid–protein interaction results in the reorganization of surfactant into intricate tubular arrays known as tubular myelin (TM) (62,72,73). Although the functions of the TM have not yet been unequivocally resolved, this form of the surfactant is superior in maintaining low surface tension, particularly in the presence of surface tension-inhibiting agents such as serum proteins (42,74). TM has previously been considered as an essential intermediate in the conversion of secreted lamellar body into the surfactant film. As SP-A knockout mice, which lack TM, form stable surfactant film (75–77), it is clear that TM is not essential for the formation of the surface active film. SP-A knockout mice function quite normally under a variety of stress conditions (76) further suggesting that, at least in these laboratory experimental conditions, TM does not provide any measurable advantage to the organism. However, a recent report suggests that DPPC clearance is defective in SP-A knockout mice under altered physiological conditions such as hyperventillation (78).

TM and other multilayer lipids often interconnect the epithelial cell layer and the surface film (79,80). This organization compartmentalizes the alveolus into small segments. It is conceivable that TM acts as a physical barrier to minimize the spread of incoming microbes and debris. TM is a rich source of SP-A (73), hence, this proteolipid complex could also facilitate the coating/opsonization of the targets. Several studies indicate that SP-A directly binds different microbes (81) and that SP-A knockout mice are defective in clearing a variety of pathogens (49). The reason for the susceptibility of SP-A deficient mice to infections is often directly attributed to the absence of interaction between SP-A and pathogens, and SP-As ability to mediate host cell immune response. Specific experiments are, however, required to differentiate the role of SP-A from TM-associated SP-A in innate immunity, *in vivo*.

Another novel lipid-related function has recently been assigned to both SP-A and SP-D by McCormack and co-workers (43). They showed that globular domains of these proteins inhibit the oxidation of lipids. It is known that the maintenance of intact lipid molecules is essential to preserve the surface-active properties of the surfactant. SP-A prevents the inactivation of surfactant film by oxidized lipids, *in vitro* (44). Detailed studies of surfactant lipids from the SP-A, SP-D, SP-A/SP-D double knockout mice are required to confirm the relevance of these new observations, *in vivo*.

Several laboratories have established that the globular head domain of SP-A interacts with DPPC in a calcium ion-dependent manner (41,70,71). As the calcium ion concentration in alveolar environment ranges between 1 and 5 mM (82), this mode of interaction between the SP-A and the lipid ligand appears to be physiologically relevant. At 150 mM NaCl salt concentration, purified human SP-A aggregates in the absence of detergents or divalent cation-chelating agents (68,69). This phenomenon suggests that SP-A may be a hydrophobic molecule. Trimeric neck/CRD fragments obtained from native SP-A (Fig. 4.2), however, do not self-aggregate under physiological buffers (68), but similar recombinant fragments can bind lipids, particularly when they are tethered together as trimers by the N-terminal segment (83). N-terminal segments appear to present all three CRDs of a single trimer to a common plane, so that the molecule binds lipid layers with a high avidity (56).

Binding of calcium to CRDs known to increase β-sheet content, and the resultant conformational change renders the globular domains resistant to proteases (68,84). Furthermore, low pH could induce SP-A or SP-A-mediated lipid vesicle aggregation (85,86). Conformational changes likely to play a critical role in the interaction between two SP-A molecules and SP-A and lipid membranes. Solving the structure of this domain with and without calcium ions by X-ray crystallography likely to provide the answers for this question (67).

The earlier studies suggest that the binding of SP-A to lipids may not simply be a hydrophobic interaction. Solid-phase binding assays suggest that SP-A binds to the acyl chains of the lipid molecules (70); however, experiments involving lipid films under near biological conditions suggest that this protein binds to the polar head region of the phospholipid molecules (71). Whether PBDs of the SP-A are partially buried into the membrane is still not completely understood.

SP-D and Lipids

In contrast to SP-A, globular domains of SP-D bind phosphatidylinositol (PI), a minor lipid component ($\sim$2%, w/w of the lipid) of the surfactant lipid (87,88). This calcium-dependent phospholipid binding ability of SP-D is similar to that of the serum collectin MBL (54,89). Studies that use mutant and chimeric proteins suggest that phospholipid-binding segment of SP-D and MBL could be interchangeable (54,90). Furthermore, it has been suggested that SP-D binds PI via the carbohydrate moiety of the glycolipid (88,90). Binding of SP-D to PI has also been considered to represent the way in which SP-D interacts with PI containing cells. SP-D binds to a nonphospholipid, glucosylceramide (55), however, biological implication of this interaction has not been completely established.

Keough and co-workers (91) examined the role of SP-D in maintaining a surface-active surfactant film. Their studies suggest that SP-D is adsorbed to lipid films primarily via hydrophobic interactions and does not significantly interfere with surface activity of surfactant, *in vitro*. Although thin layer chromatographic plate and liposome based techniques indicate that SP-D specifically interacts with PI (87,88), experiments with lipid films (91) suggest that this type of phospholipid does not affect the binding of SP-D to surfactant film. Hence, PI may not be essential for SP-D to bind to surfactant lipid films. Moreover, surfactant isolated from SP-D gene-knockout mice is similar to that of the wild-type mice and shows efficient spreading and low surface tension (39,92). SP-D, therefore, may not affect the surface-active properties of surfactant, *in vivo*.

Interestingly, SP-D mediates the generation of atypical TM-like lipid structures in the presence of increased concentrations of PI, *in vitro* (80). Although SP-A mediates the formation of long tubules with square (50 × 50 nm) cross sections, SP-D generates circular tubules with $\sim$90 nm in diameter, which show a central target-like electron density. Longitudinal sections of these atypical TM suggest that SP-D molecules span these tubules. Similar lipid structures could be detected in the surfactant secreted by cultured type II cells (80), as well as the surfactant found in the lungs of alveolar proteinosis patients (93). These examples indicate that SP-D may also play an important role in maintaining the surfactant lipid structure and improved surfactant function under certain conditions.

Although SP-D gene-knockout mice models show many phenotypes, these mice provide a clearer indication that SP-D plays an important function in the lipid homeostasis *in vivo* (39,40). Lipid-related defect includes an age-dependent accumulation of surfactant lipids and alveolar macrophages. Electron microscopy shows that although TM was detected in the large aggregate surfactant, most of the lipids existed as electron dense arrays (40). SP-D deficiency also appears to affect lipids via other mechanisms. For example, alveolar macrophages of SP-D-deficient mice generate more reactive oxygen radicals and contain oxidized lipids (94). Moreover, SP-D knockout mice show chronically inflamed lung, increased matrix metalloproteinase (MMP) expression, and progressive development of emphysema and fibrosis. Double knockout mice models suggest that neither MMPs 9, 12 nor the NADPH pathway on their own are sufficient to cause the phenotypes observed in SP-D knockout mice (95). Calculations suggest that defective clearance of lipids seen in SP-D knockout mice occurs via multiple mechanisms (92,96). In addition, a number of alveolar macrophages in the lung of SP-D deficient mice increase with increasing age and many of which become foamy. However, SP-D-mediated lipid and alveolar macrophage homeostasis have not been clearly understood.

Recent studies suggest that these alveolar macrophages show signs of apoptosis (45). Treatment of these mice with a 60 kDa SP-D(n/CRD) recombinant fragment that contains the proximal collagen-like $(Gly-X-Y)_8$ region, neck, and CRDs (Fig. 4.2), corrects the defects of the accumulation of lipids and alveolar macrophages in the lung. These results indicate that some of the important functions of this protein reside in the C-terminal portion of the molecule. Overexpression of chimeric (64,97) or mutant (98) versions of SP-D, however, failed to rescue many of the defects seen in the SP-D gene-deficient mice. Further studies are necessary to understand the protein domains that are needed to impart different functions *in vivo*. See alveolar macrophage section for more details.

B. Saccharide Ligands for Collectins

Many microbial surfaces contain repeating patterns of carbohydrate-based polymers, and the collectins are known to bind to these sugars. On the basis of the structural homology with MBL, and direct ligand binding studies, both SP-A and SP-D have been shown to bind to several hexose sugars.

Saccharide Ligands and SP-A

Although the study of C-type lectin activity of SP-A has been hampered by the propensity of this protein, from many organisms, to form massive aggregates at physiological salt and calcium concentrations, a considerable number of papers have been published on this topic. Most of the useful information, regarding the binding properties of SP-A, has been obtained from the studies with rat SP-A, which does not aggregate under these conditions (41). This body of literature suggests that SP-A binds preferentially to hexose sugars such as mannose. These results are obtained primarily from binding of the SP-A to mannosyl–BSA, mannose–agarose or mannan–agarose matrices (99,100). However, some of the recent works suggest that SP-A does not bind to the previously suggested ligands such as yeast mannan (101,102). X-ray crystallographic studies suggest that rat SP-A(n/CRD) may bind mannose (67). Hence, although CRDs of SP-A shares high homology with other known collectins, biologically relevant carbohydrate ligands that it binds have not been determined, unequivocally.

Saccharide Ligands and SP-D

Binding of SP-D to carbohydrate ligands has been characterized in detail. As this protein is soluble under physiological salt concentrations, several laboratories studied its interaction with sugars. SP-D preferentially binds glucose, maltose (di-glucose), and related hexoses. As the common form of native SP-D is a dodecamer or an asterisk like oligomer, it binds carbohydrates with very high avidity. Particularly, complexes of SP-D, or SP-D(n/CRD), formed with maltose–agarose matrices in a calcium-dependent manner are stable even at 1 M NaCl concentrations (103,104), which suggests that this lectin binds strongly to maltose–agarose matrix. Real time surface plasmon resonance (SPR) measurements show that once bound, SP-D does not disassociate easily from the yeast mannan under physiological salt conditions (104). SP-D is known to bind to fungi and allergens (101,105–107). Binding of SP-D to yeast cells appears to occur via the β1-6 linked glucans present on their surfaces (101,107).

SP-D also binds to carbohydrate moieties present on Gram-negative bacterial surface such as lipopolysaccharide (LPS) (108,109). As a single SP-D oligomeric molecule can cross link more than one bacterium, this collectin agglutinates many members from this group of bacteria (109), which thought to results in the reduction in bacterial multiplication and their enhanced clearance by phagocytes. Recent studies suggest that both SP-A and SP-D kills Gram-negative bacteria such as *Escherichia coli* by increasing membrane permeability (110). Although the agglutination ability of SP-D is dependent on the presence of collagen-like regions as well as the disulfide-bond forming N-terminal segment, the other characteristics such as the carbohydrate or bacteria-binding and killing ability of this protein resides in the globular CRDs. Hence, different domains of the protein are involved in specific functions and more than one domain participate in certain functions.

Recent reports suggest that SP-D, but not SP-A, binds to both of the Gram-positive bacterial cell wall ligands peptidoglycan (PGN) and lipoteichoic acid (LTA) (111,112). Interaction between SP-D and LTA could be competed by hexose sugars and hence, the binding appears to be mediated by lectin–carbohydrate type interactions (112). As the carbohydrate content of LTA varies among bacterial strains, it would be interesting to analyze the interaction between SP-D and LTA from different sources. Our analyses of SP-D with Gram-positive bacterial ligands also suggest that this collectin specifically interacts with both of these ligands (Nadesalingam et al., unpublished data).

Palaniyar et al. (48) recently identified that SP-D and other collectins bind nucleic acids (DNA and RNA) *in vitro* via both their collagen-like regions and globular CRDs (Fig. 4.3). This binding appears to be important *in vivo* because SP-D knockout mice accumulate DNA in the lung and anti-DNA antibodies in

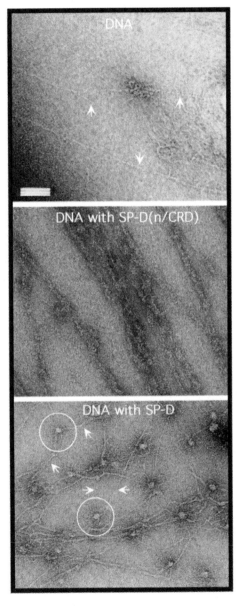

Figure 4.3 Electron micrographs showing the interaction between SP-D and DNA. Arrow, DNA; circle, oligomeric SP-D; scale bar, 50 nm.

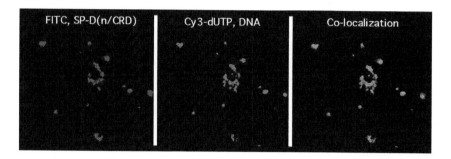

Figure 4.4 **(See Color Insert)** Co-localization of DNA and SP-D(n/CRD) on apoptotic cells. Green, FITC-labelled SP-D(n/CRD); red, dUTP-labelled DNA ends; yellow, co-localization.

the sera (47, Palaniyar et al., unpublished data). Absence of SP-D in mice shows increased accumulation of apoptotic alveolar macrophages in the lung (45) and SP-D(n/CRD) binds to apoptotic cells and colocalize with DNA (Fig. 4.4) and enhances the clearance of these dead cells from the lung (Palaniyar et al., unpublished data). These studies indicate the importance of the interaction between SP-D and DNA. Interestingly, although free DNA cause tissue inflammation, specific regions of bacterial DNA act as adjuvant and enhance immune response to several antigens *in vivo* (113). Hence, interaction between SP-D and DNA appears to have important biological significance. Detailed studies are necessary to clearly understand the interactions between SP-D and these novel ligands.

VII. Cells and Receptors

Both SP-A and SP-D bind to a variety of cells and other proteins. Some of the putative receptors are present in more than one type of cell; however, the exact nature of interactions among the ligands, collectins, receptors/binding proteins, and cells are not clearly understood.

A. Cells

Many of the cells that collectins bind are phagocytes. As SP-A and SP-D are innate immune molecules, their interactions with phagocytic cells are consistent with their proposed functions. Recent evidence indicates that these proteins also interact with cells involved in the adaptive immune system, such as lymphocytes and cells that connect the innate and adaptive immunity, that is, the dendritic cells (DCs). These interactions place the collectins as molecules that inter link these two immune systems.

Type II Cells

Although the pulmonary type II pneumocytes are the secretory cells of the alveolus, they are also professional phagocytes (114,115). Both SP-A and SP-D and other lectins are internalized and resecreted by type II cells (116,117). SP-A interacts with receptors on these cells via the collagen-like region (118) or CRDs (119) and is internalized by the coated-pit pathway (120). SP-A is also known to regulate lipid-recycling *in vitro* (41). SP-D binding to type II cells, however, does not alter the lipid-recycling, but most of the internalized SP-D is recycled via the lamellar bodies (117). Therefore, nonrelated lectins (116) as well as both SP-A and SP-D are internalized and resecreted by type II cells, but only SP-A appears to have the ability to regulate lipid-recycling. Although the effect of SP-A on type II cell and lipid-recycling has been well-established *in vitro* (41), initial characterization of SP-A knockout mouse models showed no apparent defect in lipid homeostasis (51,75). Recent experiments, however, show the relevance of SP-A in lipid clearance *in vivo*, particularly under certain stress/stimulatory conditions (78).

Alveolar Macrophages

Both SP-A and SP-D bind to monocytic cells or cell lines and alveolar macrophages (121,122). Binding of SP-D to alveolar macrophages, however, does not involve the C1q receptor (122). Although the receptors for these molecules are not clearly identified (see below), these collectins in the presence or absence of lipids are internalized and degraded by phagocytes (123,124). Hence, these results are consistent with the idea that both SP-A and SP-D are opsonins, and the phagocytes ingest them together with the foreign or dead cells or lipids. Mouse models clearly show that SP-D, but not SP-A, deficiency leads to the accumulation of lipids in macrophages (39,40). Increased lipid content in the lung could lead to its accumulation in the alveolar macrophages (125). However, whether this phenomenon is related to the phenotypes seen in the SP-D knockout mice is uncertain.

Whitsett and co-workers (50,64,97,98,126) extensively studied the abnormalities in pulmonary phenotypes by expressing several transgenic *SP-D* gene constructs in SP-D knockout mouse models. Transgenic expression of SP-D in the SP-D knockout mice under the control of doxycycline inducible lung-specific promoters provided a clear separation of SP-D-mediated phenotypes (50). Constitutive transgenic expression of rat SP-D (126) or doxycycline-based induction of *SP-D* gene at the neonatal period and its continued expression (50) corrects all the SP-D phenotypes. Turning the gene expression on in adult mice corrects the lipid and alveolar macrophage-associated phenotypes but failed to rescue the emphysema. Turning the gene expression off in the adult mice results in the appearance of all the SP-D knockout mice phenotype except that the lipid content stays low at the wild-type levels. Hence, SP-D regulates these phenotypes by different mechanisms. These results further suggest that lipid accumulation and alveolar macrophage phenotypes could be corrected by SP-D (50) or recombinant SP-D(n/CRD) fragment (45) but the emphysema may not easily be reversed by replacement of SP-D after the alteration to the airway parenchyma (50).

Polymorphonuclear Leukocyte

Both SP-A and SP-D bind polymorphonuclear leukocytes (PMNs) and act as chemoattractants [106,127–129]. Ligands opsonized by both SP-A and SP-D are preferentially phagocytosed by PMNs (106,130). LPS-mediated inflammatory changes particularly increase the amount of SP-D associated with PMNs and lung tissue (129). Once again, the receptors on this phagocyte for the collectins are not known with certainty. Like alveolar macrophages, PMNs also phagocytoze the lipids present in the lung (131) and lipid concentration may be altered by PMNs during lung injury and inflammation.

Dendritic Cells

Wright and co-workers (132,133) recently reported that collectins are involved in DC-mediated uptake and processing of antigens. It is known that immature DCs act only as phagocytes, whereas the mature DCs process foreign antigen, and present them to the adaptive immune system. SP-A and C1q inhibit DC differentiation and subsequent DC-mediated T-cell activation; however, SP-D promotes these functions. This finding represents a significant understanding of the role of SP-A and SP-D in interlinking innate and adaptive immunity (3). DCs reside exclusively in the interstitium whereas the collectins are present in the surfactant. Inflammation and lung injury leads to an increase in tissue associated SP-D, but not SP-A (129). Hence, SP-D may specifically interact with other cells including the DCs of interstitium during an insult. Surface expression of hyaluronan increases during the maturation of DCs (134) and SP-D-hyaluronan interaction (104) may be important in this function. Detailed studies are required to establish the DC-related roles of SP-A and SP-D *in vivo*.

Eosinophils, Basophils, and Mast Cells

Studies by Reid and co-workers (37,105,106,135,136) indicated the importance of lung collectins in allergy and related conditions. They showed that lung collectins block the interaction between IgE and allergens (137,138). It is well established that eosinophils, basophils, and mast cells express two receptors, FcεRI and FcεRII (CD23), and both of which bind IgE and release inflammatory mediators. Mast cells reside in mucosal and epithelial tissues and contain acidic proteoglycans and histamine-rich granules. Legation of allergens to FcεR–IgE complex induces these leukocytes to release inflammatory mediators, instantaneously. The other two leukocytes, eosinophils and basophils are derived from the same myeloid cell lineage and express FcεRs. Although eosinophils and basophils are derived from different myeloid lineages than that of mast cells, all of these leukocytes exert similar response for allergens. SP-A and SP-D blocks the binding of allergens to IgE and subsequent histamine release by basophils (137). SP-A and SP-D can also reduce the histamine release from the peripheral blood mononucleated cells isolated from asthmatic patients (139).

Eosinophil number increases drastically during allergic reaction and these cells are the major source of IL-8 at the site of allergic inflammation. SP-A inhibits the secretion of this inflammatory cytokine by eosinophils (140), suggesting that SP-A may dampen the inflammatory response. Animal models show that both SP-A and SP-D reduce IgE, blood eosinophelia, allergic response, and airway hypersensitivity (34,37). Interestingly, treatment of allergic mice with SP-A and SP-D suppresses subsequent allergic reactions. Collectin-treated mice continued to maintain low concentrations of IgE and eosinophils in the serum. Furthermore, allergen exposure leads to an immediate and dramatic ($\sim$10-fold) upregulation of SP-A and SP-D concentrations in the lung (35,36,38,136,141,142). Overexpression of allergic type (T_H2) cytokines such as IL-5 (141) and IL-13 (143) also results in the upregulation of SP-D. These findings indicate that SP-A and SP-D play important roles in maintaining surfactant that is proficient in clearing allergens. As SP-D concentration dramatically changes during allergy, this collectin likely to play a prominent role in minimizing/preventing allergic reaction.

Lymphocytes

Lymphocytes constitute $\sim$5–10% of the cells present in the lung washings, indicating the importance of these immune cells in the alveolar environment. Although the contamination of plasma and its contents with the BAL fluid during washing procedures is possible, genuine presence of these adaptive immune components have been recognized. Most of the lymphocytes detected in BAL are T-cells, which exist in a ratio of CD8 : CD4 of 1 : 1.5. Although B-cells constitute $\sim$10% of the lymphocytes present in the BAL fluid, B-lymphocyte number do not directly correlate with the concentration of antibody detected in the BAL fluid. The CD8 cytotoxic T-cells directly kill infected cells by inducing apoptosis. In contrast, T_H1 type CD4 cells secrete IFN-γ and IL-2, which are important for activating macrophages and preventing granulomatous disease such as tuberculosis. The T_H2 type CD4 cells secrete IL-4, IL-5, IL-10, and IL-13, which are important to induce antibody generation and secretion from B-lymphocytes. Current paradigm is that the shift from T_H2 to T_H1 type CD4 cells and cytokine profiles is essential to minimize pulmonary allergy and asthma (113,144).

Reid and co-workers (37,137,139,144) recognized that collectins SP-A and SP-D alleviate allergy and modulate adaptive immune response. Recent studies address the mechanisms responsible for collectin-mediated alterations in adaptive immunity (36,145–147). In addition, both SP-A and SP-D are detected in serum and SP-D concentration in plasma is highly heritable (148). It is well known that several lung diseases result in altered serum concentrations of these collectins to a significant degree (149), hence, these collectins could interact directly with lymphocytes. SP-A appears to interact with lymphocytes via the collagen-like region of the protein (150). However, the CRDs of SP-D bind to lymphocytes via lectin–carbohydrate interaction (139). Detailed understanding of potential roles of these innate immune collectins may be useful to explain some of the complex interactions among various immune pathways.

B. Receptors and/or Binding Proteins

Although SP-A and SP-D bind to a variety of phagocytes and immune-related cells, how they interact with these cells is not clearly understood. Several putative receptors that bind collectins have been isolated from the surfaces of variety of cells. Some of these receptors are specific to type II cells whereas the others are present in many cell types. In addition, SP-A and SP-D also bind to other soluble proteins or receptors.

The 32 kDa SP-A Receptor

Strayer et al. (151) identified a 32 kDa receptor for human and porcine SP-A by anti-idiotypic antibody approach. Two anti-idiotypic monoclonal antibodies were raised against the SP-A-binding regions of antibodies. Both of these antibodies recognize SP-A receptor (SPAR) and suggest that the receptor is expressed only in lungs. Sequence similarity indicates that SPAR contains transmembrane domain and hence, could act as a true receptor. These antibodies inhibit SP-A binding to type II cells, which suggests that SP-A binds to these cells primarily via the SPAR. Furthermore, SP-A binding to SPAR inhibits secretagogue-induced calcium influx into cultured type II cells and subsequent surfactant secretion (152). SP-A interaction with this receptor also appears to transduce the stimulatory signal into the cell and upregulates the concentrations and stability of surfactant protein mRNA (153). This cytokine-like function of SP-A may be related to the constitutive expression of surfactant proteins by type II cells. SP-A downregulates apoptosis of type II cells via SPAR (154,155). This specific effect is dependent on a protein kinase or PI3K activity, which suggests that this effect is a highly regulated process.

The 55 kDa SP-A Binding Protein

Stevens et al. (156) identified a 55 kDa protein as a receptor for SP-A by another auto-anti-idiotypic approach. This protein existed as a 170–200 kDa protein under nonreducing conditions, suggesting that the receptor is a homo-oligomer. It has been suggested that extracellular SP-A binds to this receptor and regulates the phagocytosis of lipids by type II cells (156,157). The antibodies against BP55 block SP-A binding to type II cells and inhibit the SP-A-mediated uptake of liposomes. This antibody, however, does not affect the secretion of SP-A by the pneumocyte suggesting that BP55 is specific for lipid uptake and directing them to nondegrading compartments of the type II cell.

The 210 kDa SP-A Receptor

Chroneos et al. (158) isolated a 210 kDa SP-A binding protein from both rat lung and U937 monocytic cell membranes by SP-A affinity chromatography. Two other proteins with 66 and 45 kDa molecular mass were also detected in some preparations. Antibody raised against 210 kDa protein saturably binds to type II cells and macrophages suggesting that this putative receptor is present on both of these cells. Antibody for the 210 kDa receptor blocked the interaction between SP-A and type II cells and abolished SP-A-mediated inhibition of surfactant secretion. Moreover, the antibodies for 210 kDa receptor inhibited the SP-A mediated uptake of *Mycobacterium bovis* (159) suggesting that this receptor is also involved in the phagocytosis of microbes. The interaction between SP-A and lymphocytes is also mediated via SP-R210 and the collagen-like region of the collectin is involved in the binding to the receptor (150).

The 86 and > 200 kDa SP-A Binding Proteins

Kresch et al. (118) used a direct affinity chromatography method to isolate SP-A binding proteins from rat lung or type II cells. They isolated at least two candidate proteins with 86 and >200 kDa native molecular mass. The >200 kDa protein complex is made of 50 kDa disulfide-linked subunits. Both 86 and 50 kDa proteins contain ~30% (w/w) N-linked carbohydrates and their peptide backbones are 60 and 35 kDa, respectively. As antibody raised against these proteins do not recognize proteins from alveolar macrophages, these SP-A-binding proteins appear to be specific for type II cells. In rats, expression of this putative receptor increases during late gestation period and again after 4–7 days post-natal period (160). The SPA-binding protein isolated by Chroneos et al. in 1996 appears to be different than the one purified by Kresch et al. (188) because the protein studied by the former group is nonreducible whereas the receptor examined by the latter group is reducible and contains glycosylated subunits.

The 200 kDa Myosin

Wright and co-workers (161) identified a major 200 kDa SP-A binding protein by SP-A affinity chromatography. This protein was identified as myosin by amino acid sequencing. SP-A directly binds myosin and enhances the uptake of this protein by alveolar macrophages. Functional relevance of this interaction remains to be determined.

The 32 kDa Annexin IV

Sohma et al. (162) isolated annexin IV as the major SP-A binding protein by SP-A-conjugated-Sepharose 4B affinity chromatography from bovine lung soluble fraction. Annexin IV is a 32 kDa lipid binding protein, however, SP-A appears to binds to this protein via calcium-dependent protein–protein interactions. Further studies suggest that calcium binding domain 3 of annexin IV and carbohydrate recognition property of SP-A are necessary for the interaction between these two proteins (163). Biological relevance of SP-A–annexin IV interactions is not completely understood.

Phagocytic Receptor for C1q

Tenner and co-workers (164) cloned C1qR(p), a 120 kDa glycoprotein that is expressed in myeloid cell lineage, platelets, and endothelial cells. C1qR(p) has a C-type lectin domain, five EGF-like domains, a transmembrane domain and a 47 amino acid long intracellular domain. Antibody against C1qR(p) blocked enhancement of phagocytosis mediated by SP-A, MBL, and C1q (164). The mouse homolog is very similar to that of human protein in terms of chromosomal location and expression profile. Later studies suggest that C1qR(p) is primarily expressed in endothelial cells and may be involved in functions other than phagocytosis (165). Recent reports, however, suggest that C1qR(p) does not bind directly to these collectins and may have other functions (33,166).

Calreticulin, a C1q Receptor

Reid and co-workers (167,168) found that a calreticulin-like protein present in the detergent-solublized Raji, U937, and human tonsil lymphocyte cells binds to C1q–Sepharose affinity matrix. Although the cC1qR migrates with different apparent molecular weight under different gel conditions (56–70 kDa), mass spectrometry indicates that it has 47 kDa molecular mass (169). Malhotra and co-workers (169) extensively studied cC1qR to determine whether this protein is identical to calreticulin. It is now known that cC1qR is calreticulin but present as different isoforms. Calreticulin is widely distributed in the cells with major concentrations in the endoplasmic reticulum. It is now known that calreticulin is present both in and out side of the plasma membranes (170) and is expressed in a wide variety of cells, including amniotic and pulmonary epithelium, B-lymphocytes, macrophages, and cell lines of myeloid origin (169). Phagocytes draw lipid membranes from organelles such as endoplasmic reticulum during the engulfment of foreign particles/pathogens (171). Calreticulin may be brought to the surface by such membrane rearrangements. As calreticulin does not contain a transmembrane domain or GPI-anchor, this protein is likely to interact with other proteins to localize itself on the plasma membranes.

The cC1qR also binds to collectins MBL, SP-A, conglutinin, and CL-43, but not to SP-D (11,169,172). Interaction between cC1qR and C1q or collectins appears to occur at the S-domain (a CUB domain) and collagen-like regions of the proteins, respectively (173). Calreticulin is a known chaperon involved in folding glycoproteins and has lectin domains (174–176). Whether the lectin activity of calreticulin is involved in the interaction with the carbohydrate moieties present on the collectins has not been clearly established. One recent report implies that calreticulin interacts with SP-D and plays a role in clearing apoptotic cells by alveolar macrophages (46).

Toll-like Receptors

Currently, many research groups are investigating the signaling pathways mediated by TLRs. TLRs are type I transmembrane proteins that contain extracellular leucine-rich repeat (LRR) domain and participate in signaling variety of microbial infections (177). Many ligands including PGN, LTA, LPS, LAM, lipoproteins, and unmethylated DNA with CpG motif activate TLRs. At least 10 TLRs are present in humans, and they appear to control immune and inflammatory response (177). Particularly, TLR-2 and -4 are related to signaling bacterial infection/clearance. Notably, TLR-2 is constitutively expressed by lung epithelial (A549) and monocytic (THP-1) cell lines (178). Furthermore, Harju et al. (179) recently showed that the expression of both TLR-2 and -4, in human lungs, are developmentally regulated, and TLR mRNA concentrations reaches a maximum after the birth of an infant. This development-dependent expression of TLR suggests that this group of receptors is important in infant life, when the adaptive immune system is not fully developed. Typically, the extracellular domains of TLRs bind various bacterial ligands. After forming complexes with other accessory binding proteins, TLRs transmit signals via their cytoplasmic Toll/Interleukin 1 receptor (TIR) domains, and this process results in the activation of NF-κB pathway (180).

A recent report suggests that SP-A can directly interact with TLR-2 and reduce the interaction between the PGN and the receptor, which results in the inhibition of PGN-induced TNF-α production by U937 monocytic cell line (111). SP-A also appears to activate NF-κB pathway and induces inflammatory cytokine TNF-α and IL-10 via TLR-4 (181). Hence SP-A may regulate inflammation and innate immune related functions via both TLR-2 and TLR-4.

CD14

Another well-studied innate immune-related receptor is the CD14. CD14 is a soluble (48 kDa) or GPI-anchored (55 kDa) glycoprotein. As CD14 does not contain a cytoplasmic domain, the presence of other receptors is envisaged for classical signal transduction process. GPI-anchored CD14 is expressed and displayed on the surface of monocytes, alveolar macrophages, DCs, and PMNs whereas the soluble form is detected both in serum and BAL (182). Both forms of the protein can induce cell signaling via AP-1 pathway (19). Interestingly, SP-A, SP-D, and MBL can bind CD14 (183,184). SP-A and MBL interact with CD14 via protein–protein interactions but SP-D binds to the carbohydrate moiety of CD14. As SP-A interacts with CD14 via its hydrophobic neck domain (183), the CRD of the protein may be available to bind bacterial ligands. It is conceivable that while all the CRDs of SP-A are interacting with microbial surface ligands, the neck regions are still available for its interaction with CD14 and subsequent signal transduction. Furthermore, CD14 directly binds many carbohydrate-based microbial polymers, hence, the protein itself is considered as a lectin (185). As CD14 binds bacterial ligands as well as collectins and acts as surface receptors on phagocytes, this receptor plays an important role in innate immune-mediated clearance of bacterial infection.

Gp-340/DMTP/Salivary Agglutinin

Holmskov et al. (186) discovered that SP-D binds gp-340. Gp-340 is present in the lung washings and alveolar macrophages and appears to decorate the membranes of the phagocytes. Cloning and further characterization of gp-340 showed that it is a glycoprotein and contains several cystine-rich scavenger receptor domains (187). Although genomic DNA sequence of gp-340 has a transmembrane coding region, such domains have not been detected at the mRNA or protein level. Therefore, whether gp-340 is a true membrane-anchored receptor or merely a SP-D-binding protein is not certain. Gp-340 (native $M_r \sim 1000$ kDa) is the pulmonary isoform of salivary agglutinin and is present not only in the lungs but also in many tissues including trachea, salivary glands, small intestine and stomach (187,188). Several other tissues also show low level of expression. In the human tracheal tissue, gp-340 is localized to Serous cells and submucosal glands and found as part of respiratory mucus gel-forming mucin MUC5AC and MUC5B (189). SP-D is secreted by goblet and Clara cells of the upper airway during allergic conditions (142). Furthermore, globular domains of SP-D bind gp-340 via protein–protein interactions in a calcium-dependent manner and this binding does not involve lectin–carbohydrate interaction (186). These findings raise the interesting possibility that binding of gp-340 to SP-D and mucins leads to localization of these proteins to mucosal surfaces. Recent reports indicate that gp-340 is secreted by both alveolar type II cells and differentiating intestinal crest cells (190). Tissue distribution of gp-340 overlaps with that of SP-D, which suggests that they may play similar role, or bind to each other, to regulate a common pathway(s). Another report suggests that SP-A also binds gp-340 (191), however, its potential role has not been further explored.

Microfibril-Associated Protein 4

Holmskov and co-workers (18) discovered that MFAP-4 is present in lung washings and can bind collagen-like regions of SP-D. This protein may be a tetramer and its globular domains are similar to that of fibrinogen. The fibrinogen-like domains each contain an RGD motif that is known to bind to integrins. Fibrinogen domains are another specialized domains that bind carbohydrate structures. Binding between MFAP-4 and SP-D, however, appears to occur via protein–protein interactions rather than carbohydrate–protein interactions. MFAP-4 appears to not to interact with the collagen-like region of native SP-D but binds to immobilized or denatured collagens (18), implying that it may bind SP-D only under specific circumstances. MFAP-4 also binds to the collagen-like regions of SP-A (192). It has been suggested that MFAP-4 may be involved in phagocyte trafficking via its interaction with integrins. Implications of the interaction between SP-D and MFAP-4 are not completely understood.

Decorin

Palaniyar and co-workers (104) discovered that SP-D interacts with decorin via both the collagen-like and the globular CRDs. Decorin is a member of the small leucine-rich proteoglycans that binds collagens, collagen-like region of C1q (193), and other extracellular matrix (ECM) components. Decorin contains a cystine-rich N-terminal segment followed by multiple LRRs, which are involved in protein–protein interactions. The decorin core (38 kDa) is predicted to fold as a C-shaped corkscrew-like molecule where amphipathic α-helices and β-sheet forms convex and concaved surfaces, respectively (194). The concave side of decorin could accommodate one collagen triple helix (194), and it is known that the hydroxylysine residue in the collagen is necessary for its interaction with decorin (195). The core protein has three potential Asn-linked carbohydrate attachment sites, that are predicted to be distributed along one side of the molecule, and a Ser-linked sulfated glycosaminoglycan (GAG) chain near the N-terminal. Asn-linked branched saccharides are highly complex and are rich in mannosyl residues whereas the GAG chain ($\sim$90 kDa) is primarily composed of dermatan sulfate ([Glucuronic or irudoic acid, N-acetyl galactosamine 4-sulfate]$_n$).

This ubiquitous proteoglycan is secreted by type II cells (196,197) and chondrocytes and detected in alveolar macrophages (198) and ECM (199). Decorin expression in lung is developmentally regulated, and in adult lung, it is confined to alveolar regions (199). Decorin binds and regulates the concentration of transforming growth factor (TGF)-β (200). Increased concentrations of TGF-β result in cell proliferation and eventual pulmonary fibrosis but transient expression of decorin in the lung alleviates the disease symptoms (201). Decorin can also induce the expression of MMP 1, 2, and 14 (202), and conversely, MMPs 2, 3, and 7 can cleave decorin under certain conditions (202,203). The CRDs of SP-D bind dermatan sulfate moiety of decorin, and decorin core peptide binds collagen-like regions of SP-D (104). Other GAGs such as heparin and hyaluronan also compete the interaction between SP-D and mannan (104), suggesting that SP-D may also bind to these ligands via its lectin domain. Detailed analysis is required to understand potential relevance of these interactions *in vivo*. SP-D deficient mice (39,40,94), and patients with low concentrations of SP-D (149), exhibit lung phenotypes that are associated with inflammation and tissue remodeling (e.g., fibrosis, emphysema). Therefore, decorin may regulate some of the phenotypes observed in *SP-D* gene deficiency.

Other Putative SP-A Binding Proteins: SP-D and C1q

Interestingly, components of classical and alternative pathways of complement are secreted by type II cells (204). Although C1q concentrations are low, higher amounts of the components that are involved in classical pathway are detected in the BAL fluid isolated from healthy volunteers (205). Alternative pathway proteins are, however, detected in low concentrations in the BAL (205). Neither SP-A nor SP-D can substitute for C1q for complement activation; however, binding of SP-A inhibits the interaction of C1q with C1r and C1s (205,206). Therefore, this interaction has been suggested to suppress the activation of complement pathway in the lung. Interestingly, some reports suggest that SP-A and SP-D bind to each other. Although an early report suggested that direct interaction of SP-A to native SP-D requires lipid component (207), later studies showed that SP-A directly binds SP-D and C1q (208). Moreover, SP-A binds C1q via nonlectin interaction and enhances the phagocytosis of C1q-coated beads by macrophages (209). These studies suggest that interaction between SP-A and C1q may minimize the inflammation in the lung and enhance the phagocytosis of opsonized particle. Interaction between SP-A and SP-D has not further been explored.

VIII. Summary and Future Directions

Although SP-A and SP-D were discovered in the pulmonary surfactant, it is becoming clear that these proteins, particularly SP-D, are present in several other tissues. Many of the ligands and receptors that these proteins interact with are consistent with their roles both in innate immunity and lipid-related functions. (1) These collectins appear to play critical roles in innate immunity and are anchored in the pulmonary surfactant. Absence of these proteins in the lung causes surfactant dysfunction, in terms of its ability to clear pathogens effectively. (2) It is also evident that these proteins, particularly SP-D, affect the lipid homeostasis *in vivo*. The firm conclusions derived from the animal studies are, however, that SP-A is essential for the formation of large aggregate TM lipid structure and SP-D is involved in lipid homeostasis. Their roles in maintaining a low surface tension, *in vivo*, are not entirely certain. (3) Although both collectins appear to be involved in allergic response and airway hypersensitivity, recent evidence suggest that SP-D plays an important role in maintaining a surfactant that is proficient in minimizing or eliminating allergy. In summary, altered levels of lung collectins will lead to dysregulation of innate immune system and lipid homeostasis and result in dysfunctional surfactant in the lung.

Several candidate receptors/binding proteins and ligands have been identified for both SP-A and SP-D in recent years. It is essential to explore the relevance of the putative ligands such as PGN, LTA, DNA, and RNA for these collectins in order to understand the signaling mechanisms involved in the clearance of microbes, apoptotic cells, and cell debris. Although putative SP-A receptors have been identified several years ago, their detailed structure and functions are not clearly understood. Understanding the relevance of the roles of putative receptors/binding proteins are far more challenging. Considerable progress has been made on the roles of gp-340. However, the detailed information on the importance of interactions between collectins and other molecules such as MFAP-4 and decorin are necessary. Other innate immune-related collectin-binding proteins/receptors such as Toll-like receptors and CD14 are only beginning to emerge. As these proteins appear to be relevant in terms of the known functions of SP-A and SP-D, further work on this area should unravel the pathways involved in regulating both innate immune and lipid related functions.

Acknowledgments

N.P. is a recipient of Wellcome Trust/CIHR Postdoctoral Fellowships.

References

1. Hamm H, Kroegel C, Hohlfeld J. Surfactant: a review of its functions and relevance in adult respiratory disorders. Respir Med 1996; 90:251–270.
2. Palaniyar N, Ikegami M, Korfhagen T, Whitsett J, McCormack FX. Domains of surfactant protein A that affect protein oligomerization, lipid structure and surface tension. Comp Biochem Physiol A Mol Integr Physiol 2001; 129:109–127.
3. Palaniyar N, Nadesalingam J, Reid KB. Pulmonary innate immune proteins and receptors that interact with Gram-positive bacterial ligands. Immunobiology 2002; 205:575–594.
4. Hakansson K, Reid KB. Collectin structure: a review. Protein Sci 2000; 9:1607–1617.
5. Fujita T. Evolution of the lectin-complement pathway and its role in innate immunity. Nat Rev Immunol 2002; 2:346–353.
6. Eggleton P, Reid KB, Tenner AJ. C1q—how many functions? How many receptors? Trends Cell Biol 1998; 8:428–431.
7. Nauta AJ, Daha MR, Kooten C, Roos A. Recognition and clearance of apoptotic cells: a role for complement and pentraxins. Trends Immunol 2003; 24:148–154.
8. Lu J, Laursen SB, Thiel S, Jensenius JC, Reid KB. The cDNA cloning of conglutinin and identification of liver as a primary site of synthesis of conglutinin in members of the Bovidae. Biochem J 1993; 292(Pt 1):157–162.
9. Holmskov U, Thiel S, Jensenius JC. Collectins and ficolins: humoral lectins of the innate immune defense. Annu Rev Immunol 2003; 21:547–578.
10. Holmskov U, Teisner B, Willis AC, Reid KB, Jensenius JC. Purification and characterization of a bovine serum lectin (CL-43) with structural homology to conglutinin and SP-D and carbohydrate specificity similar to mannan-binding protein. J Biol Chem 1993; 268:10120–10125.
11. Holmskov U, Laursen SB, Malhotra R, Wiedemann H, Timpl R, Stuart GR, Tornoe I, Madsen PS, Reid KB, Jensenius JC. Comparative study of the structural and functional properties of a bovine plasma C-type lectin, collectin-43, with other collectins. Biochem J 1995; 305(Pt 3):889–896.
12. Hansen S, Holm D, Moeller V, Vitved L, Bendixen C, Reid KB, Skjoedt K, Holmskov U. CL-46, a novel collectin highly expressed in bovine thymus and liver. J Immunol 2002; 169:5726–5734.

13. Ohtani K, Suzuki Y, Eda S, Kawai T, Kase T, Keshi H, Sakai Y, Fukuoh A, Sakamoto T, Itabe H, Suzutani T, Ogasawara M, Yoshida I, Wakamiya N. The membrane-type collectin CL-P1 is a scavenger receptor on vascular endothelial cells. J Biol Chem 2001; 276:44222–44228.

14. Ohtani K, Suzuki Y, Eda S, Kawai T, Kase T, Yamazaki H, Shimada T, Keshi H, Sakai Y, Fukuoh A, Sakamoto T, Wakamiya N. Molecular cloning of a novel human collectin from liver (CL-L1). J Biol Chem 1999; 274:13681–13689.

15. Matsushita M, Endo Y, Taira S, Sato Y, Fujita T, Ichikawa N, Nakata M, Mizuochi T. A novel human serum lectin with collagen- and fibrinogen-like domains that functions as an opsonin. J Biol Chem 1996; 271:2448–2454.

16. Lu J, Tay PN, Kon OL, Reid KB. Human ficolin: cDNA cloning, demonstration of peripheral blood leucocytes as the major site of synthesis and assignment of the gene to chromosome 9. Biochem J 1996; 313(Pt 2):473–478.

17. Matsushita M, Fujita T. The role of ficolins in innate immunity. Immunobiology 2002; 205:490–497.

18. Lausen M, Lynch N, Schlosser A, Tornoe I, Saekmose SG, Teisner B, Willis AC, Crouch E, Schwaeble W, Holmskov U. Microfibril-associated protein 4 is present in lung washings and binds to the collagen region of lung surfactant protein D. J Biol Chem 1999; 274:32234–32240.

19. Gupta D, Wang Q, Vinson C, Dziarski R. Bacterial peptidoglycan induces CD14-dependent activation of transcription factors CREB/ATF and AP-1. J Biol Chem 1999; 274:14012–14020.

20. Geijtenbeek TB, Torensma R, van Vliet SJ, van Duijnhoven GC, Adema GJ, van Kooyk Y, Figdor CG. Identification of DC-SIGN, a novel dendritic cell-specificICAM-3 receptor that supports primary immune responses. Cell 2000; 100:575–585.

21. Mitchell DA, Fadden AJ, Drickamer K. A novel mechanism of carbohydrate recognition by the C-type lectins DC-SIGN and DC-SIGNR. Subunit organization and binding to multivalent ligands. J Biol Chem 2001; 276:28939–28945.

22. Geijtenbeek TB, Van Vliet SJ, Koppel EA, Sanchez-Hernandez M, Vandenbroucke-Grauls CM, Appelmelk B, Van Kooyk Y. Mycobacteria target DC-SIGN to suppress dendritic cell function. J Exp Med 2003; 197:7–17.

23. Soilleux EJ, Morris LS, Leslie G, Chehimi J, Luo Q, Levroney E, Trowsdale J, Montaner LJ, Doms RW, Weissman D, Coleman N, Lee B. Constitutive and induced expression of DC-SIGN on dendritic cell and macrophage subpopulations *in situ* and *in vitro*. J Leukoc Biol 2002; 71:445–457.

24. King RJ, Clements JA. Surface active materials from dog lung. II. Composition and physiological correlations. Am J Physiol 1972; 223:715–726.

25. Lu J, Willis AC, Reid KB. Purification, characterization and cDNA cloning of human lung surfactant protein D. Biochem J 1992; 284(Pt 3):795–802.

26. Persson A, Chang D, Rust K, Moxley M, Longmore W, Crouch E. Purification and biochemical characterization of CP4 (SP-D), a collagenous surfactant-associated protein. Biochemistry 1989; 28:6361–6367.

27. Possmayer F. A proposed nomenclature for pulmonary surfactant-associated proteins. Am Rev Respir Dis 1988; 138:990–998.

28. Fisher JH, Mason R. Expression of pulmonary surfactant protein D in rat gastric mucosa. Am J Respir Cell Mol Biol 1995; 12:13–18.

29. Madsen J, Kliem A, Tornoe I, Skjodt K, Koch C, Holmskov U. Localization of lung surfactant protein D on mucosal surfaces in human tissues. J Immunol 2000; 164:5866–5870.

30. van Rozendaal BA, van Golde LM, Haagsman HP. Localization and functions of SP-A and SP-D at mucosal surfaces. Pediatr Pathol Mol Med 2001; 20:319–339.

31. Akiyama J, Hoffman A, Brown C, Allen L, Edmondson J, Poulain F, Hawgood S. Tissue distribution of surfactant proteins A and D in the mouse. J Histochem Cytochem 2002; 50:993–996.

32. Stahlman MT, Gray ME, Hull WM, Whitsett JA. Immunolocalization of surfactant protein-D (SP-D) in human fetal, newborn, and adult tissues. J Histochem Cytochem 2002; 50:651–660.

33. Reid KB, Colomb M, Petry F, Loos M. Complement component C1 and the collectins—first-line defense molecules in innate and acquired immunity. Trends Immunol 2002; 23:115–117.

34. Madan T, Kishore U, Singh M, Strong P, Clark H, Hussain EM, Reid KB, Sarma PU. Surfactant proteins A and D protect mice against pulmonary hypersensitivity induced by *Aspergillus fumigatus* antigens and allergens. J Clin Invest 2001; 107:467–475.

35. Haczku A, Atochina EN, Tomer Y, Chen H, Scanlon ST, Russo S, Xu J, Panettieri RA Jr, Beers MF. *Aspergillus fumigatus*-induced allergic airway inflammation alters surfactant homeostasis and lung function in BALB/c mice. Am J Respir Cell Mol Biol 2001; 25:45–50.

36. Wang JY, Shieh CC, Yu CK, Lei HY. Allergen-induced bronchial inflammation is associated with decreased levels of surfactant proteins A and D in a murine model of asthma. Clin Exp Allergy 2001; 31:652–662.

37. Strong P, Reid KB, Clark H. Intranasal delivery of a truncated recombinant human SP-D is effective at down-regulating allergic hypersensitivity in mice sensitized to allergens of *Aspergillus fumigatus*. Clin Exp Immunol 2002; 130:19–24.

38. Haley KJ, Ciota A, Contreras JP, Boothby MR, Perkins DL, Finn PW. Alterations in lung collectins in an adaptive allergic immune response. Am J Physiol Lung Cell Mol Physiol 2002; 282:L573–584.

39. Botas C, Poulain F, Akiyama J, Brown C, Allen L, Goerke J, Clements J, Carlson E, Gillespie AM, Epstein C, Hawgood S. Altered surfactant homeostasis and alveolar type II cell morphology in mice lacking surfactant protein D. Proc Natl Acad Sci USA 1998; 95:11869–11874.

40. Korfhagen TR, Sheftelyevich V, Burhans MS, Bruno MD, Ross GF, Wert SE, Stahlman MT, Jobe AH, Ikegami M, Whitsett JA, Fisher JH. Surfactant protein-D regulates surfactant phospholipid homeostasis *in vivo*. J Biol Chem 1998; 273:28438–28443.

41. McCormack FX. Functional mapping of surfactant protein A. Pediatr Pathol Mol Med 2001; 20:293–318.

42. Ikegami M, Elhalwagi BM, Palaniyar N, Dienger K, Korfhagen T, Whitsett JA, McCormack FX. The collagen-like region of surfactant protein A (SP-A) is required for correction of surfactant structural and functional defects in the SP-A null mouse. J Biol Chem 2001; 276:38542–38548.

43. Bridges JP, Davis HW, Damodarasamy M, Kuroki Y, Howles G, Hui DY, McCormack FX. Pulmonary surfactant proteins A and D are potent endogenous

inhibitors of lipid peroxidation and oxidative cellular injury. J Biol Chem 2000; 275:38848–38855.

44. Rodriguez-Capote K, McCormack FX, Possmayer F. Pulmonary surfactant protein-A (SP-A) restores the surface properties of surfactant after oxidation by a mechanism that requires the Cys6 interchain disulfide bond and the phospholipid binding domain. J Biol Chem 2003; 278:20461–20474.

45. Clark H, Palaniyar N, Strong P, Edmondson J, Hawgood S, Reid KB. Surfactant protein D reduces alveolar macrophage apoptosis *in vivo*. J Immunol 2002; 169:2892–2899.

46. Vandivier RW, Ogden CA, Fadok VA, Hoffmann PR, Brown KK, Botto M, Walport MJ, Fisher JH, Henson PM, Greene KE. Role of surfactant proteins A, D, and C1q in the clearance of apoptotic cells *in vivo* and *in vitro*: calreticulin and CD91 as a common collectin receptor complex. J Immunol 2002; 169:3978–3986.

47. Palaniyar N, Clark H, Nadesalingam J, Hawgood S, Reid KB. Surfactant protein D binds genomic DNA and apoptotic cells, and enhances their clearance, *in vivo*. Ann N Y Acad Sci 2003; 1010:471–475.

48. Palaniyar N, Nadesalingam J, Reid KB. Innate immune collectins bind nucleic acids and enhance DNA clearance, *in vitro*. Ann N Y Acad Sci 2003; 1010:467–470.

49. LeVine AM, Whitsett JA. Pulmonary collectins and innate host defense of the lung. Microbes Infect 2001; 3:161–166.

50. Zhang L, Ikegami M, Dey CR, Korfhagen TR, Whitsett JA. Reversibility of pulmonary abnormalities by conditional replacement of surfactant protein D (SP-D) *in vivo*. J Biol Chem 2002; 277:38709–38713.

51. Li G, Siddiqui J, Hendry M, Akiyama J, Edmondson J, Brown C, Allen L, Levitt S, Poulain F, Hawgood S. Surfactant protein-A—deficient mice display an exaggerated early inflammatory response to a beta-resistant strain of influenza A virus. Am J Respir Cell Mol Biol 2002; 26:277–282.

52. Crouch E, Persson A, Chang D, Heuser J. Molecular structure of pulmonary surfactant protein D (SP-D). J Biol Chem 1994; 269:17311–17319.

53. Crouch E, Chang D, Rust K, Persson A, Heuser J. Recombinant pulmonary surfactant protein D. Post-translational modification and molecular assembly. J Biol Chem 1994; 269:15808–15813.

54. Chiba H, Sano H, Saitoh M, Sohma H, Voelker DR, Akino T, Kuroki Y. Introduction of mannose binding protein-type phosphatidylinositol recognition into pulmonary surfactant protein A. Biochemistry 1999; 38:7321–7331.

55. Sano H, Kuroki Y, Honma T, Ogasawara Y, Sohma H, Voelker DR, Akino T. Analysis of chimeric proteins identifies the regions in the carbohydrate recognition domains of rat lung collectins that are essential for interactions with phospholipids, glycolipids, and alveolar type II cells. J Biol Chem 1998; 273:4783–4789.

56. Palaniyar N, McCormack FX, Possmayer F, Harauz G. Three-dimensional structure of rat surfactant protein A trimers in association with phospholipid monolayers. Biochemistry 2000; 39:6310–6316.

57. Hakansson K, Lim NK, Hoppe HJ, Reid KB. Crystal structure of the trimeric alpha-helical coiled-coil and the three lectin domains of human lung surfactant protein D. Structure Fold Des 1999; 7:255–264.

58. Kovacs H, O'Ddonoghue SI, Hoppe HJ, Comfort D, Reid KB, Campbell D, Nilges M. Solution structure of the coiled-coil trimerization domain from lung surfactant protein D. J Biomol NMR 2002; 24:89–102.

59. Voss T, Eistetter H, Schafer KP, Engel J. Macromolecular organization of natural and recombinant lung surfactant protein SP 28–36. Structural homology with the complement factor C1q. J Mol Biol 1988; 201:219–227.

60. Palaniyar N, Ridsdale RA, Holterman CE, Inchley K, Possmayer F, Harauz G. Structural changes of surfactant protein A induced by cations reorient the protein on lipid bilayers. J Struct Biol 1998; 122:297–310.

61. Palaniyar N, Ridsdale RA, Possmayer F, Harauz G. Surfactant protein A (SP-A) forms a novel supraquaternary structure in the form of fibers. Biochem Biophys Res Commun 1998; 250:131–136.

62. Palaniyar N, Ridsdale RA, Hearn SA, Heng YM, Ottensmeyer FP, Possmayer F, Harauz G. Filaments of surfactant protein A specifically interact with corrugated surfaces of phospholipid membranes. Am J Physiol 1999; 276:L631–L641.

63. Lu J, Wiedemann H, Timpl R, Reid KB. Similarity in structure between C1q and the collectins as judged by electron microscopy. Behring Inst Mitt 1993; 6–16.

64. Palaniyar N, Zhang L, Kuzmenko A, Ikegami M, Wan S, Wu H, Korfhagen TR, Whitsett JA, McCormack FX. The role of pulmonary collectin N-terminal domains in surfactant structure, function, and homeostasis *in vivo*. J Biol Chem 2002; 277:26971–26979.

65. Weis WI, Drickamer K, Hendrickson WA. Structure of a C-type mannose-binding protein complexed with an oligosaccharide. Nature 1992; 360:127–134.

66. Saitoh M, Sano H, Chiba H, Murakami S, Iwaki D, Sohma H, Voelker DR, Akino T, Kuroki Y. Importance of the carboxy-terminal 25 amino acid residues of lung collectins in interactions with lipids and alveolar type II cells. Biochemistry 2000; 39:1059–1066.

67. Head JF, Mealy T, McCormack FX, Seaton BA. Crystal structure of pulmonary surfactant protein A (SP-A). 99th International Conference, Seattle, USA, 2003.

68. Haagsman HP, Sargeant T, Hauschka PV, Benson BJ, Hawgood S. Binding of calcium to SP-A, a surfactant-associated protein. Biochemistry 1990; 29:8894–8900.

69. Haagsman HP, White RT, Schilling J, Lau K, Benson BJ, Golden J, Hawgood S, Clements JA. Studies of the structure of lung surfactant protein SP-A. Am J Physiol 1989; 257:L421–L429.

70. Kuroki Y, Akino T. Pulmonary surfactant protein A (SP-A) specifically binds dipalmitoylphosphatidylcholine. J Biol Chem 1991; 266:3068–3073.

71. Yu SH, Possmayer F. Dipalmitoylphosphatidylcholine and cholesterol in monolayers spread from adsorbed films of pulmonary surfactant. J Lipid Res 2001; 42:1421–1429.

72. Williams MC. Conversion of lamellar body membranes into tubular myelin in alveoli of fetal rat lungs. J Cell Biol 1977; 72:260–277.

73. Savov J, Wright JR, Young SL. Incorporation of biotinylated SP-A into rat lung surfactant layer, type II cells, and clara cells. Am J Physiol Lung Cell Mol Physiol 2000; 279:L118–L126.

74. Cockshutt AM, Weitz J, Possmayer F. Pulmonary surfactant-associated protein A enhances the surface activity of lipid extract surfactant and reverses inhibition by blood proteins *in vitro*. Biochemistry 1990; 29:8424–8429.

75. Korfhagen TR, Bruno MD, Ross GF, Huelsman KM, Ikegami M, Jobe AH, Wert SE, Stripp BR, Morris RE, Glasser SW, Bachurski CJ, Iwamoto HS, Whitsett JA. Altered surfactant function and structure in SP-A gene targeted mice. Proc Natl Acad Sci USA 1996; 93:9594–9599.

76. Ikegami M, Korfhagen TR, Whitsett JA, Bruno MD, Wert SE, Wada K, Jobe AH. Characteristics of surfactant from SP-A-deficient mice. Am J Physiol 1998; 275:L247–L254.

77. Ikegami M, Korfhagen TR, Bruno MD, Whitsett JA, Jobe AH. Surfactant metabolism in surfactant protein A-deficient mice. Am J Physiol 1997; 272:L479–L485.

78. Jain D, Dodia C, Bates SR, Hawgood S, Poulain FR, Fisher AB. SP-A is necessary for increased clearance of alveolar DPPC with hyperventilation or secretagogues. Am J Physiol Lung Cell Mol Physiol 2003; 284:L759–L765.

79. Schurch S, Green FH, Bachofen H. Formation and structure of surface films: captive bubble surfactometry. Biochim Biophys Acta 1998; 1408:180–202.

80. Poulain FR, Akiyama J, Allen L, Brown C, Chang R, Goerke J, Dobbs L, Hawgood S. Ultrastructure of phospholipid mixtures reconstituted with surfactant proteins B and D. Am J Respir Cell Mol Biol 1999; 20:1049–1058.

81. Crouch E, Wright JR. Surfactant proteins A and D and pulmonary host defense. Annu Rev Physiol 2001; 63:521–554.

82. Nielson DW, Lewis MB. Calcium increases in pulmonary alveolar fluid in lambs at birth. Pediatr Res 1988; 24:322–325.

83. McCormack FX, Damodarasamy M, Elhalwagi BM. Deletion mapping of N-terminal domains of surfactant protein A. The N-terminal segment is required for phospholipid aggregation and specific inhibition of surfactant secretion. J Biol Chem 1999; 274:3173–3181.

84. Sohma H, Hattori A, Kuroki Y, Akino T. Calcium and dithiothreitol dependent conformational changes in beta-sheet structure of collagenase resistant fragment of human surfactant protein A. Biochem Mol Biol Int 1993; 30:329–336.

85. McCormack FX, Stewart J, Voelker DR, Damodarasamy M. Alanine mutagenesis of surfactant protein A reveals that lipid binding and pH-dependent liposome aggregation are mediated by the carbohydrate recognition domain. Biochemistry 1997; 36:13963–13971.

86. Efrati H, Hawgood S, Williams MC, Hong K, Benson BJ. Divalent cation and hydrogen ion effects on the structure and surface activity of pulmonary surfactant. Biochemistry 1987; 26:7986–7993.

87. Ogasawara Y, Kuroki Y, Akino T. Pulmonary surfactant protein D specifically binds to phosphatidylinositol. J Biol Chem 1992; 267:21244–21249.

88. Persson AV, Gibbons BJ, Shoemaker JD, Moxley MA, Longmore WJ. The major glycolipid recognized by SP-D in surfactant is phosphatidylinositol. Biochemistry 1992; 31:12183–12189.

89. Kuroki Y, Honma T, Chiba H, Sano H, Saitoh M, Ogasawara Y, Sohma H, Akino T. A novel type of binding specificity to phospholipids for rat mannose-binding proteins isolated from serum and liver. FEBS Lett 1997; 414:387–392.

90. Ogasawara Y, McCormack FX, Mason RJ, Voelker DR. Chimeras of surfactant proteins A and D identify the carbohydrate recognition domains as essential for phospholipid interaction. J Biol Chem 1994; 269:29785–29792.

91. Taneva S, Voelker DR, Keough KM. Adsorption of pulmonary surfactant protein D to phospholipid monolayers at the air–water interface. Biochemistry 1997; 36:8173–8179.

92. Ikegami M, Whitsett JA, Jobe A, Ross G, Fisher J, Korfhagen T. Surfactant metabolism in SP-D gene-targeted mice. Am J Physiol Lung Cell Mol Physiol 2000; 279:L468–L476.

93. Takemura T, Fukuda Y, Harrison M, Ferrans VJ. Ultrastructural, histochemical, and freeze-fracture evaluation of multilamellated structures in human pulmonary alveolar proteinosis. Am J Anat 1987; 179:258–268.

94. Wert SE, Yoshida M, LeVine AM, Ikegami M, Jones T, Ross GF, Fisher JH, Korfhagen TR, Whitsett JA. Increased metalloproteinase activity, oxidant production, and emphysema in surfactant protein D gene-inactivated mice. Proc Natl Acad Sci USA 2000; 97:5972–5977.

95. Zhang L, Yoshida M, Korfhagen TR, Senior RM, Shipley JM, Shapiro SD, Whitsett JA. Development of emphysema in SP-D−/− mice is independent of MMP-12, MMP-9 and NADPH-oxidase. 99th International Conference, Seattle, USA, 2003.

96. Ikegami M, Hull WM, Yoshida M, Wert SE, Whitsett JA. SP-D and GM-CSF regulate surfactant homeostasis via distinct mechanisms. Am J Physiol Lung Cell Mol Physiol 2001; 281:L697–L703.

97. Zhang L, Hartshorn KL, Crouch EC, Ikegami M, Whitsett JA. Complementation of pulmonary abnormalities in SP-D(−/−) mice with an SP-D/conglutinin fusion protein. J Biol Chem 2002; 277:22453–22459.

98. Zhang L, Ikegami M, Crouch EC, Korfhagen TR, Whitsett JA. Activity of pulmonary surfactant protein-D (SP-D) *in vivo* is dependent on oligomeric structure. J Biol Chem 2001; 276:19214–19219.

99. Haagsman HP, Hawgood S, Sargeant T, Buckley D, White RT, Drickamer K, Benson BJ. The major lung surfactant protein, SP 28–36, is a calcium-dependent, carbohydrate-binding protein. J Biol Chem 1987; 262:13877–13880.

100. Childs RA, Wright JR, Ross GF, Yuen CT, Lawson AM, Chai W, Drickamer K, Feizi T. Specificity of lung surfactant protein SP-A for both the carbohydrate and the lipid moieties of certain neutral glycolipids. J Biol Chem 1992; 267:9972–9979.

101. Allen MJ, Voelker DR, Mason RJ. Interactions of surfactant proteins A and D with *Saccharomyces cerevisiae* and *Aspergillus fumigatus*. Infect Immun 2001; 69:2037–2044.

102. Sidobre S, Nigou J, Puzo G, Riviere M. Lipoglycans are putative ligands for the human pulmonary surfactant protein A attachment to mycobacteria. Critical role of the lipids for lectin-carbohydrate recognition. J Biol Chem 2000; 275:2415–2422.

103. Strong P, Kishore U, Morgan C, Lopez Bernal A, Singh M, Reid KB. A novel method of purifying lung surfactant proteins A and D from the lung lavage of alveolar proteinosis patients and from pooled amniotic fluid. J Immunol Methods 1998; 220:139–149.

104. Nadesalingam J, Lopez Bernal A, Dodds AW, Willis AC, Mahoney DJ, Day AJ, Reid KB, Palaniyar N. Identification and characterization of a novel interaction between pulmonary surfactant protein D and decorin. J Biol Chem 2003; 278:25678–25687.

105. Madan T, Kishore U, Singh M, Strong P, Hussain EM, Reid KB, Sarma PU. Protective role of lung surfactant protein D in a murine model of invasive pulmonary aspergillosis. Infect Immun 2001; 69:2728–2731.

106. Madan T, Eggleton P, Kishore U, Strong P, Aggrawal SS, Sarma PU, Reid KB. Binding of pulmonary surfactant proteins A and D to *Aspergillus fumigatus* conidia enhances phagocytosis and killing by human neutrophils and alveolar macrophages. Infect Immun 1997; 65:3171–3179.

107. Allen MJ, Harbeck R, Smith B, Voelker DR, Mason RJ. Binding of rat and human surfactant proteins A and D to *Aspergillus fumigatus* conidia. Infect Immun 1999; 67:4563–4569.

108. Lim BL, Wang JY, Holmskov U, Hoppe HJ, Reid KB. Expression of the carbohydrate recognition domain of lung surfactant protein D and demonstration of its binding to lipopolysaccharides of Gram-negative bacteria. Biochem Biophys Res Commun 1994; 202:1674–1680.

109. Kuan SF, Rust K, Crouch E. Interactions of surfactant protein D with bacterial lipopolysaccharides. Surfactant protein D is an *Escherichia coli*-binding protein in bronchoalveolar lavage. J Clin Invest 1992; 90:97–106.

110. Wu H, Kuzmenko A, Wan S, Schaffer L, Weiss A, Fisher JH, Kim KS, McCormack FX. Surfactant proteins A and D inhibit the growth of Gramnegative bacteria by increasing membrane permeability. J Clin Invest 2003; 111:1589–1602.

111. Murakami S, Iwaki D, Mitsuzawa H, Sano H, Takahashi H, Voelker DR, Akino T, Kuroki Y. Surfactant protein A inhibits peptidoglycan-induced tumor necrosis factor-alpha secretion in U937 cells and alveolar macrophages by direct interaction with Toll-like receptor 2. J Biol Chem 2002; 277:6830–6837.

112. van de Wetering JK, van Eijk M, van Golde LM, Hartung T, van Strijp JA, Batenburg JJ. Characteristics of surfactant protein A and D binding to lipoteichoic acid and peptidoglycan, 2 major cell wall components of Gram-positive bacteria. J Infect Dis 2001; 184:1143–1151.

113. Horner AA, Van Uden JH, Zubeldia JM, Broide D, Raz E. DNA-based immunotherapeutics for the treatment of allergic disease. Immunol Rev 2001; 179:102–118.

114. Fehrenbach H. Alveolar epithelial type II cell: defender of the alveolus revisited. Respir Res 2001; 2:33–46.

115. Mason RJ, Williams MC. Type II alveolar cell. Defender of the alveolus. Am Rev Respir Dis 1977; 115:81–91.

116. Williams MC. Uptake of lectins by pulmonary alveolar type II cells: subsequent deposition into lamellar bodies. Proc Natl Acad Sci USA 1984; 81:6383–6387.

117. Herbein JF, Savov J, Wright JR. Binding and uptake of surfactant protein D by freshly isolated rat alveolar type II cells. Am J Physiol Lung Cell Mol Physiol 2000; 278:L830–L839.

118. Kresch MJ, Christian C, Lu H. Isolation and partial characterization of a receptor to surfactant protein A expressed by rat type II pneumocytes. Am J Respir Cell Mol Biol 1998; 19:216–225.

119. Wright JR, Borchelt JD, Hawgood S. Lung surfactant apoprotein SP-A (26–36 kDa) binds with high affinity to isolated alveolar type II cells. Proc Natl Acad Sci USA 1989; 86:5410–5414.

120. Stevens PA, Wissel H, Zastrow S, Sieger D, Zimmer KP. Surfactant protein A and lipid are internalized via the coated-pit pathway by type II pneumocytes. Am J Physiol Lung Cell Mol Physiol 2001; 280:L141–L151.

121. Pison U, Wright JR, Hawgood S. Specific binding of surfactant apoprotein SP-A to rat alveolar macrophages. Am J Physiol 1992; 262:L412–L417.

122. Miyamura K, Leigh LE, Lu J, Hopkin J, Lopez Bernal A, Reid KB. Surfactant protein D binding to alveolar macrophages. Biochem J 1994; 300(Pt 1):237–242.

123. Dong Q, Wright JR. Degradation of surfactant protein D by alveolar macrophages. Am J Physiol 1998; 274:L97–L105.

124. Wright JR, Youmans DC. Degradation of surfactant lipids and surfactant protein A by alveolar macrophages *in vitro*. Am J Physiol 1995; 268:L772–L780.

125. Kramer BW, Jobe AH, Ikegami M. Exogenous surfactant changes the phenotype of alveolar macrophages in mice. Am J Physiol Lung Cell Mol Physiol 2001; 280:L689–L694.

126. Fisher JH, Sheftelyevich V, Ho YS, Fligiel S, McCormack FX, Korfhagen TR, Whitsett JA, Ikegami M. Pulmonary-specific expression of SP-D corrects pulmonary lipid accumulation in SP-D gene-targeted mice. Am J Physiol Lung Cell Mol Physiol 2000; 278:L365–L373.

127. Cai GZ, Griffin GL, Senior RM, Longmore WJ, Moxley MA. Recombinant SP-D carbohydrate recognition domain is a chemoattractant for human neutrophils. Am J Physiol 1999; 276:L131–L136.

128. Crouch EC, Persson A, Griffin GL, Chang D, Senior RM. Interactions of pulmonary surfactant protein D (SP-D) with human blood leukocytes. Am J Respir Cell Mol Biol 1995; 12:410–415.

129. Herbein JF, Wright JR. Enhanced clearance of surfactant protein D during LPS-induced acute inflammation in rat lung. Am J Physiol Lung Cell Mol Physiol 2001; 281:L268–L277.

130. Hartshorn KL, Crouch E, White MR, Colamussi ML, Kakkanatt A, Tauber B, Shepherd V, Sastry KN. Pulmonary surfactant proteins A and D enhance neutrophil uptake of bacteria. Am J Physiol 1998; 274:L958–L969.

131. Quintero OA, Wright JR. Clearance of surfactant lipids by neutrophils and macrophages isolated from the acutely inflamed lung. Am J Physiol Lung Cell Mol Physiol 2002; 282:L330–L339.

132. Brinker KG, Martin E, Borron P, Mostaghel E, Doyle C, Harding CV, Wright JR. Surfactant protein D enhances bacterial antigen presentation by bone marrow-derived dendritic cells. Am J Physiol Lung Cell Mol Physiol 2001; 281:L1453–L1463.

133. Brinker KG, Garner H, Wright JR. Surfactant protein A modulates the differentiation of murine bone marrow-derived dendritic cells. Am J Physiol Lung Cell Mol Physiol 2003; 284:L232–L241.

134. Mummert ME, Mummert D, Edelbaum D, Hui F, Matsue H, Takashima A. Synthesis and surface expression of hyaluronan by dendritic cells and its potential role in antigen presentation. J Immunol 2002; 169:4322–4331.

135. Singh M, Madan T, Waters P, Parida SK, Sarma PU, Kishore U. Protective effects of a recombinant fragment of human surfactant protein D in a murine model of pulmonary hypersensitivity induced by dust mite allergens. Immunol Lett 2003; 86:299–307.

136. Strong P, Townsend P, Mackay R, Reid KB, Clark HW. A recombinant fragment of human SP-D reduces allergic responses in mice sensitized to house dust mite allergens. Clin Exp Immunol 2003; 134:181–187.

137. Madan T, Kishore U, Shah A, Eggleton P, Strong P, Wang JY, Aggrawal SS, Sarma PU, Reid KB. Lung surfactant proteins A and D can inhibit specific IgE binding to the allergens of *Aspergillus fumigatus* and block allergen-induced histamine release from human basophils. Clin Exp Immunol 1997; 110:241–249.

138. Wang JY, Kishore U, Lim BL, Strong P, Reid KB. Interaction of human lung surfactant proteins A and D with mite (*Dermatophagoides pteronyssinus*) allergens. Clin Exp Immunol 1996; 106:367–373.

139. Wang JY, Shieh CC, You PF, Lei HY, Reid KB. Inhibitory effect of pulmonary surfactant proteins A and D on allergen-induced lymphocyte proliferation and histamine release in children with asthma. Am J Respir Crit Care Med 1998; 158:510–518.

140. Cheng G, Ueda T, Nakajima H, Nakajima A, Arima M, Kinjyo S, Fukuda T. Surfactant protein A exhibits inhibitory effect on eosinophils IL-8 production. Biochem Biophys Res Commun 2000; 270:831–835.

141. Mishra A, Weaver TE, Beck DC, Rothenberg ME. Interleukin-5-mediated allergic airway inflammation inhibits the human surfactant protein C promoter in transgenic mice. J Biol Chem 2001; 276:8453–8459.

142. Kasper M, Sims G, Koslowski R, Kuss H, Thuemmler M, Fehrenbach H, Auten RL. Increased surfactant protein D in rat airway goblet and Clara cells during ovalbumin-induced allergic airway inflammation. Clin Exp Allergy 2002; 32:1251–1258.

143. Homer RJ, Zheng T, Chupp G, He S, Zhu Z, Chen Q, Ma B, Hite RD, Gobran LI, Rooney SA, Elias JA. Pulmonary type II cell hypertrophy and pulmonary lipoproteinosis are features of chronic IL-13 exposure. Am J Physiol Lung Cell Mol Physiol 2002; 283:L52–L59.

144. Clark H, Reid KB. Structural requirements for SP-D function *in vitro* and *in vivo*: therapeutic potential of recombinant SP-D. Immunobiology 2002; 205:619–631.

145. Borron P, Veldhuizen RA, Lewis JF, Possmayer F, Caveney A, Inchley K, McFadden RG, Fraher LJ. Surfactant associated protein-A inhibits human lymphocyte proliferation and IL-2 production. Am J Respir Cell Mol Biol 1996; 15:115–121.

146. Yang S, Milla C, Panoskaltsis-Mortari A, Ingbar DH, Blazar BR, Haddad IY. Human surfactant protein A suppresses T cell-dependent inflammation and attenuates the manifestations of idiopathic pneumonia syndrome in mice. Am J Respir Cell Mol Biol 2001; 24:527–536.

147. Borron PJ, Mostaghel EA, Doyle C, Walsh ES, McHeyzer-Williams MG, Wright JR. Pulmonary surfactant proteins A and D directly suppress CD3+/CD4+ cell function: evidence for two shared mechanisms. J Immunol 2002; 169:5844–5850.

148. Husby S, Herskind AM, Jensenius JC, Holmskov U. Heritability estimates for the constitutional levels of the collectins mannan-binding lectin and lung surfactant protein D. A study of unselected like-sexed mono- and dizygotic twins at the age of 6–9 years. Immunology 2002; 106:389–394.

149. Kuroki Y, Takahashi H, Chiba H, Akino T. Surfactant proteins A and D: disease markers. Biochim Biophys Acta 1998; 1408:334–345.

150. Borron P, McCormack FX, Elhalwagi BM, Chroneos ZC, Lewis JF, Zhu S, Wright JR, Shepherd VL, Possmayer F, Inchley K, Fraher LJ. Surfactant protein A inhibits T cell proliferation via its collagen-like tail and a 210 kDa receptor. Am J Physiol 1998; 275:L679–L686.

151. Strayer DS, Yang S, Jerng HH. Surfactant protein A-binding proteins. Characterization and structures. J Biol Chem 1993; 268:18679–18684.

152. Strayer DS, Korutla L, Thomas AP. Surfactant protein-A receptor-mediated inhibition of calcium signaling in alveolar type II cells. Recept Signal Transduct 1997; 7:111–120.

153. Korutla L, Strayer DS. SP-A as a cytokine: surfactant protein-A-regulated transcription of surfactant proteins and other genes. J Cell Physiol 1999; 178:379–386.

154. White MK, Baireddy V, Strayer DS. Natural protection from apoptosis by surfactant protein A in type II pneumocytes. Exp Cell Res 2001; 263:183–192.

155. White MK, Strayer DS. Surfactant protein A regulates pulmonary surfactant secretion via activation of phosphatidylinositol 3-kinase in type II alveolar cells. Exp Cell Res 2000; 255:67–76.

156. Stevens PA, Wissel H, Sieger D, Meienreis-Sudau V, Rustow B. Identification of a new surfactant protein A binding protein at the cell membrane of rat type II pneumocytes. Biochem J 1995; 308(Pt 1):77–81.

157. Wissel H, Looman AC, Fritzsche I, Rustow B, Stevens PA. SP-A-binding protein BP55 is involved in surfactant endocytosis by type II pneumocytes. Am J Physiol 1996; 271:L432–L440.

158. Chroneos ZC, Abdolrasulnia R, Whitsett JA, Rice WR, Shepherd VL. Purification of a cell-surface receptor for surfactant protein A. J Biol Chem 1996; 271:16375–16383.

159. Weikert LF, Lopez JP, Abdolrasulnia R, Chroneos ZC, Shepherd VL. Surfactant protein A enhances mycobacterial killing by rat macrophages through a nitric oxide-dependent pathway. Am J Physiol Lung Cell Mol Physiol 2000; 279:L216–L223.

160. Poornima S, Christian C, Kresch MJ. Developmental regulation of SP-A receptor in fetal rat lung. Lung 2002; 180:33–46.

161. Michelis D, Kounnas MZ, Argraves WS, Sanford ED, Borchelt JD, Wright JR. Interaction of surfactant protein A with cellular myosin. Am J Respir Cell Mol Biol 1994; 11:692–700.

162. Sohma H, Matsushima N, Watanabe T, Hattori A, Kuroki Y, Akino T. Ca(2+)-dependent binding of annexin IV to surfactant protein A and lamellar bodies in alveolar type II cells. Biochem J 1995; 312(Pt 1):175–181.

163. Sohma H, Creutz CE, Saitoh M, Sano H, Kuroki Y, Voelker DR, Akino T. Characterization of the Ca^{2+}-dependent binding of annexin IV to surfactant protein A. Biochem J 1999; 341(Pt 1):203–209.

164. Nepomuceno RR, Henschen-Edman AH, Burgess WH, Tenner AJ. cDNA cloning and primary structure analysis of C1qR(P), the human C1q/MBL/SPA receptor that mediates enhanced phagocytosis *in vitro*. Immunity 1997; 6:119–129.

165. Fonseca MI, Carpenter PM, Park M, Palmarini G, Nelson EL, Tenner AJ. C1qR(P), a myeloid cell receptor in blood, is predominantly expressed on endothelial cells in human tissue. J Leukoc Biol 2001; 70:793–800.

166. Danet GH, Luongo JL, Butler G, Lu MM, Tenner AJ, Simon MC, Bonnet DA. C1qRp defines a new human stem cell population with hematopoietic and hepatic potential. Proc Natl Acad Sci USA 2002; 99:10441–10445.
167. Erdei A, Reid KB. The C1q receptor. Mol Immunol 1988; 25:1067–1073.
168. Erdei A, Reid KB. Characterization of C1q-binding material released from the membranes of Raji and U937 cells by limited proteolysis with trypsin. Biochem J 1988; 255:493–499.
169. Sim RB, Moestrup SK, Stuart GR, Lynch NJ, Lu J, Schwaeble WJ, Malhotra R. Interaction of C1q and the collectins with the potential receptors calreticulin (cC1qR/collectin receptor) and megalin. Immunobiology 1998; 199:208–224.
170. Zhu Q, Zelinka P, White T, Tanzer ML. Calreticulin-integrin bidirectional signaling complex. Biochem Biophys Res Commun 1997; 232:354–358.
171. Gagnon E, Duclos S, Rondeau C, Chevet E, Cameron PH, Steele-Mortimer O, Paiement J, Bergeron JJ, Desjardins M. Endoplasmic reticulum-mediated phagocytosis is a mechanism of entry into macrophages. Cell 2002; 110:119–131.
172. Malhotra R, Thiel S, Reid KB, Sim RB. Human leukocyte C1q receptor binds other soluble proteins with collagen domains. J Exp Med 1990; 172:955–959.
173. Stuart GR, Lynch NJ, Lu J, Geick A, Moffatt BE, Sim RB, Schwaeble WJ. Localisation of the C1q binding site within C1q receptor/calreticulin. FEBS Lett 1996; 397:245–249.
174. White TK, Zhu Q, Tanzer ML. Cell surface calreticulin is a putative mannoside lectin which triggers mouse melanoma cell spreading. J Biol Chem 1995; 270:15926–15929.
175. Peterson JR, Ora A, Van PN, Helenius A. Transient, lectin-like association of calreticulin with folding intermediates of cellular and viral glycoproteins. Mol Biol Cell 1995; 6:1173–1184.
176. Johnson S, Michalak M, Opas M, Eggleton P. The ins and outs of calreticulin: from the ER lumen to the extracellular space. Trends Cell Biol 2001; 11:122–129.
177. Akira S, Takeda K, Kaisho T. Toll-like receptors: critical proteins linking innate and acquired immunity. Nat Immunol 2001; 2:675–680.
178. Birchler T, Seibl R, Buchner K, Loeliger S, Seger R, Hossle JP, Aguzzi A, Lauener RP. Human Toll-like receptor 2 mediates induction of the antimicrobial peptide human beta-defensin 2 in response to bacterial lipoprotein. Eur J Immunol 2001; 31:3131–3137.
179. Harju K, Glumoff V, Hallman M. Ontogeny of Toll-like receptors Tlr2 and Tlr4 in mice. Pediatr Res 2001; 49:81–83.
180. Mushegian A, Medzhitov R. Evolutionary perspective on innate immune recognition. J Cell Biol 2001; 155:705–710.
181. Guillot L, Balloy V, McCormack FX, Golenbock DT, Chignard M, Si-Tahar M. Cutting edge: the immunostimulatory activity of the lung surfactant protein-A involves Toll-like receptor 4. J Immunol 2002; 168:5989–5992.
182. Striz I, Zheng L, Wang YM, Pokorna H, Bauer PC, Costabel U. Soluble CD14 is increased in bronchoalveolar lavage of active sarcoidosis and correlates with alveolar macrophage membrane-bound CD14. Am J Respir Crit Care Med 1995; 151:544–547.
183. Sano H, Chiba H, Iwaki D, Sohma H, Voelker DR, Kuroki Y. Surfactant proteins A and D bind CD14 by different mechanisms. J Biol Chem 2000; 275:22442–22451.

184. Chiba H, Sano H, Iwaki D, Murakami S, Mitsuzawa H, Takahashi T, Konishi M, Takahashi H, Kuroki Y. Rat mannose-binding protein A binds CD14. Infect Immun 2001; 69:1587–1592.

185. Weidemann B, Schletter J, Dziarski R, Kusumoto S, Stelter F, Rietschel ET, Flad HD, Ulmer AJ. Specific binding of soluble peptidoglycan and muramyl-dipeptide to CD14 on human monocytes. Infect Immun 1997; 65:858–864.

186. Holmskov U, Lawson P, Teisner B, Tornoe I, Willis AC, Morgan C, Koch C, Reid KB. Isolation and characterization of a new member of the scavenger receptor superfamily, glycoprotein-340 (gp-340), as a lung surfactant protein-D binding molecule. J Biol Chem 1997; 272:13743–13749.

187. Holmskov U, Mollenhauer J, Madsen J, Vitved L, Gronlund J, Tornoe I, Kliem A, Reid KB, Poustka A, Skjodt K. Cloning of gp-340, a putative opsonin receptor for lung surfactant protein D. Proc Natl Acad Sci USA 1999; 96:10794–10799.

188. Bikker FJ, Ligtenberg AJ, van der Wal JE, van den Keijbus PA, Holmskov U, Veerman EC, Nieuw Amerongen AV. Immunohistochemical detection of salivary agglutinin/gp-340 in human parotid, submandibular, and labial salivary glands. J Dent Res 2002; 81:134–139.

189. Thornton DJ, Davies JR, Kirkham S, Gautrey A, Khan N, Richardson PS, Sheehan JK. Identification of a nonmucin glycoprotein (gp-340) from a purified respiratory mucin preparation: evidence for an association involving the MUC5B mucin. Glycobiology 2001; 11:969–977.

190. Kang W, Nielsen O, Fenger C, Madsen J, Hansen S, Tornoe I, Eggleton P, Reid KB, Holmskov U. The scavenger receptor, cysteine-rich domain-containing molecule gp-340 is differentially regulated in epithelial cell lines by phorbol ester. Clin Exp Immunol 2002; 130:449–458.

191. Tino MJ, Wright JR. Glycoprotein-340 binds surfactant protein-A (SP-A) and stimulates alveolar macrophage migration in an SP-A-independent manner. Am J Respir Cell Mol Biol 1999; 20:759–768.

192. Schlosser A, Lausen M, Tornøe I, Nielsen O, Brasch F, Law A, Palaniyar N, McCormack F, Skjødt K, Holmskov U. Microfibril-associated protein 4 (MFAP-4) is present in lung washings, co-locates with elastic fibers and binds to the collagen part of surfactant protein A. Interlac 2002; 20:134.

193. Krumdieck R, Hook M, Rosenberg LC, Volanakis JE. The proteoglycan decorin binds C1q and inhibits the activity of the C1 complex. J Immunol 1992; 149:3695–3701.

194. Weber IT, Harrison RW, Iozzo RV. Model structure of decorin and implications for collagen fibrillogenesis. J Biol Chem 1996; 271:31767–31770.

195. Tenni R, Viola M, Welser F, Sini P, Giudici C, Rossi A, Tira ME. Interaction of decorin with CNBr peptides from collagens I and II. Evidence for multiple binding sites and essential lysyl residues in collagen. Eur J Biochem 2002; 269:1428–1437.

196. Maniscalco WM, Campbell MH. Transforming growth factor-beta induces a chondroitin sulfate/dermatan sulfate proteoglycan in alveolar type II cells. Am J Physiol 1994; 266:L672–L680.

197. Koslowski R, Pfeil U, Fehrenbach H, Kasper M, Skutelsky E, Wenzel KW. Changes in xylosyltransferase activity and in proteoglycan deposition in bleomycin-induced lung injury in rat. Eur Respir J 2001; 18:347–356.

198. Asakura S, Colby TV, Limper AH. Tissue localization of transforming growth factor-beta1 in pulmonary eosinophilic granuloma. Am J Respir Crit Care Med 1996; 154:1525–1530.

199. Wang Y, Sakamoto K, Khosla J, Sannes PL. Detection of chondroitin sulfates and decorin in developing fetal and neonatal rat lung. Am J Physiol Lung Cell Mol Physiol 2002; 282:L484–L490.

200. Schonherr E, Broszat M, Brandan E, Bruckner P, Kresse H. Decorin core protein fragment Leu155-Val260 interacts with TGF-beta but does not compete for decorin binding to type I collagen. Arch Biochem Biophys 1998; 355:241–248.

201. Kolb M, Margetts PJ, Galt T, Sime PJ, Xing Z, Schmidt M, Gauldie J. Transient transgene expression of decorin in the lung reduces the fibrotic response to bleomycin. Am J Respir Crit Care Med 2001; 163:770–777.

202. Schonherr E, Schaefer L, O'Connell BC, Kresse H. Matrix metalloproteinase expression by endothelial cells in collagen lattices changes during co-culture with fibroblasts and upon induction of decorin expression. J Cell Physiol 2001; 187:37–47.

203. Imai K, Hiramatsu A, Fukushima D, Pierschbacher MD, Okada Y. Degradation of decorin by matrix metalloproteinases: identification of the cleavage sites, kinetic analyses and transforming growth factor-beta1 release. Biochem J 1997; 322(Pt 3):809–814.

204. Strunk RC, Eidlen DM, Mason RJ. Pulmonary alveolar type II epithelial cells synthesize and secrete proteins of the classical and alternative complement pathways. J Clin Invest 1988; 81:1419–1426.

205. Watford WT, Ghio AJ, Wright JR. Complement-mediated host defense in the lung. Am J Physiol Lung Cell Mol Physiol 2000; 279:L790–L798.

206. Watford WT, Wright JR, Hester CG, Jiang H, Frank MM. Surfactant protein A regulates complement activation. J Immunol 2001; 167:6593–6600.

207. Kuroki Y, Shiratori M, Murata Y, Akino T. Surfactant protein D (SP-D) counteracts the inhibitory effect of surfactant protein A (SP-A) on phospholipid secretion by alveolar type II cells. Interaction of native SP-D with SP-A. Biochem J 1991; 279(Pt 1):115–119.

208. Oosting RS, Wright JR. Characterization of the surfactant protein A receptor: cell and ligand specificity. Am J Physiol 1991; 267:L165–L172.

209. Watford WT, Smithers MB, Frank MM, Wright JR. Surfactant protein A enhances the phagocytosis of C1q-coated particles by alveolar macrophages. Am J Physiol Lung Cell Mol Physiol 2002; 283:L1011–L1022.

5

Structure–Function Relationships of Hydrophobic Proteins SP-B and SP-C in Pulmonary Surfactant

JESÚS PÉREZ-GIL, ANTONIO CRUZ, and INÉS PLASENCIA

Universidad Complutense,
Madrid, Spain

I. Introduction

Decades of research on pulmonary surfactant resulted in a serious paradox that was not resolved until the mid-1980s. Seminal physiological studies had demonstrated that lack of surfactant in premature babies was the primary cause of respiratory distress syndrome associated with high morbidity and mortality. In addition, several research groups had shown that administration of an exogenous surfactant material early after birth of premature animals could prevent and largely reduce respiratory complications. Suspensions prepared using material extracted with organic solvents from animal lungs were very efficient as exogenous surfactant. Such organic extractions are routine for separation of the lipid moiety from biological samples, and hence lipids were soon recognized as essential components for the biophysical function of surfactant in the lungs. Extensive physicochemical studies from the early seventies established that the lipid composition of pulmonary surfactant appeared particularly well suited to reach and sustain very low surface tensions at low lung volumes during breathing. The main surface-active molecule in surfactant is a disaturated lecithin, dipalmitoylphosphatidylcholine (DPPC), whereas other lipid species are important to fluidize DPPC enough to facilitate its adsorption at physiological temperature into the air–liquid interface of lungs. The paradox was that no mixture of purely synthetic lipids mimicking the composition of natural surfactant worked equally well *in vivo* as exogenous surfactant. The key finding that allowed further understanding was the discovery of hydrophobic surfactant-associated proteins, now called SP-B and SP-C. These polypeptides are so hydrophobic that co-isolate with lipids in organic solvent extractions. On the other hand, they have low antigenicity and are not easily identified in routine protein assays. Therefore, until the 1980s, it was unrecognized that these proteins were present in surfactant lipid extracts.

Today, it is widely recognized that the most effective clinical surfactant preparations include hydrophobic surfactant proteins or some surfactant peptide mimics. Additional support for the importance of the hydrophobic surfactant proteins comes from the discoveries that several severe manifestations of respiratory insufficiency in neonates and infants are caused by defects on the expression of *SP-B* and/or *SP-C* genes. Extensive research during the last 15 years has provided detailed information on the structure, lipid–protein interactions, and chemico-physical behavior of SP-B and SP-C, but we still do not understand completely the specific roles of these two evolutionarily conserved proteins in alveolar spaces. Specific standardized assays to evaluate the function of either of the two proteins are not yet available, and this lack prevents development of formulations that may result in improved therapeutic surfactants.

The present chapter summarizes current working models and addresses questions on the structure–function relationships of SP-B and SP-C. Before analyzing the details on the structure and biophysical behavior of these proteins, two main considerations should be taken into account. First, what is the evolutionary importance of these two proteins in the lungs of different animal species, especially as animals adapted to air breathing? Secondly, does the importance of the proteins differ depending on whether we consider their role during normal lung function vs. their role as constituents of surfactant introduced via the trachea for treatment of lung disease?

II. Evolutionary Origin of Hydrophobic Pulmonary Surfactant Proteins

SP-B or SP-B-like proteins have been detected in most air-breathing animals including nonmammalian vertebrates such as amphibian (1), reptiles (2), or birds (3,4). The lung in most of these vertebrates consists of a set of conducting tubules and air capillaries without a real alveolar system, with gas exchange taking place directly across the respiratory epithelium via a flow-through system that does not require cyclic inspiration and expiration. At the surface of these sorts of lungs, antiglue or antiedema properties could be more important than a pure antiatelactatic effect (4). SP-B-like proteins have been detected at the epithelium of the lungs of *Neoceratodus forsteri*, considered the most ancient lungfish (5). The conservation of SP-B during evolution suggests the importance of this protein (though not necessarily to achieve a low surface tension at low lung volumes, as occurs in mammalian lungs). SP-B may be strictly required for the basic operation of creating and stabilizing an opened air–liquid interface. Structural defects in the *SP-B* gene might not be compatible with air-breathing life, what has been demonstrated at least in mammals (6,7). The presence of SP-B-related proteins has been also identified in the middle ear, again supporting a possible role of the protein to help form and maintain an air–liquid interface in various locales in the body (8). Under conditions of normal physiology, therefore, SP-B may merely facilitate trafficking of lipids both intracellularly (to assemble surfactant bilayers) and extracellularly (to enhance movement of lipids to the air–liquid interface). Interestingly, structure of mammalian SP-B is related with that of saposins (9), proteins needed in all cells to mobilize particular lipid species (sphingolipids) out of bilayers, in order to make them accessible for lipid metabolism.

In contrast with SP-B, SP-C is only present in mammals. The expression of SP-C is tightly coupled with specific differentiation of lung tissue. Furthermore, there is no protein that has known structural homology with SP-C. Altogether, these features suggest a late origin of SP-C in evolution, possibly as a solution to particular physical problems that originate with expansion and contraction of surface films during inspiration and expiration during breathing. Recent findings that will be discussed subsequently indicate that SP-C may be essential to stabilize the alveolar interface when it is compressed beyond collapse.

III. Biological vs. Clinical Engineering of Pulmonary Surfactant

The native forms of SP-B and SP-C are produced through proteolytic maturation of much larger precursors synthesized in type II pneumocytes (10). The structure of such precursors is probably optimized to facilitate the proper folding of the extremely hydrophobic sequences of SP-B and SP-C and, no less important, to protect the cell against their membrane-perturbing surface activities. Processing of these precursors to the mature proteins must be tightly coupled with the synthesis and assembly of surfactant lipid–protein complexes. Pulmonary surfactant biosynthesis in type II cells follows a complex polymorphic pathway, from the endoplasmic reticulum to specialized organelles, such as multivesicular and lamellar bodies, which are probably required to ensure packing of surfactant bilayers in a form compatible with rapid interfacial adsorption upon secretion (10,11). Many mutations of the *SP-B* and *SP-C* genes produce alterations of the primary sequence of the proteins that cause aberrant folding/processing/ assembly of the polypeptides *in vivo*, leading to lack of mature protein(s) at the airways (11). It is therefore difficult to define structural traits of the mature protein without being aware of the importance of the precursor forms required to permit the molecular and cellular mechanisms of surfactant biogenesis.

On the other hand, a variety of proteins and peptides with different sequences show, when mixed with surfactant lipids, adequate surface activities when assayed with *in vitro* or *in vivo* models. These findings qualify them as potential additives for producing efficient therapeutic surfactant preparations (12). Protein structure–function determinants for efficient surface activity might be much less restrictive when surfactant has to reach the respiratory interface from outside—as in exogenous surfactant replacement methodologies— than from inside, that is, production and secretion by the pneumocyte. Therefore, inferences from the analysis of structure–function relationships of hydrophobic surfactant proteins can be very different whether considering biological pathways of surfactant biogenesis or biophysical activity in the airspaces.

IV. Structure–Function Relationships of SP-B

Hydrophobic surfactant protein SP-B is the only protein presumed to be essential for initiation and maintenance of breathing. Homozygous mutations in the human *SP-B* gene leading to absence of SP-B at the alveoli are lethal in newborns (7,13). Mice with the *SP-B* gene knocked-out die early after birth (6). On the other hand, partial deficiencies in SP-B may cause more moderate respiratory dysfunctions (14–16). The phenotype of SP-B-deficient lungs corresponds to lungs intrinsically devoid of pulmonary surfactant, as SP-B is critically essential for surfactant assembly into lamellar bodies (17) and their later conversion, upon secretion, into the surfactant film formation at the air–liquid interface. In spite of this, we do not have details on the disposition, orientation, lipid–protein, and protein–protein interactions of SP-B in native surfactant assemblies. In fact, the molecular architecture of specialized surfactant structures, such as those in the lamellar bodies or in the ordered tubular myelin network, has still to be determined. SP-B also participates in the processing of the other hydrophobic surfactant protein, SP-C. Partially processed forms of the proSP-C precursor accumulate inside SP-B-defective pneumocytes (18), indicative of the coupling between processing and assembly of the two hydrophobic surfactant proteins, by mechanisms, that are still not completely understood.

SP-B belongs to the family of saposin-like proteins (SAPLIP), characterized by a high content of alpha-helical secondary structure and by the presence of six cysteine residues, the relative position of which in the sequence is highly preserved to form three intramolecular disulfide bridges (19–21). Figure 5.1 compares the sequence and cysteine positions of human SP-B with those of other known members of the SAPLIP folding group. Mature human SP-B has 79 amino acids and a molecular size of ∼9 kDa. Unlike the other components of the SAPLIP family, SP-B is highly hydrophobic, being only soluble in certain mixtures of polar/nonpolar organic solvents (22).

The native form of SP-B is a homodimer stabilized by an additional intermolecular disulfide bridge through a seventh cysteine (23,24). Dimer formation is not necessary for the final targeting of the protein but could be required for full surface activity of SP-B at the alveoli (25–27). Although disulfides in SP-B seem essential to ensure proper folding and assembly of SP-B in type II cells, we have demonstrated that the primary sequence of mature SP-B has the necessary structural determinants to fold in a native-like conformation even after reduction and alkylation of the cysteines (28). We propose that SP-B-mimicking polypeptides could retain enough surface-active determinants in the absence of disulfides to serve as the basis for clinical surfactant preparations. Still, optimal functional properties *in vivo* probably require the proper intra- and intermolecular disulfide connectivity.

The amino acid distribution along the sequence of SP-B supports formation of several amphipathic helical segments (22,29), common motifs in other proteins of the SAPLIP family that are implicated for the interaction of these proteins with lipids (19). Figure 5.1 shows a model in which the putative helical segments in SP-B are compared with those existing in the structure of NK-lysine, the first member of the SAPLIP family for which folding has been experimentally determined by NMR (20,23). The recently solved structure of bacteriocin (30), a bacterial protein with folding similar to that of saposins but without cysteines, is also included in this family. The high hydrophobicity of SP-B has so far prevented determination of the three-dimensional structure of this protein. The amphipathicity of the helical segments of SP-B supports a relatively superficial disposition of the protein in lipid bilayers and monolayers (31–34). The helical segments of the protein may interact primarily with the polar headgroups of the phospholipids and just slightly with their acyl chains in the hydrophobic region of the surfactant structures. However, several studies indicate that SP-B could have variable penetration into the hydrophobic core of phospholipid bilayers, depending on the method used to reconstitute lipid–protein complexes (31,35,36). A model for the structure of the SP-B dimer has been recently proposed taking into account the three-dimensional structure of the NK-lysine. According to this model, intermolecular electrostatic compensation of a couple of charges would lead to the formation of a hydrophobic core the size of which would fit a transmembrane disposition of the SP-B dimer in lipid bilayers (23) (also represented in Fig. 5.1). Although this model explains some experimental data obtained on lipid–protein interactions in samples reconstituted from purified protein and synthetic lipids, it begs the question of what is the actual lipid–protein structure

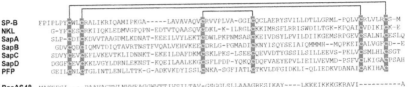

SP-B   FPIPLPYCWLCRALIKRIQAMIPKGA-----LAVAVAQVCRVVPLVA-GGICQCLAERYSVILLDTLLGRML-PQLVCRLVLRCG-M
NKL   G-YFCESCRKIIQKLEDMVGPQPN-EDTVTQAASQVCDKL-K-ILRGLCKKIMRSFLRRISWDILTGK-KPQAICVDIKICK-E
SapA   SLP-CDICKDVVTAAGDMLKDNAT-EEEILVYLEKTCDWLPKPNMSABCKEIVDSYLPVILDIIKGEMSRPGEVCSALNLCESLQ
SapB   GDVCQDCIQMVTDIQTAVRTNSTFVQALVEHVKEECQRLG-PGMADICKNYISQYSEIAIQMMMH--MQPKEICALVGFCD--E
SapC   SDVYCEVCEFLVKEVTKLIDNNKT-EKEILDAPDKMCSKLPKS-LSEECQEVVDTYGSSILSILLEEVS-PELVCSMLHLCSGT
SapD   DGGFCEVCKKLVGYLDRNLEKNST-KQEILAALEKGCSFLPDP-YQKQCDQFVAEYEPVLIEILVEVMD-PSFVCLKIGACPSAH
PFP   GEILCNLCTGLINTLENLLTTK-G-ADKVKDYISSLCNKA-SGFIATLCTKVLDFGIDKLI-QLIEDKVDANAICAKIHAC

BacAS48 MAKEFGI----PAAVAGTVLNVVEAGGWVTTIVSILTAV-GSGGLSLLAAAGRESIKAY----LKKEIKKKGKRAVI---------A

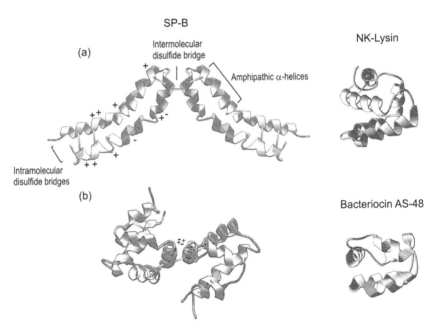

Figure 5.1 Structural models of surfactant protein SP-B, compared with some homologous folds. The primary sequence of human SP-B has been aligned above with that of the homologous proteins NK-lysin (NKL), the four human saposins (SapA, SapB, SapC, and SapD), and the amoebapore (PFP) to show the position of the cysteine residues that form equivalent disulfide bonds. The primary sequence of bacteriocin AS-48, a cyclic peptide with folding analogous to that of the saposin family but without cysteines, is also included in this family. (a) Structural model of human SP-B showing its probable alpha-helical segments, the position of the intra- and intermolecular disulfides and the charges in one of the monomers. (b) Folding model for the dimer of SP-B as proposed by Zaltash et al. (23) using the pattern determined by NMR for NK-lysin (20) indicating the position of the two salt bridges stabilizing an hydrophobic core. The folds determined experimentally for NK-lysin and bacteriocin AS-48 have been included for comparison.

as assembled *in vivo*. The analysis of the disposition and orientation of SP-B, as defined by the interaction of the proSP-B precursor with membranes, should give essential information in this regard.

The high number of basic amino acids (nine in human SP-B, with a net charge of $+7$) gives the protein a cationic character that defines a preferential interaction of the protein with acidic phospholipids, such as surfactant phosphatidylglycerol (PG), both in bilayers (33) and monolayers (37). In particular, selective interaction of SP-B with negatively charged phospholipids could be important for the formation of nonbilayer intermediates required in bilayer–monolayer transitions (38). SP-B/PG interactions have also been proposed to promote enrichment of the interfacial films with the most surface-active phospholipids, during compression (34,39,40). Although a structural model has been recently proposed using molecular dynamics simulations that suggest specific interaction of at least certain segments of SP-B with anionic PG (41), we lack experimental structural data supporting the existence of specific SP-B/PG complexes.

Partial penetration of SP-B into surfactant bilayers is probably important for the ability of the protein to produce aggregation and lipid exchange between phospholipid vesicles (36,42–44). Destabilization of surfactant bilayers by SP-B may be essential for the formation of tubular myelin and the ultimate transference of surface-active species into the surfactant monolayer (34,45). Experiments in surface balances have shown that SP-B is de-inserted/re-inserted cyclically during dynamic compression–expansion of lipid–protein films (46–48). A substantial penetration of the protein into the interface could be important during expansion, a stage in which SP-B is probably responsible for promoting insertion and re-insertion of lipid molecules from the subphase. Squeeze-out of the protein at pressures >45 mN/m may be required for the film to reach the lowest surface tensions at the end of expiration. SP-B-containing films achieve low surface tensions with less compression than needed by films made with pure phospholipids (40). At the highest surface pressures, the protein SP-B may maintain only a shallow association with the phospholipid film. Coating by SP-B of the compressed films could be the basis for SP-B to provide additional stability against collapse (49,50).

Some experiments have shown that SP-B and SP-B-mimicking peptides promote reversible two-dimensional to three-dimensional transitions, in the form of folds, buckles, and protrusions, during compression of phospholipid films (51–54). The geometry of these protrusions depends on both the phospholipid composition and the compression strategy of the films. Extensive studies on the structure of lipid–protein films during compression, by epifluorescence microscopy and recently also by atomic force microscopy, have shown that SP-B first segregates with increasing pressure at fluid regions of the films (47,50,51,55), which are also probably enriched in anionic and unsaturated phospholipid species. Extrusion of the surface film into the third dimension seems to be initiated at these protein-enriched regions when the films are further compressed (51,54). SP-B seems important to maintain the association of the extruded lipid–protein structures with the surface compressed film, what could ensure re-extension of lipid and protein during expansion (56). Potential participation of protein–protein interactions of SP-B in both the lateral segregation of regions of the film and the formation of three-dimensional protrusions has not yet been explored. These compression-driven protein-promoted structural transitions occurring in the surfactant films can be related with formation during expiration of a surfactant reservoir associated with the surface film (57). The association of surfactant layers with the pulmonary interfacial film has been shown morphologically by electron microscopy. Hydrophobic surfactant proteins, including SP-B, have been proposed to maintain the integrity of surface-associated structures, which would have an important role in (i) sustaining the structure of the compressed film at end-expiration and (ii) ensuring a rapid re-spreading of the surface-active material during inspiration.

Some evidence suggests important interactions between SP-B and the major surfactant-associated protein, SP-A. Although the presence of SP-A is not strictly required for the biophysical function of surfactant (58), SP-A improves the surface activity of lipid–protein preparations only if SP-B is present, and especially in the presence of anionic phospholipids (37,43). SP-A and SP-B also cooperate to sustain the structure of tubular myelin (44). Recent evidence also supports formation of specific SP-A/SP-B complexes in lipid–protein interfacial films (59) (Nag et al., unpublished data). The regions of SP-B for these possible specific contacts with SP-A have not yet been identified, nor has the significance of the formation of such protein–protein complexes in the assembly and molecular mechanism of surfactant, *in vivo*.

An intriguing question still under extensive research is the possible implication of SP-B in the defense activities of pulmonary surfactant at the respiratory epithelium. The structure of SP-B has significant homologies to that of other proteins with recognized antibiotic activities, such as ameobapores (9) or NK-lysine (19). Like SP-B, these analogous proteins have membrane-interacting and membrane-perturbing activities, which are the basis for their ability to disorganize the membranes of target pathogens (60). In fact, SP-B and some synthetic peptides designed from its sequence have significant microbicidal activities (61). The lethality of the lack of SP-B has not allowed so far to determine whether absence of the protein also compromises the lung's defense against pathogenic microorganisms. Analysis of the susceptibility to respiratory pathogens in animals or individuals with heterozygous mutations at the *SP-B* gene will shed light on this question.

V.   Structure–Function Relationships of SP-C

As stated earlier, SP-C is the only surfactant protein without any known structural homolog, and it is expressed strictly in the pulmonary epithelium. In spite of this, the structure–function relationships of this protein remain mostly unknown and are just now starting to be envisaged. Several cases have been described in which mutations of the *SP-C* gene are related to the occurrence of chronic familial respiratory diseases (13,62,63). In addition, an almost complete lack of SP-C has been associated in Belgian blue calves with development of neonatal respiratory distress (64). Surprisingly, mice in which the expression of their *SP-C* gene has been deleted, breathe normally after delivery (65). Later, however, these animals develop respiratory dysfunction (66), suggesting that SP-C may have a subtle but still essential role. From both patients and animal studies, SP-C deficiencies cause different forms of lung disease in different individuals (62,66), suggesting that the protein may play its role in a pleiotropic fashion with the participation of other, still unknown factors.

SP-C is isolated from lung lavage as a 35-residue polypeptide of 4 kDa molecular mass, which is co-purified with the lipids after chloroform/methanol extractions due to its extreme hydrophobicity. Its sequence is highly conserved in the species studied so far (67). This short peptide is processed in type II pneumocytes, as is the case for SP-B, from a much larger precursor. ProSP-C is a transmembrane protein of 21 kDa, in which the sequence of the mature protein serves as a membrane anchor signal. Proteolytic processing of the precursor to cleave N-terminal and C-terminal propeptides releases mature SP-C, with a type II transmembrane orientation (10,11).

The three-dimensional structure of SP-C has been determined in organic solution by NMR (68). This and other studies define two regions in the structure of SP-C (Fig. 5.2). Approximately two-thirds of the sequence forms a very regular hydrophobic alpha-helix, rich in branched aliphatic amino acids, the length of which fits the thickness of a fluid DPPC bilayer. The 10 N-terminal residues do not adopt a defined conformation in organic solvent but could form an amphipathic beta-turn in water or in membrane environments (69). In all the species studied so far, this N-terminal tail of SP-C has a cationic character and contains cysteines, usually two that are contiguous and are stoichiometrically palmitoylated (70). This post-translational modification increases, or further stabilizes, the alpha-helical conformation that probably extends, when the protein is palmitoylated, into the N-terminal segment (71). We have found that, even in the absence of acylation, the amphipathic structure of the N-terminal segment of SP-C provides a strong affinity to interact with phospholipid interfaces (72). Conformation of SP-C is very sensitive to the polarity of the environment (22,29,73). Exposure of the protein to polar solvents induces helix-to-beta structural transitions and protein aggregation, altering the surface-active properties of the protein (74). Depending on protein concentration, SP-C can form large amyloid fibrils (73,75). Synthesis and assembly of SP-C as a larger precursor in type II cells could be important to ensure the alpha-helical conformation *in vivo*. This conformation may be metastable, once the protein is processed to the mature form (76). The alpha-helical

SP-C FGIPCCPVHLKRLLIVVVVVVLIVVVIVGALLMGL

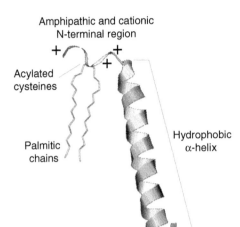

Figure 5.2 Sequence and structure of surfactant protein SP-C. The primary sequence of human SP-C and a structural model of the protein are presented, based on the three-dimensional structure determined by NMR in organic solvents (68). The two main regions of the protein, the hydrophobic highly regular alpha-helix and the N-terminal palmitoylated segment, are indicated.

conformation is considered the functional form of SP-C in alveolar spaces, a feature that should be taken into account when designing synthetic analogs of the protein as additives for clinical surfactants. In this sense, synthetic analogs of SP-C with leucines substituting for the valines of the wild-type sequence, maintains a stable monomeric helical conformation, while mimicking most of the surface-active properties of SP-C (12).

Recent experiments *in vivo* support the importance of protein–protein interactions for the assembly of SP-C and surfactant in the lungs. The transmembrane sequence of proSP-C promotes self-aggregation of the precursor that is essential for the proper intracellular trafficking of the protein (77). Homomeric association of SP-C *in vivo* could be due either to specific protein–protein interactions through the transmembrane segment or to sorting and accumulation of the protein into certain membrane domains. In this sense, lipid–protein thickness mismatch has been demonstrated to control segregation and self-aggregation of SP-C in membrane models (78). Bilayers made with surfactant lipid extracts show segregation of lipid domains at physiological temperatures (79). This could contribute to regionalize protein organization. The possibility that once processed, mature SP-C could maintain, in native surfactant, a supramolecular arrangement with functional significance needs to be explored. Interactions of SP-C with SP-B have not been detected (80).

Lipid–protein interactions of SP-C as studied in phospholipid vesicles are similar to those of other membrane integral proteins with transmembrane orientations (33,35) that are dominated by a hydrophobic alpha-helix. These interactions by themselves do not explain the ability of SP-C to promote interfacial insertion of phospholipids *in vitro* (81–83). Interfacial phospholipid adsorption probably requires simultaneous perturbation of the surface of the monolayer and associated bilayers. Accordingly, SP-C promotes exchange of phospholipids among vesicles (42). We propose that the dynamic perturbations induced by SP-C on phospholipid interfaces are mostly mediated by its N-terminal segment. As mentioned earlier, we have found that the SP-C N-terminal tail interacts and perturbs the surface of phospholipid bilayers and monolayers (69); (Plasencia and Pérez-Gil, in press). Phospholipid-interaction and perturbations induced by the N-terminal segment are stronger in the presence of anionic phospholipids (80).

Numerous studies have characterized the interfacial behavior of SP-C/lipid mixtures when deposited directly on the interface as a monolayer. At the interface, the rigid hydrophobic helix of SP-C adopts a tilted disposition (84,85) and is excluded from the ordered domains of condensed phase enriched in DPPC (47,86–88). However, it is difficult to understand how the whole hydrophobic transmembrane helix of SP-C could be transferred from surfactant bilayers in the hypohase into the air–liquid interface, *in vivo*. A more likely model might maintain the helix of SP-C inserted into the bilayers associated upon adsorption with the interfacial surfactant film. Once there, the N-terminal segment could be the only region of the protein moving dynamically between bilayers and monolayer, and contributing to the interfacial insertion of phospholipids. Scanning probe microscopy experiments have reported that SP-C promotes the association of membrane patches with interfacial phospholipid films. It is proposed that the N-terminal segment of SP-C acts as a bridge between bilayers and monolayer (89,90). SP-C could then promote formation of the surface-associated surfactant reservoir (91,92).

An interesting question, especially considering the probable participation of the N-terminal segment of the protein on surfactant activity, is the importance of palmitoylation for the function of SP-C. A recent study has shown that acylation is required to maintain the association of the N-terminal segment of SP-C with phospholipid films compressed to very high pressures (71). The covalent attachment of the palmitic chains could also be important to adjust the functional conformation of SP-C (69). Acylation may be essential for full surface activity of SP-C (93) with special relevance for the ability of SP-C to promote formation of surface-associated surfactant reservoirs (91) and to protect surfactant against inhibition by plasma proteins (94,95). Palmitoylation of SP-C could then ensure association of surfactant bilayers with the surface film at end-expiration, facilitating re-spreading of surfactant during subsequent inspirations. SP-C-promoted tight association of surfactant bilayers with the interface might also reduce the access of inhibitory proteins to the interface. These notions would be consistent with the appearance of SP-C in evolution, optimized to stabilize the airways in lungs with large tidal volumes and very high surface pressures at end-expiration. The participation of SP-C in the mechanisms described earlier would also explain why the lack of SP-C destabilizes surfactant when subjected to cyclic compression (65), ultimately leading to chronic respiratory failure (62,63). Use of nonpalmitoylated SP-C analogs to produce clinical surfactants, such as the recombinant versions of the protein included in Venticute® (96), may be efficient enough to re-establish interfacial dynamics during breathing, considering the ability of the protein to promote bilayer–monolayer transitions. However, a good SP-B analog, something which is not yet available, would probably be more efficient in this regard, considering the activities of this protein described earlier. Still, acylated SP-C forms would more likely be optimal to maintain a stable association of surfactant with the interface. This feature may be essential to resist inhibition by plasma components and may optimize formulations of exogenous surfactant for the treatment of ARDS. Future artificial surfactant should then ideally contain analogs of both proteins, SP-B and SP-C, as do the clinical surfactant preparations of natural origin used today.

A recent line of research has identified SP-C as a lipopolysacharide-binding protein (97,98). Recognition of this bacterial endotoxin is a critical step of the innate host defense system, raising the possibility that SP-C also participates in these defense mechanisms. The connection between the biophysical activities of hydrophobic surfactant proteins and their possible antipathogenic properties must be still further studied, but there appears to be an intimate relationship between these two essential functions of the respiratory epithelium.

Acknowledgments

We thank sincerely Prof. H. William Taeusch, from University of California San Francisco, for the critical reading and the comments on the chapter. Research at the laboratory of the authors is funded by the Ministry of Science and Technology and the Community of Madrid. Dr. Inés Plasencia acknowledges a Research Fellowship from Fundacion Ferrer, Barcelona, Spain.

References

1. Miller LD, Wert SE, Whitsett JA. Surfactant proteins and cell markers in the respiratory epithelium of the amphibian, *Ambystoma mexicanum*. Comp Biochem Physiol A Mol Integr Physiol 2001; 129:141–149.

2. Johnston SD, Daniels CB, Cenzato D, Whitsett JA, Orgeig S. The pulmonary surfactant system matures upon pipping in the freshwater turtle *Chelydra serpentina*. J Exp Biol 2002; 205:415–425.

3. Zeng X, Yutzey KE, Whitsett JA. Thyroid transcription factor-1, hepatocyte nuclear factor-3beta and surfactant protein A and B in the developing chick lung. J Anat 1998; 193:399–408.

4. Bernhard W, Gebert A, Vieten G, Rau GA, Hohlfeld JM, Postle AD, Freihorst J. Pulmonary surfactant in birds: coping with surface tension in a tubular lung. Am J Physiol Regul Integr Comp Physiol 2001; 281:R327–R337.

5. Power JH, Doyle IR, Davidson K, Nicholas TE. Ultrastructural and protein analysis of surfactant in the Australian lungfish *Neoceratodus forsteri*: evidence for conservation of composition for 300 million years. J Exp Biol 1999; 202:2543–2550.

6. Clark JC, Wert SE, Bachurski CJ, Stahlman MT, Stripp BR, Weaver TE, Whitsett JA. Targeted disruption of the surfactant protein B gene disrupts surfactant homeostasis, causing respiratory failure in newborn mice. Proc Natl Acad Sci USA 1995; 92:7794–7798.

7. Nogee LM, Garnier G, Dietz HC, Singer L, Murphy AM, deMello DE, Colten HR. A mutation in the surfactant protein B gene responsible for fatal neonatal respiratory disease in multiple kindreds. J Clin Invest 1994; 93:1860–1863.

8. Paananen R, Glumoff V, Sormunen R, Voorhout W, Hallman M. Expression and localization of lung surfactant protein B in Eustachian tube epithelium. Am J Physiol Lung Cell Mol Physiol 2001; 280:L214–L220.

9. Zhai Y, Saier MH Jr. The amoebapore superfamily. Biochim Biophys Acta 2000; 1469:87–99.

10. Weaver TE. Synthesis, processing and secretion of surfactant proteins B and C. Biochim Biophys Acta 1998; 1408:173–179.

11. Weaver TE, Conkright JJ. Functions of surfactant proteins B and C. Annu Rev Physiol 2001; 63:555–578.

12. Johansson J, Gustafsson M, Palmblad M, Zaltash S, Robertson B, Curstedt T. Synthetic surfactant protein analogues. Biol Neonate 1998; 74(suppl 1):9–14.

13. Whitsett JA, Weaver TE. Hydrophobic surfactant proteins in lung function and disease. N Engl J Med 2002; 347:2141–2148.

14. Dunbar AE III, Wert SE, Ikegami M, Whitsett JA, Hamvas A, White FV, Piedboeuf B, Jobin C, Guttentag S, Nogee LM. Prolonged survival in hereditary surfactant protein B (SP-B) deficiency associated with a novel splicing mutation. Pediatr Res 2000; 48:275–282.

15. Nogee LM, Wert SE, Proffit SA, Hull WM, Whitsett JA. Allelic heterogeneity in hereditary surfactant protein B (SP-B) deficiency. Am J Respir Crit Care Med 2000; 161:973–981.

16. Tryka AF, Wert SE, Mazursky JE, Arrington RW, Nogee LM. Absence of lamellar bodies with accumulation of dense bodies characterizes a novel form of congenital surfactant defect. Pediatr Dev Pathol 2000; 3:335–345.

17. Stahlman MT, Gray MP, Falconieri MW, Whitsett JA, Weaver TE. Lamellar body formation in normal and surfactant protein B-deficient fetal mice. Lab Invest 2000; 80:395–403.

18. Beers MF, Hamvas A, Moxley MA, Gonzales LW, Guttentag SH, Solarin KO, Longmore WJ, Nogee LM, Ballard PL. Pulmonary surfactant metabolism in infants lacking surfactant protein B. Am J Respir Cell Mol Biol 2000; 22:380–391.

19. Andersson M, Curstedt T, Jornvall H, Johansson J. An amphipathic helical motif common to tumourolytic polypeptide NK-lysin and pulmonary surfactant poly-peptide SP-B. FEBS Lett 1995; 362:328–332.

20. Liepinsh E, Andersson M, Ruysschaert JM, Otting G. Saposin fold revealed by the NMR structure of NK-lysin. Nat Struct Biol 1997; 10:793–795.

21. Perez-Gil J, Keogh KM. Structural similarities between myelin and hydrophobic surfactant associated proteins: protein motifs for interacting with bilayers. J Theor Biol 1994; 169:221–229.

22. Pérez-Gil J, Cruz A, Casals C. Solubility of hydrophobic surfactant proteins in organic solvent/water mixtures. Structural studies on SP-B and SP-C in aqueous organic solvents and lipids. Biochim Biophys Acta 1993; 1168:261–270.

23. Zaltash S, Palmblad M, Curstedt T, Johansson J, Persson B. Pulmonary surfactant protein B: a structural model and a functional analogue. Biochim Biophys Acta 2000; 1466:179–186.

24. Johansson J, Jornvall H, Curstedt T. Human surfactant polypeptide SP-B. Disulfide bridges, C-terminal end, and peptide analysis of the airway form. FEBS Lett 1992; 301:165–167.

25. Beck DC, Ikegami M, Na CL, Zaltash S, Johansson J, Whitsett JA, Weaver TE. The role of homodimers in surfactant protein B function *in vivo*. J Biol Chem 2000; 275:3365–3370.

26. Veldhuizen EJ, Waring AJ, Walther FJ, Batenburg JJ, van Golde LM, Haagsman HP. Dimeric N-terminal segment of human surfactant protein B [dSP-B(1–25)] has enhanced surface properties compared to monomeric SP-B (1–25). Biophys J 2000; 79:377–384.

27. Zaltash S, Griffiths WJ, Beck D, Duan CX, Weaver TE, Johansson J. Membrane activity of (Cys48Ser) lung surfactant protein B increases with dimerisation. Biol Chem 2001; 382:933–939.

28. Serrano AG, Cruz A, Rodriguez-Capote K, Possmayer F, Perez-Gil J. Intrinsic structural and functional determinants within the amino acid sequence of mature pulmonary surfactant protein SP-B. Biochemistry 2005; 44:417–430.

29. Cruz A, Casals C, Pérez-Gil J. Conformational flexibility of pulmonary surfactant proteins SP-B and SP-C, studied in aqueous organic solvents. Biochim Biophys Acta 1995; 1255:68–76.

30. Gonzalez C, Langdon GM, Bruix M, Galvez A, Valdivia E, Maqueda M, Rico M. Bacteriocin AS-48, a microbial cyclic polypeptide structurally and functionally related to mammalian NK-lysin. Proc Natl Acad Sci USA 2000; 97:11221–11226.

31. Cruz A, Casals C, Plasencia I, Marsh D, Perez-Gil J. Depth profiles of pulmonary surfactant protein B in phosphatidylcholine bilayers, studied by fluorescence and electron spin resonance spectroscopy. Biochemistry 1998; 37:9488–9496.

32. Morrow MR, Perez-Gil J, Simatos G, Boland C, Stewart J, Absolom D, Sarin V, Keough KM. Pulmonary surfactant-associated protein SP-B has little effect on acyl chains in dipalmitoylphosphatidylcholine dispersions. Biochemistry 1993; 32:4397–4402.

33. Perez-Gil J, Casals C, Marsh D. Interactions of hydrophobic lung surfactant proteins SP-B and SP-C with dipalmitoylphosphatidylcholine and dipalmitoylphosphatidyl-glycerol bilayers studied by electron spin resonance spectroscopy. Biochemistry 1995; 34:3964–3971.

34. Perez-Gil J, Keough KM. Interfacial properties of surfactant proteins. Biochim Biophys Acta 1998; 1408:203–217.

35. Shiffer K, Hawgood S, Haagsman HP, Benson B, Clements JA, Goerke J. Lung surfactant proteins, SP-B and SP-C, alter the thermodynamic properties of phospholipid membranes: a differential calorimetry study. Biochemistry 1993; 32:590–597.

36. Cruz A, Casals C, Keough KM, Perez-Gil J. Different modes of interaction of pulmonary surfactant protein SP-B in phosphatidylcholine bilayers. Biochem J 1997; 327:133–138.

37. Rodriguez-Capote K, Nag K, Schurch S, Possmayer F. Surfactant protein interactions with neutral and acidic phospholipid films. Am J Physiol Lung Cell Mol Physiol 2001; 281:L231–L242.

38. Schram V, Hall SB. Thermodynamic effects of the hydrophobic surfactant proteins on the early adsorption of pulmonary surfactant. Biophys J 2001; 81:1536–1546.

39. Veldhuizen EJ, Batenburg JJ, van Golde LM, Haagsman HP. The role of surfactant proteins in DPPC enrichment of surface films. Biophys J 2000; 79:3164–3171.

40. Nag K, Munro JG, Inchley K, Schurch S, Petersen NO, Possmayer F. SP-B refining of pulmonary surfactant phospholipid films. Am J Physiol 1999; 277:L1179–L1189.

41. Kaznessis YN, Kim S, Larson RG. Specific mode of interaction between components of model pulmonary surfactants using computer simulations. J Mol Biol 2002; 322:569–582.

42. Oosterlaken Dijksterhuis MA, van Eijk M, van Golde LM, Haagsman HP. Lipid mixing is mediated by the hydrophobic surfactant protein SP-B but not by SP-C. Biochim Biophys Acta 1992; 1110:45–50.

43. Poulain FR, Allen L, Williams MC, Hamilton RL, Hawgood S. Effects of surfactant apolipoproteins on liposome structure: implications for tubular myelin formation. Am J Physiol 1992; 262:L730–L739.

44. Williams MC, Hawgood S, Hamilton RL. Changes in lipid structure produced by surfactant proteins SP-A, SP-B, and SP-C. Am J Respir Cell Mol Biol 1991; 5:41–50.

45. Perez-Gil J. Lipid–protein interactions of hydrophobic proteins SP-B and SP-C in lung surfactant assembly and dynamics. Pediatr Pathol Mol Med 2001; 20:445–469.

46. Shanmukh S, Howell P, Baatz JE, Dluhy RA. Effect of hydrophobic surfactant proteins SP-B and SP-C on phospholipid monolayers. Protein structure studied using 2D IR and beta correlation analysis. Biophys J 2002; 83:2126–2141.

47. Nag K, Taneva SG, Perez-Gil J, Cruz A, Keough KM. Combinations of fluorescently labeled pulmonary surfactant proteins SP-B and SP-C in phospholipid films. Biophys J 1997; 72:2638–2650.

48. Taneva S, Keough KM. Pulmonary surfactant proteins SP-B and SP-C in spread monolayers at the air–water interface: I. Monolayers of pulmonary surfactant protein SP-B and phospholipids. Biophys J 1994; 66:1137–1148.

49. Ding J, Takamoto DY, von Nahmen A, Lipp MM, Lee KY, Waring AJ, Zasadzinski JA. Effects of lung surfactant proteins, SP-B and SP-C, and palmitic acid on monolayer stability. Biophys J 2001; 80:2262–2272.

50. Cruz A, Worthman LA, Serrano AG, Casals C, Keough KM, Perez-Gil J. Microstructure and dynamic surface properties of surfactant protein SP-B/dipalmitoylphosphatidylcholine interfacial films spread from lipid–protein bilayers. Eur Biophys J 2000; 29:204–213.

51. Krol S, Ross M, Sieber M, Kunneke S, Galla HJ, Janshoff A. Formation of three-dimensional protein–lipid aggregates in monolayer films induced by surfactant protein B. Biophys J 2000; 79:904–918.

52. Lipp MM, Lee KY, Zasadzinski JA, Waring AJ. Phase and morphology changes in lipid monolayers induced by SP-B protein and its amino-terminal peptide. Science 1996; 273:1196–1199.

53. Lipp MM, Lee KY, Waring A, Zasadzinski JA. Fluorescence, polarized fluorescence, and Brewster angle microscopy of palmitic acid and lung surfactant protein B monolayers. Biophys J 1997; 72:2783–2804.

54. Diemel RV, Snel MM, Waring AJ, Walther FJ, van Golde LM, Putz G, Haagsman HP, Batenburg JJ. Multilayer formation upon compression of surfactant monolayers depends on protein concentration as well as lipid composition. An atomic force microscopy study. J Biol Chem 2002; 277:21179–21188.

55. Takamoto DY, Lipp MM, von Nahmen A, Lee KY, Waring AJ, Zasadzinski JA. Interaction of lung surfactant proteins with anionic phospholipids. Biophys J 2001; 81:153–169.

56. Ding J, Doudevski I, Warriner HE, Alig T, Zasadzinski JA, Waring AJ, Sherman MA. Nanostructure changes in lung surfactant monolayers induced by interactions between palmitoyloleoylphosphatidylglycerol and surfactant protein B. Langmuir 2003; 19:1539–1550.

57. Schurch S, Green FH, Bachofen H. Formation and structure of surface films: captive bubble surfactometry. Biochim Biophys Acta 1998; 1408:180–202.

58. Korfhagen TR, Bruno MD, Ross GF, Huelsman KM, Ikegami M, Jobe AH, Wert SE, Stripp BR, Morris RE, Glasser SW, Bachurski CJ, Iwamoto HS, Whitsett JA. Altered surfactant function and structure in *SP-A* gene targeted mice. Proc Natl Acad Sci USA 1996; 93:9594–9599.

59. Taneva SG, Keough KM. Adsorption of pulmonary surfactant protein SP-A to monolayers of phospholipids containing hydrophobic surfactant protein SP-B or SP-C: potential differential role for tertiary interaction of lipids, hydrophobic proteins, and SP-A. Biochemistry 2000; 39:6083–6093.

60. Vaccaro AM, Salvioli R, Tatti M, Ciaffoni F. Saposins and their interaction with lipids. Neurochem Res 1999; 24:307–314.

61. Kaser MR, Skouteris GG. Inhibition of bacterial growth by synthetic SP-B1-78 peptides. Peptides 1997; 18:1441–1444.

62. Thomas AQ, Lane K, Phillips J III, Prince M, Markin C, Speer M, Schwartz DA, Gaddipati R, Marney A, Johnson J, Roberts R, Haines J, Stahlman M, Loyd JE. Heterozygosity for a surfactant protein C gene mutation associated with usual interstitial pneumonitis and cellular nonspecific interstitial pneumonitis in one kindred. Am J Respir Crit Care Med 2002; 165:1322–1328.

63. Nogee LM, Dunbar AE III, Wert SE, Askin F, Hamvas A, Whitsett JA. A mutation in the surfactant protein C gene associated with familial interstitial lung disease. N Engl J Med 2001; 344:573–579.

64. Danlois F, Zaltash S, Johansson J, Robertson B, Haagsman HP, van Eijk M, Beers MF, Rollin F, Ruysschaert JM, Vandenbussche G. Very low surfactant protein C contents in newborn Belgian white and blue calves with respiratory distress syndrome. Biochem J 2000; 351(Pt 3):779–787.

65. Glasser SW, Burhans MS, Korfhagen TR, Na CL, Sly PD, Ross GF, Ikegami M, Whitsett JA. Altered stability of pulmonary surfactant in SP-C-deficient mice. Proc Natl Acad Sci USA 2001; 8:8.

66. Glasser SW, Detmer EA, Ikegami M, Na CL, Stahlman MT, Whitsett JA. Pneumonitis and emphysema in *sp-C* gene targeted mice. J Biol Chem 2003; 278:14291–14298.

67. Johansson J. Structure and properties of surfactant protein C. Biochim Biophys Acta 1998; 1408:161–172.

68. Johansson J, Szyperski T, Curstedt T, Wuthrich K. The NMR structure of the pulmonary surfactant-associated polypeptide SP-C in an apolar solvent contains a valyl-rich alpha-helix. Biochemistry 1994; 33:6015–6023.

69. Plasencia I, Rivas L, Keough KMW, Pérez-Gil J. Intrinsic structural differences in the N-terminal segment of pulmonary surfactant protein SP-C from different species. Comp Biochem Physiol 2001; 129:129–139.

70. Curstedt T, Johansson J, Persson P, Eklund A, Robertson B, Löwenadler B, Jörnvall H. Hydrophobic surfactant-associated polypeptides: SP-C is a lipopeptide with two palmitoylated cysteine residues, whereas SP-B lacks covalently linked fatty aacyl groups. Proc Natl Acad Sci USA 1990; 87:2985–2989.

71. Bi X, Flach CR, Perez-Gil J, Plasencia I, Andreu D, Oliveira E, Mendelsohn R. Secondary structure and lipid interactions of the N-terminal segment of pulmonary surfactant SP-C in Langmuir films: IR reflection–absorption spectroscopy and surface pressure studies. Biochemistry 2002; 41:8385–8395.

72. Plasencia I, Rivas L, Keough KM, Marsh D, Perez-Gil J. The N-terminal segment of pulmonary surfactant lipopeptide SP-C has intrinsic propensity to interact with and perturb phospholipidbilayers. Biochem J. 2004; 377:183–193.

73. Johansson J. Membrane properties and amyloid fibril formation of lung surfactant protein C. Biochem Soc Trans 2001; 29:601–606.

74. Wustneck N, Wustneck R, Perez-Gil J, Pison U. Effects of oligomerization and secondary structure on the surface behavior of pulmonary surfactant proteins SP-B and SP-C. Biophys J 2003; 84:1940–1949.

75. Gustafsson M, Thyberg J, Naslund J, Eliasson E, Johansson J. Amyloid fibril formation by pulmonary surfactant protein C. FEBS Lett 1999; 464:138–142.

76. Zangi R, Kovacs H, van Gunsteren WF, Johansson J, Mark AE. Free energy barrier estimation of unfolding the alpha-helical surfactant-associated polypeptide C. Proteins 2001; 43:395–402.

77. Wang WJ, Russo SJ, Mulugeta S, Beers MF. Biosynthesis of surfactant protein C (SP-C). Sorting of SP-C proprotein involves homomeric association via a signal anchor domain. J Biol Chem 2002; 277:19929–19937.

78. Horowitz AD, Baatz JE, Whitsett JA. Lipid effects on aggregation of pulmonary surfactant protein SP-C studied by fluorescence energy transfer. Biochemistry 1993; 32:9513–9523.

79. Nag K, Pao JS, Harbottle RR, Possmayer F, Petersen NO, Bagatolli LA. Segregation of saturated chain lipids in pulmonary surfactant films and bilayers. Biophys J 2002; 82:2041–2051.

80. Plasencia I, Cruz A, Casals C, Perez-Gil J. Superficial disposition of the N-terminal region of the surfactant protein SP-C and the absence of specific SP-B–SP-C interactions in phospholipid bilayers. Biochem J 2001; 359:651–659.

81. Ross M, Krol S, Janshoff A, Galla HJ. Kinetics of phospholipid insertion into monolayers containing the lung surfactant proteins SP-B or SP-C. Eur Biophys J 2002; 31:52–61.

82. Perez-Gil J, Tucker J, Simatos G, Keough KM. Interfacial adsorption of simple lipid mixtures combined with hydrophobic surfactant protein from pig lung. Biochem Cell Biol 1992; 70:332–338.

83. Oosterlaken-Dijksterhuis MA, Haagsman HP, van Golde LM, Demel RA. Characterization of lipid insertion into monomolecular layers mediated by lung surfactant proteins SP-B and SP-C. Biochemistry 1991; 30:10965–10971.

84. Kruger P, Baatz JE, Dluhy RA, Losche M. Effect of hydrophobic surfactant protein SP-C on binary phospholipid monolayers. Molecular machinery at the air/water interface. Biophys Chem 2002; 99:209–228.

85. Gericke A, Flach CR, Mendelsohn R. Structure and orientation of lung surfactant SP-C and L-alpha-dipalmitoylphosphatidylcholine in aqueous monolayers. Biophys J 1997; 73:492–499.

86. Nag K, Perez-Gil J, Cruz A, Keough KM. Fluorescently labeled pulmonary surfactant protein C in spread phospholipid monolayers. Biophys J 1996; 71:246–256.

87. Kramer A, Wintergalen A, Sieber M, Galla HJ, Amrein M, Guckenberger R. Distribution of the surfactant-associated protein C within a lung surfactant model film investigated by near-field optical microscopy. Biophys J 2000; 78:458–465.

88. Bourdos N, Kollmer F, Benninghoven A, Ross M, Sieber M, Galla HJ. Analysis of lung surfactant model systems with time-of-flight secondary ion mass spectrometry. Biophys J 2000; 79:357–369.

89. von Nahmen A, Schenk M, Sieber M, Amrein M. The structure of a model pulmonary surfactant as revealed by scanning force microscopy. Biophys J 1997; 72:463–469.

90. Amrein M, Nahmen AV, Sieber M. A scanning force- and fluorescence light microscopy study of the structure and function of a model pulmonary surfactant. Eur Biophys J 1997; 26:349–357.

91. Gustafsson M, Palmblad M, Curstedt T, Johansson J, Schurch S. Palmitoylation of a pulmonary surfactant protein C analogue affects the surface associated lipid reservoir and film stability. Biochim Biophys Acta 2000; 1466:169–178.

92. Perez-Gil J. Molecular interactions in pulmonary surfactant films. Biol Neonate 2002; 81:6–15.

93. Creuwels LA, Demel RA, van Golde LM, Benson BJ, Haagsman HP. Effect of acylation on structure and function of surfactant protein C at the air–liquid interface. J Biol Chem 1993; 268:26752–26758.

94. Amirkhanian JD, Bruni R, Waring AJ, Taeusch HW. Inhibition of mixtures of surfactant lipids and synthetic sequences of surfactant proteins SP-B and SP-C. Biochim Biophy Acta 1991; 1096:355–360.

95. Amirkhanian JD, Bruni R, Waring AJ, Navar C, Taeusch HW. Full length synthetic surfactant proteins, SP-B and SP-C, reduce surfactant inactivation by serum. Biochim Biophys Acta 1993; 1168:315–320.

96. Spragg RG, Lewis JF, Wurst W, Haefner D, Baughman RP, Wewers MD, Marsh JJ. Treatment of the acute respiratory distress syndrome with rSP-C surfactant. Am J Respir Crit Care Med 2003; 20:20.

97. Augusto LA, Li J, Synguelakis M, Johansson J, Chaby R. Structural basis for interactions between lung surfactant protein C and bacterial lipopolysaccharide. J Biol Chem 2002; 277:23484–23492.

98. Augusto L, Le Blay K, Auger G, Blanot D, Chaby R. Interaction of bacterial lipopolysaccharide with mouse surfactant protein C inserted into lipid vesicles. Am J Physiol Lung Cell Mol Physiol 2001; 281:L776–L785.

Biophysics and Molecular Mechanisms

6

Chain Dancing, Super-Cool Surfactant, and Heavy Breathing: Membranes, Rafts, and Phase Transitions

KAUSHIK NAG and **SANGEETHA VIDYASHANKAR**

Memorial University of Newfoundland,
St. John's, Newfoundland and Labrador, Canada

AMIYA K. PANDA

Behala College,
Kolkata, West Bengal, India

ROBERT R. HARBOTTLE

University of Western Ontario,
London, Ontario, Canada

I. Introduction

Lung surfactant (LS) was perhaps discovered a few centuries ago by a seafarer, Fredric Marten (1671), who described LS as, "When the whales blow up water, they fling out with some fattish substance that floats up on the sea like sperm and this fat the Mallemucks (sea-gulls?) devour greedily" (1). Beyond being an item of bird feed, today we know that this material is found in all mammalian lungs (and some other parts of the body), originates in the pulmonary type-II cells, and its lack thereof or dysfunction causes "heavy" or distressed breathing (2,3). We also comprehend that the LS is complex, behaves like an extracellular membrane, although unusual in composition compared to mammalian cell membranes (3,4). The physical property of the material has been studied using various physico-chemical methodologies. The simplest of them all is Irving Langmuir's "phenomenon in (Alice's!) Flatland" (5,6). These are the studies on monolayers and some complex liquid crystalline anisotropic arrangement of molecules in soaps (7). Surfactant is defined by DeGennes in his Nobel Lecture (1991), "Surfactants allow us to protect a water surface and to generate beautiful soap bubbles which delight our children" (7).

Despite extensive research on this fascinatingly complex material from those of earlier discovery of stable bubbles in the lungs by Pattle, Von Neergard, and Clements (8), the analysis of the composition, physical properties, and function of this "fattish" material is complicated [see 1–4, 8 for reviews]. The initial studies on the composition of LS by Clements et al., suggested that the material contains significant amounts of disaturated lecithin or diaplmitoylphosphatidyl-choline (DPPC) (9), which forms stable monolayers (10) and such monolayers can be compressed to reduce the surface tension of the air–water interface to $\sim$0 mN/m (10–12). It has also been documented that the surface tension is close to this low value when measured at the alveolar air–fluid interface at end expiration (13). It was thus acceptable that owing to high contents of DPPC in LS with significant amounts of other fluid lipids, to form stable mono-molecular films which can withstand high surface pressures, the films must undergo enrichment of DPPC by selective insertion of squeeze-out of the non-DPPC (or fluid components) at an air–water interface (2,10,12). This hypothesis was agreed upon, however, not without controversies (12). The concept of near-zero surface tension was challenged as an artefact of Langmuir–Wilhelmy plate measurement, and with the concept that a solid-like, tightly packed film can abolish the "air–water" interface completely and is an air–solid interface, therefore the term "surface tension" becomes redundant (12). The lung alveoli with surfactant was envisaged to have shapes such as bucky-balls (60 carbon structures with flat faces) or a geodesic dome upon which each of the flat solid surfaces of the films reside (14,15). However, all these hypothesis are becoming phenomenally confusing owing to some recent studies which are allowing for a molecular glimpse at the structure–function and material properties of LS *in vivo* as well as *in vitro* (16–18). Surfactant from some mammals that contains low amounts of DPPC compared with their unsaturated counterparts (16:0/16:1-PC) can lower surface tension of the air–water interface to low values (18), and fluid phospholipid films made of 16:0/18:1- PC (POPC) compressed rapidly in captive bubbles can also reach such low surface tension (16,19).

Some evolving physico-chemical (20–23) as well as molecular biology methods has allowed us to look at the molecular complexity of the "super-extraordinary juice" as described by Comroe (8) in his Retrospectroscope, which is a history of initial discoveries in medical science. These evolving methods such as atomic force microscopy (AFM) (20), mass spectrometry (MS) (22), molecular dynamics simulations, and genetic knock-out studies are suggesting a picture of the lung air–water interface as more complex than previously agreed upon by "surfactologists." In addition, advances in the field of membranes, surface-interface science, and nanotechnology have recently allowed one to peak at the molecular structural arrangements of LS, membranes, and liquid crystals, thereby challenging some of the pillar concepts of the classical "behavior" of LS.

Development of some of these methods and tools also has a fascinating history of their discovery, for example those of AFM or MS. From the first visions of "touching molecules" using scanning tunneling apparatus, Binning and Rohrer (1986) stated in their Nobel lecture, "we speculated that scientist would bet cases of champagne that our first pictures of the atoms were mere computer simulations" (20). AFM uses the old gramophone record (music) playing principle of scratching a surface of polyvinyl records to produce sound with a sharp tip (those days they used "rusty nails"). When this tip is only few atoms thin, it would image (or generate sound?) atoms or molecules larger than the tip's dimension. Indeed, today we can do this, and as shown in Fig. 6.1, the terminal methyl groups of DPPC monolayers could be imaged using AFM by methods developed by Zhai and Kleijn (23), without betting on champagne. The image was obtained from scanning the surface of a DPPC film deposited on mica using an AFM. The film was deposited at surface tensions (18 dyne/cm) or packing density close to those presumed to be in the lung air–water interface.

With the advent of MS, we are already characterizing small molecular alterations in components of complex systems and soon may be able to rapidly analyze the complete "lipidome" or proteome of diseased LS (21,24–26). Recently, the surfactant proteins have also been analyzed using similar methods, and some of the lipidome of a clinically used surfactant in films could be imaged (27). The original development of electro-spray ionization MS gave "wings to molecular elephants" as stated in the recent Nobel lecture of their discoverers (21). May be soon these elephants (SP-A, -B, -C, -D) in a sea of lipidome in normal and diseased LS would be detected and mapped (27), and their complex structure–function relationships and interactions with lipids completely characterized (24,28).

With large influx of research in the detailed mechanisms of LS function, we are only beginning to glimpse at the molecular mechanisms built in evolutionarily millions of years ago in air-breathing vertebrates (29). Therefore, a comprehensive review of the structure–function property of the material taking into account the conflicting ideas will perhaps someday emerge (before the grand unified field theory, hopefully!). Thus, it is appropriate here to quote the Nobel laureate who is considered as the master of analogy, that "it is amusing to note

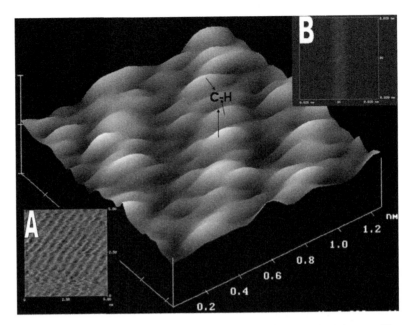

Figure 6.1 (**See color insert**) AFM image of a DPPC Langmuir–Bloggett film on mica at high surface pressure. The images were obtained by scanning the film in contact mode AFM in air at 30 Hz by methods developed by Zhai and Kleijn (23) at 5×5 nm resolution. The two-dimensional image is shown in (A) and a fast Fourier transform (FFT) of this image in (B). The FFT suggests lateral periodicity of the terminal fatty acid ends (CH_3) of the palmitoyl chains. The zoomed in three-dimensional image shows possibly either the molecular clouds of terminal fatty acyl ends of DPPC or unknown imaging artefacts (74).

that there is overlap in thought between those who study high brow string theory and description of soaps" (7). This chapter describes some of the biophysical and biochemical studies performed by us and others in understanding the complex behavior of LS with a view of events and mechanisms which can also occur in other systems, from liquid crystals, soft materials, and biological membrane. Once, we have some clues to the functioning of LS from such an analysis can we envisage LS dysfunction and physico-chemical behavior in lung disease such as in acute respiratory distress syndromes (questions regarding "severe" ones such as SARS may have to wait!) (30).

II. Membranes, Rafts, and Lung Surfactant

Perhaps, one of the most overlooked and under-cited early studies on physical properties of LS was performed by Trauble et al. (31), which allowed us a faint view of arrangements of molecules of LS in relation to the physical properties of cell membranes. This study was also interesting from the point that, certain systems such as the bacterial membranes to liquid crystalline cellular bilayers, may have some relationship to the "critical phenomenon" that can occur in LS (31,32). They suggested that "the function of the alveolar surfactant, besides the known one of reducing surface tension, is to induce critical behavior or spontaneous opening and closing of the alveoli" (31). These studies compared the physical behavior of lavaged LS with those of *Escherichia coli* membranes and suggested that both membranes show a specific molecular reorganization or "critical phenomenon" at temperatures close to its optimal function (31). This optimal behavior of LS at the physiological temperature or close to 37°C in homoeothermic mammals was documented in their studies as an induction of phase transition (31,32). The rearrangement of surfactant components was envisaged as typical restructuring or molecular aggregation in LS, which is best described as a phase transition phenomena (similar to freezing of water to ice).

Over the last decade, studies have shown that lavaged surfactant materials undergo a liquid crystalline to gel-like to other glassy phase transitions in monolayers (17,33–36) as well as in bilayers (37–39) as somewhat deducible from various model system studies of LS components (40,41). These transitions in LS occur as alteration of the lipid molecules from one chemical conformation (all-trans to trans-gauche) of tilt, hydration, accompanying volume changes to others, which can be collectively termed as "chain dancing." The transitions can be visualized or imaged as phase segregated domains of one component of LS coexisting in a sea of isotropic surrounding phase (such as ice crystals in water) (33,37). However, the organization of molecules into gel-like structures or domains may not be as simplistic as it sounds, because other transition from gel to solid-like or glass, monolayer to multilayers, lamellar to tubular structures are also observed in LS, owing to the role of the surfactant proteins (SP-A, -B, -C) and cholesterol (41).

Phase transitions in model membranes are measured as a chain melting behavior of lipids with a perturbant such as proteins, or cholesterol, under varying conditions of the membrane's environment (39). Recently, using mass spectral (MS) analysis, most mammalian surfactant was confirmed to contain significant amounts of DPPC, 1-palmitoyl-2-oleyl-phosphatidycholine (POPC or 16:0/16:0-PC), 1-pamioyl- 2-palmioleyl- PC (16:0/16:1-PC), and 1-palmitoyl-2-myristoyl PC (16:0/14:1 PC) (24,41). The latter phospholipid PMPC is also another disaturated phospholipid presents in LS, which caused the previous estimations of disaturated phosphatidycholine, in lavaged LS, some misery. In some cases, similar fatty acid chain distributions of phosphatidylglycerol (PG) has also been detected by MS. Mammalian cell membranes, however, do not contain any significant amounts of DPPC or PG. Although DPPC is the lipid of "choice" for most membrane researchers owing to its high chain melting transition temperature, biomembranes consist of mostly unsaturated phospholipids such as POPC (26) and significant amounts of cholesterol (45–48). The chain melting transition of most eukaryotic cell membranes is <0°C. Extracted lipids from such systems are cumbersome to study using physico-chemical techniques where sub-zero temperatures would be required to monitor any lipid–lipid or lipid–protein inter-actions, and as water of hydration is required in all biological systems for activity. However, what we know about the physical properties of both systems with com-pletely different compositions is that there are structured lipidic or lipid–protein aggregates present in both system at physiological temperatures whether in monolayers (14), bilayers (44–49) or some sort of tubular forms (43) at least *in vitro*. Whether these structures are large (Angstrom to micrometer) and are in equilibrium (over timescales of femto seconds to months) or transient and dynamic are still not completely resolved (49).

In case of cell membranes, functional "lipid rafts" or domains of sphingo-myelin, cholesterol, and proteins have been detected (50–55). These rafts are thought to be formed by the interactions of sphingomyelin (which has unusually high amounts of saturated fatty acyl chains) with cholesterol and may control certain functional aspects of cell membranes from signaling to disease processes (52,55). Lavaged whole surfactant as well as their lipid extracts when spread or adsorbed at an air–water interface (or in dispersions of bilayers or liposomes) shows such "raft" like structures (33–37). Recently, others have shown that the alveolar surfactant layer directly deposited on to rapidly frozen electron microscope grids suggested all sorts of layering such as bilayers as well a tubular structures associated with the air–water interface other than a simple-organized monolayer (42,43). The million dollar question about such structures and their role in surfactant do not have any answers yet, and certain physical properties of this LS compared to those of membranes may provide us with clues. In addition, if the monolayers are actually present at the lung air–water interface, they may be structured in domains as can be deducted from some *in vitro* studies. Other studies have suggested that such domains or rafts can poss-ibly align with the alveolar walls (as in a geodesic dome considered as flat) and prevent these "plaque" lined alveoli from collapsing due to the formation of rigid walls at low lung volumes (14).

III. Chain Dancing

LS lipid extract dispersions or even the lavaged material (containing all lipids and proteins) undergo a fluid to gel-like phase transition upon cooling. This transition can be monitored using various physical techniques such as differential scanning calorimetry (DSC), Fourier transform infrared (FTIR), and Raman spectroscopy (56–58). Bovine lipid extract surfactant (BLES®) is a clinically used material isolated from bovine lung lavage and contains all lipids and protein components of LS, except SP-A, SP-D and neutral lipids such as cholesterol, which are syn-thetically removed (59). This material thereby allows for specific studies to be conducted with systematic addition of the removal of components to provide for a LS model with composition close to those of LS in the lung. For example, a systematic addition of SP-A to BLES causes formation of tubular myelin. Addition of cholesterol allows for determining the role of this lipid in surfactant homeoviscous adaptations as well as a perturbant to membrane bilayer packing density or chain dancing.

The Raman spectral microscopy of BLES over the typical temperature range of the transition and typical snapshots of the surface of the dispersion obtained using a Raman spectrum at frequency change at 2880 cm^{-1} wavenumber are shown in Fig. 6.2. Raman scattering is normally obtained from the various molecular vibrations that occur in a system, when an incident wavelength of visible light is frequency shifted to a different wavenumber due to inelastic (Raman) scattering of light. The frequency shifts can then be mapped pixel by pixel from a single peak of the spectra (60,61). The peaks of the spectra [Fig. 6.2(A)] can suggest different motions of the bonds such as a C–H, C–C, and C=C stretching, scissoring, rocking, and wagging (the dogs tail!) as they

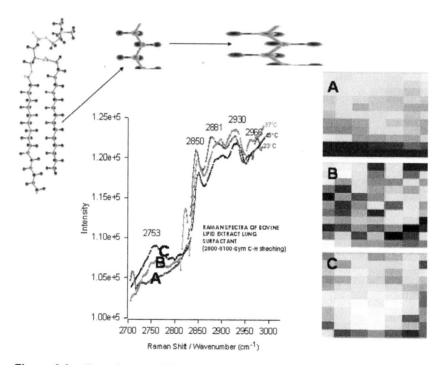

Figure 6.2 (**See color insert**) Raman spectra of BLES dispersion and spectral images obtained from the acyl CH$_2$ vibrations of DPPC undergoing phase transition. The stretching of the C–H bonds is shown in the cartoon. The three images were obtained between 23°C and 45°C from the same (10 × 15 μm) area of the dispersion and suggests change of the intensity of the symmetric stretching vibration at the center of image in (C), or a dynamic movement of the sample with such redistribution of the pixels (61). These areas may be domains of fluid lipids as suggested by others (60).

occur in the phospholipids acyl chains. These molecular vibrations can also be monitored from N–H, P–O, and other bonds from the phospholipid head group and as Amide I and II bands (N–H) of the proteins (such as SP-B/C), as also can be performed using FTIR (62,63). The snapshots of a single stretching frequency can be then mapped (or imaged) to suggest either the dynamic movement of the molecules over a region of the membrane or the specific localization of a group of molecules in a system due to phase segregation (domain coexistence). However, as these techniques generate very weak signal-to-noise ratios, the signals either need to be attenuated or sample concentration made to abnormal nonphysiological levels to obtain any conclusive results. This is also another advantage of using BLES as a sample, because it can be concentrated up to 300 mg–1 gm/mL as used in this study. Figure 6.2(A) may suggest a specific organization (aggregation) of lipids into regions of higher or lower intensities of the C–H stretching mode with change in temperature, as the images were obtained from the same microscopic region with temperature variation. This result probably suggests that surfactant in bulk phase may have some organization or domain like structure (42), as previously shown by others in other membranous systems. Recently, this method has been applied to lipids from skin-barrier dispersions and domains of cholesterol rich and poor areas have been mapped (60).

IV. Nanotubes Revisited

Although lipid organization *in vitro* of LS in films and bilayers are beginning to emerge, the situation at the lung air–water interface is filled with riddles. Surfactant is secreted as lamellar bodies (LB), which transforms into tubular myelin (TM) by unfolding or unraveling of the lamella. TM and LB are shown in the TEM images in Fig. 6.3 for rat lung lavage. The unraveling of the bilayer lamellas of an LB is suggested to occur owing to the influence of calcium and SP-A present in the lung air–water interface. However, note that in Fig. 6.3(A), the lamellar body interior seems to be unfolding into tubular structures internally. Recently, other studies of sampling the lung surfactant directly from excised lung suggest that the TM as well as lamellar structures is connected to the air–water interface, and cholesterol is sequestered in specific regions in such structures (43). *In vitro*, studies show that these peculiar nanotubular structures can be assembled at an air–water interface of type-II pneumocytes grown in culture, only if the surfaces of these culture plates are exposed to air (64).

As previously suggested, TM [Fig. 6.3(B)] are thought to be lipid–protein assemblies of SP-A, SP-B, DPPC, and POPG, and their main function is to enhance adsorption of surfactant lipids to the lung interface; it is not clear to date, if this actually is the case in the lungs. The image in Fig. 6.3(D) and (E) suggests that the TM contains loads of calcium and the center of the tubes are also loaded with soluble proteins or SP-A. Some studies have shown that TM

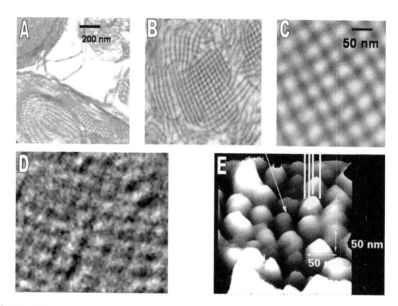

Figure 6.3 Transmission electron micrographs (A–D) and an AFM image (E) of tubular myelin in rat surfactant lavage. The TEM image in (A) shows peculiar lamellar bodies, which has TM forming inside the structure by lamellar expansion. The TM image in (D) was obtained from an unstained sample by dark field TEM, from the calcium signals (74). The AFM image was obtained from scanning the surface of an ultra thin section of embedded but unstained TEM sample, where the proteins are suggested to protrude out of the surface of such sections, and the lipidic regions depressed which allows for AFM imaging (69,91).

or only lamellar dispersion of surfactant hydrophobic fractions (without SP-A) equally enhances surface adsorption of lipids when high concentrations of materials are used in adsorption studies (65). Genetic knock-out studies of SP-A suggest that TM is absent in such lungs; however, the animal breathe normally and surface activity of such LS is not altered compared to normal (67,68). The following questions thus remain: Why is the molecular organization of the lipid protein system in the lung so intricate? Why is TM absent or significantly reduced in dysfunction and diseased lungs or in models of lung injury (67)? Why does TM form only in contact with air and not in a bulk phase of lipids and proteins at the post-secretory stage in cultured type-II cells, even when the LBs can come in contact with SP-A and calcium (64)? These unanswered questions require rigorous investigation, considering the fact that after five decades of imaging TM using electron microscopy to AFM (69) [Fig. 6.3(D and E)], we still do not comprehend why these fascinating structures are required at the air–water interface of the lung, or what their involvement is in respiration and surface activity. Genetic knock-out studies have shown that although a host of other complications arise in the lack of LS-associated proteins (SP-A, SP-C) that tubular myelin structures may not be responsible for the "surface activity" of LS, and possibly have other functions (66,70).

From such a glimpse of the lung air–water interface in the bulk, it is a distinct possibility that lipids and proteins, owing to specific interactions, produce molecular ordering, which is critical for the function of this "extraordinary juice" (8). Although we have some preliminary handle on the structure–function properties of the SPs in the interface (71), the detailed properties of the surfactant lipids can be explored at the molecular level in bulk as well as the interface owing to advances in studies of model membranes (72–74). Using methods such as giant unilamellar vesicles, we have suggested that domains of condensed or gel lipids (DPPC) can phase segregate out at or near the physiological temperature of 37°C in BLES bilayers during the phase transition (37). In addition, this study showed that the domains are coupled on both hemi-layers (monolayers) of the bilayer (37). This particular fact stands out, as it is difficult to envisage how DPPC in both monolayers can regionalize into small domains spanning the entire bilayer, when surfactant has a number of other phospholipid components possibly asymmetrically distributed in the hemi-layers. Studies on lipid extracts or whole lavage (72) from calf, porcine, bovine, and rabbit surfactants also attest to this temperature range (4,10,31,37), suggesting that surfactant at 37°C may be discretely ordered or organized, owing to its inherent composition of gel and fluid lipids.

As discussed earlier, deposited LS directly from alveolar interface of excised lungs shows these structuring in the form of layers, with underlying bilayers and tubular myelin (42,43). The X-ray diffraction of such layers suggests that the material to be phase separated into cholesterol-rich or -poor areas (43). What is amazing about this phase segregation process is that they also occur in diverse cellular membranes such as those of *E. coli* (32) as well as in kidney brush border and bacterial membranes (75) over a temperature close to the physiological temperatures of the organism, and in some cases, the domains of specific lipids or detergent resistant "rafts" could be imaged (47,48,75).

V. Physiological Correlates

The implication of surfactant being in a phase segregated form at the lung air–water interface can be directly linked to its functioning. Previous studies have suggested that this phase segregation is a critical phenomenon that may occur in most membrane systems (38,39) and causes spontaneous opening and closing of alveoli during respiration (31). For other membranous systems, the formation of lipid–protein rafts can allow for specific functional processes such as cell–cell communication, molecular signaling switches, and passage of ions (51–55). Some studies suggest that such rafts can have specific interactions with viral particles (30), and such processes could be linked to development of viral diseases (such as SARS?) in the lung. Exotic hypothesis on rafts such as relationship to development of Alzheimer's disease (76) and origin of thought processes in neural cells by opening and closing of logic circuits have been proposed (77,78). Others have suggested that such domains are formed and controlled by electro-hydrodynamics (Einstein's theories) at an air–water interface (45,46). Without delving into such esoteric mysteries, we have some preliminary evidence of functional implications and physiological correlates of the process of raft formation in LS.

Figure 6.4 shows the phase transition profiles of surfactant obtained from volume expansion of GUV liposomes [Fig. 6.4(A)], airway patency (opening) (79), and DSC chain melting profiles [Fig. 6.4(B)] of BLES over the temperature range of the transition (37). The term "lung" instead of "pulmonary" surfactant is used throughout this chapter owing to the fact that surfactant has also been detected in the upper airways (bronchioles) of the lung. However, the source of this upper airway LS is suggested to be from the terminal alveolar type-II pneumocytes. The airway surfactant is suggested to allow for easy opening of the bronchioles or millimeter size (diameter) tubes of the upper airway in the lung (79). As the bronchioles are lined with fluid/mucus, the absence of a surfactant

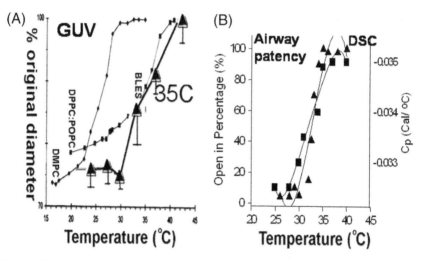

Figure 6.4   Bilayer vesicle shrinkage (A) and DSC and Airway patency (B) profiles of bovine surfactant extract. The giant uni-lamellar vesicles (GUV) shrink in diameter (A) when undergoing phase transition from fluid to gel phase upon cooling, and the midpoint of these profiles indicates the transition peak temperature as shown for BLES (34°C), and DMPC (24°C), and DPPC:POPC (35°C) is shown for comparison (37). The DSC cooling curves of BLES dispersions (37) almost overlap the airway patency (opening) profiles (79), suggesting a molecular rearrangement occurs in both systems at the same temperature regime. The airway opening profile was retraced from data published by Enhorning et al. (79).

layer would clog such microtubules with fluid and the system can be tested *in vitro* using a capillary surfactometer (79). Note the peculiar similarity (as shown in Fig. 6.4) that the temperature range for the phase transition as monitored by GUV (left panel) is similar to those of airway patency and DSC chain melting (right panel) profiles, at least for the bovine LS. At a physiological temperature of 37°C, surfactant in its most optimal condition shows maximal airway opening capability. Previous studies have shown that the surface of the BLES bilayers have gel lipids coexist with fluid lipids at this temperature (37).

As shown in Fig. 6.4(B), the liquid crystalline to gel transition in fully hydrated bilayers of BLES occurs during cooling of the material over a temperature range of 20–45°C. The peak of the transition is just below the gel to liquid crystalline chain melting transition temperature (T_m) of DPPC (41°C) bilayers. The DSC profiles suggest that the phospholipids acyl chains undergo ordering upon cooling or the molecules changing from a trans-gauche toward a more all-trans conformation (4,39). The broadness of the transition over a large temperature range suggests that the sharp decrease in acyl chain motions of DPPC is perturbed by the other components present in BLES, possibly the fluid lipids of surfactant. These profiles suggest that the DPPC acyl chains in BLES undergo conformational change from a fluid to a more solid or gel-like conformations, and the peak or T_m is close to the physiological temperature of the mammals.

VI. Supercool Surfactant

The first author of this chapter has had the daunting task of monitoring phase transition profiles from monolayers of surfactants components over the last two decades, after having had to custom build an instrument (80) for his Masters Thesis in "Biochemistry," which could make such wonderful observations at least in those decades (36,73,80–82). Every surfactant component from DPPC, PG, cholesterol, SP-A, -B, to -C (SP-D was too new) was monitored in the permutation–combination modes (82), which are also being pursued with a vengeance by others at present using far superior technology (83,84). It is amusing to note here that the natural extract of porcine lipid extract surfactant (PLE "A" S "E") behaved similar to a simple mixture of DPPC with a fluid phospholipid (dioleylphosphatidylcholine or DOPC) (85). This specific study was actually performed to monitor structures of model cellular membrane in monolayer models, rather than LS, as generous helpings of fluid lipid DOPC were used in this study (85). As there are numerous artificial and synthetic surfactants in the market in various combinations of lipids and protein components, the behavior of PLES at an air–water interface was similar to ALEC discovered by the legendary (invention of liposomes) Alex Bangham (86). Artificial lung expanding compound (ALEC^{TM}) was made with a simple mixture of phospholipids (DPPC:POPG) and is devoid of any surfactant proteins, especially SP-B and SP-C used in most of the clinically used surfactants. Although ALEC showed poorer surface activity and clinical trial success rates than other surfactants with SP-B/C, the behavior of PLES was similar to this mixture at least at an air–water interface. Studies by another group, who have systematically studied calf surfactant (17) in various combinations of cholesterol and proteins with the natural lipid extracts, convinced this author that the "laboratory assigned" roles for many of the surfactant "surface active" components including his own doctoral thesis (82) needs reexamination. The surfactant extracts behaved and had structures like none of its individual components or their mixtures but more like a system analogues to an "alloy" (82). An alloy or mixed combination of two or more elements can have physical properties, which are unique and quite different than those of its individual components. None of the phenomena such as "squeeze-out," "selective insertion," "solid-phase formation," and "DPPC-rich films at high pressures" was detectable in porcine surfactant at the air–water interface, whether they were adsorbed or solvent spread (36). It was disappointing to note that after cycling surfactant in the Langmuir surface balance, no significant quantitative loss of any of the components occurred from the surface (36).

Hall et al. have shown, by very systematic and meticulous studies, that calf surfactant behaved similar to those from porcine lungs (17,19,33). In addition, they made two fundamental observations which have changed our perceptions of how surfactant may work at the lung air–water interface, beyond those having been assigned in the laboratory. Surfactant films close to the near-zero surface tension region show the coverage of 30% DPPC-rich phase and the rest looks like fluid, suggesting the fluid lipids do not leave the monolayer, at least in the lipid extracts (17). In a separate but equally astounding study, they have also shown that a fluid phospholipids such as DMPC (above its T_m of 23°C) and POPC when compressed rapidly in monolayer in captive bubbles can sustain very high surface pressures (synonymous to a low surface tension close to 5 mN/m) similar to those of DPPC or surfactant extracts (35).

Figure 6.5 shows the surface pressure–area profiles and images of monolayers of BLES and a lipid raft mixture (sphingomyelin:POPC:cholesterol). Note that both diverse lipid mixtures show similar surface pressure (or tension)–area behavior; however, the fluorescence microscopy images of the films are quite different. The images were obtained directly from the air–water interface of a Langmuir–Wilhelmy surface balance during compression of the films. The bright or fluorescent areas are the fluid domains and the dark areas devoid of the fluorescent probe or gel domains. As BLES undergoes a fluid to condensed (gel-like) transition in films with increase in packing, there is appearance of gel domains (DPPC rich) in coexistence with fluid phase at about 15–35 mN/m (27). However, the raft mixture films contain mostly fluid lipids and show a difference in ordering of lipids into possibly liquid ordered (black regions) domains in coexistence with liquid disordered (fluid phase) at the same pressure, similar to those observed in cholesterol:fluid phospholipid mixtures (87). Recently, similar mixtures were studied in bilayers, and domains of cholesterol rich and poor

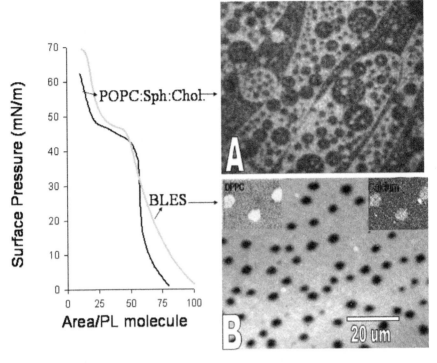

Figure 6.5 **(See color insert)** Surface pressure–area isotherms and fluorescence microscopy images of Raft lipids (A) and BLES (B) monomolecular films at 30 mN/m. The images were obtained directly from the air–water interface of a Langmuir surface balance (80), and the films were doped with low amounts of fluorescent probe NBD-PC which partitions in the fluid phase of the lipids (81). The black regions in (A) suggest liquid ordered domains and in (B) the gel (or condensed) domains. The inset in (B) is TOF-SIMS images of the condensed domains imaged from chemical fragment of DPPC (left) and calcium (right) (27). Films of BLES and Raft lipids are able to sustain high surface pressures or reduce the surface tension of the air–water interface ~5 mN/m.

phases could be imaged (48,49). These domains tended to deform the spherical bilayers [liposome], and in some cases protruded out of the plane of such layers (48). What is striking is that the surface tension–area profiles (Fig. 6.5) of these diverse systems, a system from the lung interface and the other as lipid components of a biological membrane, can both undergo ordering in two dimension at the air–water interface, and also reduce surface tension to low values. What is even more puzzling is that these "ordered" domains in both system grow in size up to a critical surface pressure of 40 mN/m (slightly above the bilayer pressures) and then disappear into a single homogenous phase as can be observed in both systems using fluorescence microscopy (36,47). This phenomenon was also observed in lipid mixtures from red blood cells (47) as well as surfactant from porcine (36), bovine (37), calf (17), and rat (72) surfactant. These observations may suggest that for a complex system like lung surfactant DPPC may not be required to reach low surface tensions, and the film may behave as a two-dimensional alloy or form peculiar phases (glass-like) which can sustain high packing densities or surface pressure.

Bilayers of some of these systems have shown phase transitions to occur in the natural membrane extract lipids around the physiological temperatures of the species, whether they contain mainly fluid lipids and cholesterol or some other gel–fluid ratio combinations as in LS (32,39,58). Recently, we have observed that surfactant from some marsupial species such as the fat-tailed Dunnart, which have significantly different proportion of gel to fluid lipid ratios compared with most mammalian LS (DPPC:fluid lipid ratios are reversed), films of these can reach low surface tension close to those of DPPC or of most other surfactants with a somewhat different sets of lipids (18). This study can almost vindicate the studies of Trauble (31) three decades ago, that respiration is a "critical phenomena," and alveolar surfactant functions beside the known one of reducing surface tension (which in turn may induce critical behavior or spontaneous opening and closing of the alveoli). Whether the critical behavior of lipid mixing has anything to do with "spontaneous opening" of alveoli is a debatable question; however, that critical phenomenon which may occur at the lung air–water interface or in biological membranes is gaining much attention due to the discovery of lipid rafts. Some studies have described this phase transition or physico-chemical behavior of surfactant (and/or membrane lipids) to suggest that these systems may exist physiologically in a "super-cool" state or phase for functioning, as those similar to material properties of glass. Glass is a super-cooled fluid, and possibly surfactant behaves like glass which shows unusual behavior distinct from either a fluid or solid. This behavior of surfactant raises more questions, than it answers such as, "What is the role of DPPC in surfactant"? In the mean time for those studying membranes, the Singer–Nicholson fluid mosaic model of cell membranes (after discovery of rafts) have also been recently revised to state that membrane systems are "dynamic yet structured" or a new "DS" model is available in the market (54).

VII. The Cholesterol Mystery

The possible role of cholesterol in altering phospholipid packing in bilayers, lipid–lipid interactions, and lipid–protein miscibility in membranes is well established (45,46,87). However, it is not clear to date what role this lipid plays in lung surfactant, and there is evidence (as well as debate) that cholesterol is an integral component of the system as it is present in significant amounts in the lung lavage. There is also a possibility that cholesterol is somehow delivered to the lungs via lipoproteins and mixes in with surfactant at the post-secretory stage. Various studies have shown that this neutral lipid can vary in amounts in surfactant during homeoviscous adaptation (29,88) and LS dysfunction (89). Although we do not know, at present, what exact functional role the material plays at the air–water interface, or its "laboratory assigned" role is surfactant film properties, cholesterol shows amazing alteration of lipid packing as related to the raft like structures and phase properties.

Figure 6.6(A) shows fluorescence images of DPPC and DPPC:cholesterol (2 mol%) binary films obtained directly from the air–water interface using fluorescence microscopy during the isothermal phase transition induced by lateral compression (1–6 in order of increasing surface pressure). Although films of DPPC [Fig. 6.6(B)] as well as such binary films reduce the surface tension of the air–water interface to 1 mN/m values, there are no major appreciable differences in the surface pressure–area profiles of the system (90). However, note the amazing difference of structures that are induced on the rafts of DPPC gel (black) domains [Fig. 6.6(B)] and the peculiar evolution of such domains (in galactic whorls!) with increase in pressure in the DPPC:cholesterol system (91). The localization of cholesterol has been suggested to be in the gel–fluid domain boundaries, and complicated theoretical as well as experimental protocols have been used to study this system exhaustively (45,46,90,91). In such

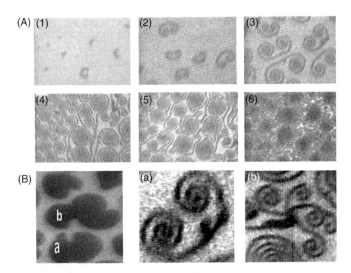

Figure 6.6 Fluorescence microscopy images of a DPPC (B) and DPPC + cholesterol (A) films. The films were imaged during progressive increase in surface pressure (1–6) from 4 to 24 mN/m, and the black regions represent the condensed and the bright areas the fluid phase (87). A typical image of the DPPC film is shown in the bottom panel. The condensed domains of DPPC show specific kidney-bean and treskillion structures, which under the influence of cholesterol becomes into the worm-like spirals and more complicated patterns fit for designs for knitting sweaters (41,90). Cholesterol acts as a line active impurity and resides at the gel–fluid domain boundaries of DPPC (44,90).

binary films, the gel domains of the phospholipid or DPPC grow not in diameter but in length. The kidney-bean shaped gel domains of DPPC turn into long-coiled worms and the three headed (treskillion?) domains into patterns "fit" for knitting designs in sweaters. In addition, the curling or spiraling of these domains follows a direction of clockwise or anticlockwise depending on the racemic or optical isomers (*R*- or *S*-DPPC) present in the system (45). The phenomenal change of the gel domain structures of DPPC induced by cholesterol may hint at processes, which are to be understood with theoretical treatment of "stripe" (hexagonal) phase formations in magnetic thin films and liquid crystals, too elusive and complicated for us to figure out [see Refs. (44,46) detailed theoretical treatment and for reviews]. What we do know, however, is that cholesterol is present in both diverse system or those in the lung surfactant and biological membranes, and its critical concentrations may control optimum structure–function properties of such systems.

Other complicated phenomenon that cholesterol may induce in surfactant film is multilayer formation. In a simple DPPC:cholesterol system, solid-like crystallites of cholesterol are observed to stack out of the plane of the films at high surface pressures (87). This phenomenon has also been speculated to occur during large cholesterol loading of arterial epithelial cell membranes, leading to atherogenesis or cardiovascular disease (hardening of the arteries by cholesterol plaques) (87). What is peculiar about films of LS model systems is that these multilayered structures can be seen to "pop" in and out (into the sub-phase?) of the films under high surface pressure close to those of the "low surface tension" regimes ($>25-5$ mN/m) or the plateaux region of the isotherm shown in Fig. 6.5 (33,34,40,83). Although these pop ups (squeeze-out) and "buckle downs" (stacks of bilayers folding in or out) can also occur in films of phospholipid systems without cholesterol, but containing SP-B and SP-C (40), this has made the understanding of the situation at the lung water interface quite grave, and cholesterol still remains a mystery to us.

As noted throughout this chapter, the physical phenomenon that may occur at the lung water interface due to the inherent interactions of its components is complex, and the classical concept of surfactant functioning may require certain revisions. In addition, the evaluation of the role of SPs in surfactant lipid organization complicates the situation even further. We know to date from genetic knock-out studies that SP-A, -C, and -D, although, cause major changes in surfactant metabolism and homeostasis, the animals can survive breathing cycles with such protein-free surfactants. Despite three decades of "laboratory testing" of surface activity of surfactant lipids with such proteins, we also do not know whether the enhancement of surface activity of LS lipids by proteins has anything to do with the animals lung air–water interface. Do these proteins have other roles, especially SP-B and SP-C in the lung, which we are not aware of? Do surfactant proteins lead to molecular organization at the lung air–water interface, which are dynamic, contains monolayer, bilayers, multilayers, tubes, and vesicles, acting as a concerted unit, as those that occur in most cellular automata? By glimpsing at such dynamic organizations from single snapshots of the lung air–water interface preserved using cooling, embedding, crushing, and under electron and X-ray beams, an illusionary image is actually being observed (as in the case of Schrodinger's cat in the box).

VIII.   Heavy Breathing: Critical Behavior Disrupted

We use the word "heavy breathing" to define lungs with dysfunctional surfactants instead of the word "difficult breathing." Numerous studies have consistently suggested that the molecular organization of lung surfactant is disrupted in a host of respiratory conditions and syndromes (89). From the time of discovery of lack of surfactant in neonatal lungs as presence of "hyaline membrane" disease to studies of structure–function properties of surfactant from ARDS, IRDS, asthma, cystic fibrosis, genetic SP-knockouts, we have some clues that the remarkable molecular arrangements of LS components may be severely disrupted in dysfunction. Earlier studies suggested that either there is a change or lack of component lipid or protein species in the dysfunctional surfactants, or this can lead to a lack of high surface activity of lavaged material from such lungs. Later studies have clearly shown that the leakage of plasma proteins into the lung interface causes impairment of surface activity as well as disruption of the ultrastructures of surfactant (65,89). Although numerous model studies on interactions of plasma protein with surfactant have shown that impairment of surface activity occurs at relatively high protein and low surfactant concentrations, it is not clear to date what the exact concentration of surfactant (5–10 mg/mL) in the alveolar airspace is, and thus model system studies with a limited concentrations of surfactants can lead to apparently confusing information at the molecular level (2). The area of studies on plasma protein inhibition of surfactant at this level is limited owing to floating membranes with lipid–protein structures are difficult to pin down (92), and this area can be treated as a "black box," considering some of the theories to explain such inhibitory role of serum proteins are simply too premature. This is mainly due to the fact that water-soluble proteins denature in the surface and such denaturations are difficult to study for complex mixtures using classical Gibbs and Langmuir isotherms (5,6). It has been shown that SP-A can reverse the effect of inhibitory plasma proteins, or in the case of oxidized surfactant (93), a situation where the surfactant lipids have been oxidized or "put out of action" ("knocked-out"?). At present, it is assumed that each of the serum proteins may inhibit surfactant by either "specific" interaction with one or other surfactant components or as a general mechanism of surface adsorption of proteins. For example, plasma proteins such as C-reactive protein can strongly bind to phosphocholine (the protein was previously called phosphorylcholine-binding protein) and thereby may inhibit the surfactant components from functioning properly (94). This protein also increases many fold in the serum and lung lavage during disease and inflammation. Other studies have suggested that albumin may compete with phospholipids for the surface during adsorption and monolayer formation. However, it is not clear why SP-A would inhibit this process, as it has minimal surface activity and probably denatures at the surface. In some studies, it was shown that SP-A can aggregate the "surface active" lipids of LS and thereby increases the adsorption rate of such lipids to a "clean" air–water interface. We, however, do not know whether in the lung, a "fresh or new monolayer" needs to be replenished ever after the neonate's first breath of air after birth and after belching out most of amniotic fluids [see Refs. (8,65,89) for detailed reviews].

Some studies have focused on trying to correlate surface tension–area profiles of surfactant from diseased lungs with those of pressure–volume curves obtained from such lungs (67). In these studies, an *ex-vivo* model is employed, such that excised lungs are made to undergo injury due to sepsis or hyperventilations and surfactant from such systems are analyzed from a compositional as well surface activity (67,68). In such models, a few significant alterations of LS are noticed, such as (1) a significant reduction of organized structures such as tubular myelin (large aggregates), (2) moderate amounts of plasma proteins in the alveolar airspace, (3) loss of surface activity of the surfactant, and (4) some compositional changes in surfactant mainly cholesterol and other phospholipids (67). This fourth factor, however, has not been completely clarified, as the phospholipid profiles of LS are not dramatically altered in some cases of lung injury, however, they may occur in others. Some studies suggest that for a situation such as cystic fibrosis, fatty acid profiles in surfactant are altered, but not the phospholipids, and the amount of SP-A and -D in such dysfunctional surfactant is changed compared with normal LS (24,95). In one of the model dysfunctional systems we have studied, it seems that all the factors mentioned above are somewhat true. In a hyperventilation injury model of rat lungs, the reduced surface activity correlate very well with the pressure–volume profiles of such lungs, or higher pressures are required to inflate such injured lungs at equivalent volumes. The interesting and conclusive fact to us is, however, that there is a dramatic reduction of organized structures in such lungs, as noted by decrease of tubular myelin, lamellar bodies, and the architecture of the adsorbed monolayer domain arrangements studied *in vitro* (67,72).

Adsorbed films of total lung lavage from hyperventilation-injured lungs have some peculiar alterations in monolayer organization or the coexisting domain structures as shown in Fig. 6.7. Figure 6.7 shows the surface topography of Langmuir–Blodgett films from a normal Fig. 6.7(A) and the hyperventilation-injured Fig. 6.7(B) surfactant imaged using AFM (96). AFM images the condensed domains as of higher elevation (7–10 Å) than the surrounding fluid phase, because the tilt of the phospholipid (DPPC) molecules in this phase is more perpendicular to the air–water interface compared with the fluid (96). This is due to the fact the molecules in the gel domains are more organized (tightly packed lipids) than the more disordered surrounding fluid phase (96) and are possibly made of DPPC which can undergo high packing densities

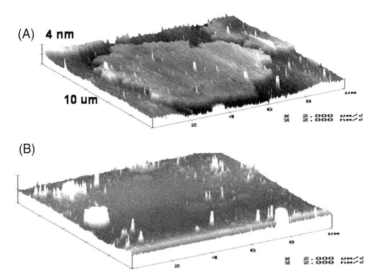

Figure 6.7 (**See color insert**) AFM images of normal (A) and hyperventilation injured (B) LS from rat lung lavage. The Langmuir–Bloggett films were deposited on mica and imaged in air. The table-like circular structures in (A) are possibly the condensed or gel domains, which are elevated 0.8 nm above the surrounding fluid phase, owing to differential tilt of the phospholipids chains (tilt-condensed phase) and packing density of the lipids in such domains (96,97). These domains are reduced in size in the injured system (B), and other large circular (smooth area in B) domains are neither gel nor fluid domains and possibly made of soluble plasma proteins (72).

(97). The higher regions (table like structure) are condensed domain of surfactant in a surrounding fluid phase (A); however, these "table-domains" (tilt condensed phase) are not distinctly observable in the dysfunctional material (B). Chemical analysis of the dysfunctional surfactant showed that the plasma protein content of such materials is almost 2–3 times higher than in the normally ventilated lungs, and the alteration of such interfacial structures is evident from the AFM image in Fig. 6.7 (B). The large diffuse domain in these dysfunctional LS may possibly be plasma protein or other cholesterol-induced fluidic domains (72).

As suggested throughout this chapter, it is perhaps not too speculative to assume that as a small amount of change in a single component (cholesterol) of surfactant can significantly alter the molecular organization of DPPC in films (Fig. 6.6) and induce critical behaviors, a change of some of these components is diseased lung could completely alter the molecular continuum and critical behaviors. Some other studies suggest that dysfunctions of surfactant can be related to proteins, which possibly disrupt the molecular structure of the surfactant continuum or network. A simple example of this is that when inhibitory proteins are added to surfactant, the surface tension–area profiles are changed (65) and also, peculiarly, the phase transition profiles are dramatically altered. One study shows that serum albumin disrupts the airway patency profiles (as in Fig. 6.3) in the same fashion as it does to the pressure–volume profiles of dysfunctional surfactant (79), and the Langmuir isotherms of films formed from such material (92).

IX. The Future

We will not delve into a conclusion as the area of LS research and the molecular mechanisms occurring in the extraordinary juice is continuously emerging, and the comprehension of the lung interface is inconclusive. Decades of research on lung surfactant from the viewpoint of membranes as well as interfaces has led us to detect certain general as well as unique and ubiquitous properties of this system. The current theory that surfactant forms floating membranes at the lung air–water interface is well established. However, nagging questions pertaining to low or near zero surface tension still persists and such values can sometimes become too low (negative surface tensions) for a good artificial surfactant with the expanding level of research on this area. Surfactant devoid of tubular myelin can reduce surface tension values equally as to those of SP-A knock-out LS as well as lipid extracts. Therefore, what is the purpose of this unique structure? Sequestration of proteins, DPPC, or some unique properties of conduction of ions or fluid hydrogen as in the case of recently synthesized carbon nanotubes? The floating membranes in the lungs are multi- and/or mono-layered or have intermediate conformations transiently visible by electron microscopy in some cases (2), and in others not so clear as they are seen as a functional syncytium (43). The hydrophobic proteins have structural similarities to saposins, which have rather quite distinct functions from surface activity. Structural homology of SP-B and -C to leucine zipper type "Velcro" motifs of ancient protein such as hemoerythrins, which carry oxygen in fluids of some marine species, may suggest some functions unknown at present (98–100). The role of SP-B and -C, although, has been assigned in laboratories to be lipid surface activity "enhancers," they also can be active as channel formers (98) and display bactericidal properties (99). SP-C has recently been shown to bind to bacterial lipopolysaccharide by specific domain, and this may have implications in surfactant dysfunction as SP-C may act as an anti-endotoxin (99). SP-C knock-out mice develop emphysema and pneumonitis and dysfunctions, which are controlled by fluid balance and possibly channel activity (70). In addition, this protein forms amyloid type fibrils (63,101) due to protein misfolding as seen in prions disease (102) and may give clues to new paradigms of lung diseases and Alzheimer and Mad Cow syndromes, where such fibrils are rampant (102). Nomenclature of these proteins as "lung surfactant associated" may change, because these (SP-A, -B, and -D) have also been detected in the gut and Eustachian tubes (103,104). Some of these studies may allow us to comprehend other "nonsurface active" functions of the proteins from channel formation for water, ions, and gas, and thereby their malfunction leading to alterations of fluid balances as detected in case of most major "channelopathy" (105,106).

The airway surfactant is also an evolving area of study, despite the debate about LS origins in the alveoli, surfactant do seem to be able to open up narrow capillary glass tubes, this optimal opening occurs at 37°C, and the process is inhibited by serum albumin (79). The compositional studies using mass spectrometry are opening up new avenues in disease detection, new lipid species are detected, and we will wait anxiously for a SP-E or Velcrin (2). The question regarding diversity of surfactant composition among various animals and the lipid–protein compositions of surfactant in ARDS, Cystic fibrosis among other lung disease is beginning to emerge; however, remains debatable until the low surface tension issue is resolved. These diverse set of inconclusive picture of LS allows us further research and debate for the next few decades; however, an integrated approach among researchers ("surfactologists") from diverse areas needs mutual recognition and acceptance to ever glimpse at the complexity of the super-extra-ordinary juice. Hopefully, at a future date, we may learn the complete evolutionary nanotechnology of the material and be much surprised to find that the "surface active material" from lungs works beyond the interfaces of our imagination.

Acknowledgments

The studies were conducted with grants from the Canadian Institute of Health Research—New Investigator (CIHR—NI) award and a Canadian Lung Association-Medical Research Council of Canada postdoctoral fellowship to K.N. A.K.P. was recipient of the BOYSCAST fellowship from the department of Science and Technology of the Government of India, and S.V. and E.S. recipients of graduate fellowships of Memorial University, and supported by a CIHR operating grant to K.N. A Canada Foundation for Innovation infrastructure grant for purchase of the AFM and Raman microspectroscope for future studies to K.N. is acknowledged. The authors would also like to thank, Drs. Kevin Keough (Chief Scientist, Health Canada), Mike Morrow and Valerie Booth (Department of Physics, Memorial University of Newfoundland), Fred Possmayer and Nils O. Petersen (University of Western Ontario), Ruud Veldhuizen and Jim lewis (Lawson Research Institute, London, Ontario), Chris Yip (University of Toronto), Derek Heyd (Ryerson University, Toronto), Louis Bagatolli (MEMPHYS, Center for Biomembrane Physics, University of Southern Denmark), Dr. Dave Bjarnson (BLES Biochemicals, London, Ontario), and Alex Bangham (UK-personal communications) for valuable discussions, insights, and laboratory facilities for the studies reported in this chapter.

References

1. Goerke J. Lung surfactant. Biochim Biophys Acta 1974; 344:241–264.
2. Goerke J. Pulmonary surfactant: functions and molecular composition. Biochim Biophys Acta 1998; 1408:79–89.

3. Scarpelli EM. Physiology of the alveolar surface network. Comp Biochem Physiol A 2003; 135:39–104.
4. Keough KMW. Physical chemistry of pulmonary surfactant in the terminal air spaces. In: Robertson B, VanGolde LMG, Batenburg JJ, eds. Pulmonary Surfactant: From Molecular Biology to Clinical Practice. Amsterdam: Elsevier, 1992:109–164.
5. Langmuir I. Two dimensional gasses, liquids and solids. Science 1936; 84:379–383.
6. Knobler CM. Seeing phenomena in flatland: studies of monolayer by fluorescence microscopy. Science 1990; 249:870–874.
7. DeGennes PG. Soft Matter (Nobel Lecture) Angwandate Chemie International Edition in English, 1992; 31:842–845.
8. Comroe JH Jr. Premature science and immature lungs. Part II, Chemical warfare and the newly born. Retrospectroscope: insights into medical discovery. Menlo Park, CA: Von Gehr Press, 1977.
9. King RJ, Clements JA. Surface active material from dog lungs II. composition and physiological correlation. Am J Physiol 1972; 223:715–726.
10. King RJ, Clements JA. Surface active material from dog lungs III: thermal analysis. Am J Physiol 1972; 223:727–733.
11. Bangham A, Morley CJ, Phillipis MC. The physical properties of an effective lung surfactant. Biochim Biophys Acta 1979; 573:552–556.
12. Bangham AD. Lung surfactant: How it does and does not work. Lung 1987; 165:17–25.
13. Schurch SJ, Goerke J, Clements JA. Direct determination of surface tension in the lungs. Proc Natl Acad Sci USA 1976; 73:4698–4702.
14. Bangham AD. Geodesic planes to facilitate the extension of alveolar liquid/air interface. Br J Anaesth 2001; 87:519–520.
15. Dorrington KL, Young JD. Development of the concept of a liquid pulmonary alveolar lining layer. Br J Anaesth 2001; 86:614–616.
16. Smith EC, Crane JM, Laderas TG, Hall SB. Metastability of a supercompressed fluid monolayer. Biophys J 2003; 85:3048–3057.
17. Piknova B, Schramm V, Hall SB. Pulmonary surfactant: phase behaviour and function. Curr Opin Struct Biol 2002; 12:487–494.
18. Possmayer F, Panda AK, Ormond C, Nag K, Postle AD, Petersen NO, Orgeig S, Daniels CB. Atypical composition and surface molecular organization of pulmonary surfactant from active and torpid fat-tailed dunnarts. Biophys J 2003; 84:310A.
19. Crane JM, Putz G, Hall SB. Rapid compression transforms interfacial monolayers of pulmonary surfactant. Biophys J 2001; 80:1863–1872.
20. Binnig G, Rohrer. Scanning tunnelling microscopy- from birth to adolescence. 1986; http://www.nobel.se/physics/laurete/1986/binnig-lecture.html.
21. Fenn JB. Electro-spray wings for molecular elephants. 2002; http//www.nobel.se/chemistry/laurete/2002/fenn-lecture.html.
22. Fenn JB, Mann M, Meng CK, Wong P, Whitehorse C. Electrospray ionization-principles and practice. Mass Spectrom Rev 1990; 9:37–70.
23. Zhai X, Kleijn J. Molecular structure of DPPC Langmuir–Blodgett monolayers studied by atomic force microscopy. Thin Solid Films 1997; 304:327–332.
24. Postle AD, Mander A, Reid KBM, Wang JY, Wright SM, Moustaki M, Warner JO. Deficient hydrophilic lung surfactant protein A and D with normal surfactant phospholipid species in cystic fibrosis. Am J Respir Cell Mol Biol 1999; 20:90–98.

25. Postle AD, Heeley EL, Wilton DC. A comparision of the molecular species compostion of mammalian lung surfactant. Comp Biochem Physiol A 2001; 129:65–73.

26. Han X, Gross RW. Global analysis of cellular lipidomes directly from crude extracts of biological samples by ESI mass spectrometry: a bridge to lipidomics. J Lipid Res 2003; 44:1071–1079.

27. Harbottle RR, Nag K, Stewart-McIntyre N, Possmayer F, Petersen NO. Molecular organization revelaed by time-of-flight secondary ion mass spectrometry of a clinically used extracted pulmonary surfactant. Langmuir 2003; 19:3698–3704.

28. Gardai SJ, Xiao Y-Q, Dickinson M, Nick JA, Voelker DR, Greene KE, Henson PM. By binding SIRPα or careticulin/CD91; lung collectins act as dual function surveillance molecules to suppress or enhance inflammation. Cell 2003; 115:13–23.

29. Daniels CB, Orgeig S. The comparative biology of pulmonary surfactant: past, present and future. Comp Biochem Physiol 2001; 129:9–36.

30. Briggs JAG, Wilk T, Fuller SA. Do lipid rafts mediate virus assembly and pseudotyping? J Gen Virol 2003; 84:757–768.

31. Trauble H, Eibl H, Sawada H. Respiration—a critical phenomenon? Naturwissenschaften 1974; 61:344–354.

32. Overath P, Trauble H. Phase transitions in cells, membranes and lipids of *Eschrichia coli*. Detection by fluorescenct probes, light scattering and dialatometry. Biochemistry 1973; 12:2625–2634.

33. Discher BM, Maloney KM, Grainger DW, Sousa CA, Hall SB. Neutral lipids induce critical behaviour in interfacial monolayers of pulmonary surfactant. Biochemistry 1999; 38:374–383.

34. Nag K, Morrow M, Keough KMW. Biophysical studies of lung surfactant. Physics in Canada: Biophysics 2004; 60:141–149.

35. Scheif WR, Meher A, Discher BM, Hall SB, Vogel V. Liquid-crystalline collapse of pulmonary surfactant monolayers. Biophys J 2003; 84:3792–3806.

36. Nag K, Perez-Gil J, Ruano M, Worthman LA, Stewart J, Casals C, Keough KMW. Phase transition in films of lung surfactant at the air–water interface. Biophys J 1998; 74:2983–2995.

37. Nag K, Pao JS, Harbottle RR, Possmayer F, Petersen NO, Bagatolli LA. Segregation of saturated chain lipids in pulmonary surfactant films and bilayers. Biophys J 2002; 82:2041.

38. Ebel H, Grabitz P, Heimbeurg T. Enthalpy and volume change in lipid membranes. I. The proportionality of heat and volume change in the lipid melting transition and its implication for the elastic constants. J Phys Chem B 2001; 105:7353–7360.

39. Heimburg T. Coupling of chain melting and bilayer structures: domains, rafts, elasticity and fusion. In: Tein HT, Ottova-Leitmannova A, eds. Planar Lipid Bilayers Membranes (BLMs) and their Applications. Elsevier: Amsterdam, Chapter 8, 2003:269–293.

40. Zasadzinski JA, Ding J, Warriner HE, Bringezu F, Waring AJ. The physics and physiology of lung surfactants. Curr Opin Colloid Interface Sci 2001; 6:506–513.

41. Veldhuizen RAW, Nag K, Orgeig S, Possmayer F. The role of lipids in pulmonary surfactant. Biochim Biophys Acta 1998; 1408:90–108.

42. Larsson M, Larsson K, Nylander T, Wollmer P. The bilayer melting transition in lung surfactant bilayers: role of cholesterol. Eur Biophys J 2003; 31:633–636.

43. Larsson M, Terasaki O, Larsson K. A solid state transition in the tetragonal lipid bilayer structure at the lung air–water interface. Solid State Sci 2003; 5:109–114.
44. McConnell HM. Structures and transition in lipid monolayers at the air–water interface. Annu Rev Phys Chem 1991; 42:171–195.
45. Radhakrishnan A, McConnell HM. Critical points in charged membranes containing cholesterol. Proc Natl Acad Sci 2002; 99:13391–13396.
46. McConnell HM, Vrljic M. Liquid–liquid immiscibility in membranes. Annu Rev Biophys Biomol Struct 2003; 32:469–492.
47. Keller SL, Pitcher WH, Huestis WH, McConnell HM. Red blood cell membrane lipids form immiscible liquids. Phys Rev Lett 1998; 81:5019–5022.
48. Veatch SL, Keller S. Separation of liquid phases in giant unilamellar vesicles of ternary mixtures of phospholipid and cholesterol. Biophys J 2003; 85: 3074–3083.
49. Veatch SL, Keller S. A closer look at the canonical 'raft mixture' in model membrane studies. Biophys J 2003; 84:725–726.
50. Edidin M. The state of lipid rafts: from model membranes to cells. Annu Rev Phys Chem 2003; 32:257–283.
51. Simons K, Ikonen E. Functional rafts in cell membranes. Nature 1997; 387:569–572.
52. Silvius JR. Role of cholesterol in lipid raft formation: lessons from lipid model system. Biochim Biophys Acta 2003; 1610:174–183.
53. Zajchowski LD, Robbins SM. Lipid rafts and little caves: compartmentalized signalling in membrane lipids. Eur J Biochem 2002; 269:737–752.
54. Vereb G, Szollosi J, Matko J, Nagy P, Farakas T, Vigh L, Matyus L, Waldmann TA, Damjanovich S. Dynamic, yet structured: the cell membrane three decades after the Singer–Nicholson model. Proc Natl Acad Sci USA 2003; 100:8053–8058.
55. Ahmed SN, Brown DA, London E. On the origin of sphingolipid/cholesterol-rich detergent–insoluble cell membranes: physiological concentrations of cholesterol and sphingolipid induced formation of a detergent-insoluble liquid-ordered lipid phase in model membranes. Biochemistry 1997; 36:10944–10953.
56. Ge Z, Brown CW, Turcotte JG, wang Z, Notter RH. FTIR studies of calcium-dependent molecular order in lung surfactant and surfactant extract dispersions. J Colloid Interface Sci 1995; 173:471–477.
57. Dluhy RA, Reilly KA, Hunt RD, Mitchell ML, Mautone AJ, Mendelsohn R. Infrared spectroscopic investigation of pulmonary surfactant: surface films transition at the air–water interface and bulk phase thermotropism. Biophys J 1989; 56:1173–1181.
58. Keough KMW, Farrel E, Cox M, Harrel G, Taeusch HW. Physical, chemical, and physiological characteristics of isolates of pulmonary surfactant from adult rabbits. Can J Physiol Pharmacol 1985; 63:1043–1051.
59. Yu S-H, Harding PGR, Possmayer F. Bovine pulmonary surfactant: chemical composition and physical properties. Lipids 1983; 18:522–529.
60. Percot A, Lafleur M. Direct observation of domains in model stratum corneum lipid mixtures by Raman microspectroscopy. Biophys J 2001; 81:2144–2153.
61. Nag K, Au H, Hyde D, Keough KMW. Raman spectral imaging and mapping of phase hetrogeneity in pulmonary surfactant dispersions. Biophys J 2003; 84(2):197a.

62. Pastrana-Rios B, Taneva S, Keough KMW, Mautone AJ, Mendelsohn R. External reflection absorption infrared spectroscopy study of lung surfactant SP-B and SP-C in phospholipid monolayers at the air–water interface. Biophys J 1995; 69:2531–2540.

63. Dluhy RA, Shanmukh S, Leapard B, Kruger P, Baatz JE. Deacylated pulmonary surfactant protein SP-C transforms from α-helical to amyloid structure via a pH-dependent mechanism: an infrared structural investigation. Biophys J 2003; 85:2417–2429.

64. Dobbs LG, Pian MS, Maglio M, Dumars S, Allen L. Maintenance of the differentiated type II phenotype by culture with an apical air surface. Am J Physiol 1997; 273:347–354.

65. Notter RH. Lung Surfactants: basic science and clinical application. Lung Biology in Health and Disease. Vol. 149. New York: Marcel Dekker Inc, 2000.

66. Ikegami M, Korfhagen TR, Whitsett JA, Bruno MD, Wer SE, Wada K, Jobe AH. Characteristics of surfactant from SP-A deficient mice. Am J Physiol 1998; 275:L247–L254.

67. Veldhuizen R, Welk B, Harbottle R, Hearn S, Nag K, Petersen N, Possmayer F. Mechanical ventilation of isolated rat lungs changes the structure and biophysical properties of surfactant. J Appl Physiol 2002; 92:1169–1175.

68. Casals C, Varela A, Ruano MLF, Valino F, Perez-Gil J, Torre N, Jorge E, Tendillo F, Castillo-Oliveres J. Increase of C-reactive protein and decrease of surfactant protein-A in surfactant after lung transplantation. Am J Respir Crit Care Med 1998; 157:43–49.

69. Nag K, Munro JG, Hearn SA, Rasmusson J, Petersen NO, Possmayer F. Correlated atomic force and transmission electron microscopy of nanotubular structures in pulmonary surfactant. J Struct Biol 1999; 126:1–15.

70. Glasser SW, Deitmer EA, Ikegami M, Na C-L, Sthalman MT, Whitsett JA. Pneumonitis and emphysema in *sp*-C gene trageted mice. J Biol Chem 2003; 278:14291–14298.

71. Perez-Gil J, Keough KMW. Interfacial properties of surfactant proteins. Biochim Biophys Acta 1998; 1408:203–217.

72. Panda AK, Nag K, Harbottle RR, Rodriguez-Capote R, Veldhuizen RAW, Petersen NO, Possmayer F. Effect of acute lung injury on structure and function of pulmonary surfactant films. Am J Respir Cell Mol Biol 2004; 30:641–650.

73. Nag K, Harbottle RR, Panda AK. Molecular architechture of a self-assembled biointerface:lung surfactant. J Surf Sci Technol 2000; 16:157–170.

74. Nag K, Panda AK, Au BH, Heyd D, Harbottle RR, Schoel M, Petersen NO, Bagtolli LA. Biophysical studies of nano-structured interfaces as models of lung surfactant membranes. Rec Res Develop Biophys 2002; 1:53–70.

75. Dietrich C, Bagatolli LA, Volovyk ZN, Thompson NL, Deri M, Jacobson K, Gratton E. Lipid rafts reconstituted in model membranes. Biophys J 2001; 80:1417–1428.

76. Pitto M, Pagani V, Masserini M, Ravasi D, Raimondo F. Membrane lipid rafts and Alzheimer's disease. Rec Res Develop Lipids 2002; 6:15–21.

77. Wallace R. Microcomputational evolution of the neural membranes. Nanobiology 1996; 4:25–37.

78. Wallace R, Price H. Neuromolecular computing: a new approach to human brain evolution. Biol Cybernetics 1999; 81:189–197.

79. Enhorning G, Hohlfeld J, Krug N, Lema G, Welliver RC. Surfactant function affected by airway inflammation and cooling: possible impact on exercise-induced asthma. Eur Respir J 2000; 15:532–538.

80. Nag K, Boland C, Rich NH, Keough KMW. Design and construction of an epifluorescence microscopic surface balance for the study of lipid phase transitions. Rev Sci Instrum 1990; 61:3425–3430.

81. Nag K, Boland C, Rich NH, Keough KMW. Epifluorescence microscopic observation of monolayer of dipalmitoylphosphatidylcholine: dependence of domain size with compression rates. Biochim Biophys Acta 1991; 1068:157–160.

82. Nag K. Association and interactions of pulmonary surfactant lipids and proteins in model membranes at the air–water interface. Ph.D. Thesis, Memorial University of Newfoundland, St. John's, Newfoundland, Canada, 1996.

83. Lipp MM, Lee KYC, Zasadzinski JA, Waring AJ. Phase and morphology changes induced by SP-B protein and its amino-terminal peptide in lipid monolayers. Science 1996; 273:1196–1199.

84. Knebel D, Sieber M, Reichelt R, Galla HJ, Amrein M. Fluorescence light microscopy of pulmonary surfactant at the air–water interface of an air-bubble of adjustable size. Biophys J 2002; 83:547–555.

85. Nag K, Keough KMW. Epifluorescence microscopic studies of monolayers containing mixtures of dioleoyl- and dipalmitoyl-phosphatidylcholine. Biophys J 1993; 65:1019–1026.

86. Bangham AD. Artificial lung expanding compound (ALEC™). In: Lasic E, Papahdojpoulos D, eds. Medical Application of Liposomes. Amsterdam: Elsevier Science, Chapter 6.2, 1998:455–472.

87. Worthman LAD, Nag K, Davis PJ, Keough KMW. Cholesterol in condensed and fluid phosphatidylcholine monolayers studied by Epifluorescence microscopy. Biophys J 1997; 72:2569–2580.

88. Lau MJ, Keough KMW. Lipid composition of lung lavage fluid from map turtles (*Malaclarys geographica*) maintained at different environmental temperatures. Can J Biochem 1981; 59:208–219.

89. Greise M. Pulmonary surfactant in health and human lung diseases: state of the art. Eur Respir J 1999; 13:1455–1456.

90. Panda AK, Hume A, Nag K, Harbottle RR, Petersen NO. Structural alterations of phospholipid film domain morphology induced by cholesterol. Indian J Biochem Biophys 2003; 40:114–121.

91. Nag K, Harbottle RR, Panda AK, Hearn SA, Petersen NO. Physiochemical mapping of phase heterogeneity in biomembrane films. Microsc Anal 2004; 18:23–25.

92. Wariner HF, Ding J, Waring AJ, Zasadzinski JA. A concentration dependent mechanism by which serum albumin inactivates replacement lung surfactants. Biophys J 2002; 82:835–842.

93. Rodriguez-Capote K, McCormack FX, Possmayer F. Pulmonary surfactant protein—A restores the surface properties of surfactant after oxidation by a mechanism that requires the Cys6 interchain disulphide bond and the phospholipid binding domain. J Biol Chem 2003; 278:20461–20474.

94. Casals C, Varela A, Ruano MLF, Valino F, Perez-Gil J, Torre N, Jorge E, Tendillo F, Castillo-Oliveres J. Increase of C-reactive protein and decrease of

surfactant protein—A in surfactant after lung transplantation. Am J Respir Crit Care Med 1998; 157:43–49.

95. Meyer KC, Sharma A, Brown R, Weatherly M, Moya F, Lewandowski J, Zimmerman JJ. Function and composition of pulmonary surfactant and surfactant-derived fatty acid profiles are altered in young adults with cystic fibrosis. Chest 2000; 118:164–174.

96. Nag K, Harbottle RR, Panda AK, Petersen NO. Atomic force microscopy of interfacial monomolecular films of pulmonary surfactant. In: Braga PC, Ricci D, eds. Atomic Force Microscopy: Biomedical Methods and Application. NJ: Humana Press, 2003:241–243.

97. Kaganer VM, Mohwald H, Dutta P. Structure and phase transition in Langmuir monolayers. Rev Mod Phys 1999; 71:779–819.

98. Oelberg DG, Xu F. Pulmaonary surfactant proteins insert cation-permeable channels in planar bilayers. Mol Genet Metabol 2000; 70:295–300.

99. Augusto LA, Li J, Sangulakis M, Johansson JJ, Chaby R. Structural basis for interactions between lung surfactant protein C and bacterial lipopolysaccharide. J Biol Chem 2002; 277:23484–23492.

100. Perez-Gil J, Keough KMW. Identical and similar amino acid sequences in the pulmonary surfactant proteins SP-B and SP-C and hemoerythrin and myohemoerytrin—an example of biochemical Velcro®. Biochem Intern 1991; 25:715–721.

101. Johansson J. Molecular determinants for amyloid fibril formation: lessons from lung surfactant protein C. Swiss Med Weekl 2003; 133:275–282.

102. Pruisner SB. Prions. (Nobel lecture) http//www.nobel.se/medicine/laureates/1997/pruisner-lecture.html.

103. Pannanan R, Glumoff V, Hallman M. Surfactant protein A and D expression in porcine Eustachian tube. FEBS Lett 1999; 452:141–144.

104. Eliakim R, Goetz GE, Rubio S, Chailey-Heu B, Shao J-S, Ducroc S, Alpers D. Isolation and characterization of surfactant like particles in rat and human colon. Am J Physiol 1997; 272:425–434.

105. Agre P, Mackinnon R. The Nobel Prize in Chemistry, 2003—Information for Public. http//www.nobel.se/chemistry/laureates/2003/public.html.

106. Jiang Y, Lee A, Cadene M, Chait BT, MacKinnon R. Crystal structure and mechanism of a calcium-gated potassium channel. Nature 2002; 417:515–522.

7

The Basis of Low Surface Tensions in the Lungs

SANDRA RUGONYI and STEPHEN B. HALL

Oregon Health & Science University,
Portland, Oregon, USA

I. Introduction

The most fundamental question concerning pulmonary surfactant is how the interfacial films that coat the alveoli achieve and sustain the very low surface tensions observed in the lungs. The low magnitude of the surface tension is now well established. Estimates based on the pressure–volume characteristics of excised lungs indicate that surface tensions reach values as low as 2–$3\,\mathrm{mN/m}$ (1). Direct measurements, using the contact angle of fluorocarbon droplets deposited in the peripheral alveoli (2), confirm surface tensions of $\sim 1\,\mathrm{mN/m}$ (3). These low surface tensions occur only in partially deflated lungs in which the surfactant films have been compressed by the shrinking alveolar surface area. After a single deflation, surface tensions remain essentially constant at these low values in static lungs for tens of minutes (1,4). A continuous compression of the films, therefore, is unnecessary to maintain the low surface tensions. These physiological observations define the unusual characteristics of the surfactant films *in situ*.

The behaviors of pulmonary surfactant in the lungs and phospholipid films *in vitro* under equilibrium conditions differ considerably. For films at increasing densities, achieved either by infinitely slow decreases in surface area or by deposition of increasing amounts of material, surface tension falls only to the equilibrium spreading tension (σ_e), which for most biological phospholipids is $\sim$25 mN/m (5). At σ_e, a phase transition occurs, and the two-dimensional film collapses to form a coexisting three-dimensional bulk phase (6). Further decreases in surface area or increases in constituents do not change the surface concentration of the monolayer but produce the formation of more bulk phase. Collapse therefore sets a fundamental limitation on the surface tension that a monolayer can achieve at equilibrium. Under non-equilibrium conditions, obtained when the interface is compressed at finite rates, surface tensions lower than σ_e can be reached. When compression of the films ceases, however, collapse returns surface tension towards equilibrium. The very low surface tensions observed in the lungs, and the persistence of those low values in static lungs for prolonged periods, indicate that rates of collapse far from equilibrium are slow and that the films exist in a metastable state.

This review considers two models that attempt to explain this metastability based on the behavior of simple films *in vitro*. The first model, referred to as the classical model, follows from the behavior of different phases within the two-dimensional film, and has been widely accepted for almost three decades. The second model, based on more recent observations on the kinetics of collapse, is referred to as the supercompressed model to emphasize an analogy to three-dimensional supercooled liquids. Both models focus exclusively on the monomolecular film itself and ignore several additional factors that might modify the behavior of the monolayer. In the lungs, for instance, the presence of additional material adjacent to the interface (7), perhaps formed during adsorption (8), might alter rates of collapse to some extent. We consider here only the fundamental behavior of the surfactant monolayer and the two known possible sources of its metastability.

II. Metastable Films of Pulmonary Surfactant

A. Classical Model

The different tendencies of films to collapse depend on their structure and therefore on the two-dimensional phases that they form. Interfacial films undergo phase transitions within the monolayer that are analogous to those that occur in bulk materials (6,9). For single chain surfactants, this phase behavior can be quite rich, with multiple phases distinguished by different degrees of order involving position, tilt, orientation, and chain elongation (10,11). For monolayers of the phosphatidylcholines, which constitute most of pulmonary surfactant, the phase diagram is simpler (12). Prior studies have identified only the gas, liquid-expanded (LE), and condensed[1] phases, which have two-dimensional characteristics analogous to the gas, liquid, and solid phases of bulk materials. At physiologically relevant temperatures and surface tensions close to σ_e, single component films of constituents from pulmonary surfactant can form only the LE and condensed phases. Below σ_e, both phases collapse. Rates for the condensed phase, however, are much slower, allowing films to deviate far from equilibrium conditions. The classical model then contends that the metastability of pulmonary surfactant *in situ* indicates the presence of a condensed film (13–15).

Formation of the condensed phase requires the presence of compounds that can adopt an ordered structure. Biological phospholipids commonly contain at least one unsaturated fatty acid, and the kink introduced by the cis double bond tends to disrupt ordered packing. Relative to disaturated compounds, unsaturated phospholipids melt from the gel to liquid-crystal phase in bilayer vesicles (16) at lower temperatures. When both transitions are readily accessible, melting temperatures in bilayers generally correlate with the condensed-to-LE transition temperature in monolayers. Early analyses, based largely on independent determination of head groups and fatty acid residues, indicated that pulmonary surfactant contains an unusually high content of disaturated phospholipids in general (17) and dipalmitoyl phosphatidylcholine (DPPC) in particular (18). More recent direct measurements of molecular species indicate that DPPC is the only constituent present in significant amounts[2] that has a bilayer melting transition above physiological temperatures and that can form the condensed phase in single-component films at 37°C. Recent determinations indicate that ~30–50% of pulmonary surfactant is DPPC (19–22).

Formation of a uniformly condensed film would require a significant change in composition. Analysis of compression isotherms suggests that to achieve the characteristics of a condensed phase, mixed phospholipid monolayers must contain >90% DPPC (23). Microscopic studies, which determine phase behavior directly, confirm that a condensed phase formed from the complete mix of surfactant phospholipids would require a DPPC content that exceeds 95% (24). The classical model then contends that relative to freshly secreted surfactant, the condensed film that functions in the lungs must be greatly enriched in DPPC (13,14).

Selective Adsorption

This enrichment could occur either by selective adsorption of DPPC (8) or by selective exclusion of other components (13–15). Selective adsorption could

---

[1]We follow here the recommendation (11) that "liquid-condensed" and "solid" phases should instead be referred to more accurately as condensed, either tilted or untilted.

[2]Dipalmitoyl phosphatidylglycerol (DPPG) forms condensed films and is present in pulmonary surfactant (18), but in amounts that represent less than a percent of the total material.

have either a thermodynamic or a kinetic basis. Both seem unlikely. A refinement based on thermodynamics could occur if DPPC had a lower σ_e than other constituents. In that case, DPPC might continue to adsorb after surface tensions had fallen to a level where insertion of other components had ceased. Experimental observations, however, suggest that σ_e is actually higher for DPPC than for other phospholipids (5). Thermodynamics therefore provides no clear basis for selective adsorption.

A mechanism for kinetic selection during adsorption is also not apparent. In contrast to classical surfactants, which adsorb as monomers, constituents in vesicles of pulmonary surfactant insert collectively into the interface (25,26). Therefore, the different components should all adsorb at the same rate. Microscopic observations on the separated phases within monolayers forming by adsorption support this contention and argue against any compositional change during adsorption at surface tensions above σ_e. Rather than revealing the uniformly condensed phase required by the classical model, fluorescence microscopy shows that at any given surface tension, films during adsorption have roughly the same ratio of LE and condensed phases as spread films that contain the complete set of surfactant constituents (27). These observations, although qualitative, argue that adsorbed films contain the full set of constituents and that different components adsorb at the same rate with no selective advantage for any particular compound.

Selective Exclusion

Enrichment of DPPC could also occur by selective exclusion of other components from the interface. Because of the insolubility of lipids in air and water (28), desorption of constituents from the films is negligible. Selective collapse, however, or squeeze-out could change the film's composition. The strongest evidence for this possibility has been the variation of surface tension during compression of mixed monolayers related to pulmonary surfactant. Surface tension remains relatively constant just below σ_e during a large change in area before compressibility[3] falls and surface tension drops more steeply (23). These results have been interpreted as demonstrating the selective exclusion at surface tensions below σ_e of constituents other than DPPC, which eventually results in a film that is sufficiently enriched in DPPC to form the condensed phase required to reach and sustain low surface tensions.

Microscopic observations on the collapse of surfactant films now link the composition of excluded material directly to phase behavior within the monolayer. Near σ_e, monolayers of pulmonary surfactant collapse to form a stacked

---

[3]Although the compressibility of a film is defined under equilibrium conditions, here we employ the same term in reference to the slope of a surface tension–area plot when the film is not in equilibrium during a dynamic compression. Similarly, although surface tension is defined at equilibrium (6), here we extend the concept to non-equilibrium conditions, recognizing that its value might include dynamic and static components.

smectic liquid-crystal (29), which is the same structure that hydrated phospholipids form in their bulk phase. Microscopy shows that like other liquid-crystalline materials (30,31), the surfactant monolayer likely flows from the interface as a continuous lamella into the collapsed stack (Fig. 7.1). The collapsed phase should therefore have the same composition as the region of the monolayer from which it is formed. Separation of a condensed phase containing only DPPC and a LE phase that collapses much more rapidly would provide the basis for selective exclusion and the formation of a film enriched in DPPC.

The phase behavior within monolayers containing extracts of pulmonary surfactant and closely related model systems provides evidence that ultimately argues against selective exclusion. Films containing the complete set of surfactant phospholipids, from which the proteins and cholesterol-containing compounds have been removed, do show the expected separation of the LE and condensed phases (24). The two phases have the necessary difference in composition, with essentially pure DPPC in the tilted-condensed (TC) domains and other constituents located in the surrounding LE film. Brewster angle microscopy also shows that the more ordered phase has the same optical anisotropy and optical thickness observed with films of pure DPPC in the TC phase. At ambient laboratory temperatures, however, the difference between collapse rates of the two phases is less than expected (32). During relatively slow compression from σ_e to low surface tensions, the ratio of areas occupied by the two phases remains essentially unchanged. Although the difference in rates of collapse might be substantial at 37°C, the behavior of the two phases at ambient laboratory temperatures suggests that a structural phase alone is insufficient to determine the ability of the films to reach low surface tensions.

Films with the complete set of constituents in surfactant extracts that specifically include the cholesterol-containing compounds also show phase separation. Both fluorescence microscopy (27,33) and Brewster angle microscopy

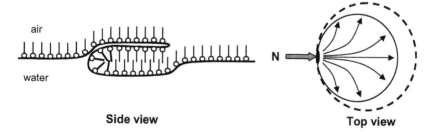

Side view   **Top view**

Figure 7.1 Mechanism of monolayer collapse for phospholipid and other liquid-crystalline surfactants. Collapsed structures grow by flow of the monolayer into a stacked bilayer to form trilayers. For pulmonary surfactant, the resulting structures have a circular shape (29), suggesting that surfactant molecules, N, enter the collapsed phase through a narrow region.

(33) demonstrate coexistence with domains of a more ordered phase that appear and grow during compression of the surfactant monolayers. The coexistence, however, is not solid–fluid as expected for the condensed and LE phases. Domains of the more ordered phase can undergo rapid changes in shape (34), indicating fluid characteristics rather than the solid behavior of the condensed phase. These domains then presumably represent a liquid-ordered phase of DPPC-cholesterol (35), comparable to the "lipid rafts" that may provide a basis for organization in cellular membranes (36,37). Under conditions at which phase separation is present at σ_e, light scattering microscopy detects collapse only from the disordered LE phase (29). The liquid-ordered and liquid-disordered phases, therefore, do show the difference in rates of collapse required for selective exclusion of different constituents.

The extent of phase separation at σ_e, however, is insufficient to provide the basis for producing a film that contains almost pure DPPC. Phase coexistence at σ_e in calf lung surfactant extract (CLSE) can be minimal or non-existent. During compression at 20°C, initial separation of two phases terminates before reaching σ_e (34). Remixing immediately follows dramatic changes in the shape of the ordered domains and in the extent of the interfacial boundary, consistent with the behavior caused by low line tension between two immiscible fluid phases close to a critical point. This remixing requires the presence of cholesterol (34). Critical points between fluid phases are now well documented in monolayers containing mixtures of cholesterol and phospholipids (38). The termination of phase coexistence above σ_e would, of course, eliminate the basis for selective exclusion.

Although the phase behavior at higher temperatures may shift to allow coexistence at σ_e, the fraction of the interface occupied by the ordered phase can be minimal. For extracts of pulmonary surfactant, the onset of phase separation at 37°C occurs only just above σ_e. Higher temperatures generally shift phase transitions to lower surface tensions, an effect that is well known for the LE–TC transition for DPPC (39). The presence of multiple additional components in surfactant films reduces transition surface tensions relative to pure DPPC by an additional 8–10 mN/m (33). The multiple components also affect the progression of the transition as well as its onset. Although the Gibbs phase rule for a single component film confines coexistence to a single surface tension, the presence of multiple components releases these constraints, and completion of the transition for films that include the surfactant phospholipids requires compression through a broad range of surface tensions (33,34). Consequently at σ_e and 37°C, the ordered phase in complete extracts of calf surfactant first appears at ~26 mN/m and occupies <4% of the interface when collapse begins (Fig. 7.2) (33). Exclusion of the LE phase would therefore require the collapse of 96% of the film. Whether the resulting liquid-ordered phase of DPPC-cholesterol would have the metastability of films in the lungs is unknown. A reduction in interfacial area of that extent, however, is physiologically unrealistic.

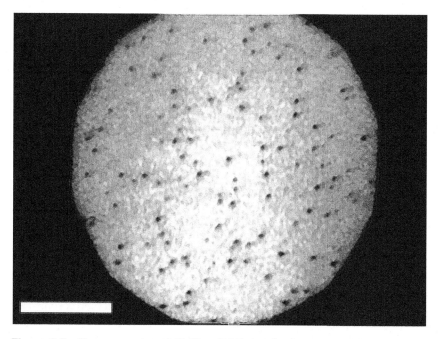

Figure 7.2   Phase separation of CLSE at 37°C visualized by fluorescence microscopy just above σ_e (33). Dark regions, which show liquid-ordered domains, account for $\sim$4% of the total interfacial area. Scale bar is 50 μm.

Although widely accepted, evidence supporting the classical model has been largely indirect. The monomolecular thickness of the film has complicated efforts using direct quantitative analysis to detect the compositional change predicted by the model. Structural evidence for the condensed phase has also been limited and inconclusive. Perhaps the strongest support for the model has simply been the absence of any film derived from pulmonary surfactant other than condensed DPPC that could replicate the behavior of films in the lungs. The supercompressed fluid model now provides one such alternative.

B.   Supercompressed Fluid Model

Although collapse of monolayers limits access to surface tensions below σ_e under equilibrium conditions, the ability of films to reach lower surface tensions during non-equilibrium compressions is well known. Like many other phase transitions, collapse of phospholipid monolayers close to σ_e begins with an energetically unfavorable process of nucleation (9,40) that can delay its onset. Nucleation events occur at a higher frequency further below σ_e and the surface tension at which collapse is first observed is lower during faster compression (6,41). After formation, subsequent growth of the nuclei occurs at finite rates. If compression is faster than collapse, then the density of the film must increase, and surface tension will fall. These considerations explain the ability of rapidly compressed films containing pulmonary surfactant or related phospholipids, which collapse just below σ_e during slow compressions, to reach the low surface tensions observed in the lungs (Fig. 7.3) (42–45).

The surfactant films *in situ* not only reach very low surface tensions but also sustain them in static lungs for prolonged periods. If collapse continued, then as soon as compression ceased, surface tensions would increase and return to σ_e. At low surface tensions, however, fluid phospholipid films become metastable. Collapse becomes remarkably slow, and fluid films containing a variety of individual phosphatidylcholines (42,45) as well as CLSE (44) achieve the metastability of films in the lungs (Fig. 7.4).

This slowing of collapse at low surface tensions, although unexpected, is analogous to the behavior of some bulk materials during cooling below a transition temperature. For those materials, rates of transformation change with decreasing temperature in the same manner that rates of collapse change with decreasing surface tension. As temperature or surface tension drops below the equilibrium value, rates of transformation initially increase to a maximum value. Further from equilibrium, however, rates decrease until they become negligible. In bulk materials, a rapid quench below a transition temperature can therefore yield metastable states for which, although the system is far from

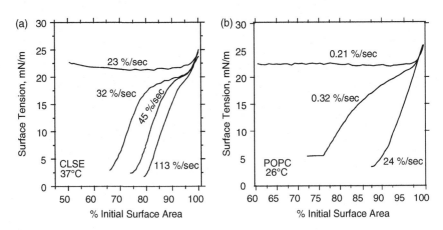

Figure 7.3 Isotherms for CLSE and POPC monolayers compressed at different rates. Similar behaviors were obtained for films of (a) CLSE at 37°C (44) and (b) POPC at 26°C (45). Slow compression of the films cannot achieve surface tensions much below a σ_e of ~25 mN/m. By increasing the rates of compression, however, very low surface tensions are obtained. The difference in area between the points at which compression starts and ends decreases with faster rates, suggesting that the extent of collapse diminishes with faster compression. Rates of compression are expressed as initial percentage decrease in area per second.

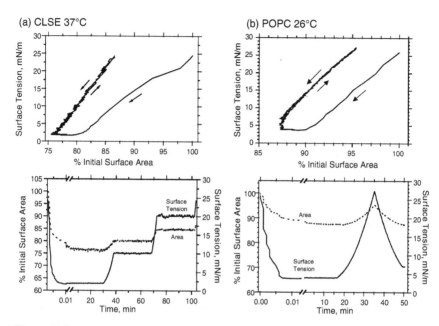

Figure 7.4 Persistent metastability of supercompressed films. Curves show surface tension–area isotherms (top) and variations of surface tension and area with time (bottom) for monolayers of (a) CLSE at 37°C (44) and (b) POPC at 26°C (45). Both films reach metastable states after a rapid compression to very low surface tensions, which can be sustained for prolonged periods without a drastic decrease in interfacial area. After a subsequent slow expansion and re-compression, the films show no evidence of further collapse.

equilibrium, rates of transformation are negligible. The formation of glasses, in which a liquid is supercooled below its freezing point to form an amorphous solid, represents such a process (46). Although the equilibrium structure is a crystal, relaxation times for the glass are extremely large, and the system is metastable. The behavior of LE monolayers, which at low surface tensions far below σ_e develop extremely slow rates of collapse, is similar, and may reflect an analogous process.

The kinetics of phase transitions are commonly summarized in transformation diagrams. For bulk materials, time–temperature–transformation (TTT) diagrams show the time at different temperatures required to transform isothermally a given fraction of the material to the new phase [Fig. 7.5(a)] (47,48). Dividing the transformed fraction by the required time yields approximate rates of transformation. TTT plots often have a C-shape such that the time for transformation reaches a minimum value at the "nose" of the diagram. This characteristic shape reflects conflicting effects of lower temperatures. The driving force for transformation increases as temperature drops below its transition value because the system is further from equilibrium. At the same time, however, molecular thermal motions, which allow individual molecules to transfer to the new phase by overcoming the activation energy for transformation, diminish at the lower temperatures. At some point, the slower molecular motions become the limiting factor in the transformation, producing rates that pass through a maximum and then decrease at temperatures below the nose.

Transformation diagrams can also be used to express the kinetics of collapse, but with surface tension for the two-dimensional films replacing temperature for the bulk materials. Time–surface tension–transformation (TσT) diagrams for isothermal monolayers show the time required at different constant surface tensions for a specific fraction of the film to collapse [Fig. 7.5(b)] (49). The extent of collapse can be measured from interfacial area, which at constant surface tension must fall because constituents are lost from the monolayer. TσT diagrams for monolayers of 1-palmitoyl-2-oleoyl phosphatidylcholine (POPC), which melts from the gel phase in bilayers at $-3°C$ (50) and which accounts for $\sim 10\%$ of pulmonary surfactant, show the same C-shape observed for bulk materials, with a maximum rate of collapse at the nose and slower rates at lower surface tensions (Fig. 7.6).

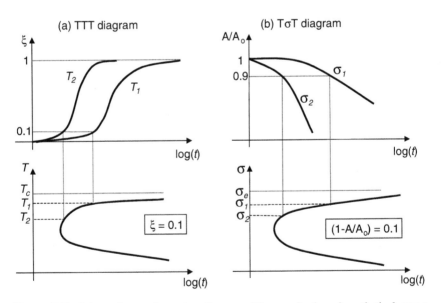

Figure 7.5 Schematic transformation diagrams. The panels show hypothetical experimental data (top) and the resulting transformation diagrams (bottom). (a) TTT plots used for bulk materials. ξ is a fixed fraction of the system transformed isothermally to the new phase at temperatures T_1 or T_2 below the transition temperature T_c. (b) TσT plot for monolayer collapse. A is interfacial area, and A_o is the value of A when surface tension first becomes constant below σ_e after a rapid compression during which collapse is negligible. The extent of collapse is measured here as a decrease in interfacial area when the film remains at constant surface tension σ_1 or σ_2 below the transition surface tension σ_e.

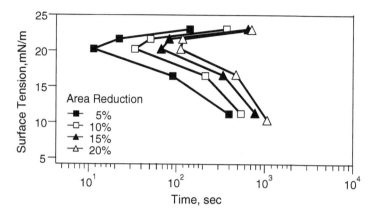

Figure 7.6 TσT diagram for POPC. The individual points show average values obtained by rapidly compressing POPC films to the different surface tensions and then keeping surface tension constant while the films collapsed. The plot then shows the time required for the area to fall by 5%, 10%, 15%, and 20%.

The similarity between TσT and TTT diagrams suggests comparable effects in the two- and three-dimensional systems. The driving force for collapse increases at surface tensions progressively further below σ_e. At the same time, increased surface concentration during compression may diminish molecular motions and increase the film's viscosity, reducing the rate at which the monolayer can flow into the collapsed structures. When eventually viscosity becomes dominant, rates of collapse pass through a maximum and then decrease despite greater deviations from equilibrium.

Transformation diagrams are particularly useful in predicting how systems will behave when collapse occurs under different conditions. TσT diagrams explain the variation of surface tension and the shape of surface tension–area isotherms during compression at different rates. Surface concentration increases, and surface tension falls, only if compression is faster than collapse. Compression slower than the maximum rate of collapse would therefore decrease surface tension only to the point at which the two processes occur at equal rates. The steep initial fall in times of transformation in the TσT diagrams (Fig. 7.6), which indicate increased rates of collapse, accurately predict the minimal change in surface tension observed over a broad range of compression rates (44,45). If compression is faster than collapse at the nose, however, surface tension would decrease continuously to low values. The TσT diagrams therefore predict a threshold rate for reaching low surface tensions that is determined by the rate of collapse at the nose. Experimental observations confirm the existence of a threshold rate required to reach low surface tensions for both CLSE and POPC (44,45), and that for POPC, the threshold rate and the maximum rate of collapse are roughly equal (45).

During compression much faster than the maximum rate of collapse, surface tension falls rapidly, the extent of collapse is limited, and isotherms show steeply declining surface tensions and low compressibilities (45). For compression only slightly faster than the threshold, at surface tensions around the nose, rates of compression and collapse are similar. Although surface concentration increases continuously, close to the nose the films collapse extensively, resulting in isotherms with relatively flat plateaus during which surface tension changes little despite significant decreases in area. At surface tensions below the nose, rates of collapse slow, and the compressibility of the film again decreases. The resulting isotherm for a LE film of POPC shows a plateau near σ_e followed by a steeply falling curve. Similar isotherms obtained for mixed lipid films that model pulmonary surfactant have previously been explained by enrichment in DPPC (23). The TσT diagrams show that the variation in rates of collapse can explain the shape of isotherms even for films with a single phosphatidylcholine and that changes in the composition of the film are unnecessary.

After reaching very low surface tension, the behavior of the films change. During subsequent expansion back to σ_e followed by recompression, rates of collapse remain quite low. Rather than passing through the same maximum that occurs during the initial compression, collapse for films of POPC simply slows as surface tension returns toward σ_e (51). Rates during the initial compression and subsequent expansion can differ by three orders of magnitude. Consequently, the metastability achieved by both POPC and CLSE at very low surface tensions persists during expansion at least to σ_e (Fig. 7.4). During compression at the same slow rates that initially produce a collapse plateau just below σ_e, films that have previously reached low surface tensions instead follow a steeply falling isotherm (44,45).

This persistent metastability is not a general characteristic of liquids supercooled to form glass. When heated, transformation rates usually increase, and crystallization frequently occurs well below the freezing temperature. For some materials, however, the onset of crystallization can be delayed at temperatures well above the glass transition for prolonged durations (52). Supercompressed films similarly do not collapse significantly even when surface tensions increase to σ_e or remain constant at values where rates of collapse during the initial compression were maximal [Fig. 7.4(a)] (44,45,51). The analogy with supercooled liquids therefore might explain the continued resistance to collapse of the monolayers during expansion from very low surface tensions.

After the initial rapid compression to low surface tensions, supercompressed films replicate most characteristics of the surfactant films *in situ*. Rates of collapse in static films are slow over the full range of surface tensions below σ_e. Cyclic changes in area that avoid expansion above σ_e or compression to surface tensions so close to zero that the films become mechanically unstable follow the same isotherm through multiple cycles with no evidence that material is lost from the monolayer (Fig. 7.4). Once formed, the supercompressed fluid films mimic the performance of surfactant films in the lungs.

The process of reaching low surface tensions does require speeds of compression that are apparently unnecessary *in situ*. Although the threshold rate required for CLSE to reach low surface tensions lies within the range that occurs during normal breathing (44), excised lungs require no comparable threshold rate of deflation to achieve normal pulmonary mechanics. Other factors could influence the behavior of surfactant films and alter the conditions required to form the metastable films. Any process that would lower rates of collapse would diminish the threshold rate required to compress the films into the metastable state. The small thickness of the liquid film that coats the alveoli, for instance, or the presence of a surface-associated reservoir formed during adsorption (8) might significantly slow collapse. These considerations, although beyond the scope of this paper, may be crucial for understanding the behavior of films in the lungs and the achievement of metastable states without substantial changes in composition.

III. Conclusions

This review discusses two models that can partially explain the behavior of surfactant films in the lungs. In the classical model, formation of films in the condensed phase, which have the highly ordered structure approaching that of a two-dimensional crystal, would require some process of refinement from the complete surfactant mixture to yield a composition containing essentially pure DPPC. Supercompressed fluid films, analogous to amorphous solids of three-dimensional materials, have no compositional constraints, but require an initial fast compression to reach the low surface tensions at which they become persistently metastable. Although condensed and supercompressed films each adequately replicate the behavior of pulmonary surfactant *in situ*, both models lack a satisfactory explanation for how the films are formed.

The temperature dependence of pulmonary mechanics should provide a basis for testing the validity of the classical model. The melting behavior of the films predicted by the two models is likely to be quite different. For the supercompressed fluid films, the restoration of rapid collapse during heating has not yet been reported. TC films of DPPC, in contrast, melt to the LE phase abruptly at discrete temperatures around 41°C and, at surface tensions below σ_e, collapse promptly (39). If low surface tensions in the lungs reflect the presence of films composed mostly of DPPC in a condensed phase, then upon melting, the films would collapse and surface tension would increase to σ_e. The larger surface tensions associated with melted films would significantly increase the pressure required to maintain the lungs at any given volume. The classical model, but probably not the supercompressed model, therefore predicts an abrupt change in pulmonary mechanics at 41°C.

Different groups that have measured the temperature dependence of pulmonary mechanics have obtained results that are strikingly different. Original reports indicated the behavior predicted by the classical model, with a sharp change in pressures just above 41°C (14,53,54). Another group, however, found only a slow increase in pressures extending over a broad range of temperatures, with no particular change around $41°C$ (55,56). These conflicting data therefore currently provide no guidance concerning which model more accurately describes the actual films in the lungs.

In summary, the supercompressed model provides an alternative mechanism not considered previously by which metastable films might form in the lungs. Our results show that rates of collapse below σ_e can reach a maximum and then become negligible at surface tensions far from equilibrium. The existence of a maximum rate of collapse at finite surface tensions below σ_e results in a threshold rate of compression above which films can attain metastable states. This characteristic is analogous to many phase transitions in bulk materials, and although not exhaustively investigated before for monolayers, it is not unique to the collapse transformation. Researchers and engineers long ago found that the kinetic behavior of phase transitions is essential in achieving materials with desired properties. Although neglected in the past, the kinetics of collapse might also have a decisive role in the behavior of films in the lungs. The supercompressed model therefore provides a means for reaching persistent metastable films that opens a new perspective in the study and understanding of pulmonary function.

Acknowledgments

This work was supported by a postdoctoral fellowship from the Pacific Mountain Affiliate of the American Heart Association (0225578Z) and by the National Institutes of Health (HL 60914).

References

1. Horie T, Hildebrandt J. Dynamic compliance, limit cycles, and static equilibria of excised cat lung. J Appl Physiol 1971; 31:423–430.
2. Schürch S, Goerke J, Clements JA. Direct determination of surface tension in the lung. Proc Natl Acad Sci USA 1976; 73:4698–4702.
3. Schürch S. Surface tension at low lung volumes: dependence on time and alveolar size. Respir Physiol 1982; 48:339–355.
4. Schürch S, Goerke J, Clements JA. Direct determination of volume- and time-dependence of alveolar surface tension in excised lungs. Proc Natl Acad Sci USA 1978; 75:3417–3421.
5. Lee S, Kim DH, Needham D. Equilibrium and dynamic interfacial tension measurements at microscopic interfaces using a micropipet technique. 2. Dynamics of phospholipid monolayer formation and equilibrium tensions at water–air interface. Langmuir 2001; 17:5544–5550.
6. Gaines GL Jr. Insoluble Monolayers at Liquid–Gas Interfaces. New York: Interscience Publishers, 1966.
7. Hills BA. The Biology of Surfactant. New York: Cambridge University Press, 1988:222–235.

8. Schürch S, Qanbar R, Bachofen H, Possmayer F. The surface-associated surfactant reservoir in the alveolar lining. Biol Neonate 1995; 67(suppl 1):61–76.
9. Defay R, Prigogine I. Surface Tension and Adsorption. New York: Wiley, 1966.
10. Knobler CM, Desai RC. Phase transitions in monolayers. Annu Rev Phys Chem 1992; 43:207–236.
11. Kaganer VM, Möhwald H, Dutta P. Structure and phase transitions in Langmuir monolayers. Rev Mod Phys 1999; 71:779–819.
12. Albrecht O, Gruler H, Sackmann E. Polymorphism of phospholipid monolayers. J Phys (Paris) 1978; 39:301–313.
13. Bangham AD, Morley CJ, Phillips MC. The physical properties of an effective lung surfactant. Biochim Biophys Acta 1979; 573:552–556.
14. Clements JA. Functions of the alveolar lining. Am Rev Respir Dis 1977; 115(6 Part 2):67–71.
15. Watkins JC. The surface properties of pure phospholipids in relation to those of lung extracts. Biochim Biophys Acta 1968; 152:293–306.
16. Huang C-H, Li S. Calorimetric and molecular mechanics studies of the thermotropic phase behavior of membrane phospholipids. Biochim Biophys Acta 1999; 1422:273–307.
17. King RJ, Clements JA. Lipid synthesis and surfactant turnover in the lungs. In: Fishman AP, Fisher AB, eds. Handbook of Physiology: A Critical, Comprehensive Presentation of Physiological Knowledge and Concepts. Section 3: The Respiratory System. Bethesda, Maryland: American Physiological Society, 1985:309–336.
18. Brown ES. Isolation and assay of dipalmitoyl lecithin in lung extracts. Am J Physiol 1964; 207:402–406.
19. Uhlson C, Harrison K, Allen CB, Ahmad S, White CW, Murphy RC. Oxidized phospholipids derived from ozone-treated lung surfactant extract reduce macrophage and epithelial cell viability. Chem Res Toxical 2002; 15:896–906.
20. Yu S, Harding PGR, Smith N, Possmayer F. Bovine pulmonary surfactant: chemical composition and physical properties. Lipids 1983; 18:522–529.
21. Kahn MC, Anderson GJ, Anyan WR, Hall SB. Phosphatidylcholine molecular-species of calf lung surfactant. Am J Physiol—Lung Cell Mol Physiol 1995; 13:L567–L573.
22. Holm BA, Wang Z, Egan EA, Notter RH. Content of dipalmitoyl phosphatidylcholine in lung surfactant: ramifications for surface activity. Ped Res 1996; 39:805–811.
23. Hildebran JN, Goerke J, Clements JA. Pulmonary surface film stability and composition. J Appl Physiol 1979; 47:604–611.
24. Discher BM, Schief WR, Vogel V, Hall SB. Phase separation in monolayers of pulmonary surfactant phospholipids at the air–water interface: composition and structure. Biophys J 1999; 77:2051–2061.
25. Schürch S, Schürch D, Curstedt T, Robertson B. Surface activity of lipid extract surfactant in relation to film area compression and collapse. J Appl Physiol 1994; 77:974–986.
26. Sen A, Hui S-W, Mosgrober-Anthony M, Holm BA, Egan EA. Localization of lipid exchange sites between bulk lung surfactants and surface monolayer: freeze fracture study. J Colloid Interf Sci 1988; 126:355–360.
27. Nag K, Perez-Gil J, Ruano ML, Worthman LA, Stewart J, Casals C, Keough KM. Phase transitions in films of lung surfactant at the air–water interface. Biophys J 1998; 74:2983–2995.

28. Smith R, Tanford C. The critical micelle concentration of L-α- dipalmitoylphosphatidylcholine in water and water–methanol solutions. J Mol Biol 1972; 67:75–83.

29. Schief WR, Antia M, Discher BM, Hall SB, Vogel V. Liquid-crystalline collapse of pulmonary surfactant monolayers. Biophys J 2003; 84:3792–3806.

30. Nikomarov ES. A slow collapse of a monolayer spread on an aqueous surface. Langmuir 1990; 6:410–414.

31. de Mul MNG, Mann JA. Multilayer formation in thin-films of thermotropic liquid-crystals at the air–water interface. Langmuir, 1994; 10:2311–2316.

32. Piknova B, Schief WR, Vogel V, Discher BM, Hall SB. Discrepancy between phase behavior of lung surfactant phospholipids and the classical model of surfactant function. Biophys J 2001; 81:2172–2180.

33. Discher BM, Maloney KM, Schief WR Jr, Grainger DW, Vogel V, Hall SB. Lateral phase separation in interfacial films of pulmonary surfactant. Biophys J 1996; 71:2583–2590.

34. Discher BM, Maloney KM, Grainger DW, Sousa CA, Hall SB. Neutral lipids induce critical behavior in interfacial monolayers of pulmonary surfactant. Biochemistry 1999; 38:374–383.

35. Discher BM, Maloney KM, Grainger DW, Hall SB. Effect of neutral lipids on coexisting phases in monolayers of pulmonary surfactant. Biophys Chem 2002; 101:333–345.

36. Edidin M. The state of lipid rafts: from model membranes to cells. Annu Rev Biophys Biomol Struct 2003; 32:257–283.

37. McConnell HM, Vrljic M. Liquid–liquid immiscibility in membranes. Annu Rev Biophys Biomol Struct 2003; 32:469–492.

38. Radhakrishnan A, McConnell HM. Critical points in charged membranes containing cholesterol. Proc Natl Acad Sci USA 2002; 99:13391–13396.

39. Crane JM, Putz G, Hall SB. Persistence of phase coexistence in disaturated phosphatidylcholine monolayers at high surface pressures. Biophys J 1999; 77:3134–3143.

40. Smith RD, Berg JC. The collapse of surfactant monolayers at the air–water interface. J Colloid Interf Sci 1980; 74:273–286.

41. Kampf JP, Frank CW, Malmstrom EE, Hawker CJ. Adaptation of bulk constitutive equations to insoluble monolayer collapse at the air–water interface. Science 1999; 283:1730–1733.

42. Goerke J, Gonzales J. Temperature dependence of dipalmitoyl phosphatidylcholine monolayer stability. J Appl Physiol 1981; 51:1108–1114.

43. Boonman A, Machiels FHJ, Snik AFM, Egberts J. Squeeze-out from mixed monolayers of dipalmitoylphosphatidylcholine and egg phosphatidylglycerol. J Colloid Interf Sci 1987; 120:456–468.

44. Crane JM, Hall SB. Rapid compression transforms interfacial monolayers of pulmonary surfactant. Biophys J 2001; 80:1863–1872.

45. Smith EC, Crane JM, Laderas TG, Hall SB. Metastability of a supercompressed fluid monolayer. Biophys J 2003; 85:3048–3057.

46. Debenedetti PG. Metastable Liquids: Concepts and Principles. Princeton, NJ: Princeton University Press, 1996.

47. Christian JW. The Theory of Transformations in Metals and Alloys: an Advanced Textbook in Physical Metallurgy. Oxford, New York: Pergamon Press, 1965.

48. Reed-Hill RE, Abbaschian R. Physical Metallurgy Principles. Boston: PWS-Kent Pub., 1992.

49. Rugonyi S, Smith EC, Hall SB. Transformation diagrams for the collapse of a phospholipid monolayer. Langmuir 2004; 20:10100–10106.

50. Davis PJ, Fleming BD, Coolbear KP, Keough KMW. Gel to liquid-crystalline transition temperatures of water dispersions of two pairs of positional isomers of unsaturated mixed-acid phosphatidylcholines. Biochemistry 1981; 20:3633–3636.

51. Smith EC, Laderas TG, Crane JM, Hall SB. Persistence of metastability after return of a supercompressed fluid monolayer to equilibrium conditions. Langmuir 2004; 20:4945–4953.

52. Courtney TH. Mechanical Behavior of Materials. New York: McGraw-Hill, 1990:330.

53. Clements JA, Trahan HJ. Effect of temperature on pressure–volume characteristics of rat lungs. Fed Proc 1963; 22:281.

54. Clements JA. The alveolar lining layer. In: De Reuck AVS, Porter R, eds. Development of the Lung. Boston: Little, Brown and Company, 1967:202–228.

55. Inoue H, Inoue C, Hildebrandt J. Temperature effects on lung mechanics in air- and liquid-filled rabbit lungs. J Appl Physiol 1982; 53:567–575.

56. Inoue H, Inoue C, Hildebrandt J. Temperature and surface forces in excised rabbit lungs. J Appl Physiol 1981; 51:823–829.

8

Surfactant and Airway Liquid Flows

DONALD P. GAVER III

Tulane University,
New Orleans, Louisiana, USA

OLIVER E. JENSEN

University of Nottingham,
Nottingham, UK

DAVID HALPERN

University of Alabama,
Tuscaloosa, Alabama, USA

I. Introduction

Our goal for this chapter is to provide an overview of research related to inter-facial phenomena and liquid-lining flows in airways. To do so, we first present the physiological significance of surface-tension-driven phenomena within the lung. Next, in order to explain the physical mechanisms that are responsible for physiological responses, we present a brief overview of fundamental surface-tension-driven interfacial phenomena that are generally responsible for liquid-lining flows. From this framework, we explore a range of different inter-facial flows that occur within pulmonary airways, and discuss the importance of surfactants on these flows.

II. Physiological Significance of Airway Lining Flows and Surface Tension in the Lung

By all accounts, Von Neergaard (1) was the first to recognize that surface tension forces are of fundamental importance in defining the mechanical characteristics of the lung. This relationship was evident after volume-cycling a lung filled with a gum arabic–saline solution, which resulted in a decrease in pressure over that required during the cycling of an air-filled lung. Von Neergaard reasoned that the absence of an air–water interface in the liquid-inflated lung caused the press-ure differences and that "in all states of expansion, surface tension was respon-sible for a greater part of lung elastic recoil than was tissue elasticity." Nearly three decades later, Pattle (2) demonstrated the stability of bubbles created in both lung edema fluid and fluid extracted from healthy lungs, suggesting that surface-active substances (surfactants) exist in the lining fluid. Shortly thereafter, Clements (3) demonstrated the surface tension/surface-area relationship of lung extracts. In 1958, Clements et al. (4) used a simple theoretical argument to suggest that this behavior could stabilize pulmonary alveoli.

Surfactant insufficiency is a significant contributor to pulmonary disease. In 1959, Avery and Mead (5) showed that surface-active material is diminished or absent in the lungs of infants with hyaline membrane disease, now known as respiratory distress syndrome (RDS). RDS results from lung immaturity at birth, which produces a high lining-fluid surface tension and a propensity for airway closure, atelectasis of portions of the lung, and inhomogeneous ventilation. Other diseases such as acute or adult respiratory distress syndrome (ARDS), though caused by other processes, can result in surfactant insufficiency that exacerbates the disease. Studies have also indicated that surfactant deficiency can play a role in asthma (6,7), though the evidence for this is inconclusive.

RDS can be treated with mechanical ventilation; however, large pressures are required to open collapsed airways and alveoli. Mechanical ventilation can cause epithelial lesions due to both the peeling apart of the epithelial surfaces during opening and the over-distension of airways (8). Positive end expiratory pressure (PEEP) is commonly applied to recruit alveoli and prevent airway closure. During PEEP, the positive pressure that exists throughout the respiration cycle keeps the airways patent and reduces the possibility of epithelial damage during inspiration. Surfactant replacement therapy (SRT) has also been shown to be effective in the short-term treatment of neonatal RDS (9,10). Here the powerful self-spreading properties of surfactants (see Marangoni-stress description in Section III) on liquid substrates are exploited to promote rapid delivery of an exogenous surfactant to the periphery of a surfactant-deficient lung. Despite the success of SRT coupled with mechanical ventilation strategies, RDS remains the fourth leading cause of death of premature infants in the United States (11).

Treatment of ARDS has been greatly revised in the last half-decade with the recognition that ventilator-induced lung injury (VILI) can result from mechanical ventilation using conventional settings (12,13). Most mechanistic investigations of VILI have pointed to damage from large lung volumes that can occur during ventilation, which can damage small airways and alveoli by tissue stretch (volutrauma) (14–17). Evidence also exists that VILI can occur at low lung volumes due to cyclic opening and closing (recruitment and derecruitment) of small airways and alveoli. It has been hypothesized that PEEP should be applied to ventilate the lung between the lower inflection point (LIP) and upper inflection point (UIP) of the pressure–volume curve, which is thought to prevent volutrauma while minimizing recruitment/derecruitment damage. Studies have confirmed that protective-ventilation strategies can be beneficial (18). Nevertheless, due to ventilation inhomogeneity, it is possible that diseased lungs will experience volutrauma and/or recruitment/derecruitment damage even under protective-ventilation scenarios.

Lining fluid dynamics may influence recruitment/derecruitment damage to the lung. Muscedere et al. (19) suggest that damage to epithelial cells results from shear stress during the peeling motion that occurs during recruitment. However, as will be described in Section IV, the stress field on these cells is quite complex and current evidence suggests that the damage is likely to be due to intra-cell variation in normal stress (the stress component directed perpendicular to the cell wall). Hubmayr (20) suggests that the dependent portion of the lung is fluid-filled, and thus has expressed doubt that recruitment/derecruitment is responsible for damage to the lung. If this is the case, damage could be caused by edema fluid and foam that fill the dependent regions of the wet lung. Thus, high pressures are required to drive foam through the airways and inflate flooded alveoli. We outline specific physiological implications of lining fluid flows prior to our exploration of the physics of these flows.

A. Airway Closure

We define airway closure as the liquid obstruction of a single bronchus (or groups of bronchi) such that no airflow can pass by the site of occlusion. In general, closure may be classified into two types. The first type of closure is called "meniscus occlusion," in which fluid spans an undeformed airway. This prevents gas exchange by producing an impediment to convection and diffusion without appreciable modification of the airway geometry. Such an occlusion is depicted in Fig. 8.1(a); an early observation was reported by Macklem et al. (21) in cats' airways with diameters of ~0.05 cm. The second type of closure, "compliant collapse," is shown in Fig. 8.1(b), and has been observed in histological investigations (22). Here, the liquid occlusion induces a transmural pressure on the airway due to surface tension forces, which buckles the walls and holds them in apposition by the adhesive properties (surface tension and viscosity) of the lining fluid (23). In both types of closure, the occlusion provides a barrier to gas exchange.

Evidence for airway closure can be seen in Phase IV of N_2 washout experiments (24), but for normal individuals airway closure does not occur to a significant degree during typical tidal breathing (25). If the lung becomes more

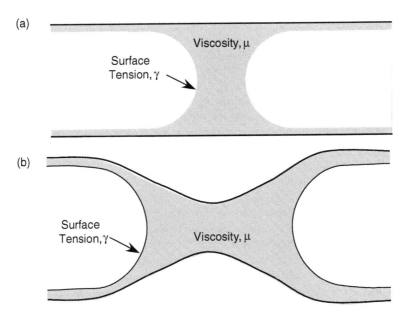

Figure 8.1 Schematic description of airway closure. (a) Meniscus occlusion. (b) Compliant collapse.

compliant, for example, due to emphysema or aging, airway closure can occur during normal tidal breathing, particularly at low lung volumes, and may define an individual's functional residual capacity (FRC). Takishima et al. (26) demonstrated that bronchi dissected free from parenchymal support were more likely to collapse than intact bronchi, indicating the importance of parenchymal tethering on the closure process. In addition, an edematous lung that has excess lining fluid can exhibit airway closure. It is common to assume that pressure above the LIP of the pressure–volume curve for patients with ARDS reflects the region where recruitment of closed airways occurs.

Ventilation inhomogeneity and ventilation/perfusion mismatch can occur if an airway remains closed for a significant portion of a tidal ventilation cycle. In addition, over-distension of patent regions of the lung can occur if positive-pressure ventilation is applied in order to attempt to reopen airways. In Sections IVA and IVB, we will explain how liquid-lining flows coupled to surfactant behavior can influence airway closure dynamics.

B. Airway Reopening

The introduction of air to a neonate's lungs and the reopening of an occluded airway are events where liquid-lining flows and interfacial phenomena can be physiologically significant. Macklem et al. (21) were the first to describe the (re)opening of airways as "gradually peeling apart the opposing walls and the liquid remaining *in situ* presumably lining that part of the bronchiole that had opened." A schematic of a reopening airway is shown in Fig. 8.2. Here, the airway is open on the left, with walls held in apposition on the right by the viscous liquid-lining fluid that "glues" the airway shut. To open the airway, a long bubble must propagate through the collapsed airway and separate the walls. On its first breath, a surfactant-deficient neonate may have trouble creating the substantial pressures needed to fully inflate the lung against the high surface tension at the surfactant-depleted air–liquid interface (27). When an RDS-neonate's lungs are inflated,

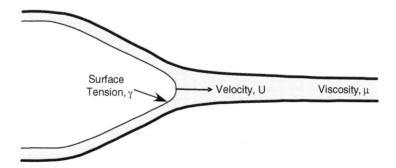

Figure 8.2 Schematic of airway re-opening. Semi-infinite bubble separates walls and penetrates viscous occlusion.

either through the infant's own effort or through mechanical ventilation, surfactant deficiency or tissue compliance may cause mechanical instability that could lead to airway closure. This may further result in atelectasis and thus decreased lung volume and hypoxemia. Yap et al. (28) demonstrated the influence of parenchymal tethering on airway reopening by modification of pleural pressure. This study showed that reopening behavior can exhibit unstable fluttering at low pleural pressure, stable peeling reopening at intermediate parenchymal tethering, and rapid "popping" open with large parenchymal tethering.

During the process of airway opening, lining fluid stresses may damage airway epithelial cells. Muscedere et al. (19) have shown that repetitive opening and closing can induce tissue damage. Tasker et al. (29) have shown that if surfactant is not deficient, repetitive reopening is not damaging; however, if surfactant deficiency exists the lung is more vulnerable to damage.

In Section IV.C, we present experimental and computational studies that explore the importance of liquid-lining flows and interfacial phenomena on reopening behavior. These studies investigate the macroscopic phenomena that determine reopening pressures, and micromechanical events that establish the mechanical stresses that can occur at the cellular level. We also explore the influence of surfactant on the reopening system. In Section IV.D, we discuss physical models for the spreading of exogenous surfactant through patent airways in SRT, and the mechanisms by which ventilation can be used to propel and disrupt liquid plugs within airways.

C. Summary

Although the damage mechanisms have not been precisely determined, it is evident that interfacial flows and fluid–structure interactions in the lung are instrumental to VILI at low lung volumes as well as the etiology of pulmonary diseases such as RDS, ARDS, and asthma. These may result in direct tissue damage, or cellular mechanotransduction related to tissue deformation, edema, inflammation, and tissue mechano-structural properties. These responses have generally been termed "biotrauma" and can elicit a host of responses in the lung including tissue remodeling (30,31), the release of cytokines (32), the up-regulation of surfactant production and release (33), and apoptosis (34,35). Some of these responses could contribute to multiple system organ failure (36).

Advances in our understanding of surfactant biophysical properties are the focus of most of this book, and thus will not be covered in detail in this chapter. Instead, we will focus on how the biophysical properties influence lining fluid flows related to disease. In the following sections, we will demonstrate that the intricate relationship between surfactant physical and chemical properties and hydrodynamic flows is central to the understanding and treatment of surfactant-related pulmonary disease.

III. Interfacial Phenomena

Before treating specific airway flows, we review briefly some of the physical laws dictating how surface tension and surfactants generate flows. Surface tension originates at a molecular level; since liquid molecules attract one another more strongly than air molecules, liquid near an air–liquid interface experiences a net force perpendicular to the interface that acts to minimize the interfacial area. A convenient way in which to characterize this force is to endow the air–liquid interface with an effective surface tension γ. Just as the tension in the skin of a balloon balances the difference in pressure between the air inside and outside the balloon, so surface tension balances the pressure jump across an air–liquid interface. Statically, this balance is expressed by the Young–Laplace equation

$$p_l - p_g = \gamma \kappa \tag{8.1}$$

where p_l is the liquid pressure; p_g, the gas pressure; and κ, the curvature of the interface, so that

$$\kappa = \pm \frac{1}{R_1} \pm \frac{1}{R_2} \tag{8.2}$$

where R_1 and R_2 are radii of curvature in orthogonal planes. Note that if the interface is convex relative to the liquid, $\kappa > 0$; if it is concave, $\kappa < 0$. For a flat interface, $\kappa = 0$; for a cylindrical interface of radius R, $\kappa = -1/R$ [Fig. 8.3(a)]; and for a spherical interface of radius R, $\kappa = -2/R$ [Fig. 8.3(b)]. In general, the curvature of an interface is more complex, as demonstrated in Fig. 8.3(c).

When the air–liquid interface assumes a shape with nonuniform κ, Eq. (8.1) implies that the pressure in the liquid will also be nonuniform. A surface-tension-driven flow will then drive the liquid from regions of high to low pressure, redistributing the liquid until κ is uniform (at least locally). This behavior is demonstrated in a 2-D example in Fig. 8.4(a).

When a surfactant adsorbs to an air–liquid interface, the intermolecular forces are modified due to the surfactant's hydrophilic head groups. This reduces the intermolecular force acting perpendicular to the interface, lowering γ by an amount dependent on the local instantaneous surfactant surface concentration Γ. Since adsorption is a dynamic diffusion-mediated process, the history of interfacial compression and expansion influences the degree of surface tension reduction. We can nevertheless regard γ as generally a decreasing function of Γ, that is, $\gamma = F(\Gamma)$ where $dF/d\Gamma \leq 0$. Thus if Γ is spatially nonuniform, then so is γ. A small surface element sitting in the air–liquid interface where a variation of Γ exists will then experience higher γ on the side where Γ is lower and vice versa. The difference in surface tension across the element exerts a net stress (called a

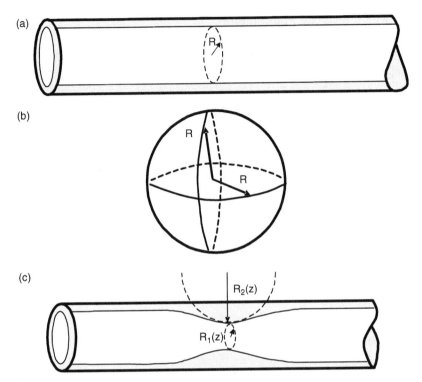

Figure 8.3 Curvature representations of different interface shapes. (a) Cylinder, $r_1 = R$, $r_2 = 0$, $\kappa = -1/R$, $p_1 - p_g = -\gamma/R$. (b) Spherical bubble, $r_1 = R$, $r_2 = R$, $\kappa = -2/R$, $p_1 - p_g = -2\gamma/R$. (c) Unduloid, $r_1 = R_1$, $r_2 = R_2$, $\kappa = -1/R_1 + 1/R_2$, $p_1 - p_g = \gamma(-1/R_1 + 1/R_2)$.

Marangoni stress, τ_M) that is tangential to the interface, directed toward the region of higher γ (and lower Γ). Thus, this tension imbalance causes the surface element to drag the viscous liquid beneath it through frictional (viscous) effects. The resulting flow, called a Marangoni flow, in which viscous drag balances surface tension gradients, leads to transport of both the liquid and the surfactant adsorbed at its surface, as illustrated in Fig. 8.4(b). Surfactant adsorbed nonuniformly to an air–liquid interface will, therefore, generate flows that drive both the liquid and the surfactant from regions of high to low surfactant concentration.

Both flow mechanisms described above (capillary and Marangoni) influence the distribution of liquids within airways and alveoli. Marangoni flows that endow surfactant monolayers with powerful self-spreading properties are discussed further in Section IVD. For the remainder of this section, we consider how airway liquids readjust under the effects of uniform surface tension when also subject to the geometric, physicochemical, and kinematic constraints imposed by nearby airway walls.

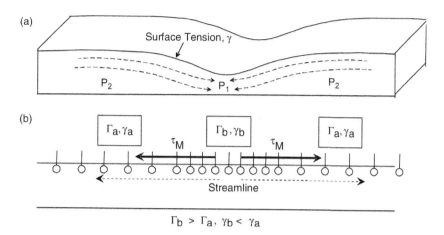

Figure 8.4   Descriptions of surface tension-driven flow. (a) Flow induced by local variation of curvature. $P_1 < P_2$, which drives a filling flow and (b) flow driven by surface tension variation along the interface. Here, the surfactant concentration Γ_b is greater than the neighboring concentration ($\Gamma_b > \Gamma_a$). This causes a local reduction of surface tension ($\gamma_b < \gamma_a$), which causes a tangential (Marangoni) stress, τ_M, that drags the top layer of fluid towards regions of higher surface tension.

A familiar example of the action of surface tension is the way in which a long cylinder of liquid spontaneously breaks up into droplets, an effect known as the Rayleigh (or capillary) instability. This can be observed during the spontaneous rupture of a thin filament of water from a faucet. This instability operates also in the situation in which a uniform, rigid cylinder (an idealized airway) is coated on its interior with an initially uniform layer of liquid [Fig. 8.5(a)]. Provided the cylinder and its lining are sufficiently long, the liquid may spontaneously readjust to a new configuration in which the air–liquid interface has lower surface area. This adjustment occurs through small disturbances to the liquid being magnified by surface-tension-driven flows. If the liquid lining is sufficiently thin, it readjusts to form a series of annular collars [Fig. 8.5(b)] separated by regions in which the liquid lining is substantially thinner, where it is ultimately controlled by long-range intermolecular or possibly electrostatic forces. The air–liquid interface of a static collar has a uniform curvature and the shape of an unduloid. If the liquid lining is sufficiently thick, however, the liquid can readjust to form isolated liquid bridges that occlude the tube [Fig. 8.5(c)], leading to the "meniscus occlusion" that is shown in Fig. 8.1(a). The liquid bridge has two hemispherical surfaces with a locally uniform curvature. This manifestation of the Rayleigh instability in the context of airway closure is discussed further in Section IV.B.

  The assumption that the liquid wets the cylinder wall, that is, liquid molecules are more strongly attracted to the wall than they are to themselves, is implicit in Fig. 8.5. In the opposite case, stronger liquid–liquid attractive forces can cause

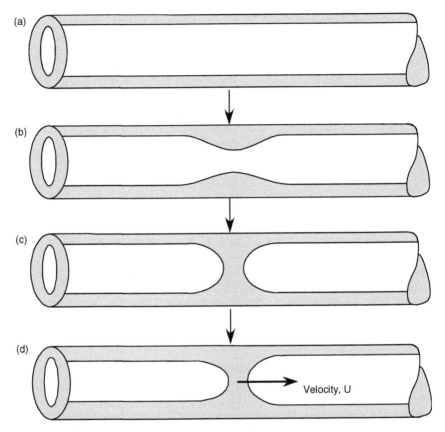

Figure 8.5 Stages of airway meniscus occlusion and motion. (a) Liquid lined tube, (b) development of an unduloid, (c) meniscus occlusion, (d) meniscus clearance (note the difference in upstream and downstream film thicknesses, which may result in a net loss of liquid to the meniscus and subsequent meniscus rupture).

a layer of liquid coating a wall to bead up spontaneously into droplets, such that the droplet's air–liquid interface meets the wall with a nonzero contact angle. [In contrast, the interfaces of the collars and bridges in Fig. 8.5(b) and (c) approach the cylinder wall tangentially, i.e., with zero contact angles.] Wetting effects are strongly dependent on material properties and can have a profound influence on the distribution of thin layers of liquid. As surfactants tend to promote wetting, it is reasonable to assume that lung liquids have small or zero contact angles on airway walls, forming macroscopic structures (such as collars or bridges) that can exist in equilibrium with neighboring ultra-thin adsorbed liquid layers. This assumption is supported by scanning electron microscopic images of rat alveoli, which show a thin continuous liquid lining adjoining deeper pools, for example, in alveolar corners (37). Regulation of liquid thickness via fluxes across the airway epithelium, controlled by either passive (osmotic) or active (e.g., ion-channel-mediated) mechanisms, is also undoubtedly significant (38,39).

Once a liquid bridge has formed in a cylinder of radius say, R, it can be displaced by blowing into one end of the cylinder. This pushes the bridge along the cylinder at speed say, U, a process described in more detail in Sections IV.C and IV.D. Since the liquid is viscous and is assumed to have a high affinity for the cylinder wall, a thin film of liquid will be deposited on the wall behind the advancing liquid bridge [Fig. 8.5(d)]. The faster the bridge moves relative to the wall, the greater the viscous forces that drag liquid out of the bridge, and the thicker the deposited film. As the flux of liquid out of the bridge increases the area of the air–liquid interface, surface tension acts to limit this flux. It does so by generating a flow that draws liquid from the cylindrical film [where $p_1 \approx p_g - \gamma/R$; Eq. (8.1)] back into the bridge (where $p_1 \approx p_g - 2\gamma/R$). The film thickness h is, therefore, determined predominantly by a balance between viscosity and surface tension, and may be expressed as $h/R = f(\text{Ca})$. Here the capillary number Ca ($=\mu U/\gamma$) is a dimensionless parameter, that is, a measure of the relative importance of viscous and surface tension forces, where μ is the liquid viscosity. The function $f(\text{Ca})$ increases with Ca, rising smoothly from $f(\text{Ca}) \approx 1.34\text{Ca}^{2/3}$ when Ca < 0.01 (when the flow is very slow and surface tension dominates) to $f(\text{Ca}) \approx 0.36$ when Ca $\gg 1$, when the flow becomes rapid enough for viscous forces to dominate surface tension (40). The notation "$\gg$" denotes "much greater than." This valve-like behavior of surface tension turns out to limit the rate at which a collapsed airway can be reopened by an advancing bubble of air (see Section IV.C). Note that another dimensionless parameter often associated with fluid flows, the Reynolds number, is generally small in peripheral-airway flows, implying that viscous forces dominate liquid inertia.

Gravity also competes with surface tension in controlling the distribution of airway liquid. The two forces are of comparable magnitude in airways with radii comparable to the capillary length $L = (\gamma/\rho g)^{1/2}$, where ρ is the density difference between liquid and air and g is the acceleration due to gravity. L is of the order of 1 mm for water in air, for example. A dimensionless parameter Bo $= R^2/L^2 = \rho g R^2/\gamma$ (the Bond number) captures the relative importance of the two effects in an airway of radius R. Generally, provided that the Bond number is very small (Bo $\ll 1$; e.g., in airways with sub-millimeter dimensions), capillary effects dominate, although slow gravity-driven flows may have a significant effect over long times.

IV. Physiological Interfacial Flows

On the basis of these observations, we now describe four related classes of airway liquid flow. We discuss how surface tension controls the distribution of airway liquid within deformable airways (Section IVA), mechanisms of airway closure and reopening (Sections IVB and IVC) and the motion of surfactant and liquid plugs along airways (Section IVD). For additional information about some of the fluid mechanical interactions that are described herein, we refer the reader to review articles by Grotberg (41,42).

A. Liquid Redistribution

There has been considerable recent interest in extending our understanding of interfacial flows in idealized systems (such as long rigid cylinders) to more realistic geometries characteristic of the lung. Focusing largely on peripheral airways and alveoli, where gravitational effects are weak and mucus-secreting cells are less common (so that the liquid lining can be represented to a crude first approximation by a single-phase Newtonian liquid), modelers and experimentalists have investigated the effects of, in particular, complex airway geometries and airway wall deformability on airway liquid redistribution.

Airway Geometry

In contrast to Fig. 8.5, airways are short, branching, and curved. Quite unlike a uniform cylinder, for which κ is uniform, the walls of real airways have curvature that is in general spatially nonuniform. We cannot expect the thin interior liquid lining of a typical airway to exist as a uniform-thickness equilibrium coating, since such a film will share the nonuniform curvature of the wall, leading to a nonuniform liquid pressure p_l [see Eq. (8.1)] which can drive flows that redistribute the liquid. Jensen (43) illustrated this in the special case of a uniformly but weakly curved tube with a thin liquid lining, for which curvature-induced pressure gradients drive the liquid lining from one side of the tube to the other (away from the center of centerline curvature). This disrupts the annular collars shown in Fig. 8.5(b), causing them to form isolated drops, drops connected by rivulets, or a single uniform rivulet, depending on the degree of tube curvature and the liquid volume. Coincidentally, identical behavior arises also in straight, liquid-lined horizontal tubes at low Bond numbers (when surface tension effects dominate gravity), illustrating how even weak gravitational effects can have profound effects on equilibrium liquid distributions. At low liquid volumes, therefore, we may expect the liquid lining of real airways generically to accumulate as rivulets running along the bottom of an airway, or along paths where the wall curvature is greatest, while the remainder of the airway wall is coated with a much thinner layer of adsorbed liquid. Understanding how rivulet distributions depend on airway geometry and gravity is important, since they provide the primary pathways for surfactant transport along airways [(44); see Section IV.D].

Airway Deformability

As indicated in Section III, surface tension causes the pressure within a liquid film coating the interior of a tube, or within a liquid bridge, to be sub-atmospheric. The higher the surface tension, or the smaller the tube radius, the lower the pressure and therefore the stronger the compressive force exerted on the tube wall. Thus in addition to driving airway closure through liquid-bridge formation [leading to meniscus occlusion, see Fig. 8.5(c) or 8.1(a) and Section IV.B]), surface tension can also lead to airway occlusion by causing the airway to collapse either locally (in the neighborhood of a liquid bridge) or globally (causing the airway to become completely flooded with liquid), leading to compliant collapse [Fig. 8.1(b)].

Halpern and Grotberg (45) used a theoretical model to show that compliant collapse in an elastic tube may occur before meniscus occlusion if surface tension is sufficiently strong compared to elastic forces in the tube wall (see Section IVB). Their model assumes that the tube and its liquid lining collapse axisymmetrically. In reality, however, elastic tubes—and airways—collapse into buckled, nonaxisymmetric configurations. In peripheral airways, the relatively inextensible epithelium and its supporting basement membrane are surrounded by a mucosal layer that in turn may be surrounded by smooth muscle. When subject to a low transmural pressure, or to external muscular compression, the epithelium buckles as the airway lumen shrinks, forming a rosette structure in which bending forces in the epithelium and basement membrane provide a significant load-bearing structure (46). The number of buckled lobes (and therefore the overall airway compliance and resistance to airflow) is controlled predominantly by the mechanical and geometrical properties of each layer of the airway wall, and so the buckling process is implicated in the remodeling of asthmatic airways [see Ref. (30,47,48)]. The liquid lining within the lumen of a buckled airway must adjust to this highly nonuniform geometry. At low liquid volumes, the liquid will accumulate where the wall curvature is greatest, namely, as rivulets in the extreme corners of each fold in the airway wall. During bronchoconstriction, however, the folds in the airways narrow, and may quickly be filled by lining fluid: the net effect is that the proportion of the lumen accessible to air may reduce rapidly, increasing resistance to airflow (49) (Fig. 8.6).

The readjustment of airway liquid to the geometry of the airway wall can also have a profound effect on overall airway mechanics, because there may be strong coupling between liquid distribution, the distribution of compressive stresses arising from low liquid pressures and airway wall shape. This has motivated recent theoretical investigations of so-called capillary-elastic instabilities in airways. Hill et al. (50), for example, computed static wall and liquid distributions in a single lobe of an axially uniform, collapsed elastic tube, showing how motion of the air–liquid interface across the neck of the lobe leads to multiple steady configurations for the same parameter values, and consequently hysteresis in the tube's pressure–volume relationship. Readjustment of the airway wall and the interior liquid may therefore contribute to pressure–volume hysteresis of an airway, and hence the whole lung. Hill et al. identified a dimensionless deformation parameter $W = \gamma R^2 / D$ that characterizes the relative importance of surface tension γ to wall flexural rigidity D and airway radius R; there remains

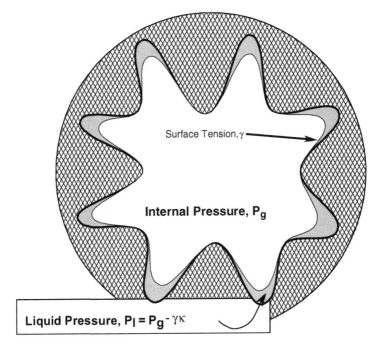

Figure 8.6 Schematic cross-section of a bronchonstricted airway demonstrating a capillary-elastic airway instability. Bronchoconstriction of the airway causes folds of the airway. These folds can fill with lining fluid that can amplify bronchoconstriction due to surface tension-induced pressures. This also reduces the portion of the lumen available for airflow, increasing airflow resistance (38,50).

considerable uncertainty in the literature over what are realistic values of W should be, however. Nevertheless, more recent theoretical models (51,52) have shown that if either the liquid volume or W is sufficiently large, a liquid-lined, axially uniform, nonaxisymmetrically buckled elastic tube can exhibit both hysteresis and compliant collapse, that is, abrupt flooding. These models complement further studies of Heil (53,54), who computed the shape and volume of the smallest static liquid bridge required to occlude a flexible tube. Together, models such as these are beginning to provide a reasonably clear picture of the static behavior of liquid-lined elastic tubes, by identifying necessary conditions for airway occlusion. Much remains to be discovered about dynamical airway readjustment, however, accounting for the effects of, for example, surfactant, airway smooth muscle constriction and active transmural fluid fluxes.

B. Airway Closure

Effective pulmonary ventilation is subject to the availability of free passageways between the mouth and the alveoli. It can be significantly hindered by closure of the small airways that cut off peripheral respiratory units. As described earlier, airway closure may arise through meniscus occlusion following a surface tension-driven instability of the liquid film that coats the inner surface of an airway [Figs. 8.1(a) and 8.5(c)]. Liquid draining from the thin film into a growing liquid plug can also induce airway wall collapse due to an increase in the pressure difference across the airway wall in the region of the obstruction, leading to compliant collapse [Fig. 8.1(b)], with the airway walls held in apposition by their liquid lining often along a considerable length of the airway. A number of theoretical and experimental studies have been undertaken to establish how factors such as pulmonary surfactant, the viscoelastic properties of the liquid film and the airway wall, airway geometry, and liquid volume influence these mechanisms of airway closure.

To test Macklem's (55) hypothesis that airway closure arises through a surface tension-induced instability of the liquid lining, Kamm and Schroter (56) experimentally simulated small airway closure using liquid-lined rigid tubes, to exclude possible compliant collapse. This study showed that there exists a minimum volume of lining fluid required for meniscus formation, and that the ratio of liquid volume to airway diameter needed to induce instability is relatively independent of airway length. Below this critical volume, the film readjusts to form stable unduloids [Fig. 8.5(b)] that do not occlude the tube. This has been confirmed through a series of theoretical studies. Dynamic unduloid formation by a thin viscous film coating the interior of a cylindrical tube of circular cross-section was described by Hammond (57) using lubrication theory, a simplified form of the governing equations of fluid mechanics that exploits the slender geometry of the liquid film. Liquid bridge formation by a thicker fluid layers was captured using extensions of Hammond's model by Gauglitz and Radke (58) (retaining an accurate expression for the film curvature) and Johnson et al. (59) (accounting also for fluid inertia). These studies identified a critical film thickness $h_c \approx 0.14R$ for meniscus formation in a cylindrical tube of radius R: below this critical thickness the film evolves to stable unduloids, above it the film becomes unstable and forms liquid bridges. Time-scales for the generation of liquid bridges were calculated to be in the order of 65 ms using realistic airway parameters (59). According to these models, meniscus occlusion in airways is most likely to occur at the end of expiration, when R is smallest and the liquid lining thickness is most likely to exceed h_c.

Since the collapsibility of airways increases peripherally (22,23), the likelihood of compliant collapse increases, and this has therefore been included in subsequent theoretical models of airway closure [45,59–63]. These share a common framework in which equations describing the time evolution of the film and wall positions are derived by applying conservation of fluid mass and momentum, again exploiting the slender geometry of the liquid lining to simplify the analysis. An equation for conservation of surfactant along the air–liquid interface may also be incorporated. Halpern and Grotberg (45) used this approach to study the coupled effects of wall compliance, liquid lining viscosity and surface tension. The results of this study demonstrated that wall flexibility enhances closure and that h_c decreases with increasing wall flexibility. Compliant collapse [Fig. 8.1(b)] was predicted for sufficiently floppy tubes or for high surface tension (i.e., for sufficiently large values of the deformation parameter W), and collapse was found to occur within a fraction of a millisecond. The studies of Heil (53,54) demonstrated the importance of nonaxisymmetric wall buckling by showing that the minimum volume required for the formation of a static liquid plug in a compliant tube can be as much as ten times smaller than the volume needed to block an axisymmetric tube. Thus a film coating a compliant tube that does not contain enough fluid to form an axisymmetric plug can nevertheless undergo a nonaxisymmetric instability leading to meniscus occlusion.

The greatest reduction in surface tension due to compression of pulmonary surfactant occurs at the end of expiration, before the interfacial surfactant has had sufficient time to desorb appreciably into the liquid bulk, a property that increases lung compliance (64). This time corresponds to that at which an airway is most likely to be prone to capillary instability. To examine theoretically how effectively surfactant stabilizes airways, Otis et al. (63) extended the model of Johnson et al. (59) by including surfactant within the film and demonstrated a stabilization effect, in that meniscus-formation times were increased by up to a factor of four [see also benchtop experiments by Cassidy et al. (65)]. These benchtop experiments were intended to investigate airway closure, using a viscous oil simulate the liquid layer coating the lung, and water as the core fluid. The viscosity ratio of these two fluids was similar to that encountered in the lung, and the density ratio of the two fluids was nearly unity in order to avoid gravitational effects. It was found that surfactant could decrease the initial growth rate of the capillary instability to 20% of the surfactant-free case. This compares favorably with theoretical estimates that predict a growth-rate decrease of $\sim$25%. They also estimated closure times, which were shown to be four times longer than the surfactant-free case. Halpern and Grotberg (60) examined the effects of surfactant in their model of a liquid-lined flexible tube, and found likewise that surfactant delayed closure times by approximately a factor of five provided the tube wall was not too compliant. The stabilizing effects of surfactant in maintaining the patency of liquid-lined tubes was also demonstrated in a benchtop system by Enhörning and coworkers (66).

Recently, Halpern and Grotberg (67) have considered the nonlinear instability of a thin film coating the inner surface of a rigid tube. These studies have been used to explore the effect of an imposed oscillatory core flow by assuming, to a first approximation, an uncoupled core-film. Lubrication theory is used to derive a nonlinear evolution equation for the position of the air–liquid interface. It is shown that if the frequency and amplitude of the core flow are sufficiently large, than the capillary instability can be saturated, that is, closure does not occur.

Surfactant-deficient neonates, who are especially prone to problems caused by airway closure, can be treated with high-frequency ventilation (HFV) which uses lower tidal volumes and higher frequencies than conventional modes of ventilation (68,69). The use of smaller volumes is beneficial since the lung parenchyma in these neonates is particularly fragile and the high peak pressures used in conventional methods of ventilation can be harmful. HFV also offers the advantage of improved carbon dioxide removal at lower pressures (70,71), and has also been used in treating adults (72–75). In order to provide some insight on how frequency and tidal volume impact airway closure, Halpern et al. (62) investigated theoretically the stability of a viscous film coating a compliant tube, including the effects of an oscillatory shear stress on the film due to the airflow. A stability analysis showed that a time-periodic shear stress could significantly dampen the fastest growing small-amplitude disturbances to the film, provided the airway wall was compliant. Furthermore, nonlinear saturation of the disturbances is possible provided the frequency and amplitude of the oscillatory shear stress are sufficiently large (61). If a liquid bridge does form via meniscus occlusion, it may be pushed along an airway by pressure drops encountered during the breathing cycle. Motion of the liquid bolus and its possible rupture are discussed in Section IV.D.

C. Airway Reopening

As described in Section III, premature neonates who are born prior to surfactant system maturity may suffer from RDS due to a deficiency in surfactant production. In contrast to healthy infants who take their first breath and open their lungs, infants with RDS cannot overcome the abnormally high resistance to airflow induced by the excessive surface tension of the lining fluid. Instead, the air–liquid interface that forms in the trachea progresses through several generations of airways, but presumably stops when the pressure drop across the air–liquid interface equals the pressure drop for a static meniscus. This pressure is proportional to the surface tension, γ, and inversely proportional to the airway radius, R [see Eq. (8.1)]. Similar situations can occur with adults suffering from obstructive lung disease such as emphysema and ARDS. The present section will outline the research studies that have investigated the complex fluid–structure interactions related to the opening of collapsed airways and the influence that surfactant plays on this system.

Benchtop Experiments

Benchtop experiments have been very useful in identifying pressure–velocity relationships for reopening of occluded airways. Classically, the static pressure drop for a hemispherical liquid interface occluding a cylindrical tube is given from Eq. (8.1) by $p_g - p_1 = 2\gamma/R$. The original investigations by Macklem (21) assumed that this pressure drop would define the reopening pressure for a closed airway. For rigid airways, this result is consistent with analysis by Bretherton (76) and experiments by Fairbrother and Stubbs (77), Taylor (78), and more recently by Hsu (79). However, these predictions may not hold for compliantly collapsed airways.

The most idealized experiments describing the opening of compliant airways have identified the modification of the pressure drop that occurs when a flaccid circular tube is allowed to flatten to a "ribbon-like" configuration where airway walls are in direct apposition as shown in Fig. 8.2 (80). In these studies, a thin-walled floppy tube coated with a viscous fluid was held open on one end to radius R, and tapered axially to a ribbon-like region entirely filled with lining fluid of initial thickness H with an applied axial tension T. When flow was applied to the gas phase, the pressure initially increased to a maximum value, then decreased as the air–liquid interface (meniscus) progressed down the tube and opened the airway at a nearly constant pressure.

When Newtonian fluids of constant surface tension are investigated, dimensional analysis of experimental data reveals an approximately universal relationship that describes the relationship between the tube radius (R), and the lining fluid properties:

$$\frac{P_{Total}}{(\gamma/R)} = 7.9 + 10.3\,Ca^{0.8} \tag{8.3}$$

Here $Ca = \mu U/\gamma$ is the capillary number introduced in Section III, representing the relative magnitudes of viscous to surface tension forces, and P_{Total} is the upstream gas-phase pressure. This result shows that a "yield pressure" of approximately $8\gamma/R$ must be overcome before any positive velocity (i.e., reopening) can occur [Fig. 8.7(a)]. A 2-D experimental model of reopening demonstrated an ~50% decrease in the yield pressure (81), indicating that the 3-D meniscus curvature increases the yield pressure. In addition, the 2-D studies demonstrated the possibility of unstable reopening at low reopening velocities (81).

Subsequent benchtop experimental investigations have identified the reopening characteristics of more complex systems. Non-Newtonian fluids that might resemble mucus were studied by Hsu and colleagues (82–84). These studies show that fluid elasticity can significantly affect the pressure–velocity relationship for reopening by inducing flow instabilities at large reopening velocity due to a sol–gel transition in the viscoelastic properties. In other studies, the effect of parenchymal tethering was investigated experimentally (85); these studies indicate that tethering stresses will reduce the airway pressure necessary to inflate a compliant airway. Thus, a reduction of tethering (e.g., emphysema) could greatly increase the airway pressure necessary to maintain airway patency.

In summary, the experimental studies demonstrate that fluid properties (particularly γ and μ) and airway mechanical properties exert profound influences upon the macroscopic pressure–velocity relationship for airway reopening. Since surfactant properties will determine the dynamic surface tension of the air–liquid

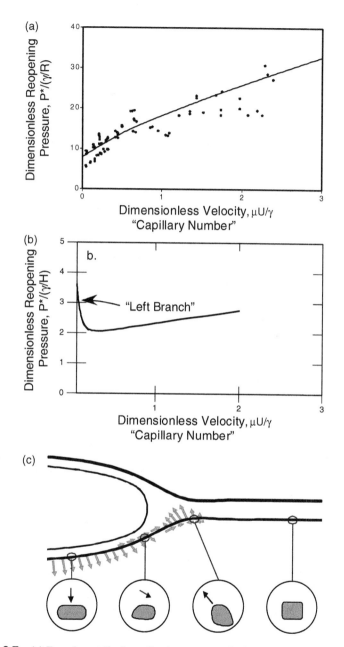

Figure 8.7 (a) Experimentally determined pressure–velocity relationship for the steady-state opening of a flexible airway. Data from Gaver et al. (80), (b) computationally-determined pressure–velocity relationship for the steady-state reopening of a compliant airway. Note the existence of a "left-branch" that is not experimentally observed, (c) stress-field for cells in the neighborhood of airway reopening.

interface, the interaction between fluid flow and surfactant transport is likely to play an important role in airway reopening, as will be demonstrated below.

Physiological Observations

Experiments to examine airway-specific reopening behavior are difficult to conduct due to the small sizes of occluded airways and the complexity of identifying the exact site of occlusion. To identify reopening phenomena for specific airways, Naureckas et al. (27) investigated the reopening of closed tantalum-coated airways. In this preparation, they were able to induce compliant collapse in 0.5–3.0 mm airways. Reopening occurred by application of a positive pressure and demonstrated a yield pressure of approximately $8\gamma/R$, consistent with the benchtop experiments of Gaver et al. (80). However, unlike the benchtop paradigm, most airways were observed to "pop" open instead of reopening at a constant velocity.

Ex vivo canine lung experiments by Yap et al. (28) and Otis et al. (86) used the alveolar capsule technique to observe the pressure signature that occurs when a collapsed peripheral airway was reopened. Yap et al., showed that if parenchymal tethering was small, airway closure would recur after reopening, resulting in an unstable low-frequency fluttering response. However, if parenchymal tethering was increased, the airway would remain patent after it was reopened (28). The studies by Otis et al., support the existence of compliant collapse as leading to airway closure and demonstrated reopening pressures that were consistent with 3-D benchtop experiments by Gaver et al. (80). Furthermore, the reopening pressure signature indicated a sequence of reopening events, suggesting either that closure exists at multiple discrete sites (as opposed to one long continuous region of collapse) or that reopening proceeds as a series of stepwise events along airway segments with a reduction in velocity at airway bifurcations.

In summary, *ex vivo* investigations not only confirm the importance of lining fluid properties on airway reopening, but also emphasize the direct coupling between interfacial phenomena and structural properties on the stability of airway reopening.

Theoretical Investigations of Fluid–Structure Interactions

Single-Airway Reopening

In order to develop a more exact understanding of reopening phenomena, a number of investigators have performed analytical and computational investigations of phenomena that are relevant to airway reopening. The first computational investigation of airway reopening was conducted to model steady reopening in a planar configuration following the 3-D benchtop experimental investigation of flaccid tube reopening (87). This study demonstrated the complex time-dependent stress field that is exerted on airway tissue as the bubble progresses to reopen the airway, as shown schematically in Fig. 8.7(c).

These stresses include the upstream pressure that is exerted on all patent airways upstream of the closure along with transient inward normal stresses and shear stresses that exist near the bubble tip. Spatial variations of these mechanical stresses may be significant to cells, as demonstrated by the recent experimental findings of Bilek et al. (88).

Recent computational investigations have been very useful in explaining reopening phenomena in more realistic situations. Heil and colleagues have performed finite-element computations of reopening that provide insight into some of the errors induced by simplification of the physiological model. For example, Heil has shown that fluid inertia can be significant if $Re/Ca > 1$, where Re is the Reynolds number that relates inertia to viscous effects (89,90). In this case, inertia leads to significant changes in the velocity and pressure fields near the bubble tip and can modify wall deformation. This may influence the wall shape, influencing the stresses exerted on airway tissue.

One curious aspect of steady-state computations is the prediction of two "branches" of the pressure–velocity response [see Fig. 8.7(b)]. At low velocities, the simulations indicate that an increase in velocity is accompanied by a counter-intuitive reduction of reopening pressure (the so-called "left" branch that results in a "pushing" motion). In contrast, the high-speed (or "peeling") branch predicts that an increase in pressure is accompanied by an increase in reopening velocity, as observed experimentally. This behavior is not an artifact of a 2-D model, as it also appears in more realistic 3-D models where the tube is collapsed into a dumbbell shape (91). However, with a nonlinear pressure-area relation such as that exhibited by a 3-D buckled tube, the negative transmural pressure where the tube is buckled can significantly decrease the air-phase pressure necessary to reopen the tube to such a degree that spontaneous reopening can occur (91).

Jensen and colleagues (92–94) have developed asymptotic mathematical models that can explain the existence of the low- and high-speed branches. This analysis divides the domain to three regimes, with the flow determined by different balances of forces in each region. The bubble-tip region acts like a low-Reynolds-number valve that determines the flow rate of the entire system. As such, the geometry and surface tension of the bubble-tip region is instrumental in determining the global behavior of the reopening system. These studies indicate that the "yield pressure" identified experimentally [see Eq. (8.3)] has a contribution both from quasistatic capillary forces [through Eq. (8.1)] and dynamic viscous pressure losses (93) and that wall permeability can introduce a further bend in the pressure–velocity curve at very low bubble speeds (94). Recently, theoretical investigations by Halpern, Jensen, and colleagues have been developed to investigate the stability of the low- and high-speed branches. This analysis shows that the low-speed (left) branch is unstable when the bubble volume flux is held constant, which may relate to the low-speed instabilities observed experimentally (81). These studies (93) also reproduce the transient overshoot in bubble pressure seen on the initiation of reopening (81,85), an event that may be physiologically significant.

Several *ex vivo* experimental investigations have suggested that airway closure may result from small segments of occlusion by a liquid bolus (28,86). This bolus could shorten during motion if the rate at which fluid volume is left on the airway wall during propagation exceeds the rate at which volume accumulates at the front of the bolus. Liquid bolus motion is discussed further in Section IV.D.

Multiple-Airway Reopening

Interesting research by Suki and colleagues has been conducted to investigate the dynamic effects of reopening multiple branches of collapsed airways. Initial theoretical models (95) assumed that airways would open at a randomly selected reopening pressure if the parent airway was patent. This relatively simple model predicts "avalanche" responses with power-law behavior that is observed for self-organized systems. This model has been improved to include the effect of airway generation on the reopening pressure (96). Subsequent experimental investigations of the slow inflation of collapsed canine lobes demonstrate "crackles" with power-law behavior similar to those of the simulations (97). Size distributions of recruited alveolar volumes, as interpreted by regional tissue elastance, is also consistent with this avalanche model (98). A similar model has been used by Bates and Irvin (99) to investigate recruitment and dere-cruitment of alveoli. This model predicts first and second pressure–volume relationships for degassed lungs that are consistent with the physiological response of injured lungs.

In these models of multiple airway reopening and alveolar recruitment, the effects of lining fluid properties and airway geometry have largely been neg-lected. Yet, the phenomena described demonstrate qualitative and quantitative behavior that is similar to physiological measurements. We suspect that at the single-airway level the airway geometry and lining-fluid properties are necessary to determine the local response of the system. This is consistent with *ex vivo* observations of the reopening of a small number of occluded airways (27,28,86). However, it appears that at multi-generational scales, the inherent inhomogeneity of the pulmonary tree structure and lining fluid properties from generation-to-generation causes a more random reopening response than one would expect from the deterministic models that are relevant for single reopening events.

Influence of Surfactant on Airway Reopening

The experimental and computational investigations described earlier have assumed a constant surface tension interface, which is not realistic if surfactant exists within the lining fluid and the interface is moving. As described in Section III, surfactant that exists within the lining fluid (with concentration C) can be transported to and from the interface (with concentration Γ), which directly modifies the interfacial surface tension by $\gamma = F(\Gamma)$ (see Section III). Pulmonary surfactant is highly insoluble, so adsorption rates are far greater than desorption rates (100–102). Nevertheless, during the motion of a bubble, the interface can assume a nonuniform surface tension that can influence the mechanical behavior of the system.

To conceptualize this interaction, consider the flow field surrounding a bubble flowing down a liquid-filled tube as shown in Fig. 8.8. Streamlines are drawn in a bubble-fixed reference frame in which flow enters from the right and exits to the left in the thin film. A recirculating region near the bubble tip occurs at low velocities. As a result, the rate of interfacial expansion/compression will vary with interfacial position. Variation of the dynamic surface tension γ can alter the pressure required to push the bubble along the tube through a modification of the pressure drop across the air–liquid interface following the Young–Laplace law [Eq. (8.1)]. The elevation of the pressure drop due to dynamic surface tension effects has been referred to as a "nonequilibrium normal stress." In addition, variation of the surface tension along the air–liquid interface creates a surface tension gradient, which allows the interface to support a shear stress τ_M that is directed from low-to-high surface tension [see Fig. 8.4(b)]. The Marangoni stress always retards bubble motion, since it typically causes the interface to act as a rigid surface.

Several investigators have studied nonequilibrium surface tension effects in nonphysiological systems. Ratulowski and Chang (103) analytically modeled trace surfactant transport and evaluated several different scenarios related to hindered transport from the bulk to the interface. Fundamentally, two processes can hinder surfactant transport: diffusion limitation in the bulk and kinetic adsorption/desorption barriers from the subphase to the interface. The diffusion barrier can be reduced through an increase in bulk concentration (C), a scenario analyzed by Stebe and Barthes–Biesel (104). Under these large-C conditions, the

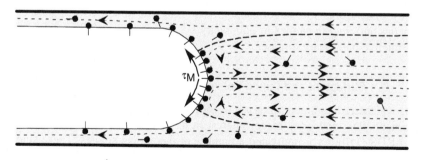

↓ represents surfactant molecule

Figure 8.8 Flow field and surfactant deposition during the steady motion of a semi-infinite bubble in a tube. τ_M represents the Marangoni-stresses that retard bubble motion due to surface tension gradients. While surfactant causes a net reduction in reopening pressure, these Marangoni stresses can modify the mechanical stresses on cells and influence reopening dynamics.

adsorption barrier will be the only limitation to surfactant transport. Therefore, equilibrium behavior at large C indicates fast adsorption properties. Recent computational investigations have explored the complex interactions that can occur during mixed-kinetics cases (105).

An analytical model used to investigate surfactant effects during airway reopening for collapsed airways was developed by Yap (106). This model assumed bulk equilibrium dynamics and investigated the effects of nonequilibrium surface tension due to interfacial sorption. This study indicates that dynamic surface tension can significantly influence airway-reopening dynamics under nonequilibrium conditions and increases the bubble pressure to values that are greater than would be expected under equilibrium surface tension conditions.

Experiments conducted to investigate dynamic surface tension effects with pulmonary surfactant have indicated that under steady reopening conditions, pulmonary surfactant maintains a surface tension that far exceeds equilibrium values (107), which will thus increase the pressure necessary to reopen pulmonary airways. So, even if highly concentrated surfactant is delivered to the airways, pressures necessary to open collapsed airways could be excessive due to adsorption limitations at the air–liquid interface. This may thus limit the efficacy of SRT (Section IV.D).

Recent studies by Gaver and colleagues have investigated whether pulsatile reopening can be used to take advantage of surfactant kinetics to reduce the pressures necessary to reopen a pulmonary airway. These studies have modified steady reopening investigations to add a small amplitude sinusoidal oscillation to the steady migration velocity (108,109). These investigations show that a small bubble-retraction phase can significantly reduce the interfacial pressure drop from that which occurs during steady motion (Fig. 8.9). However, this result was highly dependent on the amplitude and frequency of oscillation. This study underscores the importance of exploring the link between surfactant kinetics and fluid dynamics in pulmonary systems to optimize the treatment of obstructive pulmonary disease.

D. Surfactant and Liquid Delivery

The widespread and increasing use of SRT since the 1980s for the treatment of neonatal RDS, and more recent interest in its potential use in conditions such as ARDS (110), have motivated a number of theoretical studies. These studies analyze the physical mechanisms through which exogenous surfactant, delivered either as an aerosol or through an endotracheal tube, spreads to the periphery of the lung. A liquid bolus may also be delivered into the lung for other therapeutic purposes such as partial liquid ventilation and drug delivery. Different strategies may be employed in the delivery process. In some situations it may be advantageous for the bolus to be targeted to reach the alveoli or specific airway generations, whereas in other circumstances it may be more useful for the bolus to

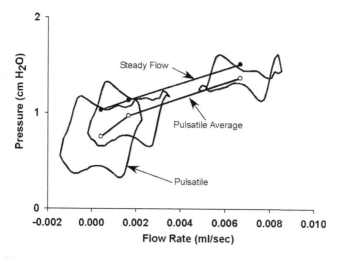

Figure 8.9 Interfacial pressure drops for steady and pulsatile motion of a semi-infinite bubble in a tube. This example demonstrates that a high-frequency (0.75 Hz) and small amplitude oscillation can reduce the average interfacial pressure drop.

spread homogeneously across many generations of airways. It may, therefore, be beneficial to blow the liquid as a plug into the airways using mechanical ventilation or to let it drain into the lung under the action of gravity and capillarity. Here, we summarize recent studies aimed at understanding the physical principles controlling surfactant-mediated and liquid-bolus flows in airways.

Surfactant-Spreading Flows

Central to the surfactant delivery process is the powerful self-spreading property of surfactant described in Section III. This is clearly illustrated by the behavior of a droplet of surfactant that is deposited on the surface of a thin layer of liquid. At the center of the droplet, where the surfactant is most concentrated, the surface tension γ is low; beyond the periphery of the droplet, γ is relatively high. The resulting gradient in surface tension generates a Marangoni stress τ_M [Fig. 8.4(b)] that acts along the free surface of the liquid, driving a vigorous spreading flow in the liquid layer. The flow carries with it surfactant that is both dissolved in the bulk and adsorbed on the air–liquid interface as a monolayer.

This self-spreading flow has some significant and unusual characteristics. First, if the monolayer is localized and the liquid layer is thin, the flow cannot extend appreciably beyond the leading edge of the monolayer, since the flow is generated by local surfactant gradients. Behind the leading edge, however, the flow is strong enough to lead to substantial deformations of the liquid layer, which thickens near the leading edge and thins near the center of the spreading droplet (111). The thinning may be severe enough to induce film rupture, leading to a dry spot forming in the film, a feature observed experimentally

(112,113) and predicted theoretically (114). At the monolayer's leading edge there can be an abrupt jump in film height, a so-called kinematic shock, the structure of which was first identified by Borgas and Grotberg (115) and which has subsequently been analyzed in considerable detail (114,116,117). Since the surfactant distribution is strongly coupled to the flow that causes it to spread, the spreading process arises through a form of nonlinear diffusion, for which the spreading rate varies with time. In special cases the spreading rate can be determined explicitly: a localized insoluble axisymmetric monolayer spreading on a thin liquid film has a radius proportional to $t^{1/4}$ at time t, for example (111,114).

Studies of this fundamental problem have provided a sound theoretical foundation upon which to develop mathematical models of surfactant-driven flows that account for features directly relevant to lung airways. Some examples are as follows. First, while the example of a spreading droplet is useful in understanding the fate of an inhaled aerosol, surfactant delivered endotracheally is likely to spread along an airway either as a continuous coating around the airway wall that spreads axially along the airway (118), or by remaining confined to regions where the liquid lining is thickest, for example, along rivulets in the liquid lining (see Section IV.B) (44), since regions where the liquid lining is either absent or extremely thin provide a substantial barrier to surfactant transport. Second, exchange of soluble surfactant between the bulk and the surface can have profound effects on spreading properties, because surfactant transport can arise through both bulk and surface convective flows, leading to enhanced film deformation (119) and flow reversal [if the surfactant adsorbs to the liquid layer's lower boundary (116)]. Third, bulk transport and wall uptake are also important concepts for surfactant-driven flows that are used to enhance drug delivery (120). If a drug is delivered as a surfactant-loaded aerosol droplet, the rapid spreading of the droplet along the airway liquid lining will carry the drug with it. Simultaneously, the droplet will dissolve in the liquid layer, increasing the area over which the drug can be absorbed by the underlying epithelium and so enhancing uptake (121). This mechanism will occur only if there are no interactions between the surfactant and drug that cause either to be inactivated (122). Fourth, in ciliated airways, spreading rates are influenced by the non-Newtonian rheology of the liquid lining, which in general has a mucous layer overlying an aqueous periciliary layer. A monolayer cannot spread over a single layer of liquid having a sufficiently high yield stress, for example, since surface tension gradients are insufficient to deform the liquid layer; however, an underlying lubricating periciliary layer does allow some spreading to take place (123).

Theoretical (124) and experimental (125) studies have identified a further effect that is potentially of great importance in SRT, namely, the interaction between delivered (exogenous) and native (endogenous) surfactant. A monolayer of exogenous surfactant, spreading by a Marangoni flow into a less concentrated monolayer of endogenous surfactant, will compress the endogenous monolayer, increasing its concentration and so reducing the surface tension gradient that drives the flow. The presence of endogenous material therefore prevents delivered surfactant from traveling as far, or as fast, as it would were the liquid layer initially uncontaminated, and reduces disturbances to the depth of the liquid layer (114,118). However, a wave of compression passes rapidly through the endogenous monolayer, causing a reduction in surface-tension-gradient to occur far ahead of the exogenous material; the more concentrated the endogenous surfactant, the more rapidly this compression wave travels. These observations may explain why a single dose of surfactant is more successful than multiple doses (using the same total volume of surfactant) (126).

Flows driven by gradients in surface tension constitute only one pathway by which exogenous surfactant, delivered as a bolus from an endotracheal tube, reaches the periphery of a surfactant-deficient lung. Independent theoretical studies of the delivery process (127,128) have identified the following likely sequence of events subsequent to the instillation of a surfactant bolus in the trachea. First, inspiratory airflow (e.g., from a ventilator) will propel the bolus distally. As it advances, it will deposit a coating film on the airway wall of thickness $h = Rf(\text{Ca})$ [(see Section III and Fig. 8.5(d)] and the bolus volume will fall until it ruptures. The pressure necessary to blow the bolus forward will depend upon the sorption characteristics of the surfactant, as well as the physical properties of the airway. This process is similar to airway reopening, discussed in Section IV.C. The instilled surfactant will then exist as a relatively thick layer of liquid coating the trachea, main stem bronchi and possibly more peripheral airways. Gravity causes this film to drain downwards into smaller airways, distributing the coating over a large surface area and reducing its thickness. As it thins, gravitational forces become weak relative to Marangoni forces (surface-tension-gradients), which drive the surfactant (and lining fluid) rapidly towards the lung periphery. The advancing monolayer is substantially diluted as it spreads over the large surface area of distal airways. In addition, models that are based on the sorption kinetics following the model of Otis et al. (100) indicate that the majority of exogenous surfactant remains trapped in the major airways (by reducing concentration gradients and thinning the airway liquid lining), although shear forces due to ventilation can help carry surfactant distally (128).

Given uncertainties in experimental estimates of liquid-lining thickness and rheology, and the difficulty of modeling delivery to an inhomogeneous lung, the theoretical models tentatively suggest that surface tension may be lowered in the lung periphery rapidly (within seconds). The system quickly approaches a near-equilibrium state in which the rate-limiting element is uptake and turnover of surfactant (both exogenous and endogenous) in the alveoli. Quasi-steady delivery of exogenous surfactant to the periphery then occurs relatively slowly, over timescales of minutes.

Liquid Bolus Transport

One means of optimizing surfactant delivery is, therefore, to ensure that the delivered bolus can be pushed as deep as possible into the lung on inspiration before it

ruptures. Understanding the conditions controlling rupture are therefore important both for SRT, therapies such as partial liquid ventilation, and for determining
when an airway occluded by a liquid bridge will reopen. The conditions most
likely to lead to the formation of a bolus during endotracheal instillation were
identified by Espinosa and Kamm (129). Once a bolus is formed, it can be propelled along an airway by an imposed pressure drop (130–132) or else by draining under gravity (133). The bolus accumulates fluid from the liquid lining ahead
of it, and loses fluid from its rear as a film coating the airway [Fig. 8.5(d)]. The
faster the bolus moves, the thicker the deposited film, and the greater the likelihood that the bolus will lose sufficient liquid volume to rupture, as has been
demonstrated experimentally (130). On the other hand, if a large quantity of
fluid is deposited, this may in turn result in subsequent airway closure due to
Rayleigh instabilities. However, slow motion will leave little surfactant behind
(due to the ultra-thin layer of fluid in the residual film), and may increase mechanical damage to the epithelial cell layer [see Bilek et al. (88)]. Thus, an optimal
rate of delivery may exist that propels surfactant to the deep lung, while protect-
ing airways from closure and mechanical stress.

The speed U at which a bolus moves is controlled by viscous dissipation in
its bulk and in narrow regions at the edge of each meniscus. Theoretical models of
slow pressure-driven bolus motion have been developed for the regime in which
surface tension controls the bolus shape, with $Ca = \mu U/\gamma \ll 1$. Howell et al.
(131) determined criteria for bolus rupture when the tube is weakly deformable
and subject to longitudinal tension. That study indicates that the critical Ca for
rupture increases with wall compliance and precursor film thickness. In turn,
there is a commensurate decrease in the pressure drop across the bolus, implying
that rupture is more likely in a more compliant tube lined with a pre-existing
thicker film. Likewise, increasing wall tension makes rupture less likely. Waters
and Grotberg (132) showed that the effect of soluble surfactant on the bolus
motion along a rigid tube, under conditions of rapid bulk diffusion and rapid
surface adsorption compared to surface advection, is (for fixed U) to increase
the pressure drop across the liquid plug and to increase the thickness of the deposited film. However the complex relationships between governing parameters indicates that the surfactant dose can be tuned to control the location of bolus rupture.
For example, with appropriate tuning, larger doses will rupture quicker and smaller
doses can persist longer and would be more likely to distribute homogeneously in
the upper airways. Weak gravitational forces in vertical tubes can also induce bolus
rupture, or cause an annular collar to snap off to form a bolus, depending on the size
of the Bond number $Bo = \rho g R^2/\gamma$ (133).

Cassidy et al. (130) have shown experimentally that at large Ca, the thickness of the deposited film may exceed the critical value h_c required for closure
(see Section IV.B), implying that delivery of a long liquid plug to peripheral
airways may be hampered if it is propelled too quickly. This study shows that
the plug velocity decreases, however, as it advances into the more distal
regions of the lung as a result of increased cross-sectional area, in a manner

that depends on the way the plug negotiates each bifurcation. Cassidy et al. (130) show that a liquid plug approaching a symmetric bifurcation divides equally into each daughter tube, but the thickness of the trailing film is smaller in the daughter tubes than in the parent tube at the same capillary number. They hypothesized that entrance (and geometrical) effects in the vicinity of the bifurcation could play an important role in explaining this difference, which current single-tube theories do not take into account. They also showed that if a liquid plug blocks one of the daughter tubes, the unblocked daughter receives a larger portion of the surfactant volume from the parent tube, and that the plug in the unblocked tube thus travels faster because of the lower resistance to flow.

Surfactant and Inhaled Particles

Finally, surfactant-driven flows are believed to play an important physiological role in driving airway surface liquid from alveoli (where endogenous surfactant is secreted) proximally into peripheral, unciliated airways, and from there to larger, ciliated airways. In this way, Marangoni forces provide a mechanism for the transport of inhaled particles, trapped in the liquid lining, from alveoli up to the lower steps of the mucociliary escalator, a process captured in an early model of steady surfactant-driven flow in a liquid-lined tube (134). Such ideas have recently been extended (135) to account for the nonuniform, periodic stretching of the airway surface that occurs during breathing, which induces concentration gradients that drive a time-averaged mean flow towards the mouth, through mechanisms dependent on the rapid adsorption but slow desorption characteristic of pulmonary surfactant (100). Predictions of transport of particles trapped in the liquid lining are complicated by observations showing that surfactant can displace trapped particles downwards, indenting the underlying epithelium (136). Substantial challenges remain to understand these and other aspects of surfactant-related flows of liquids in the lung.

V. Conclusions

The experimental and analytical models described earlier have indicated the importance of understanding the interaction among surfactant properties, fluid mechanics, and structural responses if one is to understand and develop improved treatment for obstructive pulmonary diseases related to the liquid film that coats the interior of the lung. However, the understanding of these coupled problems is still in its infancy. For example, many of the predictions are based on simple models of surfactant that ignore the interfacial molecular effects due to protein–phospholipid interactions. Recent investigations, described in other chapters, show that surfactant proteins SP-B and SP-C can dramatically influence surfactant interfacial properties. For example, studies by Zasadzinski and colleagues (137–139) demonstrate that in the presence of SP-B and SP-C a reversible folding transition can occur at monolayer collapse. This folded multilayer can provide a reservoir for reincorporation into the monolayer during interfacial expansion. Hall and his colleagues have shown that the folding dynamics are related to the rate of surface compression (140) and have explored properties of surfactant films. It is recognized that the kinetics of multilayer development and reinsertion are critical to adequate surfactant function (141–143). However, these kinetic processes are not well understood at present and must be established if we are to rationally develop adequate surfactant replacements and improved ventilation therapies.

To date, little work has been conducted to mathematically model pulmonary surfactant kinetic processes. The work by Johnson, Ingenito, Kamm, and their colleagues is capable of reproducing many features of pulmonary surfactant pressure–velocity loops and faithfully replicates several features of squeeze out that occurs if surfactant proteins are not included (100,101). Research by Krueger has included monolayer collapse and respreading mechanisms that occurs if surfactant proteins are present, but uses only basic rules for multilayer development and reinsertion dynamics (102,144). Clearly, more advanced models will be necessary in order to predict pulmonary surfactant physicochemical interactions in dynamic systems that are relevant to the lung. Further understanding of surfactant biophysical properties coupled to fluid-structure interactions may help to guide further progress in the treatment of obstructive pulmonary disease.

Acknowledgments

Donald P. Gaver III acknowledges support of this work by the National Science Foundation under Grant No. BES-9978605, NASA grant NAG3–2734, and with P20 EB001432-01. David Halpern acknowledges support from NASA grant NAG-2740. Oliver E. Jensen acknowledges support from Wellcome Trust grant 061142.

References

1. Von Neergaard K. Neue auffassungen über einen grundbegriff der atemmechanik. die retraktionskraft der lunge, abhängig von der oberflächenspannung in den alveolen: Z Gesamte Exp Med 1929; 66:373–394.
2. Pattle RE. Properties, function and origin of the alveolar lining layer: Nature 1955; 175:1125–1126.
3. Clements JA. Surface tension of lung extracts. Proceedings of the Society for Experimental Biology and Medicine 1957; 95(1):170–172.
4. Clements JA, Brown ES, Johnson RP. Pulmonary surface tension and the mucus lining of the lungs: some theoretical considerations. J Appl Physiol 1958; 12(2):262–268.
5. Avery ME, Mead J. Surface properties in relation to atelectasis and hyaline membrane disease. AMA J Dis Child 1959; 97:517–523.
6. Liu M, Wang L. Enhörning G. Surfactant dysfunction develops when the immunized guinea-pig is challenged with ovalbumin aerosol. Clin Exp Allergy 1995; 25(11):1053–1060.

7. Cheng G, Ueda T, Sugiyama K, Toda M, Fukuda T. Compositional and functional changes of pulmonary surfactant in a guinea-pig model of chronic asthma. Respir Med 2001; 95(3):180–186.

8. Robertson B. Surfactant Deficiency and Lung Injury. In: Surfactant Replacement Therapy. Alan R Liss Inc. 1989:127–144.

9. Notter RH, Finkelstein JN. Pulmonary surfactant: an interdisciplinary approach. J Appl Physiol 1984; 57(6):1613–1624.

10. Patton CD, Schulman ES. Surfactant: clinical applications. Am Fam Physician 1992; 46(1):233–236.

11. Guyer B, Hoyert DL, Martin JA, Ventura SJ, MacDorman MF, Strobino DM. Annual Summary of Vital Statistics—1998. Pediatrics 1999; 104(6):1229–1246.

12. Dos Santos CC, Slutsky AS. Invited review: mechanisms of ventilator-induced lung injury: a perspective. J Appl Physiol 2000; 89(4):1645–1655.

13. Whitehead T, Slutsky AS. The pulmonary physician in critical care-7: ventilator induced lung injury. Thorax 2002; 57(7):635–642.

14. Behnia R, Molteni A, Waters CM, Panos RJ, Ward WF, Schnaper HW, CH TSA. Early markers of ventilator-induced lung injury in rats. Ann Clin Lab Sci 1996; 26(5):437–450.

15. Savla U, Sporn PH, Waters CM. Cyclic stretch of airway epithelium inhibits prostanoid synthesis. Am J Physiol 1997; 273(5 Pt 1):L1013–L1019.

16. Oswari J, Matthay MA, Margulies SS. Keratinocyte growth factor reduces alveolar epithelial susceptibility to in vitro mechanical deformation. Am J Physiol Lung Cell Mol Physiol 2001; 281(5):L1068–L1077.

17. Tschumperlin DJ, Oswari J, Margulies AS. Deformation-induced injury of alveolar epithelial cells: effect of frequency, duration, and amplitude. Am J Respir Crit Care Med 2000; 162(2 Pt 1):357–362.

18. Amato MB et al. Effect of a protective-ventilation strategy on mortality in the acute respiratory distress syndrome. N Engl J Med 1998; 338(6):347–354.

19. Muscedere JG, Mullen JBM, Gan K, Slutsky AS. Tidal ventilation at low airway pressures can augment lung injury. Am J Respir Crit Care Med 1994; 149:1327–1334.

20. Hubmayr RD. Perspective on lung injury and recruitment: a skeptical look at the opening and collapse story. Am J Respir Crit Care Med 2002; 165(12):1647–1653.

21. Macklem PT, Proctor DF, Hogg JC. Stability of peripheral airways. Respir Physiol 1970; 8(2):191–203.

22. Hughes JMB, Rosenzweig DY, Kivitz PB. Site of airway closure in excised dog lungs: histological demonstration. J Appl Physiol 1970; 29(3):340–344.

23. Greaves IA, Hildebrandt J, Frederic J, Hoppin G. Micromechanics of the Lung. In: Fishman AP, ed. Handbook of Physiology: The Respiratory System Iii. Bethesda, MD: American Physiological Society, 1986:217–231.

24. Leff AR, Schumacker PT. Respiratory physiology: basics and applications. 1st ed. W.B. Saunders Company, 1993:198.

25. Hlastala MP, Berger AJ. Physiology of Respiration. New York City, NY: Oxford University Press, 1996:306.

26. Takishima T, Sasaki H, Sasaki T. Influence of lung parenchyma on collapsibility of dog bronchi. J Appl Physiol 1975; 38(5):875–881.

27. Naureckas ET, Dawson CA, Gerber BS, Gaver DP III, Gerber HL, Linehan JH, Solway J, Samsel RW. Airway reopening pressure in isolated rat lungs. J Appl Physiol 1994; 76(3):1372–1377.

28. Yap DY, Liebkemann WD, Solway J, Gaver DP III. Influences of parenchymal tethering on the reopening of closed pulmonary airways. J Appl Physiol 1994; 76(5):2095–2105.

29. Taskar V, John J, Evander E, Robertson B, Jonson B. Surfactant dysfunction makes lungs vulnerable to repetitive collapse and reexpansion. Am J Respir Crit Care Med 1997; 155:313–320.

30. Wiggs BR, Hrousis CA, Drazen JM, Kamm RD. On the mechanism of mucosal folding in normal and asthmatic airways. J Appl Physiol 1997; 83(6):1814–1821.

31. Swartz MA, Tschumperlin DJ, Kamm RD, Drazen JM. Mechanical stress is communicated between different cell types to elicit matrix remodeling. Proc Natl Acad Sci USA 2001; 98(11):6180–6185.

32. Tremblay L, Valenza F, Ribeiro SP, Li J, Slutsky AS. Injurious ventilatory strategies increase cytokines and c-fos m-rna expression in an isolated rat lung model. J Clin Invest 1997; 99(5):944–952.

33. Torday JS, Rehan VK. Stretch-stimulated surfactant synthesis is coordinated by the paracrine actions of Pthrp and leptin. Am J Physiol Lung Cell Mol Physiol 2002; 283(1):L130–L135.

34. Edwards YS, Sutherland LM, Murray AW. No protects alveolar type II cells from stretch-induced apoptosis: a novel role for macrophages in the lung. Am J Physiol Lung Cell Mol Physiol 2000; 279(6):L1236–L1242.

35. Sanchez-Esteban J, Wang Y, Cicchiello LA, Rubin LP. Cyclic mechanical stretch inhibits cell proliferation and induces apoptosis in fetal rat lung fibroblasts. Am J Physiol Lung Cell Mol Physiol 2002; 282(3):L448–L456.

36. Slutsky AS, Tremblay LN. Multiple system organ failure: is mechanical ventilation a contributing factor? Am J Respir Crit Care Med 1998; 157(6.1):1721–1725.

37. Bastacky J, Lee CYC, Goerke J, Koushafar H, Yager D, Kenaga L, Speed TP, Chen Y, Clements JA. Alveolar lining layer is thin and continuous: low-temperature scanning electron microscopy of rat lung. J Appl Physiol 1995; 79(5):1615–1628.

38. Yager D, Butler JP, Bastacky J, Israel E, Smith G, Drazen JM. Amplification of airway constriction due to liquid filling of airway interstices. J Appl Physiol 1989; 66(6):2873–2884.

39. Yager D, Cloutier T, Feldman H, Bastacky J, Drazen JM, Kamm RD. Airway surface liquid thickness as a function of lung volume in small airways of the guinea pig. J Appl Physiol 1994; 77(5):2333–2340.

40. Giavedoni M, FA FS. The axisymmetric and plane cases of a gas phase steadily displacing a Newtonian liquid—a simultaneous solution of the governing equations. Phys Fluids 1997; 9(8):2420–2428.

41. Grotberg JB. Pulmonary flow and transport phenomena. Annu Rev Fluid Mech 1994; 26:529–571.

42. Grotberg JB. Respiratory fluid mechanics and transport processes. Annu Rev Biomed Eng 2001; 3:421–457.

43. Jensen OE. The thin liquid lining of a weakly curved cylindrical tube. J Fluid Mech 1997; 331:373–403.

44. Williams HA, Jensen OE. Surfactant transport over airway liquid lining of nonuniform depth. J Biomech Eng 2000; 122(2):159–165.

45. Halpern D, Grotberg JB. Fluid-elastic instabilities of liquid-lined flexible tubes. J Fluid Mech 1992; 244:615–632.

46. Lambert RK. Role of bronchial basement membrane in airway collapse. J Appl Physiol 1991; 71(2):666–673.

47. Kamm RD. Airway wall mechanics. Annu Rev Biomed Eng 1999; 1:47–72.

48. Hrousis CA, Wiggs BJ, Drazen JM, Parks DM, Kamm RD. Mucosal folding in biologic vessels. J Biomech Eng 2002; 124(4):334–341.

49. Yager D, Kamm RD, Drazen JM. Airway wall liquid. sources and role as an amplifier of bronchoconstriction. Chest 1995; 107(suppl 3):105S–110S.

50. Hill MJ, Wilson TA, Lambert RK. Effects of surface tension and intraluminal fluid on mechanics of small airways. J Appl Physiol 1997; 82(1):233–239.

51. Rosenzweig J, Jensen OE. Capillary-elastic instabilities of liquid-lined lung airways. J Biomech Eng 2002; 124:650–655.

52. Heil M, White JP. Airway closure: surface-tension-driven non-axisymmetric instabilities of liquid-lined elastic rings. J Fluid Mech 2002; 462:79–109.

53. Heil M. Minimal liquid bridges in non-axisymmetrically buckled elastic tubes. J Fluid Mech 1999; 380:309–337.

54. Heil M. Airway closure: occluding liquid bridges in strongly buckled elastic tubes. J Biomech Eng-T Asme 1999; 121(5):487–493.

55. Macklem PT. Airway obstruction and collateral ventilation. Physiol Rev 1971; 51(2):368–436.

56. Kamm RD, Schroter RC. Is airway closure caused by a liquid film instability? Respir Physiol 1989; 75:141–156.

57. Hammond P. Nonlinear adjustment of a thin annular film of viscous-fluid surrounding a thread of another within a circular cylindrical pipe. J Fluid Mech 1983; 137(Dec):363–384.

58. Gauglitz PA, Radke CJ. An extended evolution equation for liquid-film break up in cylindrical capillaries. Chem Eng Sci 1988; 43(7):1457–1465.

59. Johnson M, Kamm RD, Ho LW, Shapiro A, Pedley TJ. The nonlinear growth of surface-tension-driven instabilities of a thin annular film. J Fluid Mech 1991; 233:141–156.

60. Halpern D, Grotberg JB. Surfactant effects on fluid-elastic instabilities of liquid-lined flexible tubes: a model of airway closure. J Biomech Eng 1993; 115(3):271–277.

61. Halpern D, Grotberg JB. Oscillatory shear stress induced stabilization of thin film instabilities. In: Chang HC, ed. Iutam Symposium on Non-Linear Waves in Multi-Phase Flow. Dordrecht, The Netherlands: Kluwer Academic, 2000:33–43.

62. Halpern D, Moriarty JA, Grotberg JB. Capillary-elastic instabilities with an oscillatory forcing function. In: Durban D, Pearson JRA, eds. Iutam Symposium on Non-Linear Singularities in Deformation and Flow. Dordrecht, The Netherlands: Kluwer Academic, 1999:243–255.

63. Otis DR Jr, Johnson M, Pedley TJ, Kamm RD. Role of pulmonary surfactant in airway closure: a computational study. J Appl Physiol 1993; 75(3):1323–1333.

64. West JB. Respiratory physiology—the essentials. Baltimore, MD: Williams and Wilkins, 1990.

65. Cassidy KJ, Halpern D, Ressler BG, Grotberg JB. Surfactant effects in model airway closure experiments. J Appl Physiol 1999; 87(1):415–427.

66. Liu M, Wang L, Li E, Enhörning G. Pulmonary surfactant will secure free airflow through a narrow tube. J Appl Physiol 1991; 71(2):742–748.

67. Halpern D, Grotberg JB. Nonlinear saturation of the Rayleigh instability in a liquid-lined tube. J Fluid Mech 2003; 492:251–270.

68. Johnston D, Hochmann M, Timms B. High frequency oscillatory ventilation: initial experience in 22 patients. J Paediatr Child Health 1995; 31(4):297–301.

69. Paulson TE, Spear RM, Silva PD, Peterson BM. High-frequency pressure-control ventilation with high positive end-expiratory pressure in children with acute respiratory distress syndrome. J Pediatr 1996; 129(4):566–573.

70. Hickling KG, Henderson SJ, Jackson R. Low mortality associated with low volume pressure limited ventilation with permissive hypercapnia in severe adult respiratory distress syndrome. Intensive Care Med 1990; 16(6):372–377.

71. Kallet RH, Corral W, Silverman HJ, Luce JM. Implementation of a low tidal volume ventilation protocol for patients with acute lung injury or acute respiratory distress syndrome. Respir Care 2001; 46(10):1024–1037.

72. Cartotto R, Cooper AB, Esmond JR, Gomez M, Fish JS, Smith T. Early clinical experience with high-frequency oscillatory ventilation for ards in adult burn patients. J Burn Care Rehabil 2001; 22(5):325–333.

73. Fort P, Farmer C, Westerman J, Johannigman J, Beninati W, Dolan S, Derdak S. High-frequency oscillatory ventilation for adult respiratory distress syndrome—a pilot study. Crit Care Med 1997; 25(6):937–947.

74. Mehta S, MacDonald R. Implementing and troubleshooting high-frequency oscillatory ventilation in adults in the intensive care unit. Respir Care Clin N Am 2001; 7(4):683–695.

75. Mehta S, Lapinsky SE, Hallett DC, Merker D, Groll RJ, Cooper AB, MacDonald RJ, Stewart TE. Prospective trial of high-frequency oscillation in adults with acute respiratory distress syndrome. Crit Care Med 2001; 29(7):1360–1369.

76. Bretherton FP. The motion of long bubbles in tubes. J Fluid Mech 1961; 10:166–168.

77. Fairbrother F, Stubbs AE. Studies in electroendosmosis. Part IV. The bubble-tube method of measurement. J Chem Soc 1935; 1:527–529.

78. Taylor GI. Deposition of a viscous fluid on the wall of a tube. J Fluid Mech 1961; 10:161–165.

79. Hsu SH, Hou CM. Air-liquid interfacial movement in models simulating airway reopening. Med Eng Phys 1998; 20(8):558–564.

80. Gaver DP III, Samsel RW, Solway J. Effects of surface tension and viscosity on airway reopening. J Appl Physiol 1990; 69(1):74–85.

81. Perun ML, Gaver DP III. An experimental model investigation of the opening of a collapsed untethered pulmonary airway. J Biomech Eng 1995; 117:1–9.

82. Hsu S-H, Strohl KP, Jamieson AM. Role of viscoelasticity in Tbe tube model of airway reopening I. Non-Newtonian sols. J Appl Physiol 1994; 76(6):2481–2489.

83. Hsu SH, Strohl KP, Haxhiu MA, Jamieson AM. Role of viscoelasticity in the tube model of airway reopening. II. Non-Newtonian gels and airway simulation. J Appl Physiol 1996; 80(5):1649–1659.

84. Low HT, Chew YT, Zhou CW. Pulmonary airway reopening: effects of non-Newtonian fluid viscosity. J Biomech Eng-T Asme 1997; 119(3):298–308.

85. Perun ML, Gaver DP III. Interaction between airway lining fluid forces and parenchymal tethering during pulmonary airway reopening. J Appl Physiol 1995; 79(5):1717–1728.

86. Otis DR, Petak F Jr, Hantos Z, Fredberg JJ, Kamm RD. Airway closure and reopening assessed by the alveolar capsule oscillation technique. J Appl Physiol 1996; 80(6):2077–2084.

87. Gaver DP III, Halpern D, Jensen OE, Grotberg JB. The steady motion of a semi-infinite bubble through a flexible-walled channel. J Fluid Mech 1996; 319: 25–65.

88. Bilek AM, Dee KC, Gaver DP III. Mechanisms of surface-tension-induced epithelial cell damage in a model of pulmonary airway reopening. J Appl Physiol 2003; 94(2):770–783.

89. Heil M. Finite Reynolds number effects in the Bretherton problem. Phys Fluids 2001; 13(9):2517–2521.

90. Heil M. Finite Reynolds number effects in the propagation of an air finger into a liquid-filled flexible-walled channel. J Fluid Mech 2000; 424:21–44.

91. Hazel AL, Heil M. Three-dimensional airway reopening: the steady propagation of a semi-infinite bubble into a buckled elastic tube. J Fluid Mech 2003; 478:47–70.

92. Jensen OE, Horsburgh MK, Halpern D, Gaver DP. The steady propagation of a bubble in a flexible-walled channel: asymptotic and computational models. Phys Fluids 2002; 14(2):443–457.

93. Naire S, Jensen OE. An asymptotic model of unsteady airway reopening. J Biomech Eng-T Asme 2003; 125:823–831.

94. Jensen OE, Horsburgh MK. Modeling the reopening of liquid-lined airways. In: Wall/Fluid Interactions in Physiological Flows. Collins MW, Pontrelli G, Atherton MA, eds. WIT Press, 2002.

95. Suki B, Barabasi A-L, Hantos Z, Petak F, Stanley HE. Avalanches and power-law behaviour in lung inflation. Nature 1994; 368:615–618.

96. Sujeer MK, Buldyrev SV, Zapperi S, Andrade JS, Stanley HE, Suki B. Volume distributions of avalanches in lung inflation: a statistical mechanical approach. Phys Rev E 1997; 56(3):3385–3394.

97. Alencar AM, Hantos Z, Petak F, Tolnai J, Aztalos T, Zapperis S, Andrade JS, Buldyrev SV, Stanley HE, Suki B. Scaling behavior in crackle sound during lung inflation. Phys Rev E Stat Phys Plasmas Fluids Relat Interdiscip Topics 1999; 60(4 Pt B):4659–4663.

98. Suki B, Alencar AM, Tolnai J, Asztalós T, Petak F, Sujeer MK, Patel K, Patel J, Stanley HE, Hantos Z. Size distribution of recruited alveolar volumes in airway reopening. J Appl Physiol 2000; 89(5):2030–2040.

99. Bates JH, Irvin CG. Time dependence of recruitment and derecruitment in the lung: a theoretical model. J Appl Physiol 2002; 93(2):705–713.

100. Otis DR Jr, Ingenito EP, Kamm RD, Johnson M. Dynamic surface tension of surfactant TA: experiments and theory. J Appl Physiol 1994; 77(6):2681–2688.

101. Ingenito EP, Mark L, Morris J, Espinosa FF, Kamm RD, Johnson M. Biophysical characterization and modeling of lung surfactant components. J Appl Physiol 1999; 86(5):1702–1714.

102. Krueger MA Gaver DP III. A theoretical model of pulmonary surfactant multilayer collapse under oscillating area conditions. J Colloid Interface Sci 2000; 229(2):353–364.

103. Ratulowski J, Chang H-C. Marangoni effects of trace impurities on the motion of long gas bubbles in capillaries. J Fluid Mech 1990; 210:303–328.

104. Stebe KJ, Bartes-Biesel D. Marangoni effects of adsorption–desorption controlled surfactants on the leading end of an infinitely long bubble in a capillary. J Fluid Mech 1995; 286:25–48.

105. Ghadiali SN, Gaver DP. The influence of non-equilibrium surfactant dynamics on the flow of a semi-infinite bubble in a rigid cylindrical tube. J Fluid Mech 2003; 478:165–196.

106. Yap DYK, Gaver III DP. The influence of surfactant on two-phase flow in a flexible-walled channel under bulk equilibrium conditions. Phys Fluids 1998; 10(8):1846–1863.

107. Ghadiali SN, Gaver DP. An investigation of pulmonary surfactant physico-chemical behavior under airway reopening conditions. J Appl Physiol 2000; 88(2):493–506.

108. Brennan RF, Gaver DP III. Physicochemical properties of pulmonary surfactant during pulsatile airway reopening. Faseb J 2002; 16(5):A1152.

109. Gaver DP III, Zimmer ME, Halpern D, Williams HAR. The use of pulsatile airway reopening to reduce ventilator-induced lung injury. Faseb J 2002; 16(4):A409.

110. Hohlfeld J, Fabel H, Hamm H. The role of pulmonary surfactant in obstructive airways disease. Eur Respir J 1997; 10(2):482–491.

111. Gaver DP III, Grotberg JB. The dynamics of a localized surfactant on a thin film. J Fluid Mech 1990; 213:127–148.

112. Keshgi HS, Scriven LE. Dewetting, nucleation and growth of dry regions. Chem Eng Sci 1991; 46:519–526.

113. Gaver DP III, Grotberg JB. Droplet spreading on a thin viscous film. J Fluid Mech 1992; 235:399–414.

114. Jensen OE, Grotberg JB. Insoluble surfactant spreading on a thin film: shock evolution and film rupture. J Fluid Mech 1992; 240:259–288.

115. Borgas MS, Grotberg JB. Monolayer flow on a thin film. J Fluid Mech 1988; 193:151–173.

116. Halpern D, Grotberg JB. Dynamics and transport of a localized soluble surfactant on a thin film. J Fluid Mech 1992; 237:1–11.

117. Jensen OE, Halpern D. The stress singularity in surfactant-driven flows. Part 1: viscous effects. J Fluid Mech 1998; 372:273–300.

118. Espinosa FF, Shapiro AH, Fredberg JJ, Kamm RD. Spreading of exogenous surfactant in an airway. J Appl Physiol 1993; 75(5):2028–2039.

119. Jensen OE, Grotberg JB. The spreading of heat or soluble surfactant on a thin liquid film. Physics of Fluids A 1993; 5:58–68.

120. Kharasch VS, Sweeney TD, Fredberg J, Lehr J, Damokosh AI, Avery ME, Brain JD. Pulmonary surfactant as a vehicle for intratracheal delivery of technetium sulfur colloid and pentamidine in hamster lungs. Am Rev Respir Dis 1991; 144(4):909–913.

121. Jensen OE, Halpern D, Grotberg JB. Transport of a passive solute by surfactant-driven flows. Chem Eng Sci 1994; 49:1107–1117.

122. Haitsma JJ, Lachmann U, Lachmann B. Exogenous surfactant as a drug delivery agent. Adv Drug Deliv Rev 2001; 47(2–3):197–207.

123. Craster RV, Matar OK. Surfactant transport on mucus films. J Fluid Mech 2000; 425:235–258.

124. Grotberg JB, Halpern D, Jensen OE. Interaction of exogenous and endogenous surfactant: spreading-rate effects. J Appl Physiol 1995; 78(2):750–756.

125. Bull JL, Nelson LK, Walsh JT Jr, Glucksberg MR, Schurch S, Grotberg JB. Surfactant-spreading and surface-compression disturbance on a thin viscous film. J Biomech Eng 1999; 121(1):89–98.

126. Alvarez FJ, Alfonso LF, Gastiasoro E, Lopez-Heredia J, Arnaiz A, Valls-i-Soler A. The effects of multiple small doses of exogenous surfactant on experimental respiratory failure induced by lung lavage in rats. Acta Anaesthesiol Scand 1995; 39(7):970–974.

127. Halpern D, Jensen OE, Grotberg JB. A theoretical study of surfactant and liquid delivery into the lung. J Appl Physiol 1998; 85(1):333–352.

128. Espinosa FF, Kamm RD. Bolus dispersal through the lungs in surfactant replacement therapy. J Appl Physiol 1999; 86(1):391–410.

129. Espinosa FF, Kamm RD. Meniscus formation during tracheal instillation of surfactant. J Appl Physiol 1998; 85(1):266–272.

130. Cassidy KJ, Gavriely N, Grotberg JB. Liquid plug flow in straight and bifurcating tubes. J Biomech Eng 2001; 123(6):580–589.

131. Howell PD, Waters SL, Grotberg JB. The propagation of a liquid bolus along a liquid-lined flexible tube. J Fluid Mech 2000; 406:309–335.

132. Waters SL, Grotberg JB. The propagation of a surfactant laden liquid plug in a capillary tube. Phys Fluids 2002; 14(2):471–480.

133. Jensen OE. Draining collars and lenses in liquid-lined vertical tubes. J Coll Inter Sci 2000; 221:38–49.

134. Davis SH, Liu AK, Sealy GG. Motion driven by surface tension gradients in a tube lining. J Fluid Mech 1974; 62:737–751.

135. Espinosa FF, Kamm RD. Thin layer flows due to surface tension gradients over a membrane undergoing nonuniform, periodic strain. Ann Biomed Eng 1997; 25(6):913–925.

136. Schurch S, Gehr P, Im Hof V, Geiser M, Green F. Surfactant displaces particles toward the epithelium in airways and alveoli. Respir Physiol 1990; 80(1):17–32.

137. Lipp MM, Lee KYC, Takamoto DY, Zasadzinski JA, Waring AJ. Coexistence of buckled and flat monolayers. Physical Review Letters 1998; 81(8):1650–1653.

138. Zasadzinski JA. Round-up at the bilayer corral [see comments]. Biophys J 1996; 71(5):2243–2244.

139. Zasadzinski JA, Ding J, Warriner HE, Bringezu F, Waring AJ. The physics and physiology of lung surfactants. Curr Opin Coll Int Sci 2001; 6(5–6):506–513.

140. Crane JM, Hall SB. Rapid compression transforms interfacial monolayers of pulmonary surfactant. Biophys J 2001; 80(4):1863–1872.

141. Ross M, Krol S, Janshoff A, Galla HJ. Kinetics of phospholipid insertion into monolayers containing the lung surfactant proteins SP-B or SP-C. Eur Biophys J 2002; 31(1):52–61.

142. Perez-Gil J. Molecular interactions in pulmonary surfactant films. Biol Neonate 2002; 81(suppl 1):6–15.

143. Piknova B, Schram V, Hall SB. Pulmonary surfactant: phase behavior and function. Curr Opin Struct Biol 2002; 12(4):487–494.

144. Krueger MA. Evaluation of physicochemical properties of a pulmonary surfactant analogue. In: Biomedical Engineering. Thesis. New Orleans, LA: Tulane University 1999:229.

9

Lung Surfactants: A Molecular Perspective from Computation

YIANNIS N. KAZNESSIS

University of Minnesota,
Minneapolis/St. Paul, Minnesota, USA

RONALD G. LARSON

University of Michigan,
Ann Arbor, Michigan, USA

I. Introduction

The lung epithelial cells, the alveoli, are lined with a thin liquid film that serves as a means of hydration and a host defense mechanism (1–3). Of primary biomedical importance is the surfactant component of this film, a mixture of lipids and proteins that reduces the surface tension at the air/liquid interface. This reduction stabilizes the alveoli during expiration and reduces the required work to re-expand the lung during the next respiratory cycle. Dysfunction or absence of lung surfactant (LS) results in clinically important respiratory complications in preterm infants (respiratory distress syndrome, RDS) and adults (adult respiratory distress syndrome, ARDS) (4–6). The significance of RDS among neonatal diseases and the severity of ARDS, which is one of the leading death causes in intensive care units, has led to significant efforts to identify exogenous surfactant replacement therapies (7–13). In the last few years, administration of human- or animal-derived surfactants has proven effective in treating RDS, but the potential of contamination and/or adverse immunological response to natural surfactants has shifted the interest of researchers to the development of synthetic analogs (14–17).

The rational development of design rules for synthetic LS requires the understanding of the mechanism of action of natural LS and the mode of interaction between its components. Hence, considerable effort has been invested into understanding the physicochemical principles of LS action.

The main tensoactive component and the most abundant constituent (~40%wt) of LS is the zwitterionic phospholipid dipalmitoylphosphatidylcholine (DPPC) (18,19). DPPC is an amphiphilic molecule that can pack very tightly in an insoluble monomolecular film at the air/water interface, reducing the surface tension of this interface to near zero values (0 mN/m) (20). The very low surface tension values of DPPC monolayers can enable the alveolar space to contract during expiration without collapse. However, the rheological properties of DPPC monolayers do not allow for rapid re-spreading that can follow the alveolar space expansion during inhalation (21,22). The re-spreading of DPPC monolayers can be facilitated by anionic phospholipids, such as dipalmitoylphosphatidylglycerol (DPPG), which is an important component of LS (21,23,24).

Nonetheless, in the absence of surfactant protein B (SP-B), mixtures of phospholipids inadequately mimic the pulmonary surfactant properties under dynamic conditions. In particular, SP-B has been found to be critically important for the proper respiratory function *in vivo* (25–29). This importance is substantiated by neonates suffering severe respiratory failure due to complete absence of SP-B (30–32), and by the study of transgenic mice with ablated SP-B gene expression (33). Moreover, administration of a monoclonal antibody to SP-B induced neonatal alveolar space collapse (34–36).

Insight in the mechanism of action of the protein is stemming from studies of SP-B synthetic analogs. Studies of the first 25 amino acid residues of the N-terminal of SP-B, SP-B$_{1-25}$, (FPIPL PYCWL CRALI KRIQA MIPKG) demonstrated that this peptide restores lung compliance in two animal models (37,38). SP-B$_{1-25}$, formulated in lipid mixtures of DPPC, 1-palmitoyl-2-oleylphosphatidylglycerol (POPG), and palmitic acid (69 : 22 : 9 w/w/w), greatly improves respiratory function in premature rabbits and surfactant-deficient rats (39). The structure of SP-B$_{1-25}$ was determined in POPG liposomes using Fourier transform infrared spectroscopy (40–42). These experiments predict a large α-helical content (residues 8–22), an extended β-sheet N-terminal (residues 1–7), and three conformationally random residues (residues 23–25).

Still, experiments do not provide a high-resolution picture for the relation between the sequence and the function of SP-B$_{1-25}$, and how the peptide interacts with lipid molecules. This lack of a molecular level interpretation of the interaction mechanism between the protein and lipid membranes hampers efforts to rationally improve the design of synthetic pulmonary surfactants.

A. Computer Simulations Can Provide Such a Picture

In the last decade, simulations have been successfully employed to investigate lipid bilayer membranes and the interaction among lipids, proteins, ions, and small organic molecules (43–45). Although biological membranes have been traditionally modeled as bilayers of zwitterionic lipids, primarily DPPC, the development of accurate force field potentials has recently enabled researchers to effectively simulate lipids that are ionized at physiological pH (46–48). Nowadays, simulations of hundreds of lipid molecules, for tens of nanoseconds are feasible and routinely employed (49). Such simulations can shed light on mesoscopic phenomena and allow for the development of multiscale simulation methodologies. Importantly, the great advantage of molecular mechanics simulations is the wide spectrum of properties that can be calculated from the stored positions and velocities of all the atoms. For example, structural and dynamic properties that can be calculated for the trajectory average are pair distribution functions between atoms or groups of atoms, the electron density of the system and the electron density profile of groups of atoms, the conformational and translational order of molecules, the surface tension of anisotropic systems and the diffusion/rotation relaxation times of groups of atoms. The many different properties calculated in an ensemble average can be related to the properties of a large number of different, distinct experiments. Simulations provide, thus, not only a clear atomistic picture of equilibrium systems that explains experimental findings, but also a means of connecting the results of distinct experimental observations.

Perhaps the simplest atomistic model that can capture the properties of LSs is a phospholipid monolayer. Coarse-grained models of monolayers were used until recently (50,51), when Feller and co-workers developed a molecular dynamics algorithm that samples atomistic lipid monolayer ensembles at constant surface pressure or constant surface density (52–54). This allows for the direct comparison between simulations and surface pressure/tension isotherm measurement experiments. However, the chosen geometry forces the simulation of two lipid monolayers, effectively limiting the design of simulated monolayer systems. In a recent work of ours (55,56), we simulated phospholipid monolayer systems designing a simulation cell geometry that greatly facilitates the investigation of monolayer properties (Fig. 9.1). A wall potential is applied that disallows the diffusion of water molecules in the z-direction. The wall potential can be considered as an effective finite representation of an infinite bulk system. Beglov and Roux (57) developed a rigorous theoretical framework for a solvent boundary potential that incorporates the influence of the bulk on the finite simulated system. They developed a generalized solvent boundary for a spherical

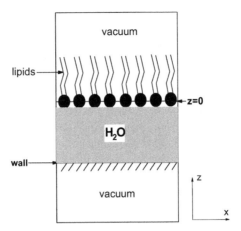

Figure 9.1 Schematic representation of the simulation geometry for a lipid monolayer.

geometry and the exact form was the result of an approximate semiempirical process. We designed the empirical wall potential, so that bulk properties would be recovered at short distances from the wall. The simulation cell is effectively periodic in the lateral x- and y-directions, as in the z-direction the size of the simulation box was arbitrarily chosen to be 200 Å.

Using this geometry, we conducted atomistic simulations of phospholipid and phospholipid/peptide systems, in order to acquire new molecular level knowledge and improve our understanding of the biomolecular phenomena involved in LS function (55,56). To build a foundation for the peptide/monolayer systems, DPPC and DPPG monolayers at the air/water interface were initially simulated in the absence of protein molecules. DPPC is zwitterionic and DPPG is anionic at physiological pH. NaCl and CaCl$_2$ water subphases were simulated at different surface densities. Detailed atomistic pair distribution functions, electron density profiles, and the surface tension were calculated for pure PC and PG monolayers and for mixtures of PC/PG systems.

Subsequently, SP-B$_{1-25}$ was added to the lipid monolayer system and its behavior simulated for a cumulative time of 20 ns (Fig. 9.2). The orientation, the position, and the secondary structure of the peptide were determined and correlated with the nature of the phospholipid and the surface density of the monolayer. The simulations clearly demonstrated that the topology and the structural integrity of the peptide are stabilized by specific interactions between residues Arg-12 and Lys-24 and DPPG head groups. A combination of electrostatic forces and stable hydrogen bond structures results in a stronger, more specific interaction of the peptide with the anionic components of lung surfactants. In DPPC, the peptide interacts with the lipid matrix through hydrophobic interactions. Specifically, the insertion sequence (residues 1–7—FPIPLPY) strongly interacts with the hydrophobic core of both kinds of lipids. This interaction has a

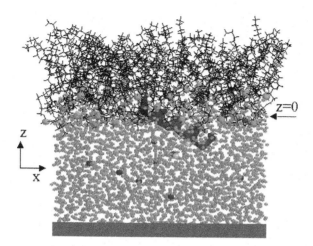

Figure 9.2 Initial configuration of SP-B$_{1-25}$ in simulated lipid monolayers. The peptide is shown with ribbon, lipids are black wire frame, water molecules are grey cpk, and sodium chloride ions with black cpk. The thick dark grey represents the repulsive wall potential.

primary role in the stabilization of SP-B in the DPPC lipid matrix, whereas it is of secondary importance in the peptide/DPPG interactions.

With this recent work of ours, we unambiguously demonstrated that simulations can provide a clear molecular level interpretation of LS phenomena. In what follows, we present a detailed description of the simulations methodology, and we describe results from previous and more recent work of ours that shed light on the molecular mechanism of LS functionality.

II. Simulations Methodology

We simulated systems of different size consisting of a periodically replicated cell containing 40 or 160 lipids spread in the xy plane (55,56). The phosphorus atoms of the lipid heads are initially positioned randomly on the xy plane at $z = 0$ with the acyl tails stretching in the positive z-direction. Around 3000 water molecules hydrate the lipid layer. Employing the geometry depicted in Fig. 9.1, the system is effectively periodic simulating an infinite system in the lateral x and y dimensions. Preequilibrated and prehydrated lipid molecules are randomly chosen from a library (58), generated by Monte Carlo simulations with a Marcelja mean field (59). Bad contacts between the lipids are reduced by systematic translations in the xy plane and rotations around the z-axis. When simulating lipid mixtures, 12 of the lipids are randomly chosen and changed from DPPC to DPPG modifying their head atoms. This gives a 7:3 ratio between zwitterionic and anionic phospholipids, close to the ratio in LSs. In the remainder of the chapter, we use the designation "PCPG" to refer to the mixtures. All of the DPPC molecules are modified to DPPG molecules for the pure DPPG systems.

In all cases, four different surface densities are simulated at 55, 60, 65, and 70 $Å^2$/lipid. The size of the simulation cell in the x- and y-directions is adjusted accordingly to accommodate 40 lipids. Subsequently, water is added in the negative z-direction. The number of water molecules ranges from 2800 to 3200 depending on the size of the simulation cell in the x- and y-directions. A weak harmonic potential applied at z approximately -30 Å, prevents the bulk water molecules from diffusing in the negative z-direction. We found that a wall potential $U_{wall} = 5/2(z_p - 3)^2$ kcal/mol, where z_p is the distance from the wall ($z_p = 0$ Å, at the wall), never allowed water molecules to diffuse, without significantly distorting the structure of the bulk water. The potential is applied for all the molecules that diffuse below the wall. The exact position of the wall potential is fine-tuned so that the density of the bulk portion of water has a value of 0.333 molecules per $Å^3$. We found that the wall effects do not propagate for more than 10 Å, allowing for an adequately large volume of water with bulk properties. In principle, there is the possibility of water molecules diffusing in the positive z-direction through the lipid monolayer to the vacuum space, but in none of the simulations was this observed.

Finally, 0.15 M NaCl is added with each ion taking the place of a randomly chosen water molecule. In addition, for the systems containing the negatively charged DPPG molecules, sodium counterions are added to neutralize the simulated system. In an additional set of 12 systems (pure DPPC, pure DPPG, and mixture of DPPC/DPPG at four different surface densities), 50 mM $CaCl_2$ was added with the 150 mM NaCl.

For the systems with the protein molecule, the monolayer is constructed following largely the protocol described by Woolf and Roux (60). The initial structure of the peptide used in the simulations was obtained from the Protein Data Bank (1DFW). This structure is the equilibrium one in a lipid monolayer as obtained by 13C-enhanced Fourier transform infrared spectroscopy (FTIR). The initial position and orientation of the peptide relative to the interfacial plane were such that the α-helical axis forms an angle of 34° with the interfacial plane, as suggested by FTIR measurements in DPPC/DPPG lipid membranes (41). We also initially positioned the Cα atom of Trp-9 on the plane of the lipid/water interface, which is at $z = 0$, in the simulation cell (41,42). To eliminate, however, any ambiguity emanating from possible starting configuration dependencies, we also simulated the peptide with starting configurations where the axis of the α-helix was perpendicular and, in a second, independent set of simulations, parallel to the interfacial plane.

With the peptide held frozen, 40 large vdW spheres were randomly positioned on the xy plane at $z = 0$. A molecular dynamics simulation of 500 ps allowed for the sphere xy positions to relax around the peptide. The phospholipids were then placed to form a monolayer with their phosphorus atoms positioned at

SP-A   SP-D   SP-D

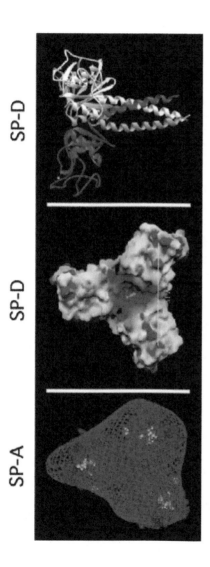

Figure 4.2 Molecular organization of CRDs of SP-A and SP-D. See Refs. (56,57) for further details.

FITC, SP-D(n/CRD)   Cy3-dUTP, DNA   Co-localization

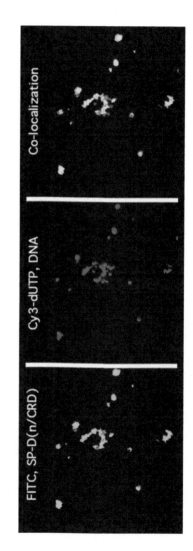

Figure 4.4 Co-localization of DNA and SP-D(n/CRD) on apoptotic cells. Green, FITC-labelled SP-D(n/CRD); red, dUTP-labelled DNA ends; yellow, co-localization.

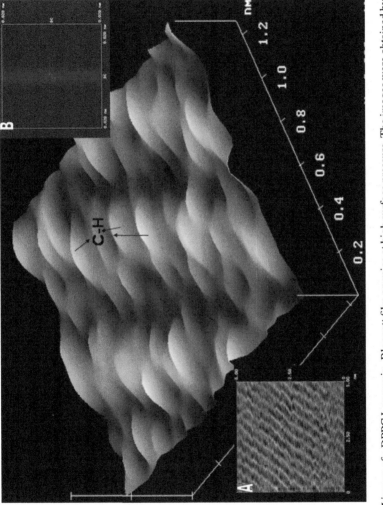

Figure 6.1 AFM image of a DPPC Langmuir–Bloggett film on mica at high surface pressure. The images were obtained by scanning the film in contact mode AFM in air at 30 Hz by methods developed by Zhai and Kleijn (23) at 5 × 5 nm resolution. The two-dimensional image is shown in (A) and a fast Fourier transform (FFT) of this image in (B). The FFT suggests lateral periodicity of the terminal fatty acid ends (CH_3) of the palmitoyl chains. The zoomed in three-dimensional image shows possibly either the molecular clouds of terminal fatty acyl ends of DPPC or unknown imaging artefacts (74).

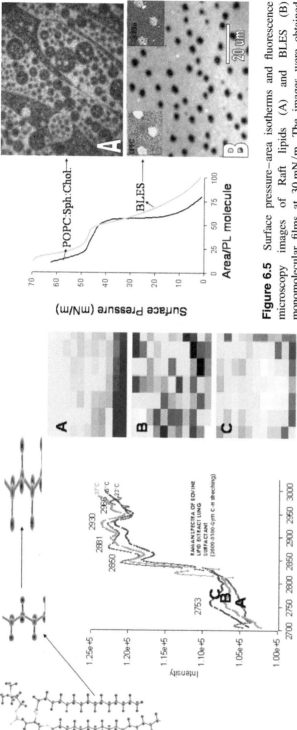

Figure 6.2 Raman spectra of BLES dispersion and spectral images obtained from the acyl CH$_2$ vibrations of DPPC undergoing phase transition. The stretching of the C–H bonds is shown in the cartoon. The three images were obtained between 23°C and 45°C from the same (10 × 15 μm) area of the dispersion and suggests change of the intensity of the symmetric stretching vibration at the center of image in (C), or a dynamic movement of the sample with such redistribution of the pixels (61). These areas may be domains of fluid lipids as suggested by others (60).

Figure 6.5 Surface pressure–area isotherms and fluorescence microscopy images of Raft lipids (A) and BLES (B) monomolecular films at 30 mN/m. The images were obtained directly from the air–water interface of a Langmuir surface balance (80), and the films were doped with low amounts of fluorescent probe NBD-PC which partitions in the fluid phase of the lipids (81). The black regions in (A) suggest liquid ordered domains and in (B) the gel (or condensed) domains. The inset in (B) is TOF-SIMS images of the condensed domains imaged from chemical fragment of DPPC (left) and calcium (right) (27). Films of BLES and Raft lipids are able to sustain high surface pressures or reduce the surface tension of the air–water interface ∼5 mN/m.

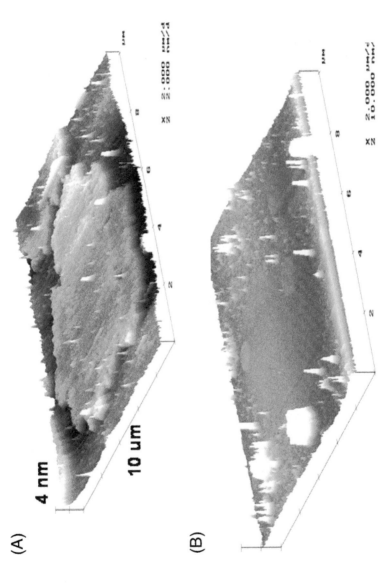

Figure 6.7 AFM images of normal (A) and hyperventilation injured (B) LS from rat lung lavage. The Langmuir–Bloggett films were deposited on mica and imaged in air. The table-like circular structures in (A) are possibly the condensed or gel domains, which are elevated 0.8 nm above the surrounding fluid phase, owing to differential tilt of the phospholipids chains (tilt-condensed phase) and packing density of the lipids in such domains (96,97). These domains are reduced in size in the injured system (B), and other large circular (smooth area in B) domains are neither gel nor fluid domains and possibly made of soluble plasma proteins (72).

the center of the vdW spheres and their tails stretching in the positive z-direction. The lipids were then translated and rotated to minimize bad contacts, defined as two heavy atoms being closer than 2.6 Å.

Altogether, each simulated system contains $\sim 12,000-14,000$ atoms, depending on the surface density of the monolayer. For the larger systems of 160 lipids, the number of atoms ranged between 50,000 and 60,000.

The program Chemistry at Harvard Molecular Mechanics (CHARMM) was used for the simulations with the PARAM26b2 parameter set (61,62). The CHARMM potential contains terms for bond lengths, bond angles, torsional angles, and improper torsional angles. Nonbonded atoms interact with a 6–12 Lennard-Jones potential. Atoms are also assigned point charges positioned at their center of mass. In the simulations, the nonbonded van der Waals interactions were smoothly switched off over a distance of 3.0 Å, between 9 and 12 Å. The electrostatic interactions are simulated using the particle mess Ewald summation with no truncation (63). A real space Gaussian width of 0.42 Å^{-1}, a B-spline order of 6, and a FFT grid of about one point per Å ($60 \times 60 \times 200$) are used. The SHAKE algorithm (64) is used to hold the hydrogen bonds fixed. The water molecules are simulated utilizing the TIP3P model (65).

After constructing the simulation cell, the energy is minimized using the adopted-basis Newton Raphson algorithm for 1000 steps. Minimization is followed by a 100 ps molecular dynamics heating period. The final temperature is 323.15 K. An equilibration period of 300 ps follows. All the systems are then simulated for 1000 ps. The constant pressure–temperature module of CHARMM is used for the simulations with a leap-frog integrator (2 fs time step). The temperature was set at 323.15 K using the Hoover temperature control with a mass of 1500 kcal ps^2 for the thermal piston. For the extended system pressure algorithm employed, all the components of the piston mass array were set to zero, resulting in constant simulation cell volume. The system's height does, however, relax in the z-direction, so that a final pressure of 0 atm is attained at equilibrium. The lateral direction pressure components obtain negative equilibrium values, because of the inhomogeneity of the system. This, in turn, gives rise to a positive monolayer surface tension, which is one of the most important properties calculated during the simulations. The surface tension calculation allows the direct comparison of the simulations with surface pressure isotherm experimental measurements.

III. Simulation Results

A. Lipid Monolayers (No Peptide)

A very interesting property calculated from the trajectories of the simulations is the surface tension of the monolayer system

$$\gamma_s = \left\langle h_z \left(P_{zz} - \frac{1}{2} \left(P_{xx} + P_{yy} \right) \right) \right\rangle$$

where the brackets indicate ensemble averages, h_z is the height of the system in the z-direction and $P_{\alpha\alpha}$ are the diagonal components of the pressure tensor, defined as

$$P_{\alpha\beta} = \frac{1}{V}\sum_{i=1}^{N}\left(\frac{p_{\alpha i}p_{\beta i}}{m_i} + r_{\alpha i}f_{\beta i}\right)$$

where V is the volume of the simulation box and the sum runs over all the N atoms in the simulation. The two terms in the sum are the kinetic and virial components of the pressure, respectively, with $p_{\alpha i}$, $r_{\alpha i}$, and $f_{\alpha i}$ being the momentum, position, and force on particle i in the α-direction. The surface tension is a measure of the anisotropy in the pressure tensor due to the inhomogeneity of the monolayer in the normal direction. Comparison of the surface tension between pure-lipid systems and lipid–peptide systems provides a clear picture of the peptide-induced disturbances in membrane structure. This calculation also allows the direct comparison between the simulations and surface pressure isotherm experimental measurements.

In Fig. 9.3, the surface pressure of DPPC, DPPG, and PCPG monolayers is plotted as a function of the area per lipid. Keeping the volume of the system fixed results in pressure fluctuations, which are of considerable magnitude for the simulated systems away from the thermodynamic limit. Nonetheless, the trends in the simulated surface pressure isotherms resemble the experimentally observed ones. Monolayers of anionic lipids exhibit higher surface pressures than zwitterionic lipids for all surface densities. There is also a general trend of decreasing surface pressure with decreased surface density.

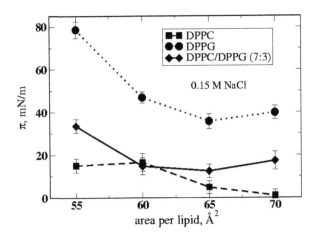

Figure 9.3 Simulated surface pressure isotherms for lipid monolayers as a function of the area per lipid.

Of course the macroscopic, experimental measurement of surface pressure is more accurate than any simulation with a finite number of molecules. The advantage of the simulations, however, is the ability to explain the observed phenomena in terms of atomic coordinates and molecular configurations. In Fig. 9.4, snapshots of DPPC monolayers at the end of the simulations are shown. The differences of monolayers at different lipid surface densities are clear. The conformational entropy of the lipid hydrocarbon chains increases with increasing the area per lipid. The integrity of the interfacial region between the lipids and the water subphase is also degraded, with increasing area per lipid, as water molecules penetrate the lipid core. We can quantify these observations by calculating the electron density of the phosphate group of the lipids as a function of the distance in the normal to the interfacial plane and by measuring the order parameter profile of acyl chains.

The electron density profile of the phosphate group of zwitterionic lipids broadens with increasing area per lipid, as more water molecules penetrate the interface (Fig. 9.5). Interestingly, the electron density profile of DPPG phosphate groups does not change appreciably with changing surface density.

Upon decreasing the DPPC surface density, there is a clear phase transition in the order parameter, which can be calculated from the Cartesian coordinates of DPPC atoms using

$$-S_{CD} = \frac{2}{3}S_{xx} + \frac{1}{3}S_{yy}$$

with each of the components calculated as

$$S_{ij} = \frac{1}{2}\langle 3\cos\theta_i \cos\theta_j - \delta_{ij}\rangle$$

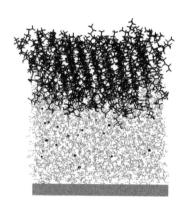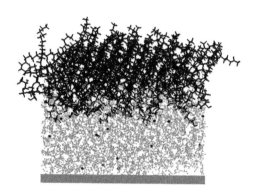

Figure 9.4 Snapshots of DPPC monolayers at the end of the simulations at 55 Å²/lipid (left) and 70 Å²/lipid (right). Lipids are shown as black wire frame, water molecules as light grey cpk, sodium and chloride ions as black cpk.

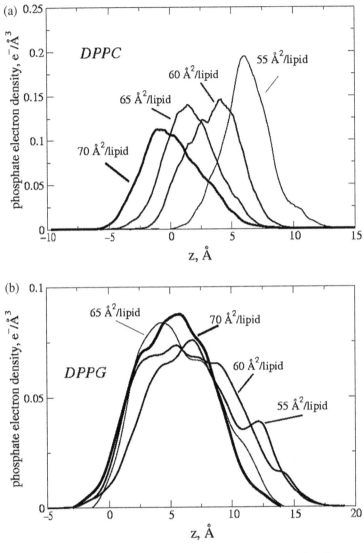

Figure 9.5 Electron density profiles of DPPC (a) and DPPG (b) phosphate groups at different surface densities [from Ref. (55), with permission].

The brackets indicate an ensemble average and θ is the angle between the carbon–hydrogen bond of the methylene and methyl groups and the monolayer normal.

DPPG hydrocarbon tails are considerably more ordered than DPPC tails at the same area per lipid, for all surface densities. There is also a more gradual increase in conformational order upon decreasing the area per lipid [Fig. 9.6(b)].

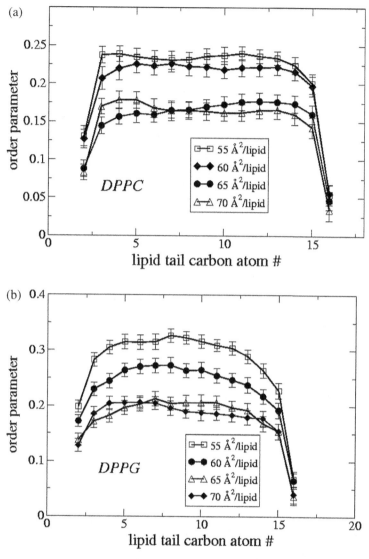

Figure 9.6 Order parameter profiles for DPPC (a) and DPPG (b) monolayers at the simulated surface densities [from Ref. (55), with permission].

An interesting observation was the formation of lateral patterns in the orientation of the acyl chains. In Fig. 9.7, a snapshot of a DPPC monolayer is shown. It is clear that interesting arrangements of acyl chains result from the simulation trajectories. It was not, however, clear whether periodic boundary conditions limit the formation of larger length scales patterns on the surface of the monolayers.

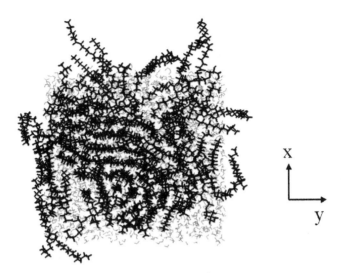

Figure 9.7 Snapshot of a DPPC monolayer (65 Å^2/lipid) at the end of the simulation. There are relatively stable patterns of concentric circles formed by the lipid acyl chains.

We have recently simulated larger monolayer systems of 160 lipids, and we are currently studying the formation of domains and the characteristics of these surface patterns shown in Fig. 9.8. Simulations can provide insight in the relationship of domain formation and physicochemical characteristic of lipid monolayers.

B. SP-B$_{1-25}$: Lipid Monolayers

The N-terminus of lung surfactant protein B, SP-B$_{1-25}$, interacts strongly with lipid monolayers. Molecular dynamics simulations clearly demonstrated the mode of interaction between the peptide and DPPC and DPPG lipids, the role of specific residues (56).

In Fig. 9.9, the distance of the Cα atom of Trp-9 from the interfacial plane is shown as a function of time for DPPC and DPPG monolayers.

At the start of the simulations, Trp-9 was placed at the interfacial plane at $z = 0$. The interfacial plane is determined by the average position of the phosphorus atoms in the z-direction. Positive deviations for the position of Trp-9 indicate that the peptide is inserting itself into the lipid core. Conversely, negative values of the distance indicate that the peptide is diffusing toward the water subphase. Clearly, the 2 ns simulations demonstrate the increased affinity of the peptide for the anionic phospholipids. This was probably expected, given the cationic character of the peptide.

The simulations allow the determination of the exact mode of interaction between the peptide and the lipid matrix. The position and orientation of SP-B

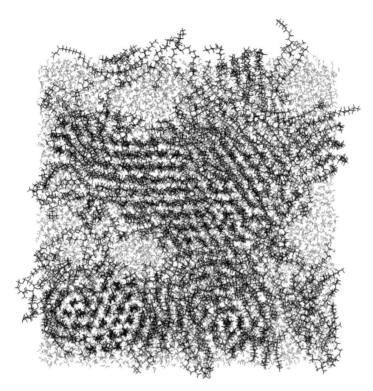

Figure 9.8   Snapshot of a DPPC monolayer with 160 lipids (65 Å^2/lipid) at the end of a 2 ns simulation. There are interesting geometrical patterns formed by the lipid acyl chains.

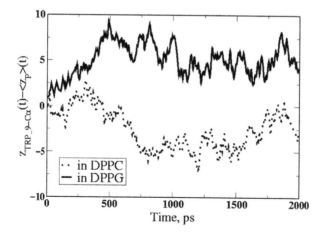

Figure 9.9   Position of the Cα atom of Trp-9 in the z-direction relative to the average phosphorus atoms position $\langle z_P \rangle$.

in DPPC is directed by hydrophobic interactions. The insertion sequence FPIPLPYC is buried in the hydrocarbon tail core of the monolayers. The amphiphilic nature of the peptide also largely determines its relative position and orientation. If the α-helical domain of the peptide is envisioned as a cylinder, the hydrophilic and hydrophobic residues are topologically partitioned in each side of the cylinder, interacting with the water subphase and the hydrocarbon core, respectively. There are apparently no highly specific interactions between peptide residues and DPPC groups. Recent longer simulations indicate some specific interactions between protein residues and the phosphate groups of DPPC lipids, but the interaction is not particularly strong. Conversely, there are very specific interactions between arginine-12 and lysine-24 and the phosphates of DPPG lipids. Calculation of pair distribution functions between the guanidinium group of arginine-12 and the phosphate of DPPG lipids clearly indicates that the interaction is strong, persisting during the simulation (Fig. 9.10). The radial distribution functions are calculated between the center of mass of the phosphate group at the lipid head group and the arginine-12 side chain terminal nitrogens (Nh1 and Nh2) or the lysine-24 side chain terminal nitrogen. Note that the pair distribution function for arginine-12 in DPPC has zero value for the first 1 nm.

The interaction between the guanidinium group of arginine-12 and the phosphate of DPPG lipids is the result of electrostatic attraction between arginine and the phosphate groups of at least two different DPPG molecules and the formation of a bidentate hydrogen bond between the hydrogen atoms of guanidinium and the oxygen atoms of the phosphate group (Fig. 9.11).

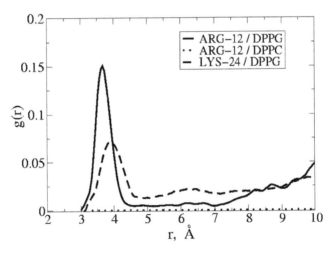

Figure 9.10 Radial distribution functions between SP-B_{1-25} residues and lipid phosphate groups.

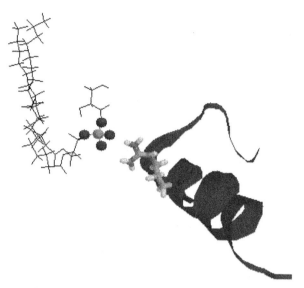

Figure 9.11 SP-B$_{1-25}$ in a DPPG monolayer at 70 Å^2/lipid. Arginine-12 interacts strongly with the phosphate group of one of the phospholipids.

This highly specific interaction between arginine-12 and lysine-24 and the phosphate groups of DPPG lipids, along with the hydrophobic interactions, which manifest themselves in a manner similar to the DPPC monolayers, stabilize the position, the orientation, and the secondary structure of the peptide in anionic lipid monolayers. The secondary structure can be monitored for the duration of the simulations by calculating the dihedral angles of the protein backbone (Fig. 9.12).

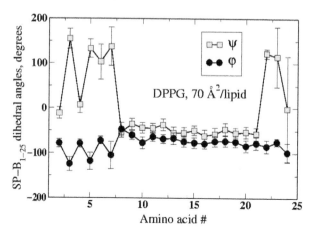

Figure 9.12 SP-B$_{1-25}$ dihedral angles φ and ψ in a DPPG monolayer.

Finally, the surface pressure of the lipid monolayer is altered upon insertion of the peptide. The simulated surface pressure of DPPC/SP-B and DPPG/SP-B monolayers behaves in the same way as experiments have indicated, that is, the surface pressure decreases considerably in DPPG monolayers, whereas there is no appreciable change for DPPC monolayers. In Fig. 9.13, the surface pressure is plotted for DPPG monolayers at different surface densities. Three systems are compared: DPPG over a water subphase with 0.15 M NaCl, DPPG over a subphase with 0.15 M NaCl and 0.05 M CaCl$_2$, and DPPG in the presence of one SP-B$_{1-25}$ molecule. Qualitatively, the simulated surface pressure is in agreement with experimental observation: calcium and SP-B result in a decrease in the surface pressure of the monolayer. Simulations are not, however, reliable enough for quantitatively accurate estimation of surface pressures, mainly because of the relatively small number of atoms simulated. The pressure components fluctuate considerably for small finite systems and adding/subtracting them to obtain the surface pressure only compounds the inaccuracies.

Nonetheless, structural properties are obtained with high accuracy, allowing comparisons with experiments. It is expected that simulations of larger systems for longer times will further reveal interesting behavior of LSs at the molecular level. Indeed, simulations can now begin to address questions about specific interactions between peptide residues and lipid components, and more work is being conducted in this area in our labs.

Recently, there has been interest in the antimicrobial character of SP-B$_{1-25}$ and studies are warranted that will determine how the sequence and the structure of the peptide not only affects the behavior of LSs but also how it confers

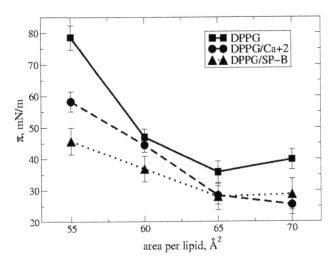

Figure 9.13 Simulated surface pressure isotherms for SP-B$_{1-25}$/lipid monolayers as a function of the area per lipid.

antimicrobial activity. Specifically, SP-B$_{1-25}$ has been not only found to lyse bacterial organisms, but was also found to possess hemolytic character. Hence, the use of SP-B$_{1-25}$ is not straightforward in LS analogs. We have initiated efforts in our lab to develop design rules for SP-B$_{1-25}$ analogs that retain the LS properties, have increased antimicrobial character but attenuated hemolytic activity. At the molecular level, this requires that any synthetic peptide should interact less with DPPC, the major component of mammalian cell membranes, and should interact more strongly with anionic lipids, which are major components of bacterial cell walls. Again the simulations provide insight, directing changes in the sequence of synthetic peptides.

IV. Conclusions

Computer simulations provide a molecular level interpretation of the experimental observations of LS monolayers. In recent work, the exact mode of interaction between SP-B$_{1-25}$ and DPPC and DPPG phospholipids was determined. The hydrophobic insertion sequence plays an important role in the position and orientation of the peptide in both DPPC and DPPG monolayers. Arginine-12 and lysine-24 stabilize the topology and the structural integrity of the peptide in DPPG monolayers through a combination of electrostatic forces and hydrogen bond structures. The peptide is largely buried in the lipid core of the DPPG monolayer. In DPPC monolayers, the peptide interacts with the lipid matrix mainly through hydrophobic interactions, although the role of more specific electrostatic interactions in currently under investigation with simulations of peptide mutants. The nonspecificity in DPPC results in increased mobility and structural flexibility for the peptide, which largely resides at the interface, interacting significantly with the water subphase. The simulation results enable us to recognize the sequence/structural elements that are the important modulators of LS activity, eventually allowing the rational development of design rules for synthetic LS analogs.

References

1. Johansson J, Curstedt T. Molecular structures and interpretations of pulmonary surfactant components. Eur J Biochem 1997; 244:675–693.
2. Notter RH, Wang Z. Pulmonary surfactant: physical chemistry, pathology, and replacement. Rev Chem Eng 1997; 13:1–118.
3. Goerke J. Pulmonary surfactant: functions and molecular composition. Biochim Biophys Acta 1998; 1408:79–89.
4. Avery ME, Mead J. Surface properties in relation to atelectasis and hyaline membrane disease. Am J Dis Child 1959; 97:517–523.
5. Taeusch HW, Ballard RA, Avery ME. Diseases of the Newborn. Philadelphia: Saunders, 1991.

6. Bernard GR, Artigas A, Brigham KL, Carlet J, Falke K. Hudson L, Lamy M, Legall R, Morris A, Spragg R. The American-European Consensus Conference on ARDS: definitions, mechanisms, relevant outcomes, and clinical trial coordination. Am J Respir Crit Care Med 1994; 149:818–824.
7. Jobe A, Taeusch HW. Surfactant Treatment in Lung Diseases. Columbus: Ross Laboratories Press, 1988.
8. Shapiro DL, Notter RH. Surfactant Replacement Therapy. New York: AR Liss, 1989.
9. Jobe AH. Pulmonary surfactant therapy. N Engl J Med 1993; 328:861–868.
10. Schwartz RM, Luby AM, Scanlon JW, Kellogg RJ. Effect of surfactant on morbidity, mortality, and resource use in newborn infants weighting 500 to 1500 g. N Engl J Med 1994; 330:1476–1480.
11. Poulain FR, Clements JA. Pulmonary surfactant therapy. West J Med 1995; 162:43–50.
12. Lachmann B. Animal models and clinical pilot studies of surfactant replacement in adult respiratory distress syndrome. Eur Respir J 1989; 3:98s–103s.
13. Nosaka S, Sakai T, Yonekura M, Yoshikawa K. Surfactant for adults with respiratory failure. Lancet 1990; 336:947–948.
14. Cohrane CG, Revak SD. Pulmonary surfactant protein B (SP-B): structure–function relationships. Science 1991; 254:566–568.
15. Revak SD, Merritt TA, Hallman M, Heldt G, La Polla RJ, Hoey K, Houghten RA, Cohrane CG. The use of synthetic peptides in the formation of biophysically and biologically active pulmonary surfactants. Pediatr Res 1991; 29:460–465.
16. Merritt TA, Kheiter A, Cohrane CG. Positive end-expiratory pressure during KL4 surfactant instillation enhances interpulmonary distribution in a simian model of respiratory distress syndrome. Pediatr Res 1995; 38:211–217.
17. Wang Y, Griffiths WJ, Curstedt T, Johansson J. Porcine pulmonary surfactant preparations contain the antibacterial peptide prophenin and a C-terminal 18-residue fragment thereof. FEBS Lett 1999; 460:257–262.
18. Holm BA, Wang Z, Egan EA, Notter RH. Content of dipalmitoyl phosphatidylcholine in lung surfactants: ramifications for surface activity. Pediatr Res 1996; 39:805–811.
19. Veldhuizen R, Nag K, Orgeig S, Possmayer F. The role of lipids in pulmonary surfactant. Biochim Biophys Acta 1998; 1408:90–108.
20. Koynova R, Caffrey M. Phases and phase transitions of the phosphatidylcholines. Biochim Biophys Acta 1998; 1376:91–145.
21. Wang Z, Hall SB, Notter RH. Dynamic surface activity of films of lung surfactant phospholipids, hydrophobic proteins, and neutral lipids. J Lipid Res 1996; 36:1283–1293.
22. Chu J, Clements JA, Cotton EK, Klaus MH, Sweet AY, Tooley WH. Neonatal pulmonary ischemia. Clinical and physiological studies. Pediatrics 1967; 40:709–782.
23. Meban C. Effect of lipids and other substances on the adsorption of dipalmitoyl phosphatidyl choline. Pediatr Res 1981; 15:1029–1031.
24. Notter RH, Holcomb S, Mavis RD. Dynamic surface properties of phosphatidylglycerol–dipalmitoyl phosphatidylcholine mixed films. Chem Phys Lipids 1980; 27:305–319.

25. Oosterlaken-Dijksterhuis MA, Haagsman HP, Van Golde LMG, Demel RA. Characterization of lipid insertion into monomolecular layers mediated by lung surfactant proteins SP-B and SP-C. Biochemistry 1991; 30:10965–10971.

26. Hall SB, Venkitaraman AR, Whitsett JA, Holm BA, Notter RH. Importance of hydrophobic apoproteins as constituents of clinical exogenous surfactants. Am Rev Respir Dis 1992; 145:24–30.

27. Yu S-H, Possmayer F. Effect of pulmonary surfactant B (SP-B) and calcium on phospholipid adsorption and squeeze-out of phosphatidylglycerol from phospholipid monolayers containing dipalmitoylphosphatidylcholine. Biochim Biophys Acta, 1992; 1126:26–34.

28. Mizuno K, Ikegami M, Chen CM, Ueda T, Jobe AH. Surfactant protein-B supplementation improves *in vivo* function of a modified natural surfactant. Pediatr Res 1995; 37:271–276.

29. Pryhuber GS. Regulation and function of pulmonary surfactant protein B. Mol Gen Metabol 1998; 64:217–228.

30. Nogee LM, DeMello DE, Dehner LP, Colten HR. Brief report: deficiency of pulmonary surfactant protein B in congenital alveolar proteinosis. N Engl J Med 1993; 328:406–410.

31. Hamvas A. Inherited surfactant protein-B deficiency. Adv Pediatr 1997; 44:369–388.

32. Nogee LM. Surfactant protein-B deficiency. Chest 1997; 111:129S–135S.

33. Clark JC, Wert SE, Bachurski CJ, Stahlman MT, Stripp BR, Weaver TE, Whitsett JA. Targeted disruption of the surfactant protein B gene disrupts surfactant homeostasis, causing respiratory failure in newborn mice. Proc Natl Acad Sci USA 1995; 92:7794–7798.

34. Robertson B, Kobayashi, T. Ganzuka M, Grossmann G, Li WZ, Suzuki Y. Experimental neonatal respiratory failure induced by a monoclonal antibody to hydrophobic surfactant-associated protein B SP-B. Pediatr Res 1991; 30:239–243.

35. Grossmann G, Suzuki Y, Robertson B, Kobayashi T, Bergren P, Li WZ, Song GW, Sun B. Pathophysiology of neonatal lung injury induced by a monoclonal antibody to surfactant protein B. J Appl Physiol 1997; 82:2003–2010.

36. Ballard PL, Nogee LM, Beers MF, Ballard RA, Planer BC, Polk L, deMello DE, Moxley MA, Longmore WJ. Partial deficiency of surfactant protein B in an infant with chronic lung disease. Pediatrics 1995; 96:1046–1052.

37. Waring AJ, Taeusch W, Bruni R. Amirkhanian J, Fan B, Stevens R, Young J. Synthetic amphipathic sequences of surfactant protein-B mimic several physicochemical and *in vivo* properties of native pulmonary surfactant proteins. Pept Res 1989; 2:308–313.

38. Bruni R, Hernandez-Juviel J, Tanoviceanu R, Walther FJ. Synthetic mimics of surfactant proteins B and C: *in vivo* surface activity and effects on lung compliance in two animal models of surfactant deficiency. Mol Gen Metabol 1998; 63:116–125.

39. Walther FJ, Hernandez-Juviel J, Gupta M, Bruni R, Waring AJ. Challenging surfactant inhibition in lavaged rats and preterm rabbits with surfactant containing synthetic surfactant peptides. Am J Respir Crit Care Med 1999; 159:A895.

40. Gordon LM, Lee KYC, Lipp MM, Zasadzinski JA, Walther FJ, Sherman MA, Waring AJ. Conformational mapping of the N-terminal segment of surfactant

protein B in lipid using ^{13}C-enhanced Fourier transform infrared spectroscopy. J Pept Res 2000; 55:330–347.

41. Gordon LM, Horvath S, Longo ML, Zasadzinski JAN, Taeusch HW, Faull K, Leung C, Waring AJ. Conformation and molecular topography of the N-terminal segment of surfactant protein B in structure-promoting environments. Protein Sci 1996; 5:1662–1675.

42. Lee KYC, Majewski J, Kuhl TL, Howes PB, Kjaer K, Lipp MM, Waring AJ, Zasadzinski JA, Smith GS. Synchrotron X-ray study of lung surfactant-specific protein SP-B in lipid monolayers. Biophys J 2001; 81: 572–585.

43. Mertz K, Roux B. Biological Membranes: A Molecular Perspective from Computation and Experiment. Boston: Birkhauser, 1996.

44. Jakobsson E. Computer simulation studies of biological membranes: progress, promise, and pitfalls. Trends Biochem Sci 1997; 22:339–344.

45. Tieleman DP, Marrink SJ, Berendsen HJ. A computer perspective of membranes: molecular dynamics studies of lipid bilayer systems. Biochim Biophys Acta 1997; 1331:235–270.

46. Forrest LR, Sansom MS. Membrane simulations: bigger and better? Curr Opin Struct Biol 2000; 10:174–181.

47. Cascales JJL, de la Torre GJ, Marrink SJ, Berendsen HJC. Molecular dynamics simulation of a charged biological membrane. J Chem Phys 1996; 104:2713–2720.

48. Bandyopadhyay S, Shelley JC, Tarek M, Moore PB, Klein ML. Surfactant aggregation at a hydrophobic surface. J Phys Chem B 1998; 102:6318–6322.

49. Lindahl E, Edholm O. Mesoscopic undulations and thickness fluctuations in lipid bilayers from molecular dynamics simulations. Biophys J 2000; 79:426–433.

50. Karaborni S, Toxvaerd S. Molecular dynamics simulations of Langmuir monolayers—a study of structure and thermodynamics. J Chem Phys 1992; 96:5505–5515.

51. Esselink K, Hilbers PAJ, van Os NM, Smit B, Karaborni S. Molecular dynamics simulations of model oil/water/surfactant systems. Colloid Surface 1994; 91:155–167.

52. Feller SE, Zhang Y, Pastor RW, Brooks RB. Constant pressure molecular dynamics simulation: the Langevin piston method. J Chem Phys 1995; 103:4613–4621.

53. Feller SE, Zhang Y, Pastor RW. Computer simulation of liquid/lipid interfaces. II. Surface tension–area dependence of a bilayer and monolayer. J Chem Phys 1995; 103:10267–10276.

54. Zhang Y, Feller SE, Pastor RW. Computer simulation of liquid/liquid interfaces. I. Theory and application to octane/water. J Chem Phys 1995; 103:10252–10266.

55. Kaznessis YN, Kim S, Larson RG. Simulations of zwitterionic and anionic phospholipid monolayers. Biophys J 2002; 82:1731–1742.

56. Kaznessis YN, Kim S, Larson RG. Specific mode of interaction between components of model pulmonary surfactants using computer simulations. J Mol Biol 2002; 322:569–582.

57. Beglov D, Roux B. Finite representation of an infinite bulk system: solvent boundary potential for computer simulations. J Chem Phys 1994; 100:9050–9062.

58. Venable RM, Zhang Y, Hardy BJ, Pastor RW. Molecular dynamics simulation of a lipid bilayer and of hexadecane: an investigation of membrane fluidity. Science 1993; 262:223–226.

59. Hardy BJ, Pastor RW. Conformational sampling of hydrocarbon and lipid chains in an orienting potential. J Comp Chem 1994; 15:208–226.
60. Woolf TB, Roux B. Molecular dynamics simulation of the gramicidin channel in a phospholipid bilayer. Proc Natl Acad Sci USA 1994; 91:11631–11635.
61. Schlenkrich M, Brickman J, MacKerell AD, Karplus M. An empirical potential energy function for phospholipids. Criteria for parameter optimization and applications. In: Merz K, Roux B, eds. Biological Membranes: A Molecular Perspective from Computation and Experiment. Boston: Birkhauser, 1996:31–81.
62. Brooks BR, Bruccoleri RE, Olafson BD, States DJ, Swaminathan S, Karplus M. CHARMM: a program for macromolecular energy, minimization, and dynamics simulations. J Comp Chem 1986; 4:187–217.
63. Essman U, Perera L, Berkowitz ML, Darden T, Lee H, Pedersen LG. A smooth particle mesh Ewald method. J Chem Phys 1995; 103:8577–8593.
64. Ryckaert JP, Ciccotti G, Berendesen HJC. Numerical integration of the cartesian equations of motion of a system with constraints: molecular dynamics of *n*-alkanes. J Comp Phys 1977; 23:327–341.
65. Jorgensen WL, Chandrasekhar J, Medura JD, Impey RW, Klein ML. Comparison of simple potential function for simulating liquid water. J Chem Phys 1983; 79:926–935.

10

Analysis of Surface Topology and Chemical Composition of Microstructures Formed in Planar Surfactant Films Under Compression

HANS-JOACHIM GALLA, STEFAN MALCHAREK, and NIKOLAUS BOURDOS*

Westfälische Wilhelms-Universität Münster,
Münster, Germany

Current affiliation: Lehrstuhl für Biophysik, Ruhr Universität Bochum, Universitätsstrasse, Bochum, Germany.

I. Introduction

The lung surfactant is a complex mixture of lipids and proteins that covers the air/water interface of type II pneumocytes in the lung. These surface active substances are necessary to lower the surface tension to a value close to zero, a basic necessity for normal breathing. There are four types of pulmonary surfactant proteins known, which can be divided into the two hydrophilic proteins SP-A and SP-D and the two hydrophobic proteins SP-B and SP-C. The hydrophobic proteins play a role in interfacial monolayer formation, formation of multilayer under compression, and reformation of the surface film on expansion.

The chemical analysis of lung lavage material shows that pulmonary surfactant mainly consists of 85–90% lipids, where not only saturated dipalmitoylphosphatidylcholine (DPPC) and unsaturated phosphatidylcholines (PCs) are predominant, but also phosphatidylglycerols (PGs), phosphatidylethanolamines (PEs), phosphatidylinositols (PIs), sphingolipids (SLs), fatty acids (FAs), and cholesterol are important components. The remaining 10–15% are proteins named surfactant proteins A,B,C, and D.

A. Film Balance and Video Enhanced Fluorescence Microscopy at the Air/Water Interface

To analyze the behavior of surfactant films at the air/water interface, we performed physical studies on the film balance with a model lipid mixture of DPPC and DPPG (4:1, molar ratio) doped with 0.4 mol% SP-C. The isotherms of this model surfactant were compared with isotherms obtained from native lung surfactant material, consisting of the natural hydrophobic lipids together with SP-B and SP-C. Both isotherms exhibit the same shape (Fig. 10.1).

Reduction of the film area leads to an increase in film pressure to a value of about 50 mN/m. On further compression, an abrupt increase in film compressibility is observed, leading to a plateau in the pressure/area diagram. The conclusion is that in the plateau region an accumulation into lamellar protrusions

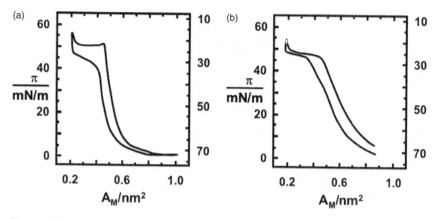

Figure 10.1 Comparison of the isotherms of (a) lipid/SP-C mixture with (b) native surfactant.

appears when the film is compressed. This phenomenon is called "squeeze-out" effect. On expansion, the excluded material respreads into the monolayer. The phase behavior and the "squeeze-out" effect of mixed films with DPPC, DPPG, and SP-C could also be observed and is quantified with fluorescence, light microscopy. Because of the lack of natural fluorescence, nitrobenzoxadiazole (NBD)-derivative is added to the system as a fluorophore at a concentration of 0.5–1 mol%. The NBD is bound to either PC or SP-C. It is important to note that the isotherm of lipid–protein mixtures is not significantly influenced by the addition of the fluorescence dye.

For excitation, a strong light is filtered and reflected at a dichroitic mirror. After the reflection, the beam is absorbed by the fluorescence dye in the lipid–protein mixture (Fig. 10.2).

The emitted light of the probe will be separated from the excitation by cut-off filters in the microscope. Images of monolayers or protrusions are taken with a camera and stored on a computer. The formation of domain structures is already observable at low surface pressure (2 mN/m) in a mixed film with DPPC/DPPG (4:1) and 0.4 mol% SP-C with fluorescence labeled phosphatidylcholine (NBD–PC). Discoidal dark domains are formed with the diameter of several micrometers and upon further compression the area covered by dark domains increase. These domains are identified as the liquid-condensed (LC) phase of pure lipid. The bright domains are thought to contain the protein, the fluorescence dye, and the lipids in the liquid-expanded (LE) phase [Figs 10.3(a–c)].

Owing to the high concentration of the dye, a self-quenching effect in the liquid phase occurs. This causes a decreasing contrast between the LC and LE domains with increasing pressure. Compared to the course of the [Figs. 10.3(a–c)], the contrast, however, reappears upon compression into the plateau region of the

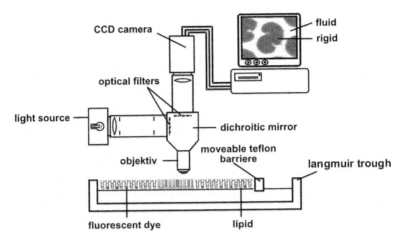

Figure 10.2 Fluorescence microscopy at the air/water interface.

isotherm [Fig. 10.3(d)]. Analysis of the images shows that the rise of the fluorescence intensity is due to the enrichment of dye molecules in the region of former LE phase and is not due to by an increasing emission of fluorescence of a single molecule.

By using statistical methods (1), mean intensities and areas of the domains were calculated. Histograms obtained from the fluorescence pictures lead to the idea that stacks of lipids bilayers are formed underneath the monolayer (Fig. 10.4). This means that the monolayer forms three-dimensional structures containing dye and lipids, which are associated with the monolayer.

According to the results of the statistical method, a model of the lung surfactant was developed (2). The multilamellar structures, so-called protrusions, are stabilized with the surfactant protein SP-C. SP-C contains a hydrophobic α-helix, which is incorporated in a bilayer. The two palmitoyl acids residues of SP-C, which are bound to two cysteins, attach the neighboring bilayers or the bilayer structures to the surface active monolayer. The monolayer lipid–protein complexes are thought to stabilize the protrusions, whereas only lipids

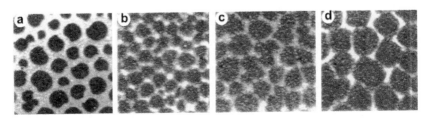

Figure 10.3 Fluorescence microscopy at the air/water interface of DPPC/DPPG/SP-C.

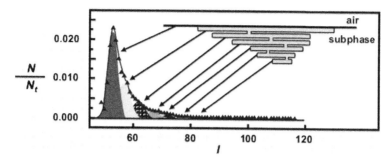

Figure 10.4 Histogram from fluorescence pictures shows the formation of distinct numbers of lipid bilayers.

remain in the liquid-condensed phase (Fig. 10.5) of the monolayer allowing maximal reduction of the surface tension.

Analyses of DPPC/DPPG/SP-C by means of scanning near-field optical microscopy (SNOM) show the formation of multilamellar structures when they are compressed. Binding a fluorescent dye to the protein leads to localization of the protein in the multilayer stacks and in the monolayer by every compression. The fluorescence intensity of the protrusion depends on the height of the protrusions (3).

II. Topological Analysis of Domains Structures

To analyze the topographical structures of the protrusions formed in DPPC/DPPG/SP-C films, scanning force microscopy (SFM) as well as scanning electron microscopy (SEM) were used. For those techniques, the film in the plateau region has to be transferred from the air/water interface to a solid support, for example mica (Fig. 10.6).

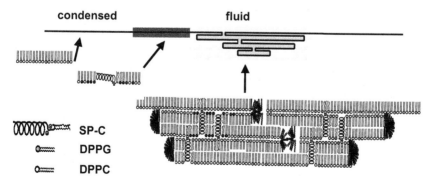

Figure 10.5 Structure of model lung surfactant.

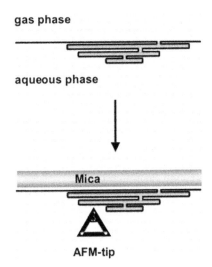

Figure 10.6   Scanning force microscopic investigation of the collapse structure.

Both techniques clearly show that our interpretation of the results obtained by the film balance technique and by fluorescence light microscopy measurements are correct and that indeed double layer protrusions are characteristic for the collapsed film in the plateau region (2,4). Figure 10.7 shows the SFM topography at the lipid/air interface for a film transferred to mica in the plateau region. Three pictures are given at different magnifications. Figure 10.7(a) and (b) taken with low resolution, shows the lamellar protrusions similar to those observed by fluorescence microscopy at the airwater interface. From high resolution SFM pictures we know that each layer is about 6 nm thick, which means that the protrusions are based on integer multiples of a lipid double layer [Figs. 10.7(c) and 10.8].

A DPPC double layer measured with the SFM under the same conditions has a thickness of 5 nm. The larger height of the lung surfactant bilayer when

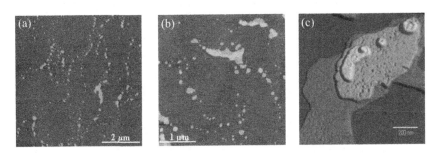

Figure 10.7   SFM topology of DPPC/DPPG/SP-C monolayer.

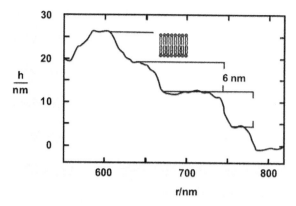

Figure 10.8 Analysis of the SFM pictures.

compared with the DPPC bilayer may be explained by the inclusion of protein and/or by significant water layers in between the lipid layers. The process of protrusions formation under compression is fully reversible. When a film is compressed to the end of the high compressibility region and is reexpanded afterwards, the protrusions will disappear.

Another technique to investigate the three-dimensional organization of lipid–peptide films at the interface is SEM. A beam of electrons scans parallel lines across the surface. Most important for this technique is the interaction of the electrons with the object. Two phenomena occur at the surface (5). On one hand, secondary electrons are emitted by the hit of the pulsed electrons with the electrons of the sample; on the other hand, high energy electrons reflect from the atomic nucleus. The emitted electrons are collected and amplified yielding a three-dimensional image of the specimen. This technique also supports the idea of protrusions of stacked lipid–peptide bilayers (Fig. 10.9).

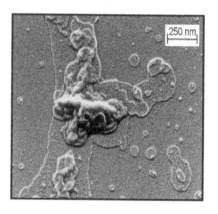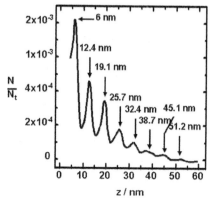

Figure 10.9 A collapsed DPPC/DPPG/SP-C film visualized by SEM (5).

III. Chemical Analysis Surfactant Composition Using Imaging Time-of-Flight Secondary Ion Mass Spectrometry

The use of fluorescence microscopy or atomic force microscopy to image lipid monolayers has the disadvantage of bearing no chemical information. For fluorescence microscopy, one also has to consider that a bulky fluorescent group is added to a molecule to visualize its lateral distribution. Such a group may affect the behavior of a thin film in many ways.

Imaging mass spectrometry (MS) is a powerful technique to analyze thin molecular overlayers on a solid substrate with respect to its chemical composition. If mass resolution is high enough, one is able to exactly assign the obtained mass to a certain molecule or atom. The MS measurements cannot be performed directly at the air/water interface but on films transferred onto a solid support. With respect to the resolution, however, MS cannot compete with force microscopy.

Here we show how to analyze phospholipid films containing SP-C by time-of-flight (TOF) MS techniques. Mass maps at different stages of film compression are presented. Our results strongly support the important role of the SP-C for respiration by stabilizing the formation of layered protrusions, and demonstrate the excellence of the applied MS techniques for the analysis of biomolecular overlayers. A special focus is put on quantitative aspects.

A. TOF-SIMS and Laser-SNMS

As we showed recently, Langmuir–Blodgett films of SP-C-containing phospholipid films could be imaged by time-of-flight secondary ion (SI) mass spectrometry (TOF-SIMS) and laser-postionized secondary neutrals (SN) mass spectrometry (laser-TOF-SNMS or laser-SNMS). By the mapping of secondary particles, we could directly visualize the domain formation and composition. Domain formation was already imaged in DPPC monolayers using TOF-SIMS, as the matrix effect allows to distinguish co-existing lyotropic phases, in which the molecules are differently packed, meaning that the chemical environment of a single molecule affects the SI formation.

TOF-SIMS and laser-SNMS spectra contain signals characteristic for DPPC and SP-C, but not for DPPG. SI and SN maps reveal domain structures in DPPC/DPPG and DPPG/SP-C films, but not in DPPC/SP-C films. In case of the SIMS images, we can distinguish between the fluid and the condensed areas due to a matrix effect, which corresponds with other imaging techniques, that is fluorescence light microscopy and SFM (Fig. 10.10).

The ternary mixture DPPC/DPPG/SP-C, transferred as partially collapsed film, shows SP-C-rich domains surrounding almost pure lipid areas, the latter of which were found by fluorescence light microscopy to be in a condensed and peptide containing domain in a fluid phase. The TOF-MS results fully accord

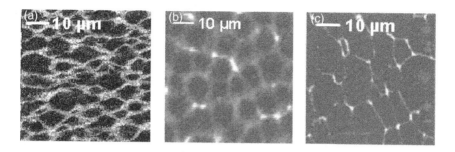

Figure 10.10   Comparison of (a) SNMS (b) fluorescence microscopy and (c) SFM.

with our earlier SFM picture of layered protrusions that serve as a compressed reservoir for surfactant material during expansion, and support the major role of the SP-C during respiration.

B.   The Principles of TOF-SIMS and Laser-SNMS Technique

The Technique

The sample or target, which consists of a gold substrate covered by a molecular Langmuir–Blodgett overlayer, is probed by an ion beam (Fig. 10.11). The impact of these primary ions triggers a collision cascade among the substrate atoms (6,7), whose energy causes the desorption of substrate atoms, overlayer molecules, and molecular fragments (Fig. 10.12); this is the sputter process. Only about 1% of the sputtered particles are ions, 99% are neutrals. The different nature of the

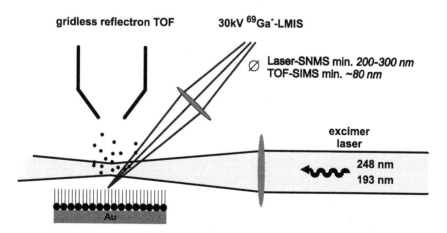

Figure 10.11   Schematic illustration of a TOF-SIMS or laser-SNMS measurement. The incident angle of the Ga primary ion beam is 45°. The desorbed particles enter either directly the analysator (SIMS) or are first ionized by a laser (SNMS).

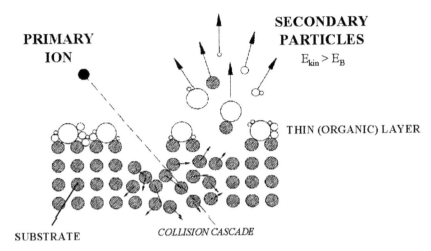

Figure 10.12 Schematic illustration of the sputter event. The impact of the primary ions induces movement among the substrate atoms. Finally, their kinetic energy is transferred to overlayer molecules: they desorb if their kinetic energy E_{kin} is greater than their binding energy E_B.

secondary particle species requires different instrumentation. The charged SI are "sucked" after desorption by an electric field of opposite charge. They enter the mass analyzer, are accelerated, and separated owing to their mass-to-charge ratio, and finally registered by a TOF detector. The SN, however, need to be ionized before they enter the analyzer. This postionization of the originally uncharged fragments is done by a laser with 193 nm wavelength.

One has to be aware that the postionization process depicts a fundamental difference between the two MS techniques. For SIMS, ionization and desorption are one process, whereas for SNMS they are two timely and spatially separated independent processes. Thus, the desorption of the SN is decoupled from the ionization process, allowing a better control of ionization by tuning of the laser wavelength.

For SIMS, because desorption and ionization are not separated, the flux or intensity of a given SI depends in a complex way on the environment in which the parental molecule is embedded. This so-called matrix effect is not defined at all and complicates the quantification of the local surface concentration of a molecule; it is possible to quantify certain simple one-component systems by an error margin of $\sim 20\%$ (8). On the other hand, the matrix effect allows to visualize co-existing phases in LB layers (9,10), taking advantage of the different SI flux in the liquid-expanded and the condensed phase. Other TOF-SIMS investigations on solid-supported LB films include stearic acid, self-assembled monolayers of thiols, polymethylacrylate, and gramicidin (11,12). Further applications are given by Bertrand and Weng (13).

The analysis of SN yields more quantitative results, as the SN are the majority of the secondary particles (14–17). Thus, if a compound is not homogeneously distributed, SN maps should mirror the proportions of its surface concentration. Laser-SNMS can also be used to distinguish co-existing phases, because concentration is higher in the condensed than in the liquid domains. However, it should be mentioned that laser-SNMS maps reveal matrix effects too, but rather than the overlayer signals the substrate signals are affected, that is, Au and trace components like Ag and Cr (18). The ionization and/or desorption of these metals seems to depend on the type of molecule covering the substrate (protein or lipid) or on the molecular density (liquid or condensed), or on both. We will not discuss this further.

The Instrumentation

The samples are placed in a vacuum chamber at pressures $<10^{-8}$ torr. The spectrometer is a combined TOF-SIMS/SNMS instrument equipped with a reflectron-type TOF analyzer, a pulsed 30 keV Ga^+ primary ion source, and an excimer laser for resonantly enhanced multiphoton postionization of neutrals, tuned at $\lambda = 193$ nm; this wavelength proved to be adequate for the analysis of amino acids and peptides (15). The device is well-suited for imaging, because it consists of a scanning optic and the Ga^+ beam can be focused to spot diameters <100 nm. The reflectron is grid-less, it accounts for transmission factors near 1, and has an improved resolution. This setup has been described in detail elsewhere (19,16) and was used earlier to study LB films of phospholipids (9,10,20) and phospholipids with SP-C (21).

TOF analyzers attain low detection limits (some fmol) and allow quasi-simultaneous and, therefore, fast detection with theoretically no upper mass limit. Actually, this limit is imposed by the desorption process; for TOF-SIMS it was found to be 15,000 atomic mass units (amu) for polymers and 4000 amu for peptides (21).

Sample Preparation

Tempax glass slides were cleaned thoroughly as described in Bourdos et al. (21). A thin layer of gold was evaporated, and the gold-covered slides were further cleaned using an organic solvent. Lipid or lipid–protein films were prepared by Langmuir–Blodgett deposition, prior to film deposition the surface was treated with argon plasma. It is crucial to have substrates being as clean as possible. A good criterion is the "missing" of silicon oil peaks at masses $73 + n \cdot 74$.

Mass Spectra

A certain area is scanned by the primary ion beam at each pixel of the digital raster, the mass signals are registered by the TOF detector. A mass spectrum is obtained by integrating SI intensities over the entire scan area after scanning it about, for instance, 100 or 200 times (one may increase the number of scans to enhance signal-to-noise ratio). To achieve high mass resolution, the PI pulse was bunched, denoting temporal compression of a 15 nm Ga^+ pulse to ~ 1 nm by time-dependent acceleration. Because the moment of the PI impact must be well-defined to serve as zero-point for the TOF measurement, short pulses enhance mass resolution. (Note: to further improve the mass resolution, almost pure ^{69}Ga is used.)

Imaging

Maps of lateral distribution of SI or SN are obtained by assigning intensities pixelwise to values of a gray scale or color map (molecular mapping). The Ga^+ beam can be focused to a minimal spot diameter of ~ 80 nm, in our experiments. However, lateral resolutions of 0.25–1 μm were obtained, corresponding to scan areas of 60×60 and 120×120 μm^2, respectively, using a raster of 128×128 or 256×256 pixels. (Note that lateral resolution is lower for SNMS measurements, only about 200–300 nm). For a better understanding of the factors determining lateral resolution [see for example Refs. (18,22,23)].

A disadvantage of bunching is the spatial spread of the PI beam, resulting into a defocused beam, which is not suitable for imaging. As a consequence, imaging had to be carried out without bunching; high mass resolution and high spatial resolution therefore contradict each other. Thus, the mapping of many mass signals was afflicted with interference between adjacent peaks, for example CH_4N^+ and $^{13}CCH_5$, both of which have the nominal mass 30 amu (CH_4N^+ is typical of peptides, whereas the latter is an isotopomer of the unspecific $C_2H_5^+$); interferences became more obvious as the mass resolution of the TOF-SIMS device was greatly enhanced over the years. But larger secondary particles, which are less intense like the two DPPC quasimolecules $(DPPC \pm H)^+$, are mapped together with their isotope clusters instead of a single peak to get a "sum image" with sufficient brightness. Except for the atomic ions like Ca^{2+}, fragments are termed "M" together with the nominal mass, so instead of $C_4H_{10}N^+$ we say M72.

Specific Features

Although TOF analyzers have no mass limit, making possible the detection of very large molecules (proteins, nucleic acids), TOF-SIMS spectra are dominated by distinct fragmentation in the so-called fingerprint region, denoting masses up to ~ 500 amu. This, too, applies to protein and lipid spectra. But if the mixture under investigation is not too complex, fingerprint signals may be utilized for the identification of large molecules that are not desorbed as whole quasimolecules, whatever the reason for this may be. Positively charged quasimolecules are for instance generated by protonation $(M + H)^+$, cationization by alkaline metals $(M + Na)^+$ or substrate atoms $(M + Au)^+$. We will only refer to positive ions here, although we also obtained negative ion spectra.

It turned out that laser-SNMS spectra hardly contain organic ions >100 amu. This is because of the large extent of fragmentation caused by the postionization and bears the shortcoming of having only a few characteristic fragments for either DPPC or SP-C. Some fragments are the same for SIMS and SNMS, like C_3H_8N (mass 58), which is formed in DPPC layers and is found as intensive peak in both types of spectra.

C. TOF-SIMS and SNMS-Investigations of DPPC/DPPG/SP-C-Films

Aim of the Investigation

Here we present results obtained by the application of surface mass spectrometry to analyze the domain structures in films consisting of the two major surfactant phospholipid components DPPC and DPPG, and their mixtures with SP-C. The collapsed ternary film is of particular interest, because protrusions with only indirectly characterized chemical composition were observed after compression, which might explain the mechanism behind the behavior of the alveolar surfactant observed during compression–expansion cycles.

Although we have presented some of our laser-SNMS results earlier (24), we focus on this special and scarcely applied technique because it is hardly known among the community of life scientists. Although the overall intensity of some SP-C fragments is very low, one obtains SN images with striking contrasts. Moreover, we show the quantitative nature of laser-SNMS by presenting some calculations by which quantitative information can be derived from SN maps.

Figures 10.13 and 10.14 show TOF-SIMS (positive SI) and Laser-SNMS spectra, respectively, of a DPPC/DPPG/SP-C film; a spectrum of a DPPC film is shown in Ref. (10), and an SP-C spectrum in Ref. (21). In Table 10.1, the most important signals are summarized. The primary ion dose density or fluence F is the PI number or PI dose per unit area (cm^2), which was applied

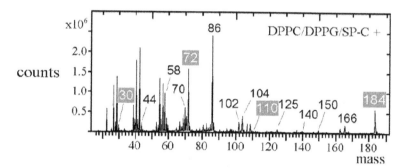

Figure 10.13 TOF-SIMS fingerprint spectrum of positive SI of a model lung surfactant composed of the dipalmitoylated phospholipids DPPC, DPPG, and the small surfactant protein C.

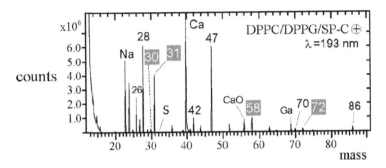

Figure 10.14   Laser-SNMS fingerprint spectrum of the model lung surfactant.

during the measurement of the respective sample. F is a measure for the damage a sample encounters during the measurement by ion bombardment, and therefore more important than the PI dose. F gives an idea whether the measurement was carried out under "static" conditions, which implies that the sample remains almost undamaged, so that one obtains constant yields

$$Y = \frac{N_S}{N_P} \qquad\qquad (10.1)$$

Table 10.1   Selection of Positive Secondary Ions and Laser SMNS Ions

		Yield ($\times 10^{-6}$)		Origin	
m/z	Sum formula	+	$\oplus$	DPPC	SP-C
18	NH_4	40	30	–	✓
26	CN	–	11,200	(✓)	✓
28	CO	–	27,800	✓*	✓
30	NO	–	10,900	–	✓
30	CH_4N	220	50	–	✓
31	P	–	36,500	✓*	–
32	S	–	200	–	✓
42	C_2H_4N	–	4,600	✓	–
44	C_2H_6N	170	100	–	✓
47	PO	–	27,300	✓*	–
58	C_3H_8N	2,200	6,400	✓	–
70	C_4H_8N	550	900	(✓)	✓
72	$C_4H_{10}N$	5,400	1,500	(✓)	✓
86	$C_5H_{12}N$	8,900	2,000	✓	✓
104	$C_5H_{14}NO$	1,700		✓	–
110	$C_5H_8N_3$	90		–	✓
184	$C_5H_{15}PNO_4$	1,850		✓	–

*Sum of all isotopomers.

where N_S is the number of the detected secondary particles and N_P is the number of PIs applied on the sample (PI dose). In case of laser-SNMS, Y is termed "sensitivity" because the intensity of a secondary particle depends not only on the conditions during desorption but also on laser parameters. Note that the yield also varies with the device: if the transmission of the analyzer is lower, Y is lower too because less particles reach the detector.

The TOF-SIMS spectrum of our model lung surfactant contains intense fingerprint fragments like M58, M72, M86, M104, and M184 each of which originates from DPPC and/or SP-C (Table 10.2). M184 is the whole polar head-group ion of DPPC. Above the fingerprint region (not shown) are the quasimolecule ions $(DPPC \pm H)^+$ (M732.5 and M734.5) and their isotope patterns, and, although yield is much lower than for the smaller fragments, the signal-to-noise ratio is excellent.

DPPG does not provide any specific positive fragment except the protonated phosphoglycerol residue M173, but this fragment has a low reproducibility and its yield is extremely low. The DPPG quasimolecule ion is present in the negative SI spectrum of the ternary film (not shown).

Because DPPC and DPPG differ in their headgroup, the mass range <200 amu can be used for the identification of DPPC: M104, M166, and

Table 10.2 Calculated Values for the Phase-Dependent Sensitivity Y^z, the Density Ratios y_1 and y_2, and the Relative Intensities i^z

Plateau	Y^{LC}	Y^{LE1}	Y^{LE2}	y_1	y_2	i^{LC}	i^{LE1}	i^{LE2}
DPPC								
M42	2,750	2,450	2,300	0.89	0.84	0.70	0.26	0.043
M58	5,000	4,350	4,100	0.87	0.82	0.70	0.26	0.043
Lipid								
$P^\oplus$	29,200	26,200	25,500	0.90	0.87	0.69	0.27	0.045
$PO^\oplus$	24,200	20,900	20,000	0.86	0.83	0.70	0.26	0.043
SP-C								
M18	20	60	75	3.0	3.8	0.40	0.49	0.11
M30	160	670	1,370	4.2	8.6	0.30	0.51	0.19
$S^\oplus$	50	90	100	1.8	2.0	0.52	0.40	0.081
M44	120	180	190	1.5	1.6	0.58	0.36	0.069
Lipid + SP-C								
$CN^\oplus$	7,200	14,000	15,750	1.9	2.2	0.50	0.42	0.082
M27	1,750	2,100	2,250	1.2	1.3	0.62	0.32	0.061
M70	570	640	650	1.1	1.1	0.64	0.30	0.054
M72	500	670	740	1.3	1.5	0.60	0.34	0.065
M86	570	600	610	1.1	1.1	0.65	0.29	0.053

Note: The values of Y^{LC}, Y^{LE1}, and Y^{LE2} should be multiplied by 10^{-6}. We considered different fragments, specific for DPPC, both phospholipids, or SP-C. Some of them can be related to lipid and protein as well.

M184 as well as other fragments listed in the table are typical of DPPC but not included in the DPPG spectrum.

SP-C forms some pronounced fragments as well; some of them interfere with DPPC fragments, like M72 and M86, emanating from valine and leucine/ isoleucine. These are $(M-45)^+$ peaks, arising from a net cleavage of the carboxylic group, and typical of amino acids. But also the small peaks M18, M30, M44, or M110 are noteworthy. M30 and M44 do not only originate from glycine and alanine, respectively, but are general constituents of peptide mass spectra (25). M110 is a (His-45) peak. The quasimolecule ion $(SP-C + H)^+$ is observed in the single-compound spectrum of SP-C (21). One has to consider that most of the N-containing secondary particles <100 amu interfere with non-specific hydrocarbons, which can be recognized by asymmetrically shaped peaks. The hydrocarbon share of such a fragment is about 10% (21).

Laser-SNMS Spectra

The neutral particle spectra are less rich in fragments being characteristic for either DPPC or SP-C. We observe a pronounced peak at mass 58, denoting C_3H_8N, which turns out to be the most intense and therefore most important DPPC signal. Further we have M31 (P) and M47 (PO), which emanate from DPPC and DPPG. Other important, although much less intense, peaks are M18, M30, and M72. These small peaks account for striking contrasts in their respective lateral distribution maps. The single-compound spectra (not shown here) shows that we can assign the small fragments M18 and M30 to SP-C, M72 to DPPC and SP-C. M26 and M28 are CO and CN, respectively, they will not be discussed. Note the strong calcium peak at mass 40 (this was a Ca-containing film). P and PO are mass peaks for both lipids, which is a remarkable difference to negative SIMS spectra (if ever, phosphorus is only desorbed as negative ion).

Images

Figures 10.15 and 10.16 show the lateral distribution maps of the TOF-SIMS and Laser-SNMS fragments, respectively, which are highlighted in the related mass spectra (Figs. 10.13 and 10.14). The two highly SP-C-specific SI M30 and M110 are mapped with high contrast, displaying high intensities in the network-like liquid-expanded small domains and low intensities in the large liquid-condensed domains. The distribution of the DPPC- as well as SP-C-based M72 is similar, but with weaker contrast. M184, the DPPC headgroup ion, is homogeneously distributed, but cannot infer homogeneous distribution of the DPPC from this finding.

The SN M30 is distributed similarly as the SP-C-specific SI (Fig. 10.16), but with much higher contrast. Not shown is the sulfur map, which has similar though much weaker contrast as M30; note that the respective mass peak is hardly seen in the spectrum. Mapping of phosphorus produces opposite contrast,

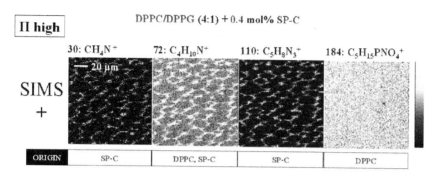

Figure 10.15 TOF-SIMS images of the ternary surfactant model system at Π = 30 mN/m. The maps show the distribution of the fragments highlighted in Fig. 10.11.

its intensity is strikingly high. P represents both phospholipids, and reveals a qualitative distribution that is expected, as its intensity is higher in the condensed domains. M58 is distributed not only similarly but also almost exactly as P, however, with weaker contrast, corresponding to the lower intensity in the spectrum. As for SIMS, the fragment M72 originates from both DPPC and SP-C, and gives a contrast similar to the respective SI image.

The equal distribution of P and M58 means that DPPC and DPPG are distributed equally, as P emanates from both phospholipids but M58 only from DPPC. As the weak but remarkable contrast of sulfur depicts, this element is obviously not found because of impurities but rather as part of the amino acids cysteine (two residues) and methionine (one residue). Considering the total amount of SP-C in the film (0.4 mol%), one can calculate the detection sensitivity; in this case it is in the sub-fmol range (40 nmol sulfur/m^2).

By both techniques TOF-SIMS and Laser-SNMS, the typical domain structure of the surfactant model film can be imaged, as shown for fluorescence microscopy or atomic force microscopy. The equal contrast of the P and M58

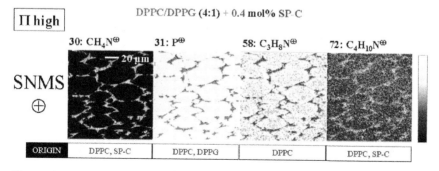

Figure 10.16 Laser-SNMS images of the ternary surfactant model system at Π = 30 mN/m. The maps show the distribution of the fragments highlighted in Fig. 10.11.

maps is remarkable. Because the latter is a molecule, one expects that it may be subject to matrix effects, but it is not. We thought that there might be at least a difference of a few percent but it is <1%.

Distribution of SP-C-Specific Fragment at Different Stages of Compression

We also present the images from our surfactant film at different stages of compression (Fig. 10.17). Again we see that results are not only similar to that obtained using atomic force microscopy and fluorescence microscopy, also for low pressure and for the plateau. We mapped the same fragment, M30 or CH_4N, as ionic and neutral species, and obtained images with similar contrasts for both techniques. We noted that this does not apply to all fragments, for instance the lipid fragment M58 is afflicted with a matrix effect as SI, showing a contrast opposite to the SN map; of course the domain structure is the same.

Determination of the Amount of SP-C Within the Fluid Domains

We present a simple calculation by means of which we are able to assess the amount of SP-C in the different film phases. We point out that this calculation does not replace a strict quantification procedure, performing calibration measurements using well-defined standards.

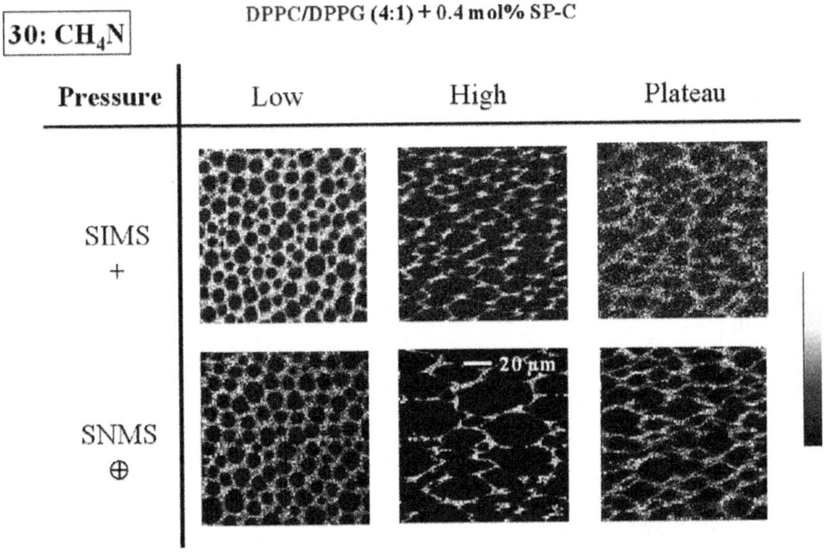

Figure 10.17 Lateral distribution of the positive and the neutral species of the SP-C fragment M30 at different film pressures. The right column shows the mapping at plateau pressure, the lateral structure closely resembles the structure obtained using fluorescence microscopy.

As a first step, we made a field analysis of the SNMS image of the plateau film (Fig. 10.17). For this we had to assess the amount of LE and LC phases in the film as follows: one can see in the M30 image that the LE domain consists of areas with different intensities; one can say it is parted into two subdomains. This is not surprising because we expect higher intensity in the parts of the film which are multilamellar. Now we binarize the images, that is, converting them into black-and-white images (Fig. 10.18) by thresholding, a common procedure in image processing. One can easily find a threshold value below which the LC domains appear black; these areas correspond to the dark patches in the M30 or M26 image. A second threshold value is used to "isolate" the brightest part of the film. Doing so, we find that the entire LC domain amounts to 67% of the film area and the LE domain to 33%. The subdomain LE1 is 5%, thus giving the LE2 area by simple subtraction, 28% (Fig. 10.18).

We now assume that M30 reflects the distribution of SP-C, M31 or P, the distribution of the phospholipids. With the phase-dependent yield Y^z and the share a^z of the area occupied by molecules in the phase z, we calculate the relative intensity i^z of a fragment in the respective phase z (= LC or LE):

$$i^z = \frac{a^z Y^z}{a^{LE} Y^{LE} + a^{LC} Y^{LC}} \tag{10.2}$$

With i^z, we can calculate the mole fraction m_p^z of SP-C in the LE or LC phase, given by

$$m_p^z = \frac{i_p^z}{i_l^z \cdot ((m_L/m_p) - 1) + i_p^z} \tag{10.3}$$

The index p denotes protein, that is, SP-C and index l the lipids. m_L and m_p are the mole fractions of the lipids and the SP-C, respectively. For the entire mixture

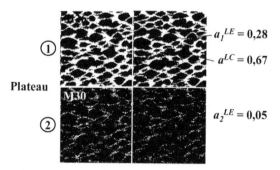

Figure 10.18 Illustration of the field analysis for the plateau film. The LE domain is divided into areas with different intensities (a_1^{LE}, a_2^{LE}), the LC share of the film is 67%. M26 is CN.

$m_L + m_p = 1$, that is, $m_p = 0.004$ and $m_L = 0.996$. Because $m_L \gg m_p$, we can use the approximation

$$m_p^z \approx \frac{m_p}{m_L} \cdot \frac{i_p^z}{i_1^z} \tag{10.4}$$

A further helpful value is the density ratio between the LE and LC phases for a given fragment $X^\oplus$, which is simply

$$y(X^\oplus) := \frac{Y^{LE}(X^\oplus)}{Y^{LC}(X^\oplus)} \tag{10.5}$$

y gives the quotient of the number of the $X^\oplus$ in the LE phase and the molecules in the LC phase. As we consider two LE phases for the plateau, 1 or 2 must be added as index.

It is remarkable that we found similar y_i values for both types of lipid fragments, indicating that DPPC and DPPG are distributed almost equally, that is, no demixing occurs. The i values tell us that $\sim70\%$ of the phospholipids are located in the LC phase, 26% in the LE1 phase, and 4% in the LE2 phase. y_1 and y_2 are similar for the lipid fragments, indicating that molecular densities do not vary much. The SP-C fragment M30 behaves differently: in the LE2 phase its density is much higher, nearly twice the LE1 phase density. This is not surprising because the LE2 phase is the domain containing the multilamellar protrusions, areas highly enriched in SP-C.

Although y_1 and y_2 are similar for the lipid fragments, the y_2 values are slightly smaller. This might point at a matrix effect, which might occur in SNMS measurements as well. However, this kind of matrix effect is different from the one discussed previously, where we said that ionization is influenced by different molecular environments. Here, in the protruded areas the molecules in the uppermost lamellae, that is, those being most far away from the substrate, are not sputtered as effectively as the molecules having direct contact with the substrate. As a consequence, intensities are lower than expected.

Using Eq. (10.4), we now calculate the mole fractions for SP-C in the LE1 and LE2 phases and obtain

$$m_p^{LE1} = 0.8 \, mol\%$$
$$m_p^{LE2} = 1.8 \, mol\%$$

One expects to find similar values, but the value for the LE2 phase is about twice as large. Perhaps the protrusion-induced matrix effect perturbs the calculation, nevertheless, the magnitude of the values seems to be quite reasonable.

The fragment CN may now be inserted to correct the obtained values. CN emerges from both DPPC and SP-C, and can be easily assigned to specific molecular groups: in DPPC it originates from the tertiary amine group —C(NH$_3$)$_3$, in SP-C it is part of the peptide bond. Our recombinant SP-C consists of 34 amino acid residues, corresponding to 33 peptide bonds, DPPC is only the origin for one CN molecule. From this one might expect that the sensitivity of the SP-C-based CN is 33 times larger than that of the DPPC-based. But it is not that simple: the sensitivity of a fragment is also proportional to the transformation probability P; we add the indices p and 1 for the SP-C-based CN and the DPPC-based CN, respectively. The ratio

$$r = \frac{P_p}{P_1} \tag{10.6}$$

can be obtained from the m^z and the i^z following a lengthy calculation which is not presented here (18). Doing this calculation for the two films below the plateau pressure (Fig. 10.17, left and middle column) in both cases we obtain a $r \approx 6$, denoting that in SP-C the fragment CN is formed with 6-fold larger probability than in DPPC. The calculation yields the same results for the LC and LE phases.

For the plateau film we obtain different values for r:

$r = 6.0$ (LC)
$r = 10.5$ (LE1)
$r = 2.1$ (LE2)

From the LC phase, we obtain the same r as for the films at lower pressure, the LE1 value is too large whereas the LE2 value is too small. This is peculiar as r must be the same for all phases. Therefore, we assume that this discrepancy is a consequence of a matrix effect, based on the formation of the multilamellar protrusions. The i^z values are given in Table 10.1.

Table 10.2 is corrected such that, i^{LE1} (P) = 0.23 (instead of 0.26) and i^{LE2} (P) = 0.068 (instead of 0.043), one obtains

$r = 6.0$ (LC)
$r = 6.0$ (LE1)
$r = 6.1$ (LE2)

It seems that the original LE2 intensity of the DPPC-based fragments is too low. We obtain the same result if we use a smaller i^{LE2} value (0.12 instead of 0.19) and a larger i^{LE1} value (0.58 instead of 0.51), respectively, for M30. Using the corrected i^z, we again calculate the mole fractions for the SP-C in the LE phases and obtain

$$m_p^{LE1} = 0.9 \, mol\%$$
$$m_p^{LE2} = 1.1 \, mol\%$$

Within the error margins (which are difficult to assess, but 10% is a good estimate), we obtain the local concentration of the SP-C in the LE phase being $\sim 1 \, mol\%$ (the LC concentration is $\sim 0.2 \, mol\%$). Obviously there is no significant difference in SP-C concentration between the two LE phases, which might also indicate that there is the same SP-C amount in each lamella of a protrusion; this is consistent with results obtained by SNOM (3). The similarity between M42/M58 and $P^{\oplus}/PO^{\oplus}$ says that there might be no selective squeeze-out of either DPPC or DPPG, which is in accordance with the result of Taneva and Keough (26): as the authors found, DPPC and DPPG are excluded from the monolayer to some extent. Another consequence of the nonselective exclusion is that the interaction between SP-C and both the lipids seems to be mainly hydrophobic.

IV. Conclusion

We have demonstrated by video enhanced fluorescence spectroscopy, scanning force microscopy, electron microscopy, and SNOM that protrusions are formed in a lipid/SP-C film under compression. This chemical phase separation allows to adapt the surface tension to the change in surface area under compression and expansion on a very low level. Laterally resolved SIMS allowed to analyse the chemical composition of this surfactant film after transfer onto a solid support. Quantification of different fragments originating from the lipids or the peptide showed that the SP-C is enriched within the fluid domains forming the reservoir. These results are true not only for the flat films obtained by the film balance technique. It was recently shown in Ref. (27) by fluorescence microscopy that these domains are also present on the curved surface of a submicrometer air bubbles formed under water on equally sized hydrophobically patterned gold surfaces. Moreover, we were able to analyse these domains on the air bubble by SFM (28). These results will be reported in Chapter 12.

Acknowledgments

We thank the Deutsche Forschungsgemeinschaft and (former Byk Gulden), who generously supported this work. Mass spectrometric work was only possible with the help of Felix Kollmer, Ralf Kamischke, and especially Alfred Benninghoven, the pioneer of surface mass spectrometry.

The results reported here were generated by former members of the group: Dr. A. v. Nahmen, Dr. M. Sieber, Ch. Loebbe, M. Ross, and in collaboration with Prof. Reichelt and Dr. M. Amrein from the Institute of Medical Physics and Biophysics.

References

1. von Nahmen A, Post A, Galla H-J, Sieber M. The phase behavior of lipid monolayers containing pulmonary surfactant protein C studied by fluorescence light microscopy. Eur Biophys J 1997; 26:359–369.
2. Galla H-J, Bourdos N, von Nahmen A, Amreim M, Sieber M. The role of pulmonary surfactant protein C during the breathing cycle. Thin Solid Films 1998; 327:632–635.
3. Kramer A, Wintergalen A, Sieber M, Galla H-J, Amrein M, & Guckenberger R. Distribution of the surfactant-associated protein C within a lung surfactant model film investigated by near-field optical microscopy. Biophys J 2000; 78:58–465.
4. Krol S, Janshoff A, Ross M, Galla H-J. Structure and function of surfactant protein B and C in lipid monolayers: a scanning force microscopy study. Phys Chem Chem Phys 2000; 2:4586–4593.
5. von Nahmen A. Strukturelle Organisation von Surfactant Protein C haltigen Phospholipid-Monoschichten an der Wasser/Luft-Grenzflaeche-ein modell des alveolaeren Surfactant. Ph.D. thesis, Westfaelische Wilhelms-Universitaet, Muenster, 1997.
6. Benninghoven A, Hagenhoff E, Niehues E. Surface MS: probing real-world samples. Anal Chem 1993; 65:630–640.
7. Benninghoven A. Chemical analysis of inorganic and organic surfaces and thin films by static time-of-flight secondary ion mass spectrometry (TOF-SIMS). Angew Chem Int Ed Engl 1994; 33:1023–1043.
8. Hagenhoff B. Sekundaerionenmassenspektrometrie an molekularen Oberflaeshen-strukturen. Ph.D. thesis, Westfaelische Wilhelms-Universitaet, Muenster, 1993.
9. Leufgen KM, Rulle H, Benninghoven A, Sieber M, Galla H-J. Imaging time-of-flight secondary ion mass spectrometry allows visualizatin and analysis of coexisting phases in Langmuir–Blodgett films. Langmuir 1996; 12:1708–1711.
10. Bourdos N, Kollmer F, Benninghoven A, Sieber M, Galla H-J. Imaging of domain structures in a one-component lipid monolayer by time-of-flight secondary ion mass spectrometry. Langmuir 2000; 16:1481–1484.
11. Hagenhoff B, Benninghoven A, Spinke J, Liley M, Knoll W. Time-of-flight secondary ion mass spectrometry investigations of self-assembled monolayers of organic thiols, sulfides, and disulfides on gold surfaces. Langmuir 1993; 9:1622–1624.
12. Hagenhoff B. Surface mass spectrometry—application to biosensor characterization. Biosensors Bioelectronics 1995; 10:885–894.
13. Bertrand P, Weng L. Time-of-flight secondary ion mass spectrometry (TOF-SIMS). Mikrochim Acta 1996; 13:167–182.
14. Schnieders A. Quantitative Surface Analysis by Laser Postionization of Sputtered Neutrals. Ph.D. thesis, Westfaelische Wilhelms-Universitaet, Muenster, 2000.

15. Terhorst M, Kampwerth G, Niehuis E, Benninghoven A. Sputtered neutrals mass spectrometry of organic molecules using multiphoton postionization. J Vac Sci Technol 1992; A10:3210–3215.

16. Kollmer F. Abbildende Nanobereichsanalyse mit der Flugzeitmassen-spektrometrie zerstaeubtere Ionen (TOF-SIMS) und Neutralteilchen (Lasen-SNMS). Ph.D. thesis, Westfaelische Wilhelms-Universitaet, Muenster, 2001.

17. Kamischke R. Abbildende TOF-SIMS und Laser-SNMS nanostrukturierter Oberflaechen. Ph.D. thesis, Westfaelische Wilhelms-Universitaet, Muenster, 2000.

18. Bourdos N. Ortsaufgeloeste massenspektrometrische Analyse von Lipid- und Lipid-Protein-Monoschichten als Modelle des alveolaren Surfactants. Ph.D. thesis, Westfaelische Wilhelms-Universitaet, Muenster, 2001.

19. Schwieters J, Cramer HG, Heller T, Juergens U, Niehuis E, Zehnpfennig J, Benninghoven A. High mass resolution surface imaging with a time-of-flight secondary ion mass spectroscopy scanning microprobe. J Vac Sci Technol 1991; A9:2864–2871.

20. Ross M, Steinem C, Galla H-J, Janshoff A. Visualization of chemical and physical properties of calcium-induced domains in DPPC/DPPS Langmuir-Blodgett layers. Langmuir 2001; 17:2437–2445.

21. Bourdos N, Kollmer F, Benninghoven A, Ross M, Sieber M, Galla H-J. Analysis of lung surfactant model systems with time-of-flight secondary ion mass spectrometry. Biophys J 2000; 79:357–369.

22. Koetter F, Benninghoven A. Secondary ion emission from polymer surfaces under Ar^+, Xe^+ and SF_5^+ ion bombardment. Appl Surf Sci 1998; 133:47–57.

23. Rulle H. Hochaufloesende Abbildungen strukturierter organischer Oberflaechen mit der Flugzeit-Sekundaerionenmassenspektrometrie (TOF-SIMS). Ph.D. thesis, Westfaelische Wilhelms-Universitaet, Muenster, 1996.

24. Bourdos N, Kollmer F, Kamischke R, Benninghoven A, Galla H-J, Sieber M. In: Benninghoven A, ed. TOF-SIMS and Laser-SNMS Characterization of Multicomponent Phospholipid Langmuir–Blodgett Layers. Amsterdam: Elsevier Science, 2000:923–926.

25. McLafferty FW. In: MacLafferty FW, Turecek FW, eds. Interpretation of Mass Spectra. California: University Science Books, 1993.

26. Taneva S-G, Keough KMW. Pulmonary surfactant proteins SP-B and SP-C in spread monolayers at the air water interface: III. Proteins SP-B plus SP-C with phospholipids in spread monolayers. Biophys J 1994; 66:1158–1166.

27. Knebel D, Sieber M, Reichelt R, Galla HJ, Amrein M. Scanning force microscopy at the air–water interface of an air bubble coated with pulmonary surfactant. Biophys J 2002; 82:474–480.

28. Knebel D, Sieber M, Reichelt R, Galla HJ, Amrein M. Fluorescence light microscopy of pulmonary surfactant at the air–water interface of an air bubble of adjustable size. Biophys J 2002; 83:547–555.

11

SP-B Peptides: Synthesis, Structure, and Surface Activity

JOSH W. KURUTZ, CHUTIMA JIARPINITNUN, TOM WITTEN, and KA YEE C. LEE

The University of Chicago,
Chicago, Illinois, USA

HAIM DIAMANT

Tel Aviv University,
Tel Aviv, Israel

ALAN J. WARING

University of California,
Los Angeles, California, USA

I. Introduction

Lung surfactant (LS), a complex mixture of lipids and proteins, lines the alveoli, and is responsible for the proper functioning of the lung (1). LS works both by lowering the surface tension inside the lungs to reduce the work of breathing and by stabilizing the alveoli through varying the surface tension as a function of alveolar volume. To accomplish this, the LS mixture must adsorb rapidly to the air–fluid interface of the alveoli after being secreted. Once at the interface, it must form a monolayer that can both achieve low surface tensions upon compression and vary the surface tension as a function of the alveolar radius. Insufficient levels of surfactant, owing to either immaturity in premature infants or disease or trauma in adults, can result in respiratory distress syndrome (RDS), a potentially lethal disease in both populations.

LS consists primarily of the saturated lipid dipalmitoylphosphatidylcholine (DPPC) and unsaturated phosphatidylcholines, significant amounts of unsaturated and anionic phospholipids such as phosphatidylglycerols (PGs), lesser amounts of anionic lipids such as palmitic acid (PA), and neutral components such as cholesterol. LS also contains four lung surfactant-specific proteins, known as SP-A, -B, -C, and -D. Of the four, SP-B and SP-C are small amphipathic proteins and exhibit high surface activities. Although the complete roles of SP-B and SP-C are not yet fully understood, they are known to be essential for the proper functioning of LS *in vivo* and in replacement surfactants for the treatment of RDS. Our laboratory has focused its attention on SP-B because it is the major protein in commercial LS replacements (2,3) and because it is critical to mammalian survival (4,5); mice lacking the SP-B gene die shortly after birth (6), whereas those lacking SP-C continue to live, albeit impaired (7).

Although SP-B is important for surfactant function, its role in LS and its important structural features are not fully understood. In LS, SP-B is a disulfide-linked homodimer of 79-residue monomers, each of which features four putative α-helices and are predicted to be amphipathic (8,9). A great deal of attention has been focused on the N-terminal 25-residue segment of SP-B, SP-B$_{1-25}$, which faithfully reproduces the functional aspects of the full-length protein. It has also been demonstrated that simple peptide sequences based on the N-terminus of SP-B possess the full-activity of the native protein (10–16). However, it is not well understood what structural features of this short peptide make it such a good mimic of the full-length SP-B.

In terms of the lipid components that constitute LS, it has been known for a long time that pure DPPC, the major lipid component in LS, can form monolayers that attain surface tensions near zero values on compression. In the context of LS, this feature of DPPC definitely helps to reduce the work of breathing. However, DPPC adsorbs and respreads slowly as a monolayer under physiological conditions, rendering itself not an ideal LS candidate (1,17–19). The unsaturated and anionic lipids present in natural LS and added to many replacement surfactants are believed to enhance the adsorption and respreading of DPPC (17–19). PA, for example, is one of the three compounds added to exogenous surfactant in Survanta (8.5% w/w; Ross Laboratory, Columbus, Ohio) and Surfactant TA (8.5% w/w; Tokyo Tanabe) used to treat premature infants with neonatal RDS.

Owing to the relatively low collapse pressure of pure fatty acid, anionic and unsaturated lipid monolayers compared with DPPC, it has been postulated that LS monolayers are refined by selective removal of lipids with low collapse pressures on repeated compression and expansion, a phenomenon known as "squeeze-out" (18,20). There is evidence that some unsaturated lipid components of LS are squeezed out of binary monolayers containing DPPC or dipalmitoyl-phosphatidylglycerol (DPPG) (18,21). However, these experiments use binary lipid mixtures that do not adequately represent the functioning LS monolayers, and have neglected the possible effects of LS proteins on monolayer behavior. Indeed, interactions between LS lipids and proteins may alter this process and remove the driving force for squeeze-out of the fluidizing components. It has been shown, for instance, that the addition of full-length SP-B or its N-terminus peptide, SP-B$_{1-25}$, to monolayers of PA results in much higher monolayer collapse pressures (lower surface tension values) than those of either PA or SP-B alone (14). Squeeze-out of the palmitoylphosphatidylglycerol (POPG) in a mixed DPPG/POPG monolayer has also been reported to be eliminated when SP-B$_{1-25}$ is present (22–24). This suggests that a synergistic effect between the anionic lipids (with low collapse pressures) and SP-B peptides may result in the retention of both the lipid and the peptide in the monolayer upon compression to high surface pressures (14,22–25).

Over the past few years, we have been interested in the structure–function relationship of SP-B peptides in the context of their surface activities in an LS-mimicking environment. A variety of SP-B peptides and peptide-mimics have been designed and synthesized for the purpose of our biophysical studies. As high-resolution structural information was not available for SP-B, we have embarked upon a nuclear magnetic resonance (NMR) study of various SP-B peptides. In this effort, we have successfully solved the structure of the truncated SP-B$_{11-25}$, thereby providing the first set of high-resolution structural data on any SP-B peptides. We have also made progress in addressing the question of how alterations in the structure of SP-B peptides may affect their ability to retain lipids with low collapse pressure in the LS mixture at high surface pressures by examining the interaction between SP-B peptides with different structural motifs and mixed DPPG/POPG monolayers. Intrigued by the reversible folding transition first observed by Zasadzinski and coworkers (22) and subsequently in our own work, we have theoretically modeled the onset of the folding instability by examining the mechanical properties of the mixed lipid–peptide film. In this chapter, we will first discuss our design and synthetic strategies for the various SP-B peptides used in our studies, and give a brief overview of our NMR efforts on SP-B peptides to date. Monolayer and fluorescence microscopy results revealing the different extent by which various SP-B peptides can prevent the squeeze-out of the unsaturated component from a mixed lipid system will be presented, and a continuum model for the folding transition will be discussed.

II. SP-B Surfactant Peptide Synthesis

As SP-B is a member of the saposin family of proteins, the rationale for selection of amino acid sequences for peptide synthesis from the full-length protein is largely based on the saposin fold (26). Saposin proteins or SAPLIP proteins (27) share several common structural and functional similarities. These similarities include a dominant amphipathic, α-helical secondary structure that facilitates functional interaction with membrane amphipathic lipids, and a disulfide connectivity that is highly conserved for all the members of the saposin family. The combination of helix–bend secondary structure with disulfide connectivity gives the mature protein a three-dimensional structure of a folded helical hairpin that optimizes the interaction of the molecule with polar lipids.

A recent residue-specific solution NMR study of the saposin protein NK-lysin (26) has helped provide a detailed structure of this class of molecule that can be used as a starting point for building a model of the full-length SP-B protein. By templating the SP-B amino acid sequence onto the NK-lysin backbone and connecting a second SP-B monomer, a theoretical model for the native SP-B homodimer has been proposed (28). A ribbon representation of one SP-B monomer backbone is shown in Fig. 11.1, with each of the domains highlighted with the corresponding amino acid sequences listed in Fig. 11.2. The N-terminal domain consists of a short proline-rich segment connected to a positively charged amphipathic α-helix by a turn and terminated at its other

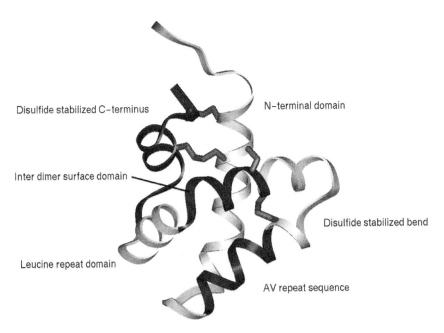

Figure 11.1   Ribbon representation of monomer of SP-B$_{1-78}$. The N-terminal domain is in light gray, the AV repeat sequence black, disulfide stabilized bend light gray, interdimer surface domain black, leucine repeat light gray, and C-terminal segment black. All disulfide connectivities are represented as dark gray tubes.

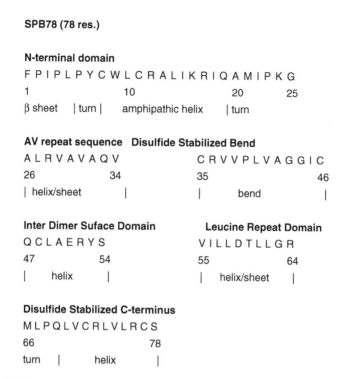

SPB78 (78 res.)

N-terminal domain

F P I P L P Y C W L C R A L I K R I Q A M I P K G
1   10   20   25
β sheet | turn | amphipathic helix | turn

AV repeat sequence Disulfide Stabilized Bend

A L R V A V A Q V   C R V V P L V A G G I C
26   34   35   46
| helix/sheet | | bend |

Inter Dimer Suface Domain   Leucine Repeat Domain

Q C L A E R Y S   V I L L D T L L G R
47   54   55   64
| helix | | helix/sheet |

Disulfide Stabilized C-terminus

M L P Q L V C R L V L R C S
66   78
turn | helix |

Figure 11.2 SP-B$_{1-78}$ synthetic amino acid sequences. The amino acid sequences are in one letter code with the sequence number and structure below the letter.

end by another turn. This amphipathic sequence is followed by a more hydrophobic segment including two valine-alanine repeats that are linked to a midsection disulfide stabilized bend sequence. The mid-section bend region is followed by a helical leucine-arginine sequence that is terminated by another turn sequence. The positively-charged amphipathic C-terminus is then connected to the N-terminal helix by two disulfide links at either end of the short helical segment. The cystine-disulfide residue spacing of the N- and C-terminal helices is highly conserved for saposin proteins including SP-B from all species that have been sequenced. Another variation of this type of structure–function strategy employed by investigators has been the synthesis of peptides of increasing length from the C-terminus of the full-length protein (29). The family of peptides produced from this synthesis is then functionally tested *in vivo* and *in vitro* to determine what minimal length is required for activity.

Solid phase synthesis of the N-terminal domain has included the first few residues, which have been hypothesized to anchor SP-B in the lipid membrane be the insertion sequence, as well as the amphipathic helical segment (10). Selection of the sequence to be synthesized has incorporated the turn components to minimize fraying of the ends of the peptide induced by removing it from the full-length protein. Our recent solution NMR studies in methanol (discussed subsequently) (30) and isotope-enchanced Fourier-transform infrared (FTIR) structural studies in POPG (31) indicate that the hydrophobic residues in the amphipathic helix stabilize the structural motif, making this domain's conformation highly conserved in the peptide and the full-length native protein. The sequence can be easily synthesized using either tert-butyloxycarbonyl (t-Boc) (10) or 9-fluorenaylmethyloxycarbonyl (Fmoc) strategies (13). Prederivatized Fmoc-gly Wang resins (p-benzyloxybenzyl alcohol) as well as low substitution of (>0.5 mmol/g) 4-hydroxymethylphenoxyacetyl-4'-methylbenzyhydrylamine resins (HMP) help to optimize the desired peptide product. Both Fmoc and t-Boc solid phase syntheses start at the C-terminal residue and sequentially add residues toward the N-terminus; the amphipathic helix is synthesized first followed by the insertion sequence. This helical segment spans from Cys-8 to Ile-21 and can be made with a yield of >85% authentic product even with single cycle FastMoc^{TM} couplings (13). However, in adding the turn and insertion sequence there is a considerable deletion of the Tyr-7 residue. Even double coupling at this position using the most common amino acid derivative Fmoc-Tyr(t-Bu)-OH (Fmoc-t-butyl-L-tyrosine) fails to enhance the addition of Tyr at this position. As this residue participates in a turn, coupling the 1–6-beta sheet to the amphipathic helix, there may be some steric hindrance of the side chain-protecting group that would interfere with the attachment of this residue. This sterically hindered coupling may be minimized by using Fmoc-Tyr(2-CLTrt)-OH (Fmoc-O-2-chlorotrityl-L-tyrosine) along with double coupling at this position.

As the SP-B$_{1-25}$ structure is largely driven by the hydrophobic residues, functional tests for polar specificity, disulfide bond formation, and attachment of fluorescent dyes and spin labels have been carried out. Polarity tests of the amphipathic helix interaction with lipids have shown that replacement of the positively charged Lys and Arg residues with the Ser residue (25) alters the interaction with lipids, but has minimal effect on the secondary structure. Similarly, the substitution of Ala for Cys to prevent the formation of disulfide linked oligomers has little effect on the structure and activity of the peptide (12). Spin label probes have also been successfully added to the N-terminus during synthesis using proxyl and nomal Fmoc coupling protocols followed by hydrofluoric acid cleavage to prevent reduction of the label (13). The spin labeled peptide can then be employed for molecular topography of the N-terminus of the peptide in liposomes (13). By substituting Ala for Cys at position 11, fluorescent labels can be selectively attached to Cys-8 provided the pH of the reaction is kept near 6.5. The dye labeled peptide can then be used to localize the peptide in surfactant lipid–peptide monolayers as a function of surface pressure by using a Langmuir trough fitted with a fluorescence microscope (32).

The N-terminal helix along with the Ala-Val mid-sequence has been synthesized using Fmoc chemistry (33). The sequence can be made using the same general guidelines for most SP-B sequences. This domain appears to show a surface pressure–concentration dependent β-sheet formation in the presence of surfactant lipids in monolayer measurements monitored by FTIR (33). These observations suggest that this element participates in peptide–peptide interactions in surfactant lipids and may have a role in specific self-association of this domain in the full-length protein.

The disulfide-stabilized bend region of SP-B (residues 35–46) has also been synthesized using Fmoc chemistry (34). In this case, the peptide was assembled on an MBHA carboxyamide resin to prevent the degradation of the C-terminal cysteine residue during cleavage from the resin. The sequence is basically a flexible loop in solvents that are used for chemical synthesis, so that it can be single coupled using an Fmoc strategy with a high yield. Although this sequence has no surface activity in lipids, understanding its folding properties provide important information for the folding of other SP-B peptides and full-length SP-B synthetic peptide into structures that resemble those of the native protein. As the mid-loop domain has cysteine residues at the N- and C-terminal positions, the proximity of these two residues is critical in the formation of the disulfide linkage that participates in stabilization of the loop segment. Determination of the distance between the two residues in various structure-promoting solvents was facilitated by attaching nitroxide spin labels to the Cys SH groups and monitoring the degree of interaction broadening. When the SP-B bend peptide was dissolved in hexafluorisopropanol or dimethylsulfoxide, there was little interaction as shown by the narrow lines of electron spin resonance (ESR) nitroxide triplet spectra. However, in trifluoroethanol (TFE) buffer the ESR spectrum showed extensive spectral line shape distortion indicative of spin–spin interactions caused by the close proximity of the two labeled Cys residues on either end of the peptide. Circular dichroism (CD) and FTIR spectra of this peptide in the TFE buffer also indicated that the segment had a strong type II turn propensity in this solvent system that would enhance the bend structure similar to that of the native SP-B protein. The formation of the disulfide bond between Cys-35 and Cys-46 further confirmed that solvent-induced folding in the bend region could be optimized in TFE buffer.

The helical sequence adjacent to the disulfide-stabilized bend domain is the region that provides the intrahomodimer interaction surface. This helical domain spanning Ile-45 to Tyr-53 has cysteine that forms a disulfide link to the Cys-48 monomer as well as the complementary Arg-52–Glu-51 ion pair that stabilizes the interaction between the monomer chains that are arranged so that their helical dipole moments are in an antiparallel fashion. This domain presents no special synthesis challenges, but the proximity of the adjacent Cys-46 in the bend region can lead to possible disulfide mismatches when these two components are part of a larger peptide construct. Since the domain has no real surfactant activity *per se* but functions as a disulfide–ion pair linkage in the parent SP-B molecule, it is only of interest as a component of larger peptides that test the specificity of homodimer formation.

The helical Leu-Leu repeat domain that encompasses Val-55 to Gly-64 is the same domain that the KL_4 peptide attempts to mimic (35). This rather simple amphipathic sequence can easily be synthesized by the solid phase approach using Fmoc or t-Boc strategies. The amphipathic nature of this sequence may help to explain its *in vitro* and *in vivo* enhancement effects on surfactant lipids (35). However, the orientation of these types of amphipathtic leucine repeat sequences in lipid multilayers suggests that this sequence does not strictly emulate the functions of full-length and truncated homodimeric SP-B peptides that include lipid mixing, formation of buckled monolayer structures, and interaction with SP-A to form tubular myelin structures.

Finally, the disulfide-stabilized C-terminal amphipathical helix domain that spans roughly from Met-66 to the C-terminal serine (synthetic peptide) or methionine (native protein) is of special interest. As the positively charged amphipathic helical sequences are associated with the C-terminus and N-terminus in the full-length SP-B protein, it can be postulated that these elements are important components for interaction with surfactant lipids. This hypothesis is further strengthened by the disulfide connectivity between the N-terminal and C-terminal domains of the mature protein. Indeed, the covalent linkage between Cys-8 and Cys-77 and Cys-11 and Cys-71 is conserved in all of the saposin protein family and suggests that the constraints imposed by the disulfide linkages may form a polar surface that enhances interaction of lipids in a specific manner. Synthesis of the C-terminal domain is straightforward using single coupling with Fmoc chemistry. However, without disulfide constraints this domain shows some concentration-dependent β-sheet formation in lipid ensembles, suggesting that helical content is driven by the amphipathic nature of the sequence as well as its N-terminal connectivity elements.

Full-length SP-B using currently available solid phase peptide synthesis technology is quite a challenge and is difficult to make in high yield. The full-length SP-B has been made starting at Ser-78, but Met-79 does not contribute significantly to the protein structure. Both Fmoc (14) and t-Boc (29) strategies have been successfully used to make full-length $SP-B_{1-78}$ sequence. In general, one employs a low substitution resin (>0.3 mmol/g) to minimize peptide–peptide interactions on the resin during synthesis. Typically, after synthesis of a major domain (20–25 residues) the synthesis is stopped and a sample is cleaved to determine the quality of the product at that point in the assembly of the peptide. Double coupling of all residues as well as extension of the coupling times is also required on a peptide of this length. Full-length SP-B is not only a challenge to synthesize but also difficult to purify by reverse phase HPLC as single amino acid deletions are eluted at the same retention times as authentic product (36). Folding of the peptide monomer into the correct disulfide format can be achieved by oxidation in 7:3 TFE/buffer that favors helix and turn conformers. However, a successful strategy for correctly folding the covalently linked homodimer is yet to be achieved.

III. NMR Structure of SP-B Peptides

To elucidate the structure of SP-B, we have chosen first to focus on the amphipathic α-helical segment at the N-terminal of the protein, SP-B$_{1-25}$. Use of this truncated version of the full-length SP-B was first reported by Bruni et al. (12). A great deal of attention has been focused on this peptide as it has been shown to faithfully reproduce the functional aspects of the full-length peptide, contains no disulfide bonds, and is more amenable to chemical synthesis than the full-length protein as described in the previous section. We have performed preliminary NMR studies with the peptide in methanol solution, endeavoring to determine the structure of this peptide. However, our spectra indicated subtle changes over the course of a week in methanol solution. The well-resolved $\varepsilon 1$ signal from Trp-9, which should be a single resonance, appeared initially as two peaks of unequal intensity. The relative intensities of these signals changed on the timescale of days, and within a week one form represented $\sim$80% of the mixture. The major difficulty this posed was that all the other peaks in the spectrum had to be treated as being duplicated, thus severely complicating the interpretation of the spectra. The cause of the duplication has not been conclusively determined, but it is most likely due to some sort of low-order oligomerization event, which is interesting because this sort of peptide–peptide association is hypothesized to be important for SP-B function (9,37). The presence of large aggregates can be discounted because both Trp-9 resonance lines are narrow, whereas one would expect the originally predominant peak to be narrow and the final peak to be broad if the peptide formed very large aggregates.

It is possible that SP-B$_{1-25}$ forms dimers under our solution conditions by disulfide bonding. However, pH was 6.9, where the cysteine side chain exists mostly in the thiol form, not the nucleophilic thiolate form, and the sample had been degassed and flushed with nitrogen, so oxidation in the NMR tube is unlikely. To probe the possible effects of oxidation, however, we have obtained an oxidation-resistant mutant peptide, SP-B$_{1-25}$(oxmut), in which Cys-8, Cys-11 and Met-21 have been changed to alanines. As noted in the previous section, the Cys to Ala mutations were first reported by Bruni et al. (12), but the inclusion of the M21A mutation is original to our laboratory. The motivation for the M21A mutation stems from our observation that some ^{1}H NMR spectra of SP-B$_{1-25}$ and, as will be discussed, SP-B$_{11-25}$, exhibited duplicate sets of peaks that could be assigned to Met-21 and neighboring residues. Each set indicated the same local structure, so we hypothesized that the duplication arose from methionine oxidation. Spectra of an SP-B$_{11-25}$ mutant in which Met-21 was replaced by norleucine, a nonstandard amino acid whose sidechain represents that of methionine where the S atom is replaced with a much less oxidizable CH$_2$ group. Alanine was chosen as the replacement residue for both cysteine and methionine not only because it has the smallest carbon-containing side chain, but also because, in free energy terms, its side chain's helical propensity (38,39) and hydrophobicity (40) are most similar to those of the sulfur-containing side chains.

As discussed in the previous section, the N-terminal hydrophobic tail of the SP-B has been postulated to be important for anchoring the peptide in the lipid monolayer by helping the peptide to insert into the lipid monolayer. We are particularly interested in the functional role of this domain and have therefore examined the structure of SP-B$_{11-25}$ peptide where the first 10 residues at the N-terminus have been eliminated. This truncated form is designed to probe the role of the first 10 residues, the so-called "insertion sequence," in the surface behavior and structure of SP-B$_{1-25}$. Secondary structure prediction algorithms, CD, and FTIR studies have suggested that SP-B$_{1-25}$ contains an amphiphilic α-helix from residues 11 through 22, and that the termini are relatively disordered (13,31). The insertion sequence is of great interest because it comprises hydrophobic residues exclusively, three of which are aromatic and three of which are rigidifying prolines.

To date, the SP-B$_{11-25}$ peptide is the SP-B peptide derivative best characterized by our laboratory. We have solved recently the NMR structure of SP-B$_{11-25}$. Here, we present the salient features of our findings; further details can be found in Kurutz and Lee (30). All NMR experiments used 1.25 mM peptide dissolved in CD$_3$OH. NMR spectra were taken at 5°C so as to enhance the signal-to-noise ratio, and were recorded on a Varian Inova 600 MHz spectrometer equipped with z-axis gradients and an RF waveform generator in the University of Chicago Biological Sciences Division NMR facility. NMR spectra were analyzed using Varian's VNMR software. Standard 2D NMR spectra were obtained for assignment and distance measurement, and resonance assignments were made with standard methods (41). Scalar-coupled spin systems were identified using double quantum filtered spectroscopy (DQCOSY, 42,43) and total correlation spectroscopy (TOCSY, 42,44) experiments, and sequential assignments were made using backbone H^N–H^N and H^N–H^α nuclear Overhauser effect spectroscopy (NOESY) cross-peaks. Sequential connectivity in the H^N–H^N and H^N–H^α regions of the NOESY spectrum is shown in Fig. 11.3. Assignment was assisted by the preliminary NMR analysis by Kumar (45). Sequential NOE contacts are also identified in Fig. 11.3. It should be noted that for some residues around Met-21, a second set of resonances were observed exhibiting identical patterns of NOE connectivity to the primary set (Fig. 11.3). To test the potential effects of oxidation on SP-B$_{11-25}$ structure and function, we obtained an oxidation resistant mutant, SP-B$_{11-25}$(oxmut), in which Cys-11 was mutated to Ala and Met-21 was changed to norleucine. Here, the sulfur atom was replaced by a methylene group. The spectra and structure of SP-B$_{11-25}$(oxmut) exhibit a single set of peaks almost identical to those of the wild-type peptide treated here (data not shown). We ascribe this duplication to the methionine oxidation, as already discussed in the SP-B$_{1-25}$ case. Similar duplications have also been observed in the NMR analysis of SP-C (46).

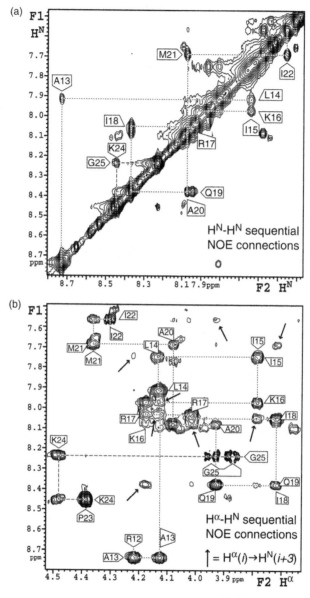

Figure 11.3 Portions of the NOESY spectrum of 1.25 mM SP-B$_{11-25}$ in CD$_3$OH, acquired at 5°C. (a) The H^N–H^N region of the NOESY spectrum, with sequential H^N(*i*)–H^N(*i* + 1) cross-peaks highlighted with dashed lines. (b) The region of the same NOESY spectrum showing H^α–H^N NOE contacts. Sequential contacts are indicated by dashed lines and flags. Important helix-indicating H^α(*i*)–H^N(*i* + 3) cross-peaks are indicated with arrows. [Reprinted with permission from Ref. (30). Copyright 2002 American Chemical Society.]

Structural characterization was accomplished by examining several qualitative structure indicators, including $^3JH^NH^\alpha$ coupling constants, NOE contact patterns, and the H^α chemical shift index (Fig. 11.4). The most significant pattern observed here is the set of NOEs between H^α signals on residues i and H^N signals on residues $i + 3$, which indicates α-helical structure (47). SP-B$_{11-25}$ exhibits such contacts from residues Arg-12 through Ile-22, as highlighted by arrows in Fig. 11.3. Other contacts supporting helical structure include $H^\alpha \rightarrow H^\beta$ $(i + 3)$ NOEs, which were also observed from residues Arg-12 through Ile-22. For each residue's H^α resonance, we calculated its chemical shift index (CSI). A group of residues exhibiting CSI $= -1$ suggests an

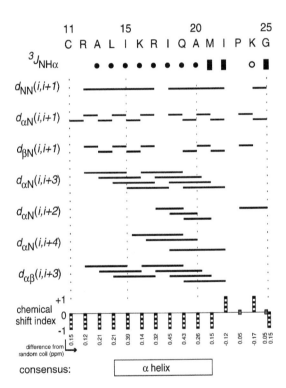

Figure 11.4 Qualitative structure indicators in SP-B$_{11-25}$, including selected NOE contact, $^3JH^NH^\alpha$ coupling constants, and chemical shift indices. Closed dots represent J-values <5.0 Hz, open circles represent J values >8.0 Hz, and vertical lines represent values between 5.0 and 8.0 Hz. $^3JH^NH^\alpha$ values <5.0 Hz generally indicate α-helical structure. The pattern of $H^\alpha(i) \rightarrow H^N(i + 3)$ and $H^\alpha(i) \rightarrow H^\beta(i + 3)$ contacts also indicates α-helical structure. The CSIs for the H^α resonances were calculated according to the method of Wishart et al. where CSI predominantly equals -1 are probably α-helical, and regions where CSI is mostly $+1$ are probably β-sheet. [Reprinted with permission from Ref. (30). Copyright 2002 American Chemical Society.]

α-helix, and a group of residues exhibiting CSI $= +1$ indicated β-sheet (48,49). The CSI values obtained indicate an helix from residue Ala-13 through Met-21.

NMR and previously published FTIR data (13,31) were translated into distance and dihedral angle restraints for use in molecular modeling. Annealing was performed and a family of accepted structures was derived (Fig. 11.5). But the annealed structures exhibit some dihedral restraint violations at Ψ(A13) and Ψ(I22), suggesting that these residues might not be best described as helical. Interpreting our data conservatively, we ascribe α-helical character to residues Leu-14 through Met-21. Our molecular models show that the distribution of polar sidechains is not uniform but bimodal on one side of the helix, leaving a small gap opposite the more hydrophobic face. We hypothesize that this enables the peptide to extend its cationic side chains farther than if the distribution were uniform, thus facilitating interaction with slightly more distant anionic portions of headgroups in the lipid monolayer.

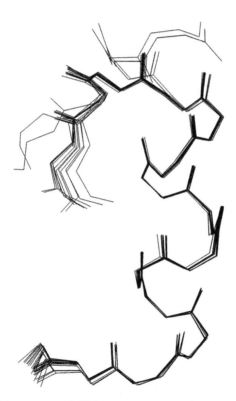

Figure 11.5 Backbone traces of 17 lowest-energy annealed structures for SP-B$_{11-25}$. Structures were aligned to minimize heavy-atom differences among residues Ile-14 through Met-21 and the corresponding atoms of the lowest energy structure. [Reprinted with permission from Ref. (30). Copyright 2002 American Chemical Society.]

IV. Effect of SP-B Peptides on LS Monolayer Collapse

As pointed out in Section I, recent reports have demonstrated that the squeeze-out of lipids with low collapse pressures from a mixed lipid system can be eliminated when SP-B peptides are present (14,22–24). To better understand how the presence of cationic SP-B peptides prevents such squeeze-out events and to delineate how the structure of a given SP-B peptide affects its ability to retain anionic lipid components in the mixed monolayer, we have employed a home built Langmuir trough/fluorescene microscope setup to study the general phase behavior and collapse mechanics of DPPG/POPG monolayers in the presence of various SP-B peptides. Details of the experimental apparatus have been described elsewhere (50). Briefly, the homebuilt Teflon Langmuir trough is equipped with two identical mobile Teflon barriers which allow for symmetric compression of the monolayers spread at the interface. Ultrapure Milli-Q water was used as the subphase, and the temperature was kept at 30°C for all experiments through a control station comprising thermoelectric units joined to a heat sink. A resistively heated indium tin oxide-coated glass plate was placed over the trough to minimize dust contamination, air currents, and evaporative losses. The trough is positioned on translation stages that permit scanning along the x, y, and z directions. This assembly is fixed to a custom-built microscope stage for simultaneous fluorescence microscopy. In fluorescence microscopy, a small mole fraction (1 mol%) of probe (lipid-linked Texas-Red DHPE) is incorporated in the monolayer, and contrast between coexisting phases is made possible by the preferential partitioning of probe molecules into less-ordered phases owing to steric hindrances. Images from the fluorescent microscope are collected using a silicon intensified target camera and recorded onto Super VHS-formatted videotape for analysis. This technique allows one to detect the influence of the peptide on lipid monolayers, and to pinpoint the location and structure of three-dimensional collapsed phases in LS systems. By fluorescently labeling the LS peptide with a probe different from that of the lipid, one can also perform dual-probe experiments to identify the location of protein in the lipid matrix, and determine the partitioning of protein between phases.

The effect of SP-B$_{1-25}$ on the collapse behavior of lipid films has been probed in our laboratory. Surface pressure–area isotherms of the lipid mixture 3:1 DPPG/POPG were measured with concurrent fluorescence microscopy in the presence and absence of SP-B$_{1-25}$ (51). In the absence of protein, compression of the mixed monolayer at 30°C results in a system exhibiting coexistence of a condensed and a disordered phase until the surface pressure reaches ∼47 mN/m (see curve in Fig. 11.6). Beyond this pressure, the POPG-rich disordered phase becomes squeezed out, with complete elimination of the disordered phase achieved at ∼50 mN/m (Fig. 11.7). This region appears as a "plateau" on the isotherm because large reductions in area induce changes in the monolayer without significantly increasing the surface pressure. Monolayer collapse occurs at ∼56 mN/m and follows a

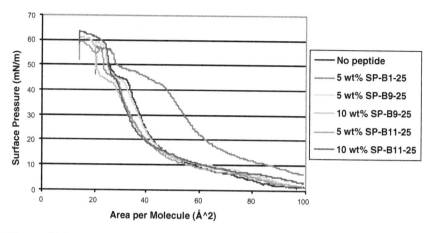

Figure 11.6 Isotherms of 3:1 DPPG/POPG film without any SP-B peptide, with 5 wt% SP-B$_{1-25}$, 5 wt% SP-B$_{9-25}$, 10 wt% SP-B$_{9-25}$, 5 wt% SP-B$_{11-25}$, and 10 wt% SP-B$_{11-25}$. Surface pressure is in mN/m and area per molecule is in Å^2.

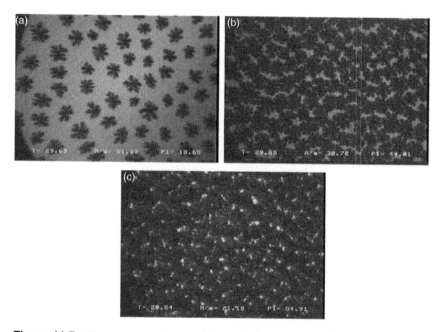

Figure 11.7 Fluorescence microscopy images of a 3:1 DPPG/POPG mixture with 1 mol% TR-DHPE monolayer on pure water at 30°C, showing (a) the fluid/condensed coexistence with the condensed phase exhibiting dark, flower-like structure, (b) tightly packed condensed phase at the start of the plateau region of the isotherm, and (c) the detachment of globular structures formed during compression through the plateau region; the squeezed-out materials do not readsorb to the monolayer upon expansion. The lateral size of the image is 240 μm.

mechanism in which bright globules form on the monolayer then detach from it, irreversibly meandering into the subphase.

When as low as 5 wt% SP-B$_{1-25}$ is included in the monolayer, the liftoff of the isotherm occurs at a higher area per molecule. This shift of the isotherm to the right clearly indicates that the peptide is taking up position at the interface. The two-phase coexistence is retained until collapse, suggesting that SP-B$_{1-25}$ eliminates squeeze-out in this lipid system. The plateau region begins at a lower surface pressure when this peptide is present, 43 mN/m, and continues through ~49 mN/m (see curve in Fig. 11.6). Bright structures form in the disordered regions on the peptide-containing monolayer, but they do not detach from it, as they do in the pure lipid system. These brighter structures in the interstitial regions are likely multilayer formation similar to those first reported in Lipp et al. (22). SP-B$_{1-25}$ also raises the collapse pressure slightly to ~59 mN/m, and significantly changes the collapse mode from irreversible vesiculation and detachment to reversible folding (Fig. 11.8). Expansion of the film results in efficient respreading of material from the folds.

To explore the effect of the insertion sequence on collapse, we compared the effects of SP-B$_{1-25}$ to those of the truncated peptides SP-B$_{9-25}$ and SP-B$_{11-25}$, in which the insertion sequence has been deleted (51). SP-B$_{9-25}$ includes Trp-9, which is significant because tryptophans have been proposed to play a major role in protein–lipid interactions (52,53). SP-B$_{9-25}$, examined at 5 wt% peptide concentration raises the collapse pressure of the lipid film slightly to ~58 mN/m (curve in Fig. 11.6), but fails to shift the collapse mechanism to folding. This peptide also lowers the beginning of the plateau region to ~43 mN/m, above which the morphology of the film resembles that of the peptide-free film; the plateau terminates at 47 mN/m. At 5 wt% SP-B$_{9-25}$, the film collapses by vesiculation featuring tubular structures that detach from the disordered regions and are irreversibly lost to the subphase [Fig. 11.9(a)]. When this peptide is present at 10 wt%, collapse occurs with folds in addition to vesicles [Fig. 11.9(b)].

SP-B$_{11-25}$ also induces changes in the film behavior relative to the peptide-free film. At 5 wt%, it lowers the plateau region to 43–47 mN/m, as observed with SP-B$_{9-25}$, and it increases the collapse pressure to ~60 mN/m (see curve in Fig. 11.6). Like SP-B$_{9-25}$, 5 wt% SP-B$_{11-25}$ induces globules to form from the disordered phase during the plateau region of compression, after which they detach from the film, but reversible folds are also observed upon collapse (Fig. 11.10), unlike the fold-free collapse in the presence of 5 wt% SP-B$_{9-25}$. Compression of the 10 wt% SP-B$_{11-25}$-containing film yielded a smaller plateau region than the isotherm taken with 5 wt% peptide, ranging from ~43 to 46 mN/m. During the plateau segment of compression, bright patches were observed to form from the disordered phase, but they did not detach to go into the subphase. These patches were similar to those found at the plateau region when 5 wt% of SP-B$_{1-25}$ was present. The collapse pressure is elevated to ~63 mN/m when 10 wt% SP-B$_{11-25}$ is present, and collapse occurs by

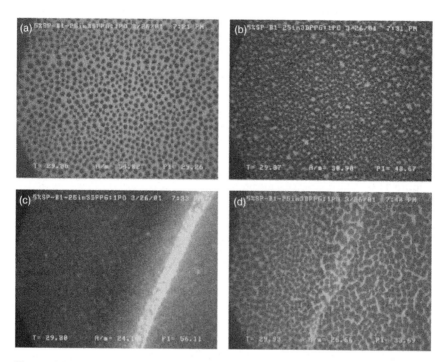

Figure 11.8 Fluorescence miscroscopy images of 5 wt% SP-B$_{1-25}$ in 3:1 DPPG/ POPG/1 mol% TR-DHPE monolayer on pure water at 30°C, showing (a) the preferential partitioning of the peptide into the POPG-rich fluid phase and the formation of smaller DPPG-rich dark domains with higher number density (compared to the case without SP-B$_{1-25}$). (b) The retention of the POPG-rich fluid phase in the monolayer through the plateau region. (c) The formation of long length-scale folded structures at collapse. (d) The folds unzip upon expansion and the materials in the folds get reincorporated reversibly into the monolayer. The lateral size of the image is 240 μm.

reversible folding without detachment of vesicles. Thus, the collapse behavior of 10 wt% SP-B$_{11-25}$ is more similar to that of 5 wt% SP-B$_{1-25}$ than to that of 10 wt% SP-B$_{9-25}$.

Comparisons of the peptides' effects on collapse shed some light on the importance of the insertion sequence and Trp-9. The primary effect of SP-B$_{1-25}$ is to shift the collapse mechanism from irreversible vesiculation to reversible folding. Reversible folding can also be induced somewhat by 10 wt% SP-B$_{9-25}$ and as little as 5 wt% SP-B$_{11-25}$. Note that the concentrations of the truncated peptides necessary for meaningful levels of folding are significantly higher than those required for SP-B$_{1-25}$ to have the same effect. This requirement is magnified when considering concentrations based on mole percent. Thus, the insertion sequence appears to improve the probability that the monolayer will collapse by folding. It should be pointed out that the

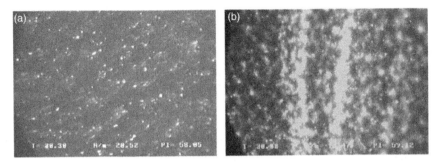

Figure 11.9 Fluorescence microscopy images of (a) 5 wt% and (b) 10 wt% of SP-B$_{9-25}$ in 3:1 mol/mol DPPG/POPG/1 mol% TR-DHPE monolayer on pure water at 30°C, showing (a) the detachment of the squeezed-out strucutre in the plateau region when 5 wt% SP-B$_{9-25}$ is present. (b) The film collapses via both squeeze-out and fold formation when 10 wt% SP-B$_{9-25}$ is present. The lateral size of the image is 240 μm.

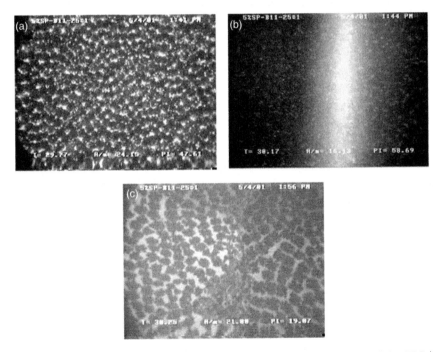

Figure 11.10 Fluorescence microscopy images of a 5 wt% SP-B$_{11-25}$ in 3:1 DPPG/POPG/1 mol% TR DHPE monolayer on pure water at 30°C, showing the film collapses via both (a) squeeze-out and (b) fold formation, and (c) the folds open up and the materials reincorporate reversibly into the monolayer upon expansion. The lateral size of the image is 240 μm.

compression isotherms for the truncated peptides strongly resemble that of the pure lipid system, suggesting that they do not occupy much area in the film. In contrast, the SP-B$_{1-25}$ isotherm is markedly shifted to the right of the lipid-only isotherm below ~50 mN/m, indicating that this peptide takes up space between the lipids at the air–water interface (Fig. 11.6). Thus, it appears that residues 1–8 and/or 1–10 are essential for interacting with the hydrophobic lipid tails in order to ensure a folding mode of collapse. The differences between SP-B$_{9-25}$ and SP-B$_{11-25}$ are more subtle and require further rigorous study to explain fully.

V. Elastic Theory of LS Monolayers

Our fluorescence microscopy work has demonstrated that the presence of adequate amount of SP-B peptides can alter the mode of monolayer collapse from irreversible vesiculation to reversible folding. For the systems we have studied, collapse via folding only occurs when the monolayer exhibits a biphasic structure, that is, when two phases are in coexistence. An intriguing question is how one can theoretically understand the onset of the folding instability observed. In this section, we briefly review the theory of the structure and instability of model LS monolayers. A more detailed presentation can be found elsewhere (54,55).

A. The Monolayer as an Elastic Sheet

As has been shown in the previous section, both the lateral structure (i.e., domain pattern) of the monolayer and its three-dimensional structures (folds) are found in experiments to be of micron size, much larger than the molecular scale. This justifies a continuum description of the monolayer as an elastic sheet. There are various experimental indications that LS monolayers may be at biphasic coexistence during a large portion of the compression–expansion cycle (22,23,50,56). In setting up a theoretical model to understand the driving force for the folding transition observed experimentally, we need, therefore, to consider a *heterogeneous* sheet. Indeed, we shall see that heterogeneity plays a key role in determining the three-dimensional structure and stability of the monolayer.

Another experimental fact to bear in mind is that the two sides of the monolayer are not identical—on one side there are lipid headgroups facing an aqueous phase whereas on the other there are hydrocarbon tails facing air. This asymmetry implies a natural tendency of the monolayer to bend, that is, a *spontaneous curvature* (57). Apart from the molecular source (i.e., different packing of lipid heads and tails), the spontaneous curvature can also have an electrostatic contribution (58). Both contributions typically amount to a radius of curvature of the order of a few nanometers. Opposing bending is the air–water interfacial tension, which progressively decreases upon monolayer compression from

~72 mN/m (the tension of the bare interface at room temperature) at low lipid surface density to only a few mN/m at monolayer collapse.

Thus, we are led to consider as a minimum model for the LS monolayer a heterogeneous elastic sheet with bending rigidity K, surface tension γ, and spontaneous curvature c_0 that has differing values, c_{01} and c_{02}, in the two types of domains. The bending rigidity of a highly compressed lipid monolayer is typically a few hundred times the thermal energy $k_B T$, where k_B is the Boltzmann constant and T is the absolute temperature (59). One can also consider differing values of K for the two types of domains involved, yet the results remain qualitatively the same (54). We are about to consider elastic deformations of such a sheet, whose energy is much larger than both $k_B T$ and the gravitational cost of the consequent contortion of the water surface (55). The model is therefore static and purely elastic, neglecting thermal fluctuations and gravitational effects.

The elastic parameters K and γ define a new length, $\lambda = (K/\gamma)^{1/2}$, which determines the lateral extent of elastic deformations. For the earlier mentioned values we get λ of order a few nanometers. Thus, both $(c_0)^{-1}$ and λ are of nanometer scale, much smaller than the domain size (tens of microns). In addition, the typical width of domain boundaries is also not larger than a few molecules. This statement is true for any biphasic structure far from a critical point, a condition under which our experiments were conducted. Hence, we can focus on a single domain boundary and assume that it is straight, sharp, and separates two very large phases, as illustrated in Fig. 11.11(a). Such a simplified structure, which is uniform in the direction parallel to the boundary, can be conveniently parametrized by its local angle $\theta(s)$ with respect to a reference plane at arc-length s from the boundary [Fig. 11.11(b)]. The elastic energy of the monolayer (per unit length of boundary) is then a function of the topography $\theta(s)$:

$$g[\theta(s)] = \int_{-\infty}^{\infty} ds \left[\left(\frac{1}{2} K \left(\frac{d\theta}{ds} \right)^2 - K c_0 \frac{d\theta}{ds} \right) + \gamma (1 - \cos \theta) \right] \qquad (11.1)$$

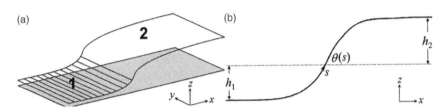

Figure 11.11 (a) Sketch of a biphasic monolayer in the vicinity of a domain boundary. (b) The monolayer topography is parametrized by the angle $\theta(s)$ which made with a reference plane at arc-length s from the boundary.

In Eq. (11.1) the first two terms are the bending energy due to deviations of the local mean curvature $c(s) = d\theta/ds$ from the spontaneous curvature c_0, whereas the last term is the tensile energy associated with deviation from a flat state.

B. Mesa Topographies

The static shape of the monolayer in the vicinity of a domain boundary is the one that minimizes Eq. (11.1). The somewhat surprising result is that, as long as the domains differ in their elastic parameters (i.e., $c_{01} \neq c_{02}$), the sheet will always be inflected in the vicinity of the domain boundary. This implies that domains of different phases, owing to the different materials properties, have different heights. In other words, the biphasic structure is accompanied by a three-dimensional topography of "mesas". The total height difference can be obtained from the following simple arguement, without explicitly minimizing Eq. (11.1). Far away on one side of the boundary the monolayer is subjected to a torque $Kc_{01} - \gamma h_1$ [Fig. 11.11(b)]. Similarly, far away on the other side acts a different torque of $Kc_{02} + \gamma h_2$. For the monolayer to remain stationary these torques must balance each other, hence,

$$h = h_1 + h_2 = \frac{K(\delta c_0)}{\gamma} = \lambda^2(\delta c_0) \tag{11.2}$$

where $\delta c_0 = c_{01} - c_{02}$. The height difference h increases with the contrast in spontaneous curvature δc_0, rigidity K, and compression (i.e., decrease in γ). For moderate compression, where γ is equal to a few tens mN/m, h should be minute, typically not larger than a few angstroms, yet at high compression ($\gamma \sim 1$ mN/m), it may reach a few nanometers. As a result of these small values, and because of the fluidity of the interface, mesas have not yet been decisively observed, even though hints of possible existence of these mesas have been observed (60,61).

In order to obtain the topography in more detail, we should minimize Eq. (11.1) with respect to $\theta(s)$ while requiring that the monolayer be flat far away from the domain boundary, $\theta(s \to \pm\infty) = 0$, and continuous at the boundary, $\theta(s = 0^-) = \theta(s = 0^+) = \theta_0$. The resulting topography is given by (54,55)

$$\tan\frac{\theta(s)}{4} = \tan\frac{\theta_0}{4}\exp\left(-\frac{|s|}{\lambda}\right), \quad \sin\frac{\theta_0}{2} = \frac{\lambda(\delta c_0)}{4}. \tag{11.3}$$

Upon compression (decreasing γ and increasing λ) the inflection becomes sharper and higher, subsequently developing a stable overhang, as illustrated in Fig. 11.12.

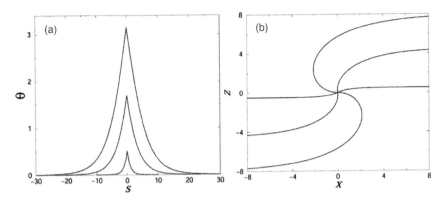

Figure 11.12 (a) Angle profiles (in radians) near a domain boundary as compression is increased. The curves are obtained from Eq. (11.3) using the values (from bottom to top) $\lambda(\delta c_0) = 1$, 3, and 4. The uppermost curve is the critical profile. (b) The corresponding topographies. All lengths are in units of $(\delta c_0)^{-1}$.

C. Instability

As is readily seen in Eq. (11.3), when $\lambda(\partial c_0) > 4$, that is,

$$\gamma < \gamma_c = \frac{1}{16} K(\delta c_0)^2 \tag{11.4}$$

the solution obtained for the monolayer topography becomes invalid. This marks an instability whereupon the resistance of the monolayer to further compression vanishes. Note that this elastic instability occurs at *positive surface tension*—an unusual effect brought about by heterogeneity and spontaneous curvature.

At instability the monolayer in the vicinity of the domain boundary is expected to undergo a shape transformation to another state, which is determined by factors outside this simple elastic model (e.g., the observed localized folds). In fact, we expect the new state to become energetically favorable, in practice, before the instability condition [Eq. (11.4)] is reached, thus making the transition abrupt (first-order) rather than continuous (second-order).

One mechanism that has been recently suggested as a driving force for fold formation is monolayer–monolayer adhesion into a bilayer (59). In homogeneous monolayers the formation of a fold through adhesion requires overcoming nucleation barriers much higher than $k_B T$. Thus, the mesa topography in a biphasic monolayer and its elastic instability could provide a way to reduce and eliminate these barriers. This supports the conjecture that a biphasic structure of the LS monolayer is a necessary condition for its efficient folding upon compression, as indeed seems to be indicated in experiments (50,56).

References

1. Shapiro DL, Notter RH, ed. Surfactant Replacement Therapy. New York: Liss, 1989.
2. Suresh GK, Soll RF. Current surfactant use in premature infants. Clin Perinatol 2001; 28(3):671–694.
3. Milligan DW, Ainsworth SB. Animal-derived or synthetic surfactant for the treatment of neonatal respiratory distress syndrome: a review. Acta Paediatr 2001; 436(suppl 90):25–27.
4. Hamvas A, Cole FS, deMello DE, Moxley M, Whitsett JA, Colten HR, Nogee LM. Surfactant protein B deficiency: antenatal diagnosis and prospective treatment with surfactant replacement. J Pediatr 1994; 125(3):356–361.
5. Tryka AF, Wert SE, Mazursky JE, Arrington RW, Nogee LM. Absence of lamellar bodies with accumulation of dense bodies characterizes a novel form of congenital surfactant defect. Pediatr Dev Pathol 2000; 3(4):335–345.
6. Weaver TE, Beck DC. Use of knockout mice to study surfactant protein structure and function. Biol Neonate 1999; 76(suppl 1):15–18.
7. Glasser SW, Burhans MS, Korfhagen TR, Na CL, Sly PD, Ross GF, Ikegami M, Whitsett JA. Altered stability of pulmonary surfactant in SP-C-deficient mice. Proc Natl Acad Sci USA 2001; 98(11):6366–6371.
8. Hawgood S, Derrick M, Poulain F. Structure and properties of surfactant protein B. Biochim Biophys Acta 1998; 1408(2–3):150–160.
9. Beck DC, Ikegami M, Na CL, Zaltash S, Johansson J, Whitsett JA, Weaver TE. The role of homodimers in surfactant protein B function *in vivo*. J Biol Chem 2000; 275(5):3365–3370.
10. Waring A, Taeusch W, Bruni R, Amirkhanian J, Fan B, Stevens R, Young J. Synthetic amphipathic sequences of surfactant protein-B mimic several physico-chemical and *in vivo* properties of native pulmonary surfactant proteins. Pept Res 1989; 2(5):308–313.
11. Takahashi A, Waring A, Amirkhanian J, Fan B, Taeusch H. Structure–function relationships of bovine pulmonary surfactant proteins: SP-B and SP-C. Biochim Biophys Acta 1990; 1044:43–49.
12. Bruni R, Taeusch HW, Waring AJ. Surfactant protein B: lipid interactions of synthetic peptides representing the amino-terminal amphipathic domain. Proc Natl Acad Sci 1991; 88(8):7451–7455.
13. Gordon LM, Horvath S, Longo ML, Zasadzinski JA, Taeusch HW, Faull K, Leung C, Waring AJ. Conformation and molecular topography of the N-terminal segment of surfactant protein B in structure-promoting environments. Protein Sci 1996; 5(8):1662–1675.
14. Lipp MM, Lee KYC, Zasadzinski JA, Waring AJ. Phase and morphology changes induced by SP-B protein and its amino-terminal peptide in lipid monolayers. Science 1996; 273(5279):1196–1199.
15. Lee KYC, Majewski J, Kuhl TL, Howes PB, Kjaer K, Lipp MM, Waring AJ, Zasadzinski JA, Smith GS. Synchrotron X-ray study of lung surfactant specific protein SP-B in lipid monolayers. Biophys J 2001; 81:572–585.
16. Gupta M, Hernandez-Juviel JM, Waring AJ, Walther FJ. Function and inhibition sensitivity of the N-terminal segment of surfactant protein B (SP-B1-25) in preterm rabbits. Thorax 2001; 56(11):871–876.

17. Mathialagan N, Possmayer F. Low-molecular weight hydrophobic proteins from bovine pulmonary surfactant. Biochim Biophys Acta 1990; 1045:121.

18. Cockshutt A, Absolom D, Possmayer F. The role of palmitic acid in pulmonary surfactant: enhancement of surface activity and prevention of inhibition by blood proteins. Biochim Biophys Acta 1991; 1085:248–256.

19. Longo M, Waring A, Zasadzinski JA. Lipid bilayer surface association of lung surfactant protein SP-B, amphipathic segment detected by flow immunofluorescence. Biophys J 1992; 63:760–773.

20. Pastrana-Rios B, Flach C, Brauner J, Mautone A, Mendelsohn R. A direct test of the "squeeze-out" hypothesis of lung surfactant function. External reflection FT-IR at the air/water interface. Biochemistry 1994; 33:5121–5127.

21. Egberts J, Sloot H, Mazure A. Minimal surface tension, squeeze-out and transition temperatures of binary mixtures of dipalmitoylphosphatidylcholine and unsaturated phospholipids. Biochim Biophys Acta 1989; 1002:109–113.

22. Lipp MM, Lee KYC, Zasadzinski JA, Waring AJ. Coexistence of buckled and flat monolayers. Phys Rev Lett 1998; 81:1650–1653.

23. Takamoto DY, Lipp MM, Nahmen Av, Lee KYC, Waring AJ, Zasadzinski JA. Interaction of lung surfactant proteins with anionic phospholipids. Biophys J 2001; 81:153–169.

24. Ding J, Takamoto DY, Nahmen Av, Lipp MM, Lee KYC, Waring AJ, Zasadzinski JA. Effects of lung surfactant proteins SP-B and SP-C and palmitic acid on monolayer stability. Biophys J 2001; 80:2262–2272.

25. Longo M, Bisagno A, Zasadzinshi J, Bruni R, Waring A. A function of lung surfactant protein SP-B. Science 1993; 261:453–456.

26. Liepinsh R, Andersson M, Ruysschaert J-M, Otting G. Saposin fold revealed by the NMR structure of NK-lysin. Nat Struct Biol 1997; 4:793–795.

27. Munford RS, Sheppard PO, O'Hara PJ. Saposin-like protein (SAPLIP) carry out diverse functions on a common backbone structure. J Lipid Res 1995; 36:1653–1663.

28. Zaltash S, Palmblad M, Curstedt T, Johansson J, Persson B. Pulmonary surfactant protein B: a structural model and a functional analogue. Biochim Biophys Acta 2000; 1466:179–186.

29. Sarin VK, Gupta S, Leung TK, Taylor VE, Ohning BL, Whitsett JA, Fox JL. Biophysical and biological-activity of a synthetic 8.7-kDa hydrophobic pulmonary surfactant protein SP-B. Proc Natl Acad Sci USA 1990; 7:2633–2637.

30. Kurutz JW, Lee KYC. NMR structure of lung surfactant peptide SP-B11-25. Biochemistry 2002; 41(30):9627–9636.

31. Gordon LM, Lee KYC, Lipp MM, Zasadzinski JA, Walther F, Sherman MA, Waring AJ. Conformational mapping of the N-terminal segment of surfactant protein B in lipid using ^{13}C-enhanced Fourier transform infrared spectroscopy. J Pept Res 2000; 55:330–347.

32. Lipp MM, Lee KYC, Waring AJ, Zasadzinski JA. Design of a fluorescence, polarized fluorescence, and Brewster angle microscope/Langmuir trough assembly for the study of lung surfactant monolayers. Rev Sci Instrum 1997; 68(6):2574–2582.

33. Dieudonne D, Mendelsohn R, Farid RS, Flach CR. Secondary structure in lung surfactant SP-B peptides: IR and CD studies of bulk and monolayer phases. Biochim Biophys Acta 2001; 1511:99–112.

34. Waring A, Faull K, Leung C, Chang-Chien, Mercado P, Taeusch W, Gordon LM. Synthesis, secondary structure and folding of the bend region of lung surfactant protein B. Pept Res 1996; 9:28–39.

35. Cochrane C, Revak S. SP-B: Structure-function relationships. Science 1991; 254:566–568.

36. Walther FJ, Hernandez-Juviel J, Bruni R, Waring AJ. Protein composition of synthetic surfactant affects gas exchange in surfactant-deficient rats. Pediatr Res 1998; 43:666–673.

37. Veldhuizen EJA, Waring AJ, Walther FJ, Batenburg JJ, Van Golde LMG, Haagsman HP. Dimeric N-terminal segment of human surfactant protein B [dSP-B(1-25)] has enhanced surface properties compared to monomeric SP-B(1-25). Biophys J 2000; 79:377–384.

38. Myers JK, Pace CN, Scholtz JM. Helix propensities are identical in proteins and peptides. Biochemistry 1997; 36:10923–10929.

39. Pace CN, Scholtz JM. A helix propensity scale based on experimental studies of peptides and proteins. Biophys J 1998; 75:422–427.

40. Roseman MA. Hydrophilicity of polar amino acid side-chains is markedly reduced by flanking peptide bonds. J Mol Biol 1988; 200:513–522.

41. Wüthrich K. NMR of Proteins and Nucleic Acids. New York: John Wiley & Sons, 1986.

42. Cavanagh J, Fairbrother WJ, Palmer AG Jr, Skelton NJ. Protein NMR Spectroscopy: Principles and Practice. San Diego, California: Academic Press, Inc., 1996.

43. Piantini U, Sorenson OW, Ernst RR. Multiple quantum filters for elucidating NMR coupling networks. J Am Chem Soc 1982; 104:6800–6801.

44. Davis DG, Bax A. Assignment of complex ^{1}H NMR spectra via two-dimensional homonuclear Hartmann–Hahn spectroscopy. J Am Chem Soc 1985; 107:2820–2821.

45. Kumar S. Conformational Analysis of a Synthetic Fragment of Lung Surfactant Apolipoprotein B [Master of Science]. Minneapolis, MN: University of Minnesota, 1992:111.

46. Johansson J, Szyperski T, Curstedt T, Wuthrich K. The NMR structure of the pulmonary surfactant-associated polypeptide SP-C in an apolar solvent contains a valyl-rich alpha-helix. Biochemistry 1994; 33(19):6015–6023.

47. Wüthrich K, Billeter M, Braun W. Polypeptide secondary structure determination by nuclear magnetic resonance observation of short proton–proton distances. J Mol Biol 1984; 180(3):715–740.

48. Wishart DS, Sykes BD, Richards FM. The chemical-shift index—a fast and simple method for the assignment of protein secondary structure through NMR-spectroscopy. Biochemistry 1992; 31(6):1647–1651.

49. Merutka G, Dyson HJ, Wright PE. "Random coil" ^{1}H chemical shifts obtained as a function of temperature and trifluoroethanol concentration for the peptide series GGXGG. J Biomol NMR 1995; 5(1):14–24.

50. Gopal A, Lee KYC. Morphology and collapse transitions in binary phospholipid monolayers. J Phys Chem B 2001; 105:10384–10354.

51. Jiarpinitnun C. Biophysical Characterization of Lung Surfactant Protein B and its Mutant Engineered Peptides [Bachelor of Science]. Chicago: The University of Chicago, 2000.

52. Killian JA, von Heijne G. How proteins adapt to a membrane-water interface. Trends Biochem Sci 2000; 25:429–434.

53. Yau WM, Wimley WC, Gawrisch K, White SH. The preference of tryptophan for membrane interfaces. Biochemistry 1998; 37:14713–14718.

54. Diamant H, Witten TA, Gopal A, Lee KYC. Unstable topography of biphasic surfactant monolayers. Europhys Lett 2000; 52(2):171–177.

55. Diamant H, Witten TA, Ege C, Gopal A, Lee KYC. Topography and instability of monolayers near domain boundaries. Phys Rev E 2001; 061602.

56. Piknova B, Schief WR, Vogel V, Discher BM, Hall SB. Discrepancy between phase behavior of lung surfactant phospholipid and the classical model of surfactant function. Biophys J 2001; 81:2172–2180.

57. Safran SA. Statistical Thermodynamics of Surfaces, Interfaces and Membranes. New York: Addison-Wesley, 1994.

58. Wurger A. Bending elasticity of surfactant films: The role of the hydrophobic tails. Phys Rev Lett 2000; 85(2):337–340.

59. Guttman GD, Andelman D. Electrostatic interactions in 2-component membranes. J Phys II 1993; 3(9):1411–1425.

60. Schief WR, Touryan L, Hall SB, Vogel V. Nanoscale topographic instabilities of a phospholipid monolayer. J Phys Chem B 2000; 104(44):7388.

61. Schief WR, Hall SB, Vogel V. Spatially patterned static roughness superimposed on thermal roughness in a condensed phospholipid monolayer. Phys Rev E 2000; 62:6831–6837.

12

Structure and Function of the Molecular Film of Pulmonary Surfactant at the Air–Alveolar Interface: The Role of SP-C

MATHIAS AMREIN

University of Calgary,
Alberta, Calgary, Canada

D. KNEBEL

JPK-Instruments AG,
Berlin, Germany

M. G. HAUFS

Ruhr-Universität Bochum,
Bochum, Germany

I. Basic Considerations

A. Function and Composition of Pulmonary Surfactant

The molecular film of pulmonary surfactant (PS) offsets the surface tensions of the hydrated lung epithelia to the air and thereby provides stability to the lung. In a condition of a dysfunctional surfactant, on the other hand, the surface tension will be high throughout the lung. As a consequence, the alveoli will merge with the small airways. As a result, gas exchange area is lost and lung injury may occur. In addition to providing stability to the lung, the reduction in surface tension reduces the work of breathing. The work required to inflate the lung upon inspiration is proportional to the actual surface tension of the interface and, hence, strongly reduced by the interfacial film.

PS is secreted by the alveolar type II epithelial cells (1–3). Neutral phosphatidylcholines (PC) represent 80% of its mass. Half of the PC is the disaturated dipalmitoylphosphatidylcholine (DPPC). A 5–10% is the negatively charged phosphatidylglycerols (PG) (4). In addition to its unique lipid composition, PS is distinct by two water-soluble (SP-A and SP-D) and two hydrophobic surfactant-associated proteins (SP-B and SP-C). The latter two are permanently associated with the lipids of PS because of their high amount of hydrophobic amino acid side chains. They play a major role in the surface activity of surfactant. SP-A and SP-D are mainly ascribed a function in host defense, but SP-A has also been shown to have a remarkable effect on the surface activity of PS (5). SP-B is a member of the saposin-like family of peptides (molecular mass 17 kDa) (6,7) with five positively charged amino acid side chains at physiological pH. One intermolecular disulfide bond leads to the predominant form of homodimers. The tertiary structure may closely resemble NK-lysin because of the high similarity (8). There appear to be five amphipatic helices (i.e., the helices are distinct by a highly hydrophobic face on the one side and a hydrophilic face on the other side of the helix-axis). SP-B associates with the vesicles of the mulitvesicular bodies of pulmonary epithelial type II cells. This putatively leads to vesicle lysis and reorganization and, finally, multilamellar bodies. They are the excretion forms of PS.

The other one of the two hydrophobic surfactant proteins, SP-C, is composed of 35 amino acids (molecular mass ~4 kDa) in the case of human surfactant. Two palmitoyl groups are covalently linked to the two cysteine residues located in the N-terminus region. The C-terminus region (amino acids 13–35) contains exclusively hydrophobic amino acids. CD- as well as IR-spectroscopy revealed that the protein occurs predominantly in an α-helical secondary structure under physiological conditions. The ternary structure of SP-C in an organic solvent, and in micellar solution, was studied by 2D ^{1}H NMR (9,10). The hydrophobic C-terminus region was a highly regular α-helix (amino acids 9–34). The conformation of the hydrophilic N-terminus part, as well as the conformation of the palmitoyl-groups, was flexibly disordered.

A highly preserved primary structure of SP-C in evolution and its confinement to the alveolar type II cells suggest a very specific and vital function of the peptide (11). However, knockout mice that are homozygous for an inactivated *SP-C* gene are viable at birth and similar to wild-type mice in lung morphology, growth, reproduction, and duration of life (12–14). Complete deficiency of SP-B, on the other hand, leads to an ineffective PS. As a result, it is lethal at birth (15–17). These results suggest an important role for SP-B but not for SP-C. However, SP-B deficient organisms suffer also from a dysfunctional SP-C, whereas SP-B is not affected by SP-C deficiency, that is, SP-B knockout mice are functionally dysfunctional for both hydrophobic proteins. This is explained by the pattern of processing of SP-C proprotein. ProSP-C is inserted in the membranes of the vesicles of the multivesicular bodies of the pulmonary epithelial type II cells. Proteolytic cleavage is required on both the N-terminus and the C-terminus end of the peptide (18) and, hence, on the outer and inner side of the vesicles. Putatively, the proteases are localized in the lumen of the multivesicular body and only have access to the C-terminus of the SP-C proprotein but not to the N-terminus inside the vesicles. Cleavage of the N-terminus propeptide of SP-C is therefore dependent on the lysis of the vesicles by SP-B (19). Hence, SP-C may still play an important role in the functional lung, but its function being replaceable by SP-B in the case of SP-C deficiency.

B. Surface Activity of PS

The surface activity of a substance describes its ability to form a molecular film at an interface and thereby reduce the surface tension of this interface. The resulting remainder surface tension of the interface is obtained by subtracting the pressure excerpted by the film (film pressure) from the surface tension of the interface in absence of the molecular film (free interface). The surface tension of a free air–water interface is $\sim$70 mN/m.

First, the surface activity of PS is characterized by its rate of adsorption from the aqueous phase to the air–liquid interface and the according reduction in surface tension. The rate of adsorption is representative for the ability of the surfactant to spread to the newly formed interface during the first breath after birth and to replenish the interfacial film if matter has been lost or inactivated. Secondly, it depicts the change of the surface tension upon the reduction or expansion in interfacial area as it occurs during the breathing cycle. PS shows a very distinct surface activity: from its secretion form (tubular myelin), it adsorbs very quickly to the air–aqueous interface to form a tightly packed molecular film. As the area of the alveolar interface decreases upon the expiration, the molecules become even more tightly packed at the interface and the film pressure rises further. At end expiration, the film pressure offsets the surface tension of the free air–buffer interface. The actual surface tension changes from 30 mN/m at total lung capacity to $\sim$20 mN/m at 80% of total lung capacity, and to $\sim$0 mN/m at residual lung capacity (20). The film is also distinct by its high-mechanical strength (21).

C. Adsorption of Phospholipids

The study of the surface activity has identified the phospholipids as the primary surface tension lowering components. They impart many of the required properties to the interfacial film. DPPC plays the major role in this function both for its abundance in PS and for its properties (2,3). Consequently, DPPC is mass-wise the major component in any of the surfactant replacement products used to compensate a deficient surfactant to date. A significant amount of PG or, in some cases, phosphatidylinositols (PI) suggest an important role for either one or both of these negatively charged phospholipids. For a number of minor lipid components, the function at the air–liquid interface is yet to be established. The role of each of the lipid components as far as known has recently been comprehensively reviewed (22,23).

Phospholipids are well accommodated at an air–aqueous interface, where they form a monomolecular film. The hydrophilic head-groups are immersed in the aqueous phase, whereas the hydrophobic aliphatic tails are directed toward the air. They adsorb from the aqueous phase to the air–liquid interface until the equilibrium surface tension is reached (e.g., 25 mN/m for DPPC at 37°C at a concentration of 1 mg/mL in the aqueous phase). At this point, no net new matter moves into the interface because it has become energetically too costly to squeeze itself into the film that had already formed.

Although the equilibrium surface tension is comparable for many phospholipids, the time needed to reach it can differ very much among different lipid species, specific compositions of mixed substances, and molecular organization of these substances in the aqueous phase. There are several factors that affect the rate of adsorption. First, the matter has to diffuse from the bulk-aqueous phase to the interface. However, in the lung, diffusion might play a minor role, as the aqueous layer is very thin (in the micrometer range). When the alveoli become inflated, this layer is stretched-out and vice versa upon deflation. The surfactant matter in the aqueous phase occurs in aggregates of comparable dimensions to the thickness of the aqueous lining. The matter may therefore be forced into close contact to the interface rather than diffuse to it.

The aggregates of surfactant are composed of unilamellar vesicles, multilamellar vesicles, or embody some specific structure such as tubular myelin. All of these structures are based on lipid bilayers. The unsaturated lipids (i.e., containing double-bonds in their aliphatic tails) form fluid bilayers, whereas a bilayer of the fully saturated DPPC is in the more condensed gel-phase at physiological temperature. Its hydrophobic tails can align and densely pack, because of the absence of double-bonds. Bilayers of purely DPPC insert into the interface very slowly when compared with structures formed by unsaturated lipids, as they are less likely to break up and rearrange in a monolayer than some bilayer in a fluid state. Adding unsaturated lipids to DPPC therefore increases the rate of adsorption.

Another reason for the slow adsorption of DPPC layers may be the strong hydration shell that emanates from the zwitterionic head-groups. It prevents two adjacent layers of DPPC (e.g., a partial monolayer at the air–liquid interface and a vesicle below it) to come close and fuse (24). Hence, there is a high potential energy barrier that must be overcome, before the matter from the bulk aqueous phase can adsorb to the interface. On the other hand, charged lipid layers of PG or PI, for example, repel each other. Their head-group charge attracts counter-ions to form a diffuse layer of increased ion concentration close by (electrical double layer). If the electrical double layers of two adjacent lipid layers start to overlap, they become repelled due to an osmotic stress. However, unlike the hydration shell, the electrical double layer is strongly diminished by the presence of (divalent) ions. A physiological amount of divalent cations is sufficient for these interfaces to come into close contact and fuse. Adding charged phospholipids augments the rate of adsorption of surfactant to the air–liquid interface. However, note that any adsorption of lipid mixture is highly inferior when compared with surfactant extracted from natural sources or reconstituted surfactant containing one or both of the hydrophobic surfactant proteins (discussed subsequently).

As the space per molecule at the air–water interface becomes less during the process of adsorption, fully saturated lipids, such as DPPC, pack into an increasingly well-ordered condensed phase, very much like they were in the condensed gel-phase in the bilayer. Unsaturated lipid species remain in the less-ordered liquid expanded phase. In the case of mixed films of saturated and unsaturated lipids, the saturated lipids segregate into densely packed crystalline areas, surrounded by the more fluid unsaturated components.

D. Compression of Phospholipids

The minimum surface tension obtained after adsorption, the equilibrium surface tension, is insufficient to stabilize the lung at end expiration. The required further reduction is brought about by compression of the film upon the expiration. As the film pressure increases, the surface tension becomes more reduced. It is decisive for a functional surfactant film to sustain a high film pressure without collapsing. Films from unsaturated lipids dissolve into the aqueous phase already at a relatively low film pressure. Hence, although the fluid lipids increase the rate of adsorption, they are detrimental to a high film pressure as required in the lung. Saturated lipids, on the other hand, can usually sustain a higher film pressure. They become increasingly well ordered into a solid phase. However, at some point, these films crack like a plate under compression. The matter lost from the interface upon this incidence forms multiple stacks of lipid bilayers. When the film is now relaxed, this matter does not spread again readily to the air–liquid interface.

DPPC is the only major component in PS, capable to sustain a film pressure high enough to reduce the surface tensions close to zero in a pure film. Only 10–12% of area reduction is sufficient to lower surface tension from equilibrium to ~1 mN/m. Furthermore, the film remains at this low surface tension for hours, whereas most other lipid films return to their respective equilibrium surface tension in a short period of time. These properties are very close to the situation found in the lung with respect to the low surface tension achieved, the area reduction required to achieve it, and the stability over time (20). On the basis of this evidence, a surface monolayer highly enriched in DPPC has commonly been assumed to be responsible for the critical reduction in surface tension in the lung and an almost exclusive DPPC layer at the air–liquid interface at end expiration as predicted (1).

However, DPPC alone is not sufficient to account for the function of PS for reasons in addition to discussed earlier: it adsorbs too slowly to the air–liquid interface to be effective during the first breath after birth and collapses irreversibly when it is over-compressed or mechanically agitated (21). Moreover, the surface tension of a monomolecular film of DPPC increases rapidly to an un-physiological high surface tension, when the interfacial area is expanded as much as the lung's interface during deep breathing ($\sim$30%). This is because the spacing between the molecules becomes too large, and the adsorption of new matter from the water phase is too slow to fill the gaps in the timeframe of breathing cycle. All of these reasons do not yet preclude that a monolayer of purely DPPC might form each time toward end expiration. The fluid components that help the adsorption, on the one hand, but prevent a high film pressure as required in the lung, on the other hand, may become excluded from the film upon compression. However, there is apparently not enough DPPC present in the lung to cover the lung's interface completely at end expiration (25). Hence, there must be a film that accommodates non-DPPC components, even unsaturated lipids, at all times at the interface and at the same time allows for a surface tension close to zero.

We will highlight the interaction of SP-C with phospholipids to form such film and discuss its structure and function in the light of the earlier-described requirements for a functional surfactant. We will also introduce recently developed methods to study this and related problems.

II. The Role of SP-C for the Structure–Function Relationship of PS

A. Methods

The film structures formed by models of PS, as well as surfactant extracts, are conveniently studied by microscopy. Fluorescence light microscopy (FLM) may be performed directly at the air–aqueous interface of a Langmuir-trough by placing a microscope objective closely over the films. For high-resolution microscopy, including atomic force microscopy AFM, spatial resolved mass spectrometry, and near field optical microscopy, films are commonly prepared at the air–aqueous interface of a Langmuir-trough and thereafter transferred onto a solid support at different states of compression (26–34).

Although the transfer for the high-resolution techniques arrest the films in their state prior to transfer, FLM at the air–aqueous interface of a Langmuir-trough allows observing dynamic changes such as they occur on compression and decompression of the films. However, there are substantial limitations of this technique with regard to PS: compression rates that would reflect breathing are not possible, because the quick motion of the movable barrier would agitate the large interface; some film area moves out of the field of view of the microscope, as soon as the film is compressed or decompressed, respectively; a high film pressure is often not sustainable on a Langmuir-trough, because the film creeps over the walls and the barrier of the trough. This is particularly the case with many natural and artificial PS systems. Moreover, the film balance represents a planar lipid film, whereas the alveolar monolayer is strongly curved.

For these reasons, we performed FLM and AFM at the air–aqueous interface of air-bubbles (Fig. 12.1). Bubbles have earlier been recognized to be highly advantageous for the evaluation of the surface activity of PS under dynamic conditions (21,35) and now proved to eliminate the earlier-mentioned limitations in microscopy too. The static picture of the molecular structure of surfactant was thus complemented by a dynamic view of how the film organizes, when matter becomes adsorbed to the interface from the aqueous phase, and how the film rearranges, when the interface is compressed thereafter (36,37). A model surfactant of DPPC, dipalmitoyl-phosphatidylglycerol (DPPG), and recombinant SP-C was used. This mixture has proven to reflect many aspects of natural surfactant (38–40) and allows to discuss some of the earlier-raised questions and requirements for a functional surfactant. The model proved also particularly useful for the evaluation of the novel microscopical techniques employed.

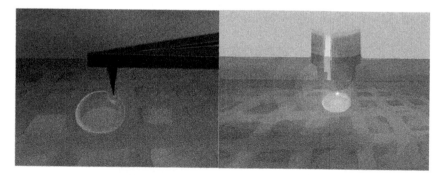

Figure 12.1 Experimental setup of the microscopy at an air–buffer interface (AFM, left; FLM, right). Air bubbles in the range of 50–500 μm in diameter were submersed in buffer. They were anchored to hydrophobic areas on an elsewhere hydrophilic mica support. The interfacial film formed from vesicles, injected into the buffer. The film was viewed from above by either the probe of the AFM or across the immersion light microscope objective. For FLM, the sample was contained in an airtight chamber and the pressure adjusted to increase or decrease the size of the bubble.

B. Vesicle Adsorption

The adsorption of surfactant to the interface has to be rapid to be effective in the lung. The model system used proved effective in that respect and an interfacial film would form immediately when the concentration was high and the aqueous phase stirred (i.e., in the range of 1 mg phospholipid/mL). However, to be able to study the film formation within an observable timeframe, vesicles were also added to a buffer at low concentration and the aqueous phase not stirred. In the presence of Ca^{2+}, the vesicles aggregated to clusters of several micrometers in size even before a film at the interface formed (Fig. 12.2). The clusters often adhered to the bubble surface. In the absence of Ca^{2+}, no clusters formed, and also no visible film formed. This demonstrates the role of the earlier-described reduction of the electrical double layer repulsion by Ca^{2+}, which then allows the negatively charged vesicles to come close to each other and cluster (24). When Ca^{2+} was removed from the buffer, the clusters in the aqueous phase disintegrated. Hence, the vesicles were merely aggregated.

A film formation from large aggregates is important for the proper function of surfactant in the lung. New surfactant matter is delivered to the interface much faster in large clusters than would be through the diffusion limited adsorption of small vesicles. This observation is in line with adsorption studies of surfactant extracts (25,41). The surface tension decreased in discrete steps (adsorption clicking) rather than continuously. The authors assessed the co-operative insertion of up to 10^{14} lipid molecules per single step. Note that unlike SP-C, SP-B leads to an irreversible fusion of vesicles.

C. Film Formation

In an early stage, the film at the air–water interface of the bubble consisted of condensed (dark) patches of lipids that diffused like rafts in a fluid, fluorescent

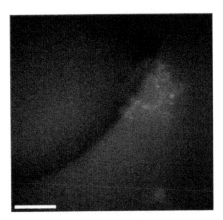

Figure 12.2 Optical section across an air-bubble, after vesicles were allowed to adsorb. In the presence of Ca^{2+}, the vesicles formed clusters. They adhered to the bubble. The bar corresponds to 25 μm.

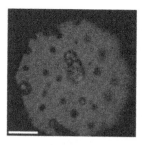 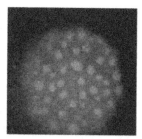 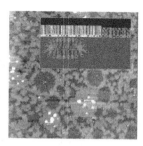

Figure 12.3 FLM (left and center, the bar corresponds to 25 μm) of the film upon formation from vesicles. Condensed lipid rafts (dark) diffused in a fluid matrix that contained also the fluorescent dye. Rafts often contained a bright spot, more and more commonly observed with increasing adsorption time. Sometimes, the condensed rafts became fully covered by this bright matter and the contrast appeared reversed (center). AFM (right) showed that the bright spots or areas in the FLM images consisted of additional lipid bilayers, adherent exclusively to condensed areas (inset). Note that in the AFM image, the fluid areas of the film constituted the lowest topographical level (darkest shade of gray). The condensed regions were thicker by a fraction of a nanometer (intermediate shade of gray). The bilayer areas, displayed as white regions, rise ~5 nm above the level of the condensed areas.

matrix (Fig. 12.3). Note that in the case of films of a single lipid-species, two coexisting phases, liquid expanded and liquid condensed are indicative of a phase transition of first order, such as melting or evaporation. In the case of the mixed film under investigation, the coexistence of two phases could be additionally attributed to the segregation of the different components with some component being condensed and some other component still being in a fluid state. We found earlier that the fluid phase contains the SP-C and a fraction of the lipids in addition to the fluorescent dye; the condensed phase consists of purely lipid (26,38).

Most interestingly, many of the condensed patches had additional lipid bilayers attached to them. Sometimes, all of the condensed rafts were fully covered by at least one additional lipid bilayer. In the light microscope, they appeared as bright areas inside the condensed rafts; the AFM exposed their height of ~5 nm and multiples thereof (42). Often, the vesicular aggregates adhered to these double layers, indicating that the adsorption of vesicles takes place in the condensed phase (Fig. 12.3). This may result from a specific interaction of the two palmitoyl groups of the SP-C with the monolayer. They may specifically insert themselves in the condensed areas of the monolayer as the first step of the adsorption of new matter from vesicles. Thereby, they may act as a hydrophobic anchor that ensures a tight contact of the bilayers to the monolayer. This function has also been demonstrated by observing the film pressure of a purely lipid film on a film balance upon the adsorption of vesicles that also contained SP-C (42). When the vesicles were added to the subphase under

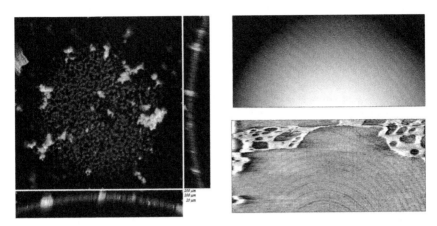

Figure 12.4   (Left) Data set from a laser scanning confocal FLM of the top part of a bubble after the adsorption of the model surfactant system has been completed. There are polygonal lipid patches that are surrounded by a protein-rich rim. In addition to the film at the air–water interface, there are large clusters of vesicular matter that are tightly anchored to the bubble surface. Apparently, the film is formed from these extended clusters. (Top right) AFM topography of a similar specimen (25 μm × 12 μm; gray scale: 2 μm). (Bottom) After subtraction of the nearly spherical shape of the bubble (gray scale: 10 nm), there are two distinct levels of height with the elevated region of ∼4–5 nm above the lower area. The concentric rings visible in the lower area are center in the apex of the bubble. They are most probably due to the capillary waves.

conditions, where fusion of the vesicles with the monolayer was not taking place (i.e., in absence of calcium ions), the film pressure rose nevertheless. This increase in surface pressure was not observed, when the two palmitoyl groups had been removed from SP-C beforehand. It is interesting to note that palmitoyl groups also constitute the lipid-anchor of many of the proteins, associated with sphingolipid rafts in the outer leaflet of cell membranes. There also the association is specifically with the condensed, fully saturated lipids of the rafts (43). This points to the general role of palmitoyl groups to anchor proteins specifically to condensed regions of lipid layers.

Although the palmitoyl groups of the SP-C are apparently associated with the condensed lipids of the first monolayer at the air–water interface, the helical part of the SP-C is known to span lipid bilayers in a fluid state, but is excluded from bilayers in the condensed gel-phase (9). Hence, SP-C may cross-link the condensed monolayer of saturated lipids to fluid bilayers that can also contain unsaturated lipids. It is tempting to believe that in the lung, where unsaturated lipids make up a substantial amount of the surfactant lipids, SP-C also causes sorting, directing the unsaturated lipids to the bilayers and the saturated lipids to the monolayer. A full coverage of the monolayer with saturated lipids may be, in fact, prerequisite for the low surface tension of the interface observed in the lung.

D. Equilibrium Structure

Upon completion, the film did no longer change its appearance and all of the film motion became arrested. The interfacial tension in equilibrium state of the model system, and of natural surfactant extract, is known to be ~20 mN/m, a value found in the lung at ~80% of total lung capacity. Monomolecular areas were surrounded by layered protrusions. The layered protrusions were based on multiples of lipid bilayers. SP-C promotes the reversible formation of these protrusions. Attaching a fluorescent dye to the protein allows the localization of its lateral distribution with high resolution by means of scanning near-field optical microscopy (SNOM) (Fig. 12.5). The protein is included within the bilayers with the content per unit area being proportional to the height of the stacks, that is, each SP-C molecule is associated with a distinct number of lipid molecules (44).

The local formation of lipid bilayer structures and multiples thereof is a characteristic of the specific model surfactant system used here and of any other functional surfactant. It depends on the presence of SP-C or SP-B or both. Similar structures have, in fact, been found with films containing SP-B instead of SP-C or animal lung extract, containing both proteins (45,46) and also in surfactant extract.

Lipp et al. (46) have demonstrated that in the case of SP-B, these multi-layered areas had a dramatic effect on the stability of the films and that now even unsaturated lipids could be incorporated in the surface film without hampering its ability to reach a very low surface tension. The films also proved to be exceptionally cohesive and would rather form macroscopic folds than collapse. Interestingly, hydrophobic-extract surfactant from bovine lung lavage also revealed the formation of a monolayer phase in equilibrium with a lamellar phase

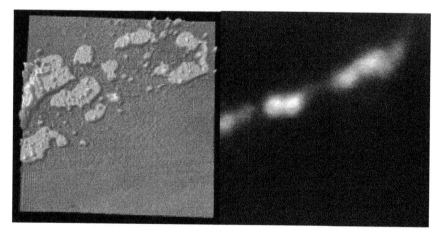

Figure 12.5 (Left) AFM topography of the model system (3D representation, 2.5 μm × 2.5 μm). (Right) SNOM: the bilayer areas contain the fluorescent SP-C (2.5 μm × 2.5 μm).

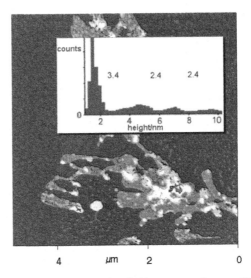

Figure 12.6 AFM topography of bovine lipid extract surfactant. The extract contains the lipids as well as SP-B and SP-C, but not the hydrophilic SP-A and SP-D. The surfactant was spread from buffer to the air–water interface of a Langmuir-trough, until the equilibrium surface tension was reached. Thereafter, it was adsorbed onto freshly cleaved mica by Langmuir–Blodgett transfer. As a common motif with the model system described here and SP-B containing model systems, there were monolayer areas, intercepted by multilamellar regions. The histogram (inset) reveals the height of these elevations. Interestingly, they seem to include also half of a lipid bilayer.

(Fig. 12.6). The monolayer showed distinct levels of height, $\sim$0.5 nm apart. This suggests the incorporation of saturated (long) and unsaturated (short) lipids within these areas, locally separated into small domains. The lamellar phase showed clearly distinct levels of height including 2.4, 3.4 (Fig. 12.6), and 4.2 nm (data not shown). This indicated that many of its components separated into distinct domains in the lamellar areas as well. Like the SP-B containing model system employed by Lipp et al., natural lipid extract surfactant can be compressed to achieve a very low surface tension and is exceptionally cohesive (21). These properties conceivably rely on the same principles. However, this has not yet been demonstrated by microscopy due to the difficulty for compressing natural surfactant films beyond equilibrium surface tension on a Langmuir-trough. It will be a matter of investigation by the earlier-described novel microscopy at the air–water interface of an air-bubble.

The ability to accommodate unsaturated lipids at the alveolar interface, the high-mechanical stability, and coherence are important properties of the surfactant film, based on its unique structure. In the next section, we describe yet another important aspect of surfactant function that is also based on the interplay of a monomolecular and a multilamellar phase. We have been using the earlier described model system of SP-C, DPPC, and DPPG, then expanded and compressed the films upon breathing at the interface of a bubble.

E. Expansion and Compression

Once an equilibrium film had formed at the interface, it was expanded (by expanding the bubble) by ~30% to reflect the situation of deep breathing. The expanded film showed no internal motion and, hence, was still in a condensed state. The bubble was then decreased incrementally to its original size and observed by FLM. Upon compression, the fluorescent rims became broader, and the dark areas became smaller (Fig. 12.7). This was indicative of a transition of the condensed monolayer phase into a (bright) multilamellar phase. This process was reversible.

The expansion and compression cycle demonstrates the function of the SP-C to build up a surface-associated reservoir that guaranties a full molecular coverage of the interface, when the interface is increased. It mediates the motion of the lipids forth and back between the monolayer and bilayer phases. The more the film becomes compressed, the more of the surfactant matter is "stored" in single and multiple lipid bilayers. The fluorescent areas exhibit several distinct levels of brightness, reflecting the number of bilayers stacked on top of each other. Our results are consistent with surface-activity studies by the captive bubble technique of a comparable system (21). After *de novo* formation of an interfacial film, Schurch et al., found that the matter associated with the interface was sufficient to cover up to six times the original area, depending on the presence of SP-C (these films consisted of PG/DPPC and had a SP-C content of 1% w/w). Hydrophobic-extracts of surfactant from natural sources had formed a reservoir of at least two additional monolayers after adsorption.

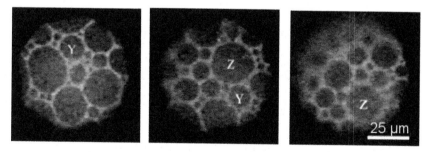

Figure 12.7   Three FLM micrographs from a video sequence of a compression cycle of an air-bubble. The diameter of the bubble is decreased and, hence, the surface film compressed [from left (100%) to right (75%)]. A fluorescent mesh becomes increasingly broader upon compression to the debit of the dark domains. This is indicative of the formation of more and more multilamellar structures in the bright areas that act as a surface-associated reservoir. Note that the area in view slightly moved in direction from the upper to the lower part of the image. The letters denote common domains in the film.

In summary, the high mechanical strength, cohesiveness, and ability to adjust to a strongly variable interfacial area of the molecular film of PS at the air–alveolar interface depend on a unique structure of a lipid monolayer in equilibrium with multilamellar areas and are conveyed to the film by SP-B or SP-C or both.

Acknowledgments

We acknowledge Drs. S. Schurch and J. Bruch for valuable discussions, Dr. M. Schoel for careful corrections, Drs. A. Bitterman for drawing Fig. 12.1, A. Wintergalen for preparing the specimen to obtain Fig. 12.3 (right), U. Kubitschek for his collaboration to obtain Fig. 12.4 (left), A. Kramer for Fig. 12.5 (right), and S. Kroll for preparing the specimen to obtain Fig. 12.6. The experimental work was supported by the IMF (Innovative Medizinische Forschung) at the University of Münster, Germany (grant nos.: RE-1-5-II/ 96-16 and RE-1-5-II/97-26) and the DFG (grant nos.: SFB 424, Si 670, and AM III/3-1).

References

1. Bangham AD, Morley CJ, Phillips MC. The physical properties of an effective lung surfactant. Biochim Biophys Acta 1979; 573:552–556.
2. Brown ES. Isolation and assay of dipalmitoyl lecithin in lung extracts. Am J Physiol 1964; 207:402–406.
3. Notter RH, Tabak SA, Mavis RD. Surface properties of binary mixtures of some pulmonary surfactant components. J Lipid Res 1980; 21:10–22.
4. Shelley SA, Balis JU, Paciga JE, Espinoza CG, Richman AV. Biochemical composition of adult human lung surfactant. Lung 1982; 160:195–206.
5. Schurch S, Possmayer F, Cheng S, Cockshutt AM. Pulmonary SP-A enhances adsorption and appears to induce surface sorting of lipid extract surfactant. Am J Physiol 1992; 263:L210–L218.
6. Patthy L. Homology of the precursor of pulmonary surfactant-associated protein SP-B with prosaposin and sulfated glycoprotein 1. J Biol Chem 1991; 266:6035–6037.
7. Hawgood S, Derrick M, Poulain F. Structure and properties of surfactant protein B. Biochim Biophys Acta 1998; 1408:150–160.
8. Andersson M, Curstedt T, Jornvall H, Johansson J. An amphipathic helical motif common to tumourolytic polypeptide NK-lysin and pulmonary surfactant polypeptide SP-B. FEBS Lett 1995; 362:328–332.
9. Johansson J, Szyperski T, Curstedt T, Wüthrich K. The NMR structure of the pulmonary surfactant-associated polypeptide SP-C in an apolar solvent contains a valyl-rich α-helix. Biochemistry 1994; 33:6015–6023.
10. Johansson J, Szyperski T, Wüthrich K. Pulmonary surfactant-associated polypeptide SP-C in lipid micelles: CD studies of intact SP-C and NMR secondary structure determination of dipalmitoyl-SP-C (1–17). FEBS Lett 1995; 362:261–265.

11. Hatzis D, Deiter G, deMello DE, Floros J. Human surfactant protein-C: genetic homogeneity and expression in RDS; comparison with other species. Exp Lung Res 1994; 20:57–72.

12. Conkright JJ, Bridges JP, Na CL, Voorhout WF, Trapnell B, Glasser SW, Weaver TE. Secretion of surfactant protein C, an integral membrane protein, requires the N-terminal propeptide. J Biol Chem 2001; 276:14658–14664.

13. Glasser SW, Detmer EA, Ikegami M, Na CL, Stahlman MT, Whitsett JA. Pneumonitis and emphysema in sp-C gene targeted mice. J Biol Chem 2003; 278:14291–14298.

14. Ikegami M, Weaver TE, Conkright JJ, Sly PD, Ross GF, Whitsett JA, Glasser SW. Deficiency of SP-B reveals protective role of SP-C during oxygen lung injury. J Appl Physiol 2002; 92:519–526.

15. Nogee LM, deMello DE, Dehner LP, Colten HR. Brief report: deficiency of pulmonary surfactant protein B in congenital alveolar proteinosis. N Engl J Med 1993; 328:406–410.

16. Clark JC, Weaver TE, Iwamoto HS, Ikegami M, Jobe AH, Hull WM, Whitsett JA. Decreased lung compliance and air trapping in heterozygous SP-B-deficient mice. Am J Respir Cell Mol Biol 1997; 16:46–52.

17. Clark JC, Wert SE, Bachurski CJ, Stahlman MT, Stripp BR, Weaver TE, Whitsett JA. Targeted disruption of the surfactant protein B gene disrupts surfactant homeostasis, causing respiratory failure in newborn mice. Proc Natl Acad Sci USA 1995; 92:7794–7798.

18. Vorbroker DK, Profitt SA, Nogee LM, Whitsett JA. Aberrant processing of surfactant protein C in hereditary SP-B deficiency. Am J Physiol 1995; 268:L647–L656.

19. Weaver T, Conkright J. Function of surfactant proteins B and C. Annu Rev Physiol 2001; 63:555–578.

20. Schurch S. Surface tension at low lung volumes: dependence on time and alveolar size. Respir Physiol 1982; 48:339–355.

21. Schurch S, Green FH, Bachofen H. Formation and structure of surface films: captive bubble surfactometry. Biochim Biophys Acta 1998; 1408:180–202.

22. Veldhuizen R, Nag K, Orgeig S, Possmayer F. The role of lipids in pulmonary surfactant. Biochim Biophys Acta 1998; 1408:90–108.

23. Veldhuizen EJ, Batenburg JJ, van Golde LM, Haagsman HP. The role of surfactant proteins in DPPC enrichment of surface films. Biophys J 2000; 79:3164–3171.

24. Israelachvili JN. Intermolecular and Surface Forces. London: Academic Press, 1997.

25. Goerke J, Clements JA. Alveolar surface tension and lung surfactant. In: Handbook of Physiology. The Respiratory System. Mechanics of Breathing, Vol. 3. Am Physiol Soc 1986:247–261.

26. Bourdos N, Kollmer F, Benninghoven A, Ross M, Sieber M, Galla HJ. Analysis of lung surfactant model systems with time-of-flight secondary ion mass spectrometry. Biophys J 2000; 79:357–369.

27. Lee MM, Green FH, Roth SH, Karkhanis A, Bjarnason SG, Schurch S. Sulfuric acid aerosol induces changes in alveolar surface tension in the guinea pig but not in the rat. Exp Lung Res 1999; 25:229–244.

28. Ding J, Takamoto DY, von Nahmen A, Lipp MM, Lee KY, Waring AJ, Zasadzinski JA. Effects of lung surfactant proteins, SP-B and SP-C, and palmitic acid on monolayer stability. Biophys J 2001; 80(5):2262–2272.

29. Lee KYC, Lipp MM, Takamoto DY, Zasadzinski JA, Waring AJ. Collapse mechanism in lung surfactant system. Abstr Pap Am Chem Soc 1998; 216:288-COLL.

30. Perez-Gil J, Nag K, Taneva S, Keough KM. Pulmonary surfactant protein SP-C causes packing rearrangements of dipalmitoylphosphatidylcholine in spread monolayers. Biophys J 1992; 63:197–204.

31. Nag K, Taneva SG, Perez-Gil J, Cruz A, Keough KM. Combinations of fluorescently labeled pulmonary surfactant proteins SP-B and SP-C in phospholipid films. Biophys J 1997; 72:2638–2650.

32. Nag K, Perez-Gil J, Cruz A, Rich NH, Keough KM. Spontaneous formation of interfacial lipid–protein monolayers during adsorption from vesicles. Biophys J 1996; 71:1356–1363.

33. Grunder R, Gehr P, Bachofen H, Schurch S, Siegenthaler H. Structures of surfactant films: a scanning force microscopy study. Eur Respir J 1999; 14:1290–1296.

34. Amrein M, von Nahmen A, Sieber M. A scanning force- and fluorescence light-microscopy study of the structure and function of a model pulmonary surfactant. Eur Biophys J 1997; 26:349–357.

35. Enhorning G. A pulsating bubble technique for evaluating pulmonary surfactant. J Appl Physiol 1977; 43:198–203.

36. Knebel D, Sieber M, Reichelt R, Galla HJ, Amrein M. Fluorescence light microscopy of pulmonary surfactant at the air–water interface of an air bubble of adjustable size. Biophys J 2002; 83:547–555.

37. Knebel D, Sieber M, Reichelt R, Galla HJ, Amrein M. Scanning force microscopy at the air–water interface of an air bubble coated with pulmonary surfactant. Biophys J 2002; 82:474–480.

38. Nahmen von A, Post A, Galla HJ, Sieber M. The phase behavior of lipid monolayers containing pulmonary surfactant protein C studied by fluorescence light microscopy. Eur Biophys J 1997; 26:359–369.

39. Nahmen von A, Schenk M, Sieber M, Amrein M. The structure of a model pulmonary surfactant as revealed by scanning force microscopy. Biophys J 1997; 72:463–469.

40. Post A, Nahmen AV, Schmitt M, Ruths J, Riegler H, Sieber M, Galla HJ. Pulmonary surfactant protein C containing lipid films at the air–water interface as a model for the surface of lung alveoli. Mol Membr Biol 1995; 12:93–99.

41. Schurch S, Schurch D, Curstedt T, Robertson B. Surface activity of lipid extract surfactant in relation to film area compression and collapse. J Appl Physiol 1994; 77:974–986.

42. Wintergalen A. Lungensurfactant Protein C vermittelte Vesikelfusion an der Wasser-Luft–Grenzfläche: Ausbildung von Multischichtstrukturen zur Anpassung der Oberflächenspannung Ph.D. dissertation, WWU Muenster, Muenster, 1999.

43. Simons K, Toomre D. Lipid rafts and signal transduction. Nat Rev Mol Cell Biol 2000; 1:31–39.

44. Kramer A, Wintergalen A, Sieber M, Galla HJ, Amrein M, Guckenberger R. Distribution of the surfactant-associated protein C within a lung surfactant model film investigated by near-field optical microscopy. Biophys J 2000; 78:458–465.

45. Krol S, Ross M, Sieber M, Kunneke S, Galla HJ, Janshoff A. Formation of three-dimensional protein–lipid aggregates in monolayer films induced by surfactant protein B. Biophys J 2000; 79:904–918.

46. Lipp MM, Lee KYC, Takamoto DY, Zasadzinski JA, Waring AJ. Coexistence of buckled and flat monolayers. Phys Rev Lett 1998; 81:1650–1653.

13

Analysis of SP-C Function Using Transgenic and Gene Targeted Mice

STEPHAN W. GLASSER and THOMAS R. KORFHAGEN

Cincinnati Children's Hospital Medical Center,
Cincinnati, Ohio, USA

I. Introduction

Experiments that use genetically modified mice are providing new insights into the molecular basis of pulmonary developmental disorders (neonatal surfactant deficiency) and diseases that result from injury, environmental exposures, or hereditary defects. Broadly speaking, such preplanned alterations can be classified as gain- or loss-of-function. Gain-of-function is usually performed by the permanent insertion of a modified DNA construct that has been microinjected into the fertilized mouse egg. The injected DNA inserts randomly into the genome (transgene) and if it is inserted into an active region of chromatin, the biological activity of the transgene can be assessed. Transgenic mice have been used to identify candidate promoter regions of lung-specific genes that direct tissue and cell-specific patterns of expression. Lung-specific promoters, in turn, are being used to direct high-level expression of effector molecules such as growth factors, cytokines, or transcription factors to define their biological function (1–3). Loss-of-function is usually accomplished by targeted gene inactivation (gene targeting). Gene targeting is accomplished by homologous recombination into the native gene of a mutated gene producing an inactive allele. Gene inactivation is accomplished in pluripotent embryonic stem (ES) cells, and mice generated from the modified ES cells develop in the absence of the targeted gene product. Functional consequence of the gene inactivation can be determined in the resultant knockout mice and the role of the inactivated gene product inferred (4). The goals of this chapter are to summarize how *in vivo* analysis of the pulmonary surfactant protein C (*SP-C*) gene has been used to (1) characterize genomic sequences that direct developmental and type II cell-specific gene expression and (2) model interstitial lung disease (ILD) related to recently identified familial deficiencies of SP-C.

II. SP-C Structure and Function

SP-C is one of the two hydrophobic surfactant proteins that promotes the surface active properties of surfactant phospholipid films. The mature form of SP-C associated with alveolar surfactant is a 35 amino acid peptide that is proteolytically processed from either 191 or 197 amino acid proprotein produced by alternative mRNA splicing. The hydrophobic domain of mature SP-C spans residues 13–28 and contains an extended polyvaline domain (5,6). NMR studies of SP-C structure model SP-C as an α-helical peptide from residues 9–34 such that SP-C spans a lipid bilayer (7). The hydrophobicity of SP-C is enhanced by palmitoylation of cysteine residues at positions 5 and 6 with a minor fraction palmitoylated at lysine 11. Some species (dog, mink) have a single palmitoyl modification at cysteine 6. This unusual combination of an extended hydrophobic helical domain and dipalmitoylated short amino terminus, accounts for the lipid associating properties of SP-C. Evidence suggests that SP-C alters phospholipid surface film activity by disruption of acyl chain packing (8,9). SP-C enhances *in vivo* surfactant function as well. Surfactant phospholipid preparations, supplemented with SP-C as the only protein, were effective in restoring lung compliance in surfactant depleted rodent lung models of acute lung injury (10).

SP-C functions may extend beyond the predicted role in dynamic lung compliance. New experiments suggest that SP-C may have an immunoprotective function in alveolar homeostasis. Lipid associated SP-C was shown to efficiently bind bacterial lipopolysaccharide (LPS) (11). SP-C binding was specific and occurs via the lipid A component of LPS (12). Optimal SP-C–LPS interaction is complex, requiring the amino and carboxy domains of SP-C (13). It is not known whether the binding of SP-C to LPS facilitates LPS presentation to immune surveillance cells or whether SP-C functions to sequester LPS from contact with immune cells thus suppressing inflammatory stimuli from inhaled microbial LPS.

III. *SP-C* Gene Structure and Expression

The human and mouse *SP-C* gene sequences are highly conserved reflecting the near invariant SP-C peptide sequence reported for several species. The *SP-C* gene is compact and part of an unusual locus. The mouse *SP-C* gene is 3.2 kb long, whereas the human *SP-C* gene is only 2.7 kb in length. The *SP-C* gene is organized in six exons with the mature SP-C airway peptide encoded by exon 2 (14,15). With both species, the *SP-C* gene ends directly adjacent to the presumptive promoter region and first exon of the *BMP-1* gene, which encodes procollagenase C. Sequence homology between the two *SP-C* genes ends abruptly at the 3′ boundary of SP-C leading into the BMP-1 promoter region. The loss of sequence homology beyond the final exon on the two *SP-C* genes suggested that essential transcriptional control sequences would be located in 5′ flanking DNA.

SP-C gene expression is detected only in the lung. *In situ* hybridization studies from mice and humans demonstrate that *SP-C* gene expression is initiated at the earliest stages of lung development (16,17). SP-C mRNA is detected over distal epithelial cells of the primitive airways. SP-C expression is sustained at the advancing edge of tubules as they progressively branch throughout development, whereas SP-C expression is extinguished in the established proximal epithelium. Ultimately SP-C mRNA is detected only in type II cells of the mature lung. In contrast, SP-A and SP-B expressions are detected in both bronchiolar and alveolar type II cells with SP-A expression also in tracheal gland cells. Because SP-C alone is expressed exclusively in type II cells, SP-C has served as a type II cell marker in disease or during injury. The *SP-C* gene has been similarly used as a model gene to define components of transcription that are selective for the type II cell.

IV. SP-C Transgenes Identify Regions that Specify Pulmonary Epithelial Cell Expression

Initial attempts to identify genomic regions that confer lung-specific expression tested 3.7 kb of the human SP-C promoter, which was the largest segment of available DNA. Transgenic mice were generated with 3.7 SP-C directing expression of a diphtheria toxin A (DTA) reporter gene or a bacterial chloramphenicol acetyl transferase (CAT) reporter gene. The 3.7 SP-C–DTA founder mice died of respiratory failure at birth (18). The lungs of 3.7 SP-C–DTA mice had different degrees of lung pathology varying from type II cell injury to severe disruption of distal lung morphogenesis. This finding indicated that 3.7 kb SP-C promoter directed organ-specific production of the DTA toxin. By linking the same 3.7 SP-C promoter to a neutral reporter gene (CAT), the specificity of transgene expression could be monitored without disturbing lung morphogenesis. The pattern of 3.7 SP-C–CAT expression closely paralleled endogenous SP-C expression. CAT mRNA was detected by *in situ* hybridization early in embryonic lung development in distal airway epithelial cells following the proximal to distal migration of airway growth (15,16). In the adult lung, 3.7 SP-C–CAT transgene expression did not precisely recapitulate endogenous SP-C expression. CAT mRNA was present focally over alveolar epithelial cells. The number of alveolar sites of transgene expression was less than for SP-C and varied between different 3.7 SP-C–CAT transgenic lines (19). These findings suggest that the site of transgene integration may influence the extent of type II cell expression and that there may be as yet unrecognized differences in the transcriptional capability of type II cells. High levels of 3.7 SP-C–CAT mRNA were also detected along the bronchiolar epithelium, distinct from the alveolar restricted pattern of SP-C mRNA [Fig. 13.1(a–d)]. The discordance in human 3.7 SP-C transgene and in normal SP-C expression could reflect species sequence difference in the two promoters, altering recognition of cis-acting element(s) that precisely regulate SP-C transcription. Alternatively, the human promoter might simply not contain cis-active elements necessary to suppress bronchiolar expression. When the mouse *SP-C* gene was cloned, the regions upstream of the promoter were sequenced and compared to the human 3.7 kb sequence. The mouse and human 5′ regions were highly divergent, supporting the explanation that species differences in nucleotide sequence or configuration of cis-active elements account for the discordant expression. Three regions of sequence homology were maintained between human and murine SP-C–DNA. The homologous regions of the human 3.7 kb sequence were distributed over 4.8 kb of the mouse DNA. Near-sequence identity exists in the proximal region of homology that extends to −318 bp of the TATA elements. The two distal regions of reduced homology are located from −3.9 to −3.6 kb and from −1.9 to −1.5 kb of the promoter. Two additional SP-C promoter studies have been completed. Transgenic mice were made with deletions of the 3.7 SP-C promoter and also with the mouse 4.8 kb homolog of the human 3.7 kb promoter. When the original 3.7 kb was shortened to 0.6 kb, CAT reporter expression was still lung specific, but at very low levels of activity (19). The reduced level of *in vivo* expression from the 0.6 kb SP-C promoter demonstrated that an enhancer element was located in the deleted upstream region of DNA. An attractive hypothesis is that one or both of the distal regions of homologous sequence represent the enhancer. *In vitro* transient and stable transfection

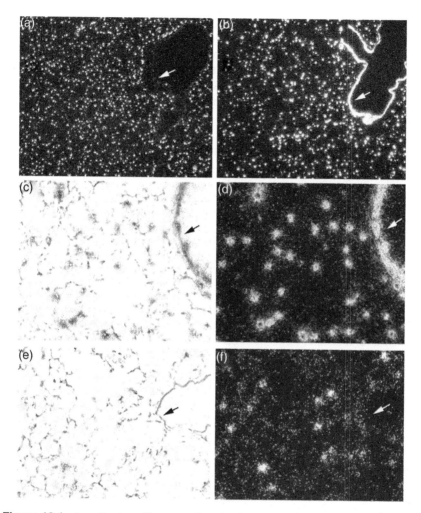

Figure 13.1 Localization of human and murine SP-C transgene expression *in vivo*. The cellular sites of human 3.7 kb and murine 4.8 kb SP-C promoter activity in transgenic mouse lung were determined using CAT antisense riboprobes. The pattern of endogenous *SP-C* gene expression was determined using an SP-C antisense riboprobe. Dark field images for SP-C and 3.7 SP-C–CAT expression are shown at low magnification in (a) and (b), respectively. The 3.7 SP-C–CAT expression is detected in a pattern similar to the type II cell-specific expression of SP-C seen in (a), but is also detected along bronchiolar epithelium (arrows). (e) and (f) illustrate the alveolar specificity of mouse 4.8 kb promoter activity at high magnification. Bronchoalveolar expression of the human 3.7 SP-C–CAT transgene is shown in (d), whereas only alveolar specific sites of expression are detected in 4.8 SP-C–CAT lung (f). Corresponding bright field images (c and e) are presented for identification of morphological structures. Arrows indicate bronchiolar structures in paired dark–bright field panels. (a) and (b) were photographed at 4× magnification. (c–f) were photographed at 20× magnification.

experiments suggest that the distal enhancer activity is chromatin dependent. Finer deletions of the human SP-C promoter mapped an essential region of lung expression to within the -215 bp promoter region. Analysis of the proximal region *in vitro* has identified multiple transcription factors that stimulate SP-C promoter activity. The murine 4.8 kb SP-C promoter directs high level of lung specific CAT reporter activity similar to the human 3.7 SP-C promoter. Using *in situ* hybridization, the 4.8 SP-C–CAT transgenic mice expression was shown to be alveolar cell specific [Fig. 13.1(e) and (f)]. This finding confirms that the bronchiolar expression in human 3.7 SP-C–CAT transgenic mice resulted from altered arrangement or misrecognition of the human cis-active elements by the mouse transcriptional apparatus. Continued *in vivo* functional mapping of cell-specific control elements coupled with *in vitro* promoter transactivation studies will provide a powerful approach to define how type II cell-specific transcription is achieved.

V. Altered Expression of SP-C and Familial ILD in Humans

Abnormalities of SP-C have been recently related to familial forms of ILD. ILD covers several distinct forms of disease that have diverse clinical and pathological features. The underlying cause(s) of an adult ILD is often obscure and is also referred to as idiopathic interstitial pneumonia (IIP). The characteristic features common to the various forms of ILD include cellular infiltrates (predominantly monocytic cells), alveolar wall thickening, type II cell hyperplasia with alveolar remodeling, and overt fibrosis in some cases. Familial ILD in children is associated with high mortality. Examples of familial ILD have been described where the disease is associated with the absence of SP-C or mutations in the *SP-C* gene that produce a truncated proSP-C peptide. A sibship of a mother and her two children who were severely affected by ILD were reported, who lacked mature SP-C in alveolar lavage and tissue levels of proSP-C were reduced (20). These findings suggest that the lack of mature SP-C in the alveolus may result in ILD/IIP. Interestingly, no mutation was found in the *SP-C* gene of these individuals, suggesting that there is a regulatory defect either in an essential transcription factor or in the SP-C promoter region resulting in reduced SP-C transcription. Quantitative RNA analysis was not obtained from the affected individuals. The finding of reduced SP-C expression emphasizes the need for ongoing transcriptional studies using transgenic mice to characterize regulatory elements that might be altered in human SP-C disease.

Distinct from the simple absence of mature SP-C, mutations in the *SP-C* gene have been identified which alter the carboxy terminus region of proSP-C. The first report of an *SP-C* gene mutation associated with ILD found that a single base pair mutation of the intron 4 splice site results in exon 4 deletion and loss of 37 amino acids (21). This truncated proSP-C is misprocessed and accumulates in type II cells, whereas no mature SP-C is found in alveolar lavage. A separate kindred has been identified which include 14 affected adults and children diagnosed with forms of ILD (22). A single base pair mutation in exon 5 substitutes a glutamine for a leucine at position 188 of proSP-C. The severity of disease and age of diagnosis were highly variable between family members with three individuals diagnosed in the early months of life. Expression of the altered proSP-C *in vitro* was toxic to tissue culture cells. Thus, the associated ILD may stem from accumulation of a misfolded protein and resulting cell injury rather than the simple absence of the airway form of SP-C. Expression of altered SP-C *in vivo* in transgenic mice supports the concept that human ILD is associated with misprocessing of proSP-C. Transgene expression of just the mature form of SP-C in the lung resulted in severe disruption of lung morphogenesis (23). This finding is consistent with the requirement for precise intracellular routing and processing of SP-C. Although it is unlikely that all familial ILD is due to a genetic deficiency of SP-C, the current findings suggest a broader principle that familial ILD may often result from accumulation of an unknown misfolded protein in airway epithelial cells.

VI. SP-C Knockout Mice as a Model of ILD

In order to discern the role of SP-C in lung function, the *SP-C* gene was inactivated by conventional gene targeting techniques. Exon 2, which encodes the mature SP-C airway peptide cells, was interrupted by insertion of a neomycin resistance gene (24). This modified *SP-C* gene was used to produce targeted ES cells which in turn were used to ultimately generate mice carrying the insertional inactivated *SP-C* gene. Mice homozygous for the targeted disruption did not produce mature SP-C mRNA or corresponding protein. The initial knockout mouse model was generated on an outbred (Swiss/Black) genetic background. Mild abnormalities in pulmonary mechanics and *in vitro* surfactant function were detected. No histological changes were seen in young adult mice, but infrequent small cell infiltrates and subtle parenchymal changes were seen in old (>9 months) outbred SP-C−/− mice.

The variation in severity of human SP-C deficiency among affected individuals had suggested that unknown genetic or environmental influences affect the SP-C deficient phenotype. Experimentally, the phenotype of a mutation can often be enhanced by breeding the mutation onto inbred strains of mice where genetic variation is reduced (25,26). When the SP-C−/− allele was bred onto the 129/Sv inbred strain of mice, SP-C−/− mice had poor reproduction and developed a progressive interstitial pneumonitis (27). The extent of pulmonary injury was variable within the lungs of individual SP-C−/− 129/Sv mice. Cell infiltrates consisted of mixed granulocytes and macrophages in young mice, whereas macrophages were the principle cell type found in alveolar spaces of adult SP-C−/− mice. Extensive interstitial and peribronchiolar lymphocytic infiltrates were seen in a significant portion of adult SP-C−/− mice. In adults, the macrophage accumulation often resulted in areas of consolidation, whereas other adjacent cell free regions showed dramatic alveolar disruption similar in appearance to emphysema [Fig. 13.2(a–c)]. The parenchymal region with dense cell infiltrates showed the most extensive remodeling characterized by a mix of areas of dramatic septal thickening and type II cell hyperplasia. Thickened septae stained intensely with Masson's trichrome stain, indicating that lack of SP-C−/− also led to collagen disposition and regional fibrosis [Fig. 13.2(d)]. Areas of airspace loss were associated with a more complex remodeling that included reduction in the alveolar elastin fiber

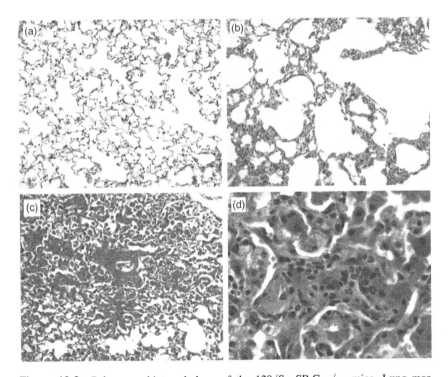

Figure 13.2 Pulmonary histopathology of the 129/Sv SP-C−/− mice. Lung morphology of an age-matched wild-type 129/Sv mouse is shown in (a). (b) and (c) depict variable changes seen in SP-C−/− mice. The extensive loss of alveoli and cellular thickening of residual alveolar structures is shown in (b). Macrophages and lymphocytic cells are associated with the thickened interstitium, but are not free in airspaces. An area of extensive cellular infiltration throughout airspaces is shown in (c). Areas of remodeling are evident in the dense cellular structures left and central in (c). Aberrant remodeling is indicated by morphology and trichrome staining in (d). Dense blue staining identifies extensive collagen deposition and fibrosis extending throughout. (a–c) were photographed at 10× magnification and (d) at 20× magnification.

network and a fibroblast to myofibroblast transformation identified by α-smooth muscle actin staining. This heterogeneity is consistent with the variable clinical and histopathological diagnosis for SP-C deficient family members. An important extension of these studies will be to identify genetic modifier loci and gene products that would be targets for therapeutic intervention.

Because the abnormalities in the SP-C$-/-$ lung increased with age, matrix metalloproteinosis (MMP) activity was assessed as an underlying cause of alveolar destruction. MMP activity was measured in the supernatant of cultured macrophages using gel zymography. Gelatinase activity was detected from SP-C$-/-$ macrophage media that was consistent with the molecular weight of MMP-2 and MMP-9. Virtually no activity was detected in SP-C$+/+$ media. The enhanced production of MMP-2 and MMP-9 probably contributes to selective degradation of alveolar extracellular matrix.

Signaling events which initiate cell influx and activation are unknown, but may result from LPS binding activity of SP-C. If a role for alveolar SP-C is to bind and sequester LPS from alveolar epithelial cells, then epithelial cells of SP-C$-/-$ mice may be exposed to increased LPS stimulus and produce a cytokine-mediated response that recruits the immune cells seen in SP-C$-/-$ mice. The SP-C$-/-$ mice were maintained in a microisolator barrier facility and free from detectable infection, but normal flora may provide sufficient LPS to induce inflammation. This reasoning predicts that SP-C$-/-$ mice will have an enhanced response to LPS or pathogen challenge. Consistent with this hypothesis of increased cytokine signaling is a marked airway epithelial cell dysplasia observed in SP-C$-/-$ mice. Mucus cell transformation is observed histologically, and cells are Alcian Blue and mucin (MUC5A/C) positive. Thus, SP-C influences gene expression outside the alveolus, suggesting soluble mediator signaling. Goblet cell transformation is known to be induced by several cytokines via altered EGFR signaling. The implication is that although SP-C expression is restricted to the alveolus, the release of soluble mediators into the alveolar extracellular fluid mediates the changes in proximal epithelial cell phenotype.

VII. Abnormalities in Surfactant Composition and Function with SP-C Deficiency

Because SP-C enhances the surface properties of surfactant phospholipids, it is possible that the lack of mature SP-C in the airspace could alter surfactant function eventually producing an injury that progresses to ILD. Lung mechanics were impaired in the SP-C$-/-$ 129/Sv mice, but this finding may simply reflect the significant pneumonitis which was established by the time lung compliance measurements were obtained. Surfactant from the SP-C$-/-$ 129/Sv mice has not been evaluated for altered *in vitro* surface activity. SP-B levels were unaltered in the SP-C$-/-$ mice and may be sufficient to sustain surfactant function. Other alterations of surfactant that may affect function include composition, distribution, and intracellular forms of surfactant. Lipid abnormalities in SP-C$-/-$ 129/Sv mice include a two-fold elevation in lung phospholipid content as well as unusual lipid inclusions in pulmonary vessels and interseptal lipofibroblasts. Despite these ultrastructural differences, the distinctive multi-vesicular and lamellar bodies of type II cells appear unaltered, suggesting that the intracellular assembly of surfactant is intact. The functional consequences of the observed lipid imbalance have not been linked to a lipid storage disease or chronic lung disease.

VIII. Utility of Current SP-C Mouse Models to Explore Pathogenic Mechanisms and Therapy for Familial ILD

The complex molecular events that precipitate ILD are likely to be different when the underlying defects are mutations that alter proSP-C structure vs. expression defects of diminished proSP-C or absence of mature SP-C. Transgenic mice that mimic the human proSP-C mutations can be used to dissect changes in proSP-C processing, vesicular trafficking, or unfolded protein response stress as causes of SP-C associated ILD. Conditionally, activated lung promoters can now be used to regulate the timing and levels of mutant proSP-C expression in order to avoid confounding developmental changes that result from perinatal overexpression generated with the original 3.7 SP-C promoter. The SP-C knockout or null mouse can be used to investigate whether SP-C deficient ILD originates from environmental inflammation by determining whether SP-C$-/-$ mice have an exaggerated response to microbial or LPS challenge. The SP-C deficient mice should also be useful to determine whether exogenous replacement of SP-C/phospholipid mixture is sufficient to prevent onset or inhibit progression of SP-C deficient disease. It is conceivable that SP-C fulfills a chaperone function in movement of surfactant material, as suggested from adenoviral SP-C expression in SP-C$+/+$ vs. SP-C$-/-$ type II cells (28). If SP-C has a specific chaperone function then exogenous treatment should reduce the injury. Alternatively, if the disease results from a misrouting of mutant SP-C, SP-C restoration may not ameliorate the disease. The challenge will be to use the transgenic and gene knockout models to differentiate intra-cellular from extracellular roles for SP-C in ILD.

Acknowledgment

The authors would like to acknowledge Dr. Jeffrey Whitsett for review and editing of the manuscript. This work has been supported by NIH grants HL50046, HL61646 (SWG), and HL58795 (TRK).

References

1. Glasser SW, Korfhagen TR, Wert SE, Whitsett JA. Transgenic models for study of pulmonary development and disease. Am J Physiol Lung Cell Mol Physiol 1994; 267:L489–L497.
2. Whitsett JA, Glasser SW. Targeting gene expression to the lung. In: Brigham KL, Lenfant C, eds. Gene Therapy for Diseases of the Lung Series in Lung Biology in Health and Disease. Vol. 104. New York: Marcel Dekker, 1997:193–208.
3. Whitsett JA, Glasser SW, Tichelaar JW, Perl A, Clark JC, Wert SE. Transgenic models for study of lung morphogenesis and repair. Chest 2001; 120:27S–30S.
4. Bronson SK, Smithies D. Altering mice by homologous recombination using embryonic stem cells. J Biol Chem 1994; 269:27155–27158.
5. Weaver TE, Conkright JJ. Functions of surfactant proteins B and C. Annu Rev Physiol 2001; 63:555–578.
6. Johansson J. Structure and properties of surfactant protein C. Biochim Biophys Acta 1998; 1408:161–172.
7. Johansson J, Szyperski T, Curstedt T, Wuthrich K. The NMR structure of SP-C in an apolar solvent contains a valyl-rich a helix. Biochemistry 1994; 33:6015–6023.
8. Horowitz AD, Elledge B, Whitsett JA, Baatz JE. Effects of lung surfactant proteolipid SP-C on the organization of model membrane lipids: a fluorescence study. Biochim Biophys Acta 1992; 1107:44–54.
9. Nag K, Perez-Gil J, Cruz A, Keough KM. Fluorescently labeled pulmonary surfactant protein C in spread phospholipid monolayers. Biophys J 1996; 71:246–256.
10. Davis AJ, Jobe AH, Hafner D, Ikegami M. Lung function in premature lambs and rabbits treated with a recombinant SP-C surfactant. Am J Respir Crit Care Med 1998; 157:553–559.
11. Augusto L, Le Blay K, Auger G, Blanot D, Chaby R. Interaction of bacterial lipopolysaccharide with mouse surfactant protein C inserted into lipid vesicles. Am J Physiol 2001; 281:L776–L785.
12. Augusto LA, Li J, Synguelakis M, Johansson J, Chaby R. Structural basis for interactions between lung surfactant protein C and bacterial lipopolysaccharide. J Biol Chem 2002; 277:23484–23492.
13. Augusto LA, Synguelakis M, Johansson J, Pedron T, Girard R, Chaby R. Interaction of pulmonary surfactant protein C with CD14 and lipopolysaccharide. Infect Immun 2003; 71:61–67.
14. Glasser SW, Korfhagen TR, Perme CM, Pilot-Matias TJ, Kister SE, Whitsett JA. Two *SP-C* genes encoding human pulmonary surfactant proteolipid. J Biol Chem 1988; 263:10326–10331.
15. Glasser SW, Korfhagen TR, Bruno MD, Dey C, Whitsett JA. Structure and expression of the pulmonary surfactant protein-*SP-C* gene in the mouse. J Biol Chem 1990; 265:21986–21991.
16. Wert SE, Glasser SW, Korfhagen TR, Whitsett JA. Transcriptional elements from the human SP-C gene direct expression in the primordial respiratory epithelium of transgenic mice. Dev Biol 1993; 156:426–443.
17. Khoor A, Stahlman MT, Gray ME, Whitsett JA. Temporal-spatial distribution of SP-B and SP-C proteins and mRNAs in the developing respiratory epithelium of the human lung. J Histochem Cytochem 1994; 42:1187–1199.

18. Korfhagen TR, Glasser SW, Wert SE, Bruno MD, Daugherty CC, McNeish JD, Stock JL, Potter SS, Whitsett JA. Cis-acting sequences from a human surfactant protein gene confer pulmonary-specific gene expression in transgenic mice. Proc Natl Acad Sci USA 1990; 87:6122–6126.

19. Glasser SW, Burhans MS, Eszterhas SK, Bruno MD, Korfhagen TR. Human *SP-C* gene sequences that confer lung epithelium-specific expression in transgenic mice. Am J Physiol 2000; 278:L933–L945.

20. Amin RS, Wert SE, Baughman RP, Tomashefski JF Jr, Nogee LM, Brody AS, Hull WM, Whitsett JA. Surfactant protein deficiency in familial interstitial lung disease. J Pediatr 2001; 139:85–92.

21. Nogee LM, Dunbar AE, Wert SE, Askin F, Hamvas A, Whitsett JA. A mutation in the surfactant protein C (*SP-C*) gene associated with interstitial lung disease. N Engl J Med 2001; 344:573–579.

22. Thomas AQ, Lane K, Phillips J III, Prince M, Markin C, Speer M, Schwartz DA, Gaddipati R, Marney A, Johnson J, Roberts R, Haines J, Stahlman M, Loyd JE. Heterozygosity for a surfactant protein C gene mutation associated with usual interstitial pneumonitis and cellular nonspecific interstitial pneumonitis in one kindred. Am J Respir Crit Care Med 2002; 165:1322–1328.

23. Conkright JJ, Na CL, Weaver TE. Overexpression of surfactant protein-C mature peptide causes neonatal lethality in transgenic mice. Am J Respir Cell Mol Biol 2002; 26:85–90.

24. Glasser SW, Burhans MS, Korfhagen TR, Na C, Sly PD, Ross GF, Ikegami M, Whitsett JA. Altered stability of pulmonary surfactant in SP-C deficient mice. Proc Natl Acad Sci USA 2001; 98:6366–6371.

25. Kallapur S, Ormsby I, Doetschman T. Strain dependency of TGFbeta1 function during embryogenesis. Mol Reprod Dev 1999; 52:341–349.

26. Doetschman T. Interpretation of phenotype in genetically engineered mice. Lab Anim Sci 1999; 49:137–143.

27. Glasser SW, Detmer EA, Ikegami M, Na CL, Stahlman MT, Whitsett JA. Pneumonitis and emphysema in *SP-C* gene targeted mice. J Biol Chem 2003; 278:14291–14298.

28. Conkright JJ, Bridges JP, Na C, Voorhout WF, Trapnell B, Glasser SW, Weaver TE. Secretion of surfactant protein C, an integral membrane protein, requires the N-terminal propeptide. J Biol Chem 2001; 276:14658–14664.

14

Alternative Functions of SP-B and SP-C

DAVID G. OELBERG

Eastern Virginia Medical School and Children's Hospital of
  The King's Daughters,
Norfolk, Virginia, USA

I. Introduction

Reduction of surface tension created by alveolar air–liquid interfaces is a primary function of pulmonary surfactant (PS). Of the four apoproteins associated with PS, SP-B, and SP-C are necessary and sufficient for reduction of alveolar surface tension (1). This occurs through the transformation, stabilization, and recycling of the phospholipid surface film. Although the other two apoproteins, SP-A and SP-D, support surface film homeostasis, they are not necessary for normal gas exchange (2), and their primary functions appear related to host defense and anti-inflammation (3).

Neonatal respiratory distress syndrome occurs in premature newborns born with insufficient pools of endogenous PS. Administration of exogenous PS to newborns suffering respiratory distress syndrome has revolutionized treatment by permitting ventilation of atelectatic lungs. Morbidity and mortality have been reduced. Available as both synthetic and natural preparations of PS, the most effective PS preparations are those containing either natural or recombinant SP-B and/or SP-C or those containing analogues thereof (4–8). These successes have led to the treatment of other pulmonary disorders caused by insufficient or dysfunctional PS, such as adult respiratory distress syndrome (9–11), aspiration syndromes (12,13), and pneumonia (12,14). Observations from clinical trials and animal models investigating some of these disorders have shown improvements that are attributable to direct regulation of inflammation. These secondary contributions of immunomodulation are unexplained on the sole basis of surface tension reduction.

The regulation of pulmonary inflammation is particularly important in the treatment of adult respiratory distress syndrome, meconium aspiration syndrome, and pneumonia. The release of proteases and production of oxygen radicals by pulmonary neutrophils are key injurious mechanisms in the development of both chronic lung disease following neonatal respiratory distress syndrome and acute pulmonary disorders in older children and adults (15). Over the past two decades, multiple *in vivo* investigations have demonstrated the anti-inflammatory effect of PS administration upon ventilated or acutely injured lungs during human disease or through use of animal models (16–18). However, these studies have failed to distinguish between direct anti-inflammatory effects of PS and indirect effects of PS on immune system components that are mediated through improved pulmonary function, reduced barotrauma, and/or decreased hyperoxia. To distinguish between the direct and indirect effects of PS on immune responses, *in vitro* responses of activated cellular components have been compared with or without pre-exposure to exogenous PS. Excluding PS preparations containing SP-A or SP-D, pre-exposures to preparations containing SP-B and SP-C have demonstrated decreased neutrophil adherence, aggregation, chemotaxis, respiratory burst, and elastase production following physiologic activation (19–23). Among other immunologic cell lines, cytokine release, immunoglobulin production, and cell proliferation are decreased in lymphocytes (24). Phagocytosis is decreased in monocytes (25). Differentiating between SP-B and SP-C effects on immune responses, SP-B appears to promote the secondary immune response by lymphocytes (26) and inhibit the lipopolysaccharide-induced nitric oxide response by alveolar macrophages (27). In contrast, SP-C promotes bacterial lipopolysaccharide recognition through direct binding to the molecule (28). These studies, when viewed in light of the clinical benefits of natural PS containing surfactant proteins, strongly support immunomodulatory roles for the surfactant apoproteins SP-B and SP-C.

The purpose of this chapter is to first review clues from the literature suggesting an electrophysiologic mechanism underlying the proposed immunomodulatory functions of SP-B/C. Secondly, I will support some of these clues by presenting ongoing observations from my laboratory defining these mechanisms.

II. Clues from the Biophysical Characteristics of SP-B and SP-C

By their very hydrophobic structures, both SP-B and SP-C are expected to directly interact with cellular plasma membranes. As one of the most hydrophobic molecules secreted by cells (29), SP-C is composed of 35 amino acids. Sixty-nine percent of its amino acids is hydrophobic, and overall hydrophobicity is increased by palmitoylation of cysteines at positions 5 and 6. The SP-C molecule is 37 Å long, and its structure is dominated by a rigid α-helix over positions 9–34. This α-helical segment spanning 23 Å is sufficiently long to span the hydrophobic domain of plasma membrane bilayers (30,31). It has been observed by FTIR spectroscopy that upon interaction with bilayers, the SP-C molecule inserts by spanning the bilayer in the α-helical configuration (32). Coupled with the observation that SP-C spans bilayers with a 24° tilt (33), SP-C appears well suited to comprise part of an oligomeric channel complex (32). In contrast, its propensity to exist in monomeric state within lipid bilayer (34) limits its suitability for channel formation in pure form. As will be discussed later, SP-C might complex with other SP-C molecules to form a channel oligomer. Although the occurrence of SP-C and SP-B complexes that form oligomeric channel structures has not been described, the possibility exists.

With 79 amino acids in the final SP-B monomer, SP-B is a larger peptide than SP-C. Fifty-two percent of its amino acids is hydrophobic, and it contains several basic amino acids providing a net charge of +5 (35). Approximately, half of the molecule conforms to the α-helical configuration, but, in contrast to the transmembrane orientation of SP-C in lipid bilayer, FTIR spectroscopy indicates that SP-B interacts with bilayers by shallow anchoring at the membrane surface (36). It is, therefore, limited in its suitability as a complete channel protein because of its parallel alignment with the bilayer axis that does not provide transmembrane access. Other characteristic features of the three-dimensional structure include three intramolecular sulfhydryl bridges between cysteine residues that stabilize the molecule's helical structures and support propensity for oligomeric formation as dimeric structures (35). Despite formation of homodimers, SP-B complexes do not transverse the bilayer membrane as intact channel proteins. However, as will be discussed shortly, SP-B is structurally related to a group of peptides known as saposin-like proteins (SAPLIP), and some SAPLIPs do demonstrate channel function.

III. Clues from the Channel Activities of Amyloid-Forming Peptides

By virtue of its relative thermodynamic instability in the α-helical conformation, SP-C has been included among a group of amyloid-forming peptides that potentially induce disease through the deposition of amyloid and/or insertion of channel activities (37,38). It is recognized for some of these peptides that subtle mutations may occur causing additional instability of the peptide (39). Destabilization of the amyloid-forming proteins in the α-helical conformation causes unfolding of the α-helix, intermolecular bonding among monomers through β-linkages, irreversible formation of stable β-sheets, and deposition of the β-sheets as amyloid fibrils (40). On the basis of the origin of the parent protein, deposition of these abnormal amyloid fibrils causes a wide range of chronic diseases. Within the central nervous system, encephalopathies caused by deposition of β-amyloid peptide, prion protein, or α-synuclein include Alzheimer's disease, Creutzfeldt–Jakob disease, or Parkinson's disease, respectively (41–44). In the liver, deposition of α_1-antitrypsin amyloid deposits causes hepatitis and cirrhosis (45).

With respect to SP-C, spontaneous destabilization from the less stable α-helical conformation to the more stable β-sheet structure parallels that of other amyloid-forming peptides. This is certainly true of SP-C in a mixed organic solvent environment where α-helical SP-C undergoes irreversible β-sheet transformation to insoluble aggregates (46). When analyzed, organic extracts of bovine lung lavage contain SP-C in dimeric form ($[SP-C]_2$) (47). Whereas 46% of monomeric SP-C is in α-helical structure, $<7\%$ of $[SP-C]_2$ is α-helical, and 82% is in β-sheet structure. In contrast to the estimated 23–25 Å length of SP-C, $[SP-C]_2$ is estimated to be 36 Å long. It is hypothesized, though not demonstrated, that $[SP-C]_2$ traverses the membrane bilayer configured with three or more other $[SP-C]_2$ units in a β-barrel structure resembling that of porins (47). If present within the membrane in this configuration, SP-C homodimers might be capable of channel activity. Although the clinical significance of $[SP-C]_2$ or SP-C deposition as insoluble amyloid fibrils in healthy lung remains unclear, deposition of SP-C in an insoluble β-sheet conformation has been identified in the rare lung disease known as pulmonary alveolar proteinosis (48). The reason(s) for increased deposition of the insoluble β-sheet conformer in pulmonary alveolar proteinosis is not known, but it appears likely that in healthy lungs, transformation of normal SP-C from the α-helical to β-sheet conformation as either [SP-C]$_2$ or insoluble amyloid does occur without clinically apparent consequences (48–51). Analogous to α_1-antitrypsin liver disease, pulmonary alveolar proteinosis might occur following mutations or conditions that promote increased transformation of SP-C α-helical conformers to β-sheet conformers. In this regard, decreased palmitoylation of the SP-C molecule is associated with pulmonary alveolar proteinosis (44), and decreased palmitoylation accelerates transition of monomeric α-helical SP-C to soluble, polymeric aggregates considered intermediate to the formation of insoluble amyloid fibrils (52). The relationship between monomeric SP-C, [SP-C]$_2$, and SP-C-derived amyloid fibrils remains unclear; however, the conversion of human [SP-C]$_2$ (recovered from patients with pulmonary alveolar proteinosis) by mouse lung to monomeric SP-C (53) suggests that [SP-C]$_2$ is distinct from amyloid fibril. It is conceivable that [SP-C]$_2$ serves as a reversible, intermediate structure in the pathway to irreversible amyloid formation.

Analogous to pulmonary alveolar proteinosis that is caused by normally secreted SP-C, insulin-independent type II diabetes mellitus is caused by normally secreted amylin (54,55). Amylin (also known as islet amyloid polypeptide) is an amyloid-forming peptide secreted by the pancreas. Direct cytotoxicity of amylin and increased pancreatic deposition of amyloid are both likely contributors to the pathogenesis of type II diabetes.

The relevance of this discussion about amyloid-forming peptides to a possible channel-mediated, anti-inflammatory action of SP-C is that many of the amyloid-forming peptides, particularly those that inhibit leukocytes or induce cytotoxicity, insert ion channels in bilayer membranes. Amylin (56), fragments of β-amyloid peptide (57) and prion protein (58), and other amyloid peptides (59) have each been shown to insert gated, ion channel conductances in artificial, planar lipid bilayers, thereby excluding receptor-mediated activity. These intact or fragmented peptides are characteristically small (21–40 amino acids), hydrophobic molecules with α-helical structures that are hypothesized to form channels through refolding of monomers (37,60). Following refolding of monomeric peptides, aggregation of monomers into β-sheet structures is believed to provide one route to the formation of ion channels. Aggregate structures constituting amyloid pores and capable of membrane conductance may represent intermediate structures in the transition of amyloid-forming peptides from α-helical monomers to amyloid fibrils (61). I hypothesize that the same refolding occurs for a fraction of SP-C monomers that are transitioning from the α-helical structure to the SP-C fibril formation.

The conductances and ion selectivities of amyloid peptide channels vary among peptides. Peptide structure, lipid bilayer composition, and ionic strength of the bathing solutions influence variances (50–57). Most channels are cation-selective. Permeability to anions is limited, and single channel conductances are generally < 100 pS. Voltage dependencies and rectification are uncommon, and identified channel blockers are limited. Tris, aluminum, Zn^{2+}, Cu^{2+}, and Cd^{2+} provide blockage of β-amyloid peptide channels (62–64).

In addition to the receptor-independent, channel insertion by amyloid peptides in artificial membranes, these peptides also are observed to insert channels *in vivo*. Following insertion of channels, depolarization of cells or dissipation of ionic gradients initiates cytotoxic or inhibitory pathways through disruption of cytosolic Ca^{2+} (37,55). Specifically, β-amyloid peptide, prion protein, and amylin each induces cytosolic Ca^{2+} rise in neurons through channel insertion (65). β-Amyloid peptide inserts K^+ and Ca^{2+} channels in neural cells that cause release of internal Ca^{2+} stores (66,67). In neutrophil-like HL-60 cells, β-amyloid peptide initiates cytosolic Ca^{2+} elevations through a pertussis toxin-sensitive, G protein-mediated pathway. Similar to β-amyloid peptide, prion protein also activates neutrophils, lymphocytes, and monocytes through release of internal Ca^{2+} stores via a pertussis toxin-sensitive pathway (68). Pertussis toxin-sensitive G proteins also mediate amylin effects on pancreatic cells (69,70). As will be presented later in this chapter, the effects of SP-B and SP-C upon neutrophils are also observed to depolarize neutrophils and release internal Ca^{2+} stores through a channel-mediated and pertussis toxin-sensitive pathway. Initiation of pertussis toxin-sensitive, G protein pathways by receptor-independent pathways is not unique to amyloid peptides as another channel-forming peptide, aerolysin, releases Ca^{2+} from internal stores by similar G protein pathways (71).

Although not directly germane to our consideration of SP-C and other amyloid-forming peptides as channel proteins, it is notable that many of the amyloid peptides are included in a family of proteins known as serpins. Serpins are serine protease inhibitors. Serine proteases are active in inflammatory, complement, coagulation, and fibrinolytic cascades, and serpins influence these cascades through inhibition of proteolytic activities. Although SP-C is excluded as a serpin by its nonhomologous amino acid sequence with the serpin shutter domain (38), SP-C is observed to inhibit fibrinolysis and surfactant degradation that occurs by serine proteases (72–74). Hence, an alternative mechanism by which SP-C may modulate alveolar inflammation is through direct inhibition of proteolysis, perhaps via binding to the protease as observed for serpins (75).

IV. Clues from the Channel Activities of SAPLIPs

Through its homologous structure, SP-B has been classified as a SAPLIP (76,77). The characteristic, polypeptide motif of this protein superfamily is defined by sequences of hydrophobic amino acids and six cysteine residues that give rise to three intradomain, disulfide bonds. SAPLIPs are typically small (<80 amino acids) polypeptides, and three-dimensional structures include four to five α-helical bundles stabilized by the disulfide bonds. Among the different family members of SAPLIP, functions are varied, and disruption of disulfide bonds eliminates functional activities for most of the proteins (78,79).

Relevant to SP-B's possible channel activity, the two most important SAPLIP members are the pore-forming lysins and amoebapores. The lysins include human granulysin and porcine NK-lysin, both released by cytolytic, T lymphocytes. The amoebapores include toxins secreted by parasites *Entamoeba histolytica* and *Naegleria fowleri* (80). Although both lysins and amoebapores insert pores in planar lipid bilayers (81,82), the pores created by lysins cause direct membrane disruption, whereas those created by amoebapores induce discrete channel conductances. Membrane lysis is hypothesized to occur through binding of a helix-loop-helix structure to membrane, penetration of membrane, and electroporation of membrane bilayer via high electrostatic potential (77,78,83). Penetration of bilayer membrane in a transverse configuration crossing the bilayer is not portrayed. The antibacterial activity of lysin is created by permeabilization of Gram-positive and Gram-negative bacteria, fungi, and mycobacteria. However, the toxins are not hemolytic, and cytotoxicity toward human cells is limited (77). In contrast, channel insertion by amoebapores is hypothesized to occur through formation of four antiparallel, α-helix bundles transversing the bilayer (75,84). Disease is caused by resulting cytotoxicity toward mammalian cells (85).

While comparing SP-B with lysins and amoebapores, SP-B functionally resembles the lysins because a synthetic analog of SP-B (SP-B$_{1-78}$) also inhibits bacterial growth *in vitro*. Moreover, cytotoxicity by SP-B toward mammalian cells is unlikely (86). This pattern of functioning that resembles lysins is consistent with the structured model of interaction that occurs between lysins and bilayer membranes. Both SP-B and lysins interact with bilayer membranes superficially with only limited penetration. This contrasts with amoebapores that cross the bilayer in a channel configuration and cause cytotoxicity. On the basis of these observations, it is unlikely that SP-B as a monomer or homologous oligomer initiates channel activity. If SP-B does participate in membrane conductance, it would be expected to occur in association with other peptides or lipids.

V. Observed Cation Channel Insertion by SP-B/C in Planar Lipid Bilayers

Clues from the literature summarized in Sections III–V strongly suggest that SP-B/C is capable of inducing ion conductance in plasma membrane through creation of channel activity. Of the two apoproteins, SP-C would be chosen as the best candidate for channel activity through its transmembrane orientation in lipid bilayers. However, SP-C is less likely to form oligomeric channel complexes than SP-B, and SP-B might participate in channel activity through organization of SP-B/C channel complexes. To test the hypothesis that SP-B and/or SP-C insert channel activity in plasma membrane, artificial membranes were experimentally created by employing planar lipid bilayers (Fig. 14.1).

A. Electrophysiology of Planar Lipid Bilayers

Planar lipid bilayers were created by painting phospholipids dissolved in decane across an aperture (250 μm diameter) separating cis and trans compartments of buffered salt solutions (87). A film of phosphatidylethanolamine:phosphatidylserine (50:50) was painted across the aperture, while immersed in buffered 50–500:50–500 mM (cis:trans) salt solution composed of sodium, potassium, or choline chloride salts. Electrical measurements were made by way of agar bridges connecting $Ag^+/AgCl$ electrodes to cupped solutions of electrolyte on either side of the bilayer. Centrally located areas of thinned film (50–100 μm diameter) constituted the bilayer with capacitances of ~200 pF and resistances >100 Ω/cm^2. The bilayer mimics the lipid component of native plasma membrane both structurally and electrically. The hydrophobic interior blocks conductance of charged ions, thus providing high electrical resistance to current even in the presence of electrical potential gradients. In the absence of inserted channel

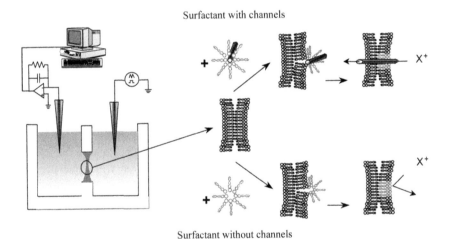

Surfactant with channels

Surfactant without channels

Figure 14.1 The planar lipid bilayer experimental model tests insertion of channel activity. This cartoon depicts two compartments of salt solution connected by an aperture across which the biconcave phospholipid bilayer is painted. The computer-driven electronics permit clamping of voltage across the bilayer, while concurrently measuring passage of current. Arrows point to exploded views of the biconcave phospholipid bilayer. Surfactant is depicted as a ring-like structure of phospholipid molecules with (top path) or without (bottom path) channel-forming protein. If surfactant contains channel-forming proteins, then cation X^+ will be conducted through the bilayer. Otherwise, cation conductance will not occur.

proteins, the bilayer, like native plasma membrane, is an excellent insulator but poor conductor of electrical charge.

Following stabilization of the lipid bilayer, channel activity was sought by exposing bilayers to potential channel proteins from the cis chamber, and holding the trans chamber at virtual ground by a patch clamp amplifier that measured current, while clamping voltage across the bilayer (87). Membrane capacitance was manually nulled. Under these conditions and at holding potentials greater than the reversal potential (E_{rev}), incorporation of a cation-selective channel was represented by positive current fluctuations. Upon identification of gated current activity across the bilayer, single channel slope conductance (g_s) was calculated from the equation $g_s = dI(V)/dV$, where $dI(V)$ is the measured single channel current at an applied potential (V). Channel rectification was indicated by loss of linearity over the I/V slope. Cation/anion selectivity of a channel was determined from the applied holding potential at which current activity was absent (E_{rev}) calculated by the Goldman–Hodgkin–Katz equation.

B. Channel Activity Inserted by Commercial Surfactant Containing SP-B and SP-C

SP-B/C were provided experimentally to the bilayer by suspending commercially available surfactant preparation, Survanta®, in the cis chamber at dilutions of 0.03–0.3%. As a control, commercial preparation lacking surfactant protein, Exosurf®, was suspended similarly in separate experiments. Within 5–20 min of adding Survanta to the stirred cis chamber, current conductance was typically induced in the lipid bilayers. Under both symmetrical (50:50 or 500:500 mM) and asymmetrical (500:50 mM) NaCl and KCl conditions, conductance at a given holding potential exhibited gating between two levels of current with sharp transitions between open and closed states characteristic of single channel activity (Fig. 14.2). Slope conductances averaged 39 ± 6 pS (mean $\pm$ SE) [Fig. 14.3(a)]. Observed E_{rev} for preparations employing asymmetric cis:trans salt compositions confirmed that current was carried by both monovalent cations, Na^+ and K^+ [Fig. 14.3(a)]. Randomly occurring dwell times within open and closed states also defined single channel activity, as opposed to simple diffusion or carrier-mediated transport [Fig. 14.3(b)]. Examining average open probability (P_o) as a function of the applied holding potential, dependence of P_o upon voltage was not observed. Among observed conductances for Na^+ and K^+, small predilection for K^+ was observed, based on the change in E_{rev} ($P_K/P_{Na} = 1.3$). Divalent cation conductance was not observed in the presence of symmetrical 50 mM $CaCl_2$ or $MgCl_2$ and absence of monovalent cations. Channel blockade did not occur in the presence of amiloride (1 mM), Ba^{2+} (6 mM), or Gd^{3+} (1 mM), and channel rectification was not observed [Fig. 14.3(a)]. Channel insertion was promoted by increased concentrations of beractant (0.3–1%), application of higher holding potentials (± 50–70 mV), and mechanical stirring of the cis compartment. These conditions presumably increased channel

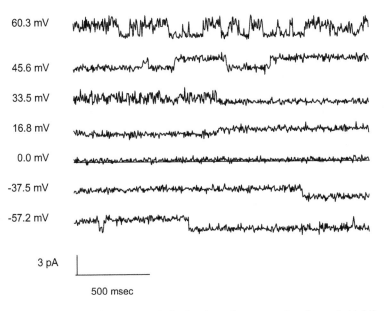

60.3 mV

45.6 mV

33.5 mV

16.8 mV

0.0 mV

-37.5 mV

-57.2 mV

3 pA

500 msec

Figure 14.2 Survanta incorporated single channel currents in planar lipid bilayer. Bilayer was symmetrically cast between 50:50 mM (cis:trans) NaCl buffered solutions. Intact Survanta (0.03%) was added to the cis chamber. Single channel currents were recorded at indicated holding potentials. Current openings were indicated by upward deflections at positive potentials and downward deflections at negative potentials. [Figure reproduced from Oelberg and Xu (87).]

insertion by promoting fusion of channel-forming components with the planar bilayer.

In contrast to observed channel insertion by Survanta containing SP-B and SP-C, Exosurf lacking SP-B and SP-C did not initiate channel activity at any time. These studies provided the first electrophysiological evidence that PS containing SP-B and SP-C has the potential to insert monovalent cation channels in plasma membrane. The observed 39 pS monovalent, cation conductance resembles the 40 pS conductance of amyloid peptide channels (Section III) (50–57) and other α-helical proteins forming cation channels as pentameric clusters (88).

C. Channel Activity Inserted by Extracted SP-B and SP-C

To control for possible lipid or non-SP-B/C contributions to the observed channel activity, SP-B and SP-C were extracted from Survanta and introduced to the lipid bilayer either directly or following reconstitution with lipids mimicking natural PS. SPs were extracted by modified Folch extraction (89) and were isolated by column extraction (90). One-dimensional SDS-PAGE was performed

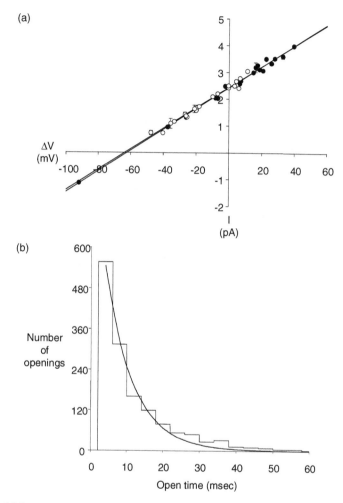

Figure 14.3 (a) During three experiments, data were combined for analysis of current–voltage relationships created by Survanta single channel activities. Bilayers were cast between 500:50 mM (cis:trans) buffered NaCl (closed circles) and KCl (open circles). E_{rev} equaling -62 and -64 mV, respectively, confirm that channels were selective for monovalent cations Na^+ and K^+. Slope conductances averaged 38 pS. (b) The time constant determined from open channel time distributions at $+70$ mV was 8 ms. [Figure reproduced from Oelberg and Xu (87).]

for identification of extracted proteins as SP-B and SP-C (Fig. 14.4) (91). Direct introduction of extracted SPs to the lipid bilayer was performed prior to casting the lipid bilayer. By this approach, extracted SPs from fraction 26 were mixed directly with bilayer phospholipids phosphatidylethanolamine: phosphatidylserine (50:50) in $CHCl_3$ providing a 1:1000 (w/w) protein:lipid mixture. Solvent

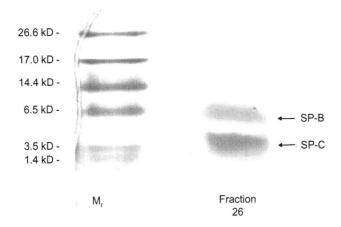

Figure 14.4 SPs extracted from Survanta (fraction 26) were compared with standard proteins (M_r) by SDS-PAGE. Protein bands at 3 and 6 kDa correspond to SP-C and SP-B, respectively. [Figure reproduced from Oelberg and Xu (87).]

was removed, the dried protein:lipid residue was redissolved in decane (20 mg/mL), and the bilayer (containing SPs by direct addition) was cast. By the second approach, extracted SPs were reconstituted with phospholipids (protein:lipid ratio = 5:1000) dipalmitoylphosphatidylcholine, phosphatidylglycerol, and phosphatidic acid (7:2:1) resembling those of intact PS. The reconstituted SPs were then suspended in the cis chamber at a dilution of 0.03–0.3%. In separate experiments lacking SPs, dipalmitoylphosphatidylcholine, phosphatidylglycerol, and phosphatidic acid (7:2:1) were added to the cis chamber at the same dilutions.

By both methods of introducing extracted SPs to lipid bilayers, SPs inserted selective cation channels of uniform conductances [Fig. 14.5(a)] similar to those inserted by intact Survanta. Slope conductances following direct addition and reconstitution were 37 and 39 pS, respectively [Fig. 14.5(b)]. Observed E_{rev} during 500:50 mM NaCl conditions confirmed cation selectivity nearly identical ($E_{rev} = -58$ mV) to that of intact PS + SP (data not shown). Na$^+$ was selectively conducted over larger cation, choline$^+$ ($P_{choline}/P_{Na} = 0.5$), and voltage dependence was not observed. Amiloride had no effect on activity, and channel rectification was not apparent [Fig. 14.5(b)].

In the absence of extracted SPs, reconstituting lipids, such as dipalmitoylphosphatidylcholine, phosphatidylglycerol, and phosphatidic acid, alone did not induce channel activity when presented to lipid bilayers. The failure of reconstituting lipids lacking SP-B and SP-C to initiate channel activity demonstrates that SPs are critical to channel formation. These experiments did not clarify the relative contributions of SP-B and/or SP-C to channel activity. The possibility that channel activities were caused by an unidentified contaminant in the employed

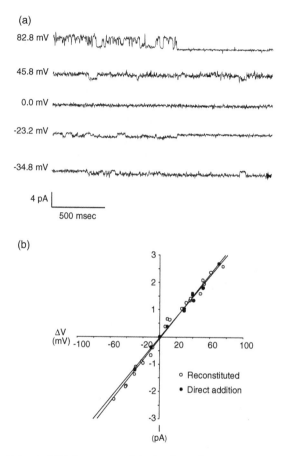

Figure 14.5 Extracted SPs incorporated single channel currents in planar lipid bilayer. (a) An aliquot of fraction 26 mixed directly with phosphatidylethanolamine: phosphatidyl-serine (50:50) prior to casting bilayer between 50:50 mM (cis:trans) NaCl inserted single channel currents at indicated holding potentials. (b) Current–voltage relationships of single channels inserted by extracted SPs in symmetric bilayers (50:50 mM NaCl). SPs inserted in bilayers by prior reconstitution with lipids (open circles) or by direct addition (closed circles). [Figure reproduced from Oelberg and Xu (87).]

buffer solutions, Survanta preparation, casting bilayer lipids, or reconstituting lipids cannot be fully excluded. However, the likelihood of this possibility is very low for the following reasons. Channel activity was not observed in the absence of SPs that were presented as either intact Survanta or extracted SPs. Analyses of the Survanta and extracted SPs have failed to identify components other than the identified lipids and hydrophobic proteins (90,92). These observations over several months combined with repeated demonstration of uniform channel properties employing several different batches of the supplied Survanta limit the probability of a contaminating channel protein.

VI. Observed Neutrophil Depolarization and G Protein-Mediated Calcium Mobilization by Surfactant with SP-B/C

Prior *in vitro* observations employing the planar lipid bilayer model confirmed that SP-B/C insert monovalent, cation channels into artificial plasma membrane. Whether the same would occur employing intact, living cells remained undetermined. To address this question for an early respondent of the inflammatory cascade, neutrophils were selected for exposure to PS ± SP. Evidence of channel insertion in neutrophils by PS ± SP would address the first question, while raising equally important questions about the pathophysiologic significance of these investigations.

It is well recognized that selected bacterial toxins with conductance properties resembling those of SP-B/C insert channels into neutrophils and cause membrane depolarization (71,93,94). Associated with membrane depolarization, some investigators also observe changes in intracellular calcium activities or changes in functional activation of the neutrophils (71,95,96). Collectively, on the basis of these observations, it was predicted that SP-B/C would insert similar channels into neutrophils, cause membrane depolarization, and alter intracellular calcium activity.

A. Surfactant with SP-B/C Depolarize Neutrophils

To examine the effect of SP-B/C on neutrophil membrane potential, human neutrophils were exposed to 1% Survanta, 1% Exosurf, or control buffer for 3 min, then washed and resuspended in physiologic buffer (23). Although it was desired to simultaneously monitor membrane potential for possible change at the time of initial surfactant exposure, turbidity created by suspended surfactant prevented monitoring by any of the available single wavelength, potential-sensitive indicators. Hence, neutrophils were pre-exposed to surfactant and washed before adding potential-sensitive dye, $diOC_5(3)$ (225 nM), to the neutrophil suspension. Because membrane potential changes at the time of $diOC_5(3)$ addition were expected to have occurred or be progressing, spectrofluorometric measurements were postponed until fluorescence had stabilized. Stabilization of fluorescence indicated completion of any membrane potential change induced by surfactant or control buffer exposures. To qualitatively assess the extent of membrane potential change that occurred following exposures, depolarization was extended by exposure to either 50 mM KCl or 1 μM gramicidin-D.

By this approach, it was observed that prior exposure of neutrophils to Survanta decreased extended membrane depolarizations by 50 mM KCl and 1 μM gramicidin-D exposures 28 and 32 mV, respectively, relative to control (23).

In contrast, prior exposure to Exosurf had no effect on the extended depolarizations. These results confirmed that 1% Survanta containing SP-B/C depolarizes neutrophils ~40%. Continued experimentation comparing the depolarizing efficacy of 1% Survanta with 10 μM gramicidin-D followed by washing and extended depolarization by 150 mM KCl confirmed 30–40% depolarization by Survanta and gramicidin-D under these conditions. The failure to detect >30–40% depolarization by 10 μM gramicidin-D following exposure and subsequent washing of neutrophils (when 100% depolarization would be expected) suggests that depolarization prior to washing and measurement may have been >40%. Likewise, Survanta may also induce more complete depolarization masked by the washing of neutrophils and by the delayed membrane potential measurement.

B. Surfactant with SP-B/C Induces Transient Ca²⁺ Activity

To determine the possible effect of surfactant-mediated membrane depolarization on neutrophil calcium activities, neutrophils were loaded with dual wavelength, fluorescent Ca^{2+} probe fura2. Fura2 was loaded by incubating (37°C in the dark, 5% CO_2, 45 min) neutrophils with 2 μM fura2-AM (the methyl ester form of fura2), sedimenting neutrophils, and then washing twice to remove non-incorporated, extracellular fura2-AM. After resuspending neutrophils in buffer, cells were examined for fluorescence at excitation wavelengths of 340 and 380 nm and at emission wavelength of 510 nm. Maximum (R_{max}) and minimum (R_{min}) fura2 fluorescence ratios were calculated by adding 0.1% Triton followed by 20 mM EGTA, respectively, to cells in the spectrofluorometer. Neutrophil cytosolic [Ca^{2+}] values were then calculated from the equation:

$$[Ca^{2+}] = K_d \left[\frac{R - R_{min}}{R_{max} - R} \right] \beta$$

where R is the ratio of the 340 nm/380 nm fluorescence, R_{min} the minimal ratio of 340 nm/380 nm fluorescence, R_{max} the maximal ratio of 340 nm/380 nm fluorescence, β is the ratio of 380 nm fluorescence under Ca^{2+}-free/Ca^{2+}-saturated conditions, and K_d the dissociation constant for Ca^{2+} binding to fura2, based on calibration curves from our laboratory (23,97). Experiments were performed in both calcium-supplemented and calcium-free physiologic buffers. Calcium-free buffer was prepared by adding 30 μM EGTA to buffer.

Exposure of neutrophils to 1% Survanta rapidly induced transient peaking of cytosolic [Ca^{2+}] (Fig. 14.6). Within 60 s of Survanta addition (closed circles), [Ca^{2+}] peaked and was followed by prompt return toward baseline over the next 120 s. The observation of this internal [Ca^{2+}] response in the absence of extracellular Ca^{2+} strongly suggested that intracellular Ca^{2+} stores provide the source for cytosolic [Ca^{2+}] peaking. In separate experiments employing buffer with extracellular Ca^{2+} (1.6 mM), results resembled those in Fig. 14.6 (data not shown).

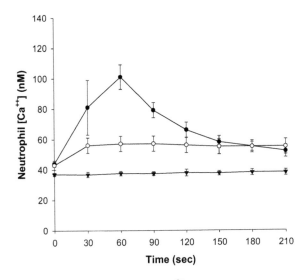

Figure 14.6 Survanta initiated neutrophil [Ca^{2+}] response. Neutrophils suspended in Ca^{2+}-free buffer were exposed to 1% Survanta (closed circles), 1% Exosurf (open circles), or 1% purified phospholipids (closed triangles) at time zero. [Ca^{2+}] response was monitored over time. Data are expressed as mean ± SEM values ($n = 4$).

In contrast to the effect of Survanta, exposure to 1% Exosurf (open circles) induced minimal change in neutrophil [Ca^{2+}] (Fig. 14.6). Likewise, exposure of neutrophils to 1% phospholipids (composed of phospholipids more closely resembling the phospholipid content of Survanta than those of Exosurf) failed to increase neutrophil [Ca^{2+}] (closed triangles). The negligible Ca^{2+} response to Exosurf or phospholipids implied that SP-B and/or SP-C are necessary for the observed neutrophil Ca^{2+} response.

To provide additional support for a causal relationship between Survanta and the Ca^{2+} response by neutrophils, the dose effect of Survanta on the magnitude of intracellular neutrophil Ca^{2+} response was examined. At concentration as low as 0.2%, Survanta induced release of cytosolic Ca^{2+} in Ca^{2+}-free buffer (data not shown). Release was not observed at lower concentrations, and concentrations >1% could not be examined because of excessive optical interference. However, between 0.1% and 1% concentrations, dose dependency was observed by a logarithmic response of neutrophil [Ca^{2+}] to [Survanta] (magnitude of Ca^{2+} peak = 53.07 + 20.64 {ln[Survanta]}, $R^2 = 0.93$).

It is hypothesized that the effect of Survanta upon neutrophil [Ca^{2+}] is mediated by insertion of monovalent cationic channels into plasma membrane, dissipation of transmembrane, monovalent, cation (i.e., Na$^+$ and K$^+$) gradients, and collapse of electrochemical potential gradients, thereby causing membrane depolarization. To test for the dependency of Ca^{2+} response upon pre-existing membrane polarization, Survanta-induced membrane depolarization was prevented by depolarizing neutrophils prior to Survanta exposure. Substituting extracellular 150 mM KCl (Fig. 14.7, open circles) for extracellular NaCl (closed circles), neutrophils were depolarized prior to Survanta exposure. Prior depolarization by KCl blocked any Ca^{2+} response to Survanta (Fig. 14.7).

C. Pertussis Toxin Inhibits Surfactant-Induced Ca^{2+} Changes

Others' observations that pore-forming toxins depolarize neutrophils and induce Ca^{2+} changes by a G protein-mediated pathway prompted our testing for pertussis toxin sensitivity (71). G protein-activated, internal Ca^{2+} store release is the proposed pathway, and current results remain consistent with this proposal. To test for G protein activation, suspended neutrophils were incubated with or without pertussis toxin (50 ng/mL) (90 min, darkness, 37°C, 5% CO_2) (71) before loading with fura2 and exposing to 1% Survanta or 1 μM fMLP. fMLP is a physiologic activator of neutrophils, and G protein dependence is limited at the dose employed. Under these conditions, pertussis toxin significantly inhibited the neutrophil Ca^{2+} response to Survanta by 74% [Fig. 14.8(a) and (b)]. Ca^{2+} response to fMLP was minimally affected as predicted.

VII. Observed Inhibition of Neutrophil Activation by Surfactant with SP-B/C

As discussed earlier in Section I, surfactant preparations containing SP-B and SP-C inhibit multiple neutrophil functions including adherence, aggregation,

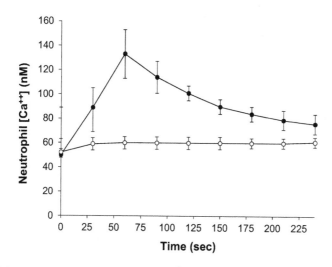

Figure 14.7 Prior depolarization blocks Ca^{2+} response. Prior to exposure of neutrophils to 1% Survanta at time zero, neutrophils were depolarized by suspension in Ca^{2+}-free KCl buffer (open circles). Neutrophils suspended in Ca^{2+}-free NaCl buffer served as a control (closed circles). $[Ca^{2+}]$ response was monitored over time. Data are expressed as mean ± SEM values ($n = 4$).

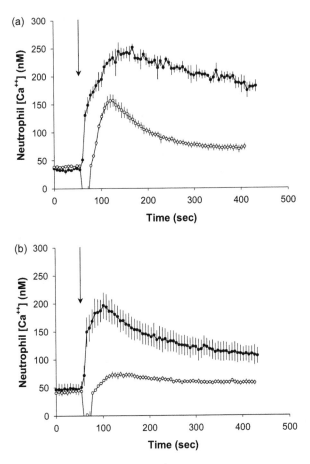

Figure 14.8 Pertussis toxin inhibits the Ca^{2+} response to Survanta. Neutrophils were activated with (b) or without (a) prior exposure to pertussis toxin. At the arrow (60 s) either 1 μM fMLP (closed circles) or 1% Survanta (open circles) was added, and Ca^{2+} responses were monitored. Data are expressed as mean ± SEM values (*n* = 4).

chemotaxis, respiratory burst, and elastase production following physiologic activation (19–23). In light of our prior observations, it was hypothesized that surfactant induces a Ca^{2+} response and that subsequent physiologic activation requiring a repeated Ca^{2+} response is reduced.

To investigate this hypothesis, neutrophils were exposed to 1% Survanta, 1% Exosurf, or buffer (control) for 3 min, washed, and resuspended in buffer. Neutrophil function was tested either by activating neutrophils with phorbol ester, PMA (29 ng/mL), and measuring neutrophil adherence, or by activating with formyl peptide, fMLP (1 μM), and measuring neutrophil aggregation subsequent to surfactant exposure (23). By these experiments, I observed that exposure of neutrophils to Survanta both decreased adherence to plastic induced by PMA and decreased aggregation induced by fMLP [Fig. 14.9(a) and (b)]. Exposure to Exosurf did not decrease neutrophil function relative to control buffer. Adherence to plastic induced by PMA decreased 39% following Survanta exposure [control: $77 \pm 3\%$ (mean $\pm$ SE) adherence; Exosurf: $77 \pm 9\%$ adherence; Survanta: $47 \pm 5\%$ adherence; $p < 0.05$ PS + SAP vs. control or PS-SAP] [Fig. 14.9(a)]. Survanta exposure also decreased subsequent aggregation induced

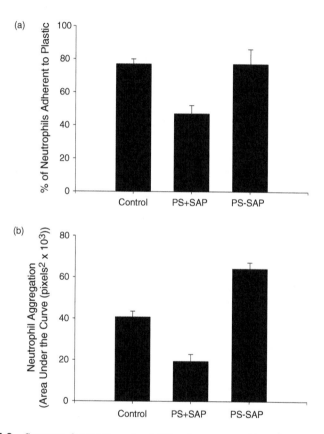

Figure 14.9 Survanta decreases neutrophil function measured by adherence and aggregation. (a) Neutrophils were exposed to 1% Survanta, 1% Exosurf, or buffer (control) (3 min, 24°C), placed on tissue-culture wells and stimulated by phorbol ester (20 ng/mL). Adherence was measured by MPO activity and expressed as the percentage of total MPO activity present in adherent neutrophils. Data are expressed as mean $\pm$ SE values ($n = 4$). (b) Neutrophils were exposed to 1% Survanta, 1% Exosurf, or buffer (control) (3 min, 24°C), washed, and resuspended in buffer. After formyl peptide (1 μM) stimulation, aggregation response was monitored for 3 min. Aggregation is expressed by area under the response curve (pixel^2). Data are expressed as mean $\pm$ SE values ($n = 4$). [Figure reproduced from Chacon-Cruz et al. (23).]

by fMLP 53% [control: 40688 ± 2744 pixels^2; PS-SAP: 64024 ± 3024 pixels^2; PS + SAP: 19308 ± 3476 pixels^2; $p < 0.05$ PS + SAP vs. control or PS-SAP] [Fig. 14.9(b)]. The significantly increased aggregation response to fMLP following Exosurf exposure was not further investigated.

To examine the effect of surfactant on the Ca^{2+} response of neutrophils following physiologic activation, neutrophil $[Ca^{2+}]$ was monitored after exposing neutrophils first to surfactant and then to formyl peptide. Figure 14.10 demonstrates how Survanta suppresses the Ca^{2+} response to formyl peptide activation. Under control conditions, stimulation of neutrophils with fMLP (1 μM) induced a rapid increase in $[Ca^{2+}]$ followed by slow decay (Fig. 14.10, closed circles). Pre-exposure to 1% Survanta followed by fMLP stimulation had little effect upon the early $[Ca^{2+}]$ peaking response at 30 s (Fig. 14.10, open circles), but a more rapid fall in $[Ca^{2+}]$ was observed after peaking occurred. On basis of the area under the $[Ca^{2+}]$ response curve, neutrophil $[Ca^{2+}]$ responses to fMLP were suppressed 49% by Survanta [control: 511 ± 40 nM min; Exosurf: 405 ± 28 nM min; Survanta: 264 ± 22 nM min; $p < 0.05$ Survanta vs. control or Exosurf].

The fMLP-stimulated $[Ca^{2+}]$ response of neutrophils occurs in two or more phases (98). Because initial release of internal Ca^{2+} stores (producing the early $[Ca^{2+}]$ peak) is accompanied by subsequent Ca^{2+} influx across neutrophil

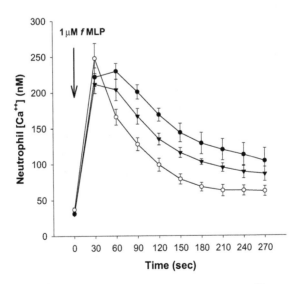

Figure 14.10 Survanta decreases the formyl peptide-induced $[Ca^{2+}]$ response in neutrophils. Neutrophils were exposed to 1% Survanta (open circles), 1% Exosurf (closed triangles), or buffer (control, closed circles) (3 min, 24°C), washed, and resuspended in buffer. Formyl peptide (1 μM) was added, and $[Ca^{2+}]$ response was monitored. Data are expressed as mean ± SE values ($n = 5$). [Figure reproduced from Chacon-Cruz et al. (23).]

plasma membrane, and because the early $[Ca^{2+}]$ peak appeared unaffected by Survanta in Fig. 14.10, subsequent experiments were designed to determine whether Survanta exposure modified Ca^{2+} influx into activated neutrophils. Accordingly, fura2-loaded neutrophils were exposed to Survanta, Exosurf, or buffer, washed, and resuspended in buffer without Ca^{2+} plus 30 μM EGTA (to provide a Ca^{2+}-free buffer with minimal excess EGTA). In the presence of the Ca^{2+}-free buffer, the peak $[Ca^{2+}]$ response to fMLP stimulation was not significantly altered by either of the experimental conditions including Survanta or Exosurf exposure (Fig. 14.11). However, in comparison with the $[Ca^{2+}]$ rise and decay following fMLP stimulation in the presence of external Ca^{2+} (Fig. 14.10), decays of $[Ca^{2+}]$ in the absence of external Ca^{2+} over 60–210 s were equally accelerated under all three experimental conditions (Fig. 14.11). The accelerated decays of neutrophil $[Ca^{2+}]$ under all conditions were consistent with expected decreases of Ca^{2+} influx in the absence of extracellular Ca^{2+}. Subsequently, $CaCl_2$ (5 mM) was returned to all three suspending external buffers at 210 s (Fig. 14.11). As expected, neutrophil $[Ca^{2+}]$ rose promptly in all three conditions, consistent with Ca^{2+} influx. However, the magnitude of $[Ca^{2+}]$ increase in Survanta-exposed neutrophils (Fig. 14.11, open circles), as determined by the area under the curve, was 39% less than those of control and Exosurf-exposed cells [control: 275 ± 11 nM min; Exosurf: 243 ± 19 nM min; Survanta:

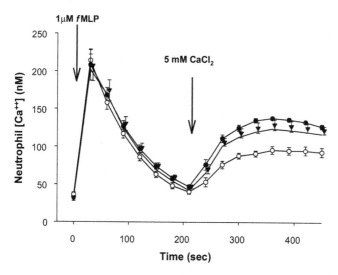

Figure 14.11 Survanta suppresses Ca^{2+} influx in neutrophils. Neutrophils were exposed to 1% Survanta (open circles), 1% Exosurf (closed triangles), or buffer (control, closed circles) (3 min, 24°C), washed, and resuspended in buffer without Ca^{2+} plus 30 μM EGTA. Formyl-peptide (1 μM) was added, and $[Ca^{2+}]$ response was monitored. After 210 s, $CaCl_2$ (5 mM) was added. Data are expressed as mean ± SE values ($n = 5$). [Figure reproduced from Chacon-Cruz et al. (23).]

167 ± 19 nM min; $p < 0.05$ Survanta vs. control or Exosurf]. This last set of experiments demonstrates that Survanta blocks Ca^{2+} entry into neutrophils following fMLP stimulation. I speculate that this blockade is related to neutrophil depolarization by Survanta.

VIII. Conclusions

Multiple clues from the literature support proposals that (1) PS exerts multiple actions within lung unexplained by surface tension reduction and (2) hydrophobic apoproteins SP-B and SP-C, in particular, are structurally well-suited to contribute to channel protein complexes. Experiments from my laboratory demonstrate that (1) SP-B/C insert monovalent cation channels in artificial membrane and (2) PS preparation containing SP-B/C depolarizes neutrophils, releases Ca^{2+} from internal stores by a G protein-activated and polarization-dependent pathway, blocks Ca^{2+} entry to recognized physiologic stimulants, and alters subsequent neutrophil responses. I speculate that SP-B/C insert monovalent cationic channels into neutrophil membranes causing cell depolarization and G protein-mediated release of intracellular Ca^{2+} stores. Ongoing membrane depolarization, blockade of Ca^{2+} entry from external sources, and depletion of internal Ca^{2+} stores reduce neutrophil capacity for subsequent physiologic response. This surfactant-initiated cascade of events modulates the response of human neutrophils during inflammation to improve clinical outcomes in patients with respiratory distress syndromes. Although the commercially available surfactant preparations currently available do not contain the other two major surfactant apoproteins, native SP-A and SP-D are believed to play important roles in local lung defense by enhancing chemotaxis, opsonizing bacteria, enhancing macrophage function, and stimulating antibody production (3). Hence, it would appear that in addition to reducing surface tension, native PS shares both pro- and anti-inflammatory properties. For this reason, it is considered that in the course of pulmonary disease, a balance is sought between the two immunomodulatory arms of surfactant to address both invading microorganisms and over-exuberant host inflammatory responses. It is exciting to contemplate that the promotional effect of surfactant upon fluid clearance is also related to cation channel insertion in neonatal alveolar membranes. However, supporting evidence remains limited (99,100). Continued investigation of channel insertion by SP-B/C may refine current therapeutic applications of surfactant in the lung, while stimulating novel applications to nonpulmonary diseases.

References

1. Jobe AH, Ikegami M. Biology of surfactant. Clin Perinatol 2001; 28:655–669.
2. Ikegami M, Jobe AH, Whitsett J et al. Tolerance of SP-A deficient mice to hyperoxia or exercise. J Appl Physiol 2000; 89:644–648.

3. Crouch E, Wright JR. Surfactant proteins A and D and pulmonary host defense. Annu Rev Physiol 2001; 63:521–554.

4. Halliday HL. Overview of clinical trials comparing natural and synthetic surfactants. Biol Neonate 1995; 67:32–47.

5. Revak SD, Merritt TA, Cochrane CG et al. Efficacy of synthetic peptide-containing surfactant in the treatment of respiratory distress syndrome in preterm infant rhesus monkeys. Pediatr Res 1996; 39:715–724.

6. Davis AJ, Jobe AH, Hafner D, Ikegami M. Lung function in premature lambs and rabbits treated with a recombinant SP-C surfactant. Am J Respir Crit Care Med 1998; 157:553–559.

7. Robertson B, Johansson J, Curstedt T. Synthetic surfactants to treat neonatal lung disease. Mol Med Today 2000; 6:119–124.

8. Walther FJ, Hernandez-Juviel JM, Mercado PE, Gordon LM, Waring AJ. Surfactant with SP-B and SP-C analogues improves lung function in surfactant-deficient rats. Biol Neonate 2002; 82:181–187.

9. Wilson DF, Zaritsky A, Bauman LA et al. Instillation of calf lung surfactant extract (calfactant) is beneficial in pediatric acute hypoxemic respiratory failure. Members of the Mid-Atlantic Pediatric Critical Care Network. Crit Care Med 1999; 27:188–195.

10. Gregory TJ, Steinberg KP, Spragg R et al. Bovine surfactant therapy for patients with acute respiratory distress syndrome. Am J Respir Crit Care Med 1997; 155:1309–1315.

11. Wiswell TE, Smith RM, Katz LB et al. Bronchopulmonary segmental lavage with Surfaxin (KL_4-surfactant) for acute respiratory disteress syndrome (ARDS). Am J Respir Crit Care Med 1999; 160, 1188.

12. Lotze A, Mitchell BR, Bulas DI, Zola EM, Shalwitz RA, Gunkel JH. Multicenter study of surfactant (beractant) use in the treatment of term infants with severe respiratory failure. Survanta in Term Infants Study Group. J Pediatr 1998; 132:40–47.

13. Soll RF, Dargaville P. Surfactant for meconium aspiration syndrome in full term infants. Cochrane Database Syst Rev 2000; 2, CD002054.

14. Herting E, Gefeller O, Land M, van Sonderen L, Harms K, Robertson B. Surfactant treatment of neonates with respiratory failure and group B streptococcal infection. Members of the Collaborative European Multicenter Study Group. Pediatrics 2000; 106:957–964.

15. Henson PM. Johnston BR. Tissue injury in inflammation. Oxidants proteinases and cationic proteins. J Clin Invest 1987; 79:669–674.

16. Merritt TA, Cochrane CG, Hallman M et al. Reduction of lung injury by human surfactant treatment in respiratiry distress syndrome. Chest 1983; 83:27S–31S.

17. Ikegami M, Weaver TE, Conkright JJ et al. Deficiency of SP-B reveals protective role of SP-C during oxygen lung injury. J Appl Physiol 2002; 92:519–526.

18. Ikegami M, Jobe AH. Injury responses to different surfactants in ventilated premature lamb lungs. Pediatr Res 2002; 51:689–695.

19. Suwabe A, Otake K, Yakuwa N, Suzuki H, Ito M, Tomoike H, Saito Y, Takahashi K. Artificial surfactant (surfactant TA) modulates adherence and superoxide production of neutrophils. Am J Respir Crit Care Med 1998; 158:1890–1899.

20. Ahuja A, Oh N, Chao W, Spragg RG, Smith RM. Inhibition of the human neutrophil respiratory burst by native and synthetic surfactant. Am J Respir Cell Mol Biol 1996; 14:496–503.

21. Finck CM, Hodell MG, Marx WH, Paskanik AM, McGraw DJ, Lutz CJ, Gatto LA, Picone AL, Nieman GF. Endotoxin-stimulated alveolar macrophage recruitment of neutrophils and modulation with exogenous surfactant. Crit Care Med 1998; 26:1414–1418.

22. Tegtmeyer FK, Gortner L, Ludwig A, Brandt E. *In vitro* modulation of induced neutrophil activation by different surfactant preparations. Eur Respir J 1996; 9:752–757.

23. Chacon-Cruz E, Buescher ES, Oelberg DG. Surfactant modulates calcium response of neutrophils to physiologic stimulation via cell membrane depolarization. Pediatr Res 2000; 47:405–413.

24. Bartmann P, Gortner L, Pohlandt F, Jaeger H. *In vitro* lymphocyte functions in the presence of bovine surfactant and its phospholipid fractions. J Perinat Med 1992; 20:189–196.

25. Speer CP, Gotze B, Curstedt T, Robertson B. Phagocytic functions and tumor necrosis factor secretion of human monocytes exposed to natural porcine surfactant (Curosurf). Pediatr Res 1991; 30:69–74.

26. van Iwaarden JF, Claassen E, Jeurissen SHM, Haagsman HP, Kraal G. Alveolar macrophages surfactant lipids and surfactant protein B regulate the induction of immune response via the airways. Am J Respir Cell Mol Biol 2001; 24:452–458.

27. Miles PR, Bowman L, Rao KMK, Baatz JE, Huffman L. Pulmonary surfactant inhibits LPS-induced nitric oxide production by alveolar macrophages. Am J Physiol Lung Cell Mol Physiol 1999; 276:L186–L196.

28. Augusto L, Le Blay K, Auger G, Bkanot D, Chaby R. Interaction of bacterial lipo-polysaccharide with mouse surfactant protein C inserted into lipid vesicles. Am J Physiol Lung Cell Mol Physiol 2001; 281:L776–L785.

29. Kabore AF, Wang WJ, Ruso SJ, Beers MF. Biosynthesis of surfactant protein C: characterization of aggresome formation by EGFP chimeras containing propeptide mutants lacking conserved cysteine residues. J Cell Sci 2000; 114:293–302.

30. Johansson J, Szyperski T, Curstedt T, Wüthrich K. The NMR structure of the pulmonary surfactant-associated polypeptide SP-C in an apolar solvent contains a valyl-rich alpha-helix. Biochemistry 1994; 33:6015–6023.

31. Montal M. Molecular anatomy and molecular design of channel proteins. FASEB J 1990; 4:2623–2635.

32. Vandenbussche G, Clercx A, Curstedt T, Johansson J, Jornvall H, Ruysschaert JM. Structure and orientation of the surfactant-associated protein C in a lipid bilayer. Eur J Biochem 1992; 203:201–209.

33. Pastrana B, Mautone AJ, Mendelsohn R. Fourier transform infrared studies of secondary structure and orientation of pulmonary surfactant SP-C and its effect on the dynamic surface properties of phospholipids. Biochemistry 1991; 30:10058–10064.

34. Horowitz AD, Baatz JE, Whitsett JA. Lipid effects on aggregation of pulmonary surfactant protein SP-C studied by fluorescence energy transfer. Biochemistry 1993; 32:9513–9523.

35. Weaver TE, Conkwright JJ. Function of surfactant proteins B and C. Annu Rev Physiol 2001; 63:555–578.

36. Vandenbussche G, Clercx A, Clercx M, Curstedt T, Johansson J, Jornvall H, Ruysschaert JM. Secondary structure and orientation of the surfactant protein

SP-B in a lipid environment. A Fourier transform infrared spectroscopy study. Biochemistry 1992; 31:9169–9176.

37. Johansson J. Membrane properties and amyloid fibril formation of lung surfactant protein C. Biochem Soc Trans 2001; 29:601–606.

38. Kourie JI, Henry CL. Ion channel formation and membrane-linked pathologies of misfolded hydrophobic proteins: the role of dangerous unchaperoned molecules. Clin Exp Pharm Physiol 2002; 29:741–753.

39. Lomas DA, Carrell RW. Serpinopathies and the conformational dementias. Nat Rev 2002; 3:759–768.

40. Jimenez JL, Guijarro JI, Orlova E et al. Cryo-electron microscopy structure of an SH3 amyloid fibril and model of the molecular packing. EMBO J 1999; 18:815–821.

41. Blanchard BJ, Konopka G, Russell M, Ingram VM. Mechanism and prevention of neurotoxicity caused by beta-amyloid peptides: relation to Alzheimer's disease. Brain Res 1997; 776:40–50.

42. Walker LC, Bian F, Callahan MJ, Lapinski WJ, Durham RA, LeVine H. Modeling Alzheimer's disease and other proteopathies *in vivo*: is seeding the key? Amino Acids 2002; 23:87–93.

43. Prusiner SB. Molecular biology of prion diseases. Science 1991; 252:1515–1522.

44. Goldberg M, Lansbury PTJ. Is there a cause-and-effect relationship between α-synuclein fibrillization and Parkinson's disease? Nat Cell Biol 2000; 2:E115–E119.

45. Lomas DA, Evans DL, Finch TJ, Carrell RW. The mechanism of Z α_1-antitrypsin accumulation in the liver. Nature 1992; 357:605–607.

46. Szyperski T, Vandenbussche G, Curstedt T et al. Pulmonary surfactant-associated polypeptide C in a mixed organic solvent transforms from a monomeric alpha-helical state into insoluble beta-sheet aggregates. Protein Sci 1998; 7:2533–2540.

47. Baatz JE, Smyth KL, Whitsett JA, Baxter C, Absolom DR. Structure and functions of a dimeric form of surfactant protein SP-C: a Fourier transform infrared and surfactometry study. Chem Phys Lipids 1992; 63:91–104.

48. Gusatfsson M, Thyberg J, Naslund J, Eliasson E, Johansson J. Amyloid fibril formation by pulmonary surfactant protein C. FEBS Lett 1999; 31:138–142.

49. Kallberg Y, Gustafsson M, Persson B, Thyberg J, Johansson J. Prediction of amyloid fibril-forming proteins. J Biol Chem 2001; 276:12945–12950.

50. Shanmukh S, Howell P, Baatz JE, Dulhy RA. Effect of hydrophobic surfactant proteins SP-B and SP-C on phospholipid monolayers. Biophys J 2002; 83:2126–2141.

51. Hosia W, Johansson J, Griffiths WJ. Hydrogen/deuterium exchange and aggregation of a polyvaline and polyleucine alpha-helix investigated by matrix-assisted laser desorption ionization mass spectrometry. Mol Cell Proteomics 2002; 1:592–597.

52. Gustafsson M, Griffiths WJ, Furusjo E, Johansson J. The palmitoyl groups of surfactant protein C reduce unfolding into a fibrillogenic intermediate. J Mol Biol 2001; 310:937–950.

53. Li Z, Suzuki Y, Kurozumi M, Shen H, Duan C. Removal of a dimeric form of surfactant protein C from mouse lungs: its acceleration by reduction. J Appl Physiol 1998; 84:471–478.

54. de Konig EJP, Morris ER, Hofhuis FMA et al. Intra- and extracellular amyloid fibrils are formed in cultured pancreatic islets of transgenic mice expressing human islet amyloid polypeptide. Proc Natl Acad Sci USA 1994; 91:8467–8471.

55. Hayden MR Tyagi SC. "A" is for amylin and amyloid in type 2 diabetes mellitus. J Pancreas 2001; 2:124–139.

56. Mirzabekov TA, Lin M, Kagan BL. Pore formation by the cytotoxic islet amyloid peptide amylin. J Biol Chem 1996; 271:1988–1992.

57. Mirzabekov T, Lin MC, Yuan WL et al. Channel formation in planar lipid bilayers by a neurotoxic fragment of the beta-amyloid peptide. Biochem Biophys Res Commun 1994; 202:1142–1148.

58. Kourie JI, Culverson A. Prion peptide fragment PrP[106–126] forms distinct cation channel types. J Neurosci Res 2001; 62:120–133.

59. Kourie JI, Shorthouse AA. Properties of cytotoxic peptide-formed ion channels. Am J Physiol Cell Physiol 2000; 278:C1063–C1087.

60. Hirakura Y, Yiu WW, Yamamoto A, Kagan BL. Amyloid peptide channels: blockade by zinc and inhibition by congo red (amyloid channel block). Amyloid 2000; 7:194–199.

61. Lashuel HA, Hartley D, Petre BM, Walz T, Lasbury PT. Amyloid pores from pathogenic mutations. Nature 2002; 418:291.

62. Arispe N, Pollard HB, Rojas E. Zn^{2+} interaction with Alzheimer amyloid beta protein calcium channels. Proc Natl Acad Sci USA 1996; 93:1710–1715.

63. Arispe N, Rojas E, Pollard HB. Alzheimer disease amyloid beta protein forms calcium channels in bilayer membranes: blockade by tromethamine and aluminum. Proc Natl Acad Sci USA 1993; 90:567–571.

64. Mirzabekov TA, Lin MC, Yuan WL et al. Channel formation in planar lipid bilayers by a neurotoxic fragment of the beta-amyloid peptide. Biochem Biophys Res Commun 1994; 202:1142–1148.

65. Kawahara M, Kuroda Y, Arispe N, Rojas E. Alzheimer's beta-amyloid human islet amylin and prion protein fragment evoke intracellular free calcium elevations by a common mechanism in a hypothalamic GnRH neuronal cell line. J Biol Chem 2000; 275:14077–14083.

66. Chung S, Lee J, Joe EH, Uhm DY. Beta-amyloid peptide induces the expression of voltage dependent outward rectifying K^+ channels in rat microglia. Neurosci Lett 2001; 300:67–70.

67. He LM, Chen LY, Lou XL, Qu AL, Zhou Z, Xu T. Evaluation of beta-amyloid peptide 25–35 on calcium homeostasis in cultured rat dorsal root ganglion neurons. Brain Res 2002; 939:65–75.

68. Diomede L, Sozzani S, Luini W et al. Activation effects of a prion protein fragment [PrP-(106–126)] on human leucocytes. Biochem J 1996; 320:563–570.

69. Silvestre RA, Salas M, Garcia-Hermida O, Fontela T, Degano P, Marco J. Amylin (islet amyloid polypeptide) inhibition of insulin release in the perfused rat pancreas: implication of the adenylate cyclase/cAMP system. Regul Pept 1994; 50:193–199.

70. Wang F, Permert J, Ostenson CG. Islet amyloid polypeptide regulates multiple steps in stimulus-secretion coupling of beta cells in rat pancreatic islets. Pancreas 2000; 20:264–269.

71. Krause KH, Fivaz M, Monod A, van der Goot FG. Aerolysin induces G-protein activation and Ca^{2+} release from intracellular stores in human granulocytes. J Biol Chem 1998; 273:18122–18129.

72. Gunther GA, Bleyl H, Seeger W. Apoprotein-based synthetic surfactants inhibit plasmic cleavage of fibrinogen *in vitro*. Am J Physiol 1933; 265:L186–L192.

73. Seeger W, Grube C, Gunther A. Proteolytic cleavage of fibrinogen: amplification of its surfactant inhibitory capacity. Am J Respir Cell Mol Biol 1993; 9:239–247.

74. Liau DF, Yin NX, Huang J, Ryan SF. Effects of human polymorphonuclear leukocyte elastase upon surfactant proteins *in vitro*. Biochim Biophys Acta 1996; 1302:117–128.

75. Augusto LA, Synguelakis M, Johansson J, Chaby R. Structural basis for interactions between lung surfactant protein C and bacterial lipopolysaccharide. J Biol Chem 2002; 277:23484–23492.

76. Munford RS, Sheppard PO, O'Hara PJ. Saposin-like proteins (SAPLIP) carry out diverse functions on a common backbone structure. J Lipid Res 1995; 36:1653–1663.

77. Vaccaro AM, Salvioli R, Tatti M, Ciaffoni F. Saposons and their interaction with lipids. Neurochem Res 1999; 24:307–314.

78. Andreu D, Carreno C, Linde C, Boman HG, Andersson M. Identification of an antimycobacterial domain in NK-lysin and granulysin. Biochem J 1999; 344:845–849.

79. Ernst WA, Thoma-Uszynski S, Teitelbaum R et al. Granulysin, a T cell product, kills bacteria by altering membrane permeability. J Immunol 2000; 165:7102–7108.

80. Herbst R, Ott C, Jacobs T et al. Pore-forming polypeptides of the pathogenic protozoan *Naegleria fowleri*. J Biol Chem 2002; 277:22353–22360.

81. Ruysschaert JM, Goormaghtigh E, Homble F, Andersson M, Liepinsh E, Otting G. Lipid membrane binding of NK-lysin. FEBS Lett 1998; 425:341–344.

82. Keller F, Hanke W, Trissl D, Bakker-Grunwald T. Pore-forming protein from *Entamoeba histolytica* forms voltage- and pH-controlled multi-state channels with properties similar to those of the barrel-stave aggregates. Biochim Biophys Acta 1989; 982:89–93.

83. Miteva M, Andersson M, Karshikoff A, Otting G. Molecular electroporation: a unifying concept for the description of membrane pore formation by antibacterial peptides exemplified with NK-lysin. FEBS Lett 1999; 462:155–158.

84. Nickel R, Ott C, Dandekar T, Leippe M. Pore-forming peptides of *Entamoeba dispar*. Eur J Biochem 1999; 265:1002–1007.

85. Zhai Y, Saier MH. The amoebapore superfamily. Biochim Biophys Acta 2000; 1469:87–99.

86. Kaser MR, Skouteris GG. Inhibition of bacterial growth by synthetic SP-B$_{1-78}$ peptides. Peptides 1997; 18:1441–1444.

87. Oelberg DG, Xu F. Pulmonary surfactant proteins insert cation-permeable channels in planar bilayers. Mol Genet Metab 2000; 70:295–300.

88. Grove A, Iwamoto T, Montal MS, Tomich JM, Montal M. Synthetic peptides and proteins as models for pore-forming structure of channel proteins. Methods Enzymol 1992; 207:510–525.

89. Bligh EG, Dyer WJ. A rapid method of total lipid extraction and purification. Can J Biochem Physiol 1959; 37:911–917.

90. Takahashi A, Fujiwara T. Proteolipid in bovine lung surfactant: its role in surfactant function. Biochem Biophys Res Comm 1986; 135:527–532.

91. Schagger H, von Jagow G. Tricine-sodium dodecyl sulfate-polyacrylamide gel electrophoresis for the separation of proteins in the range from 1 to 100 kDa. Anal Biochem 1987; 166:368–379.

92. Whitsett JA, Weaver TE. Pulmonary surfactant proteins: implications for surfactant replacement therapy. In: Shapiro DL, Notter RH, eds. Surfactant Replacement Therapy. New York: Alan R. Liss, 1989:71–89.

93. Seligmann BE, Gallin EK, Martin DL, Shain W, Gallin JI. Interaction of chemotactic factors with human polymorphonuclear leukocytes: studies using a membrane potential-sensitive cyanine dye. J Memb Biol 1980; 52:257–572.

94. Di Virgilio F, Lew DP, Andersson T, Pozzan T. Plasma membrane potential modulates chemotactic peptide-stimulated cytosolic free Ca^{2+} changes in human neutrophils. J Biol Chem 1987; 262:4574–4579.

95. Matsumoto T, Takeshige K, Minakami S. Spontaneous induction of superoxide release and degranulation of neutrophils in isotonic potassium medium: the role of intracellular calcium. J Biochem 1986; 99:1591–1596.

96. Pittet D, Di Virgilio F, Pozzan T, Monod A, Lew DP. Correlation between plasma membrane potential and second messenger generation in the promyelocytic cell line HL-60. J Biol Chem 1990; 265:14256–14263.

97. Hansen CA, Monck JR, Williamsons JR. Measurement of intracellular free calcium to investigate receptor-mediated calcium signaling. Methods Enzymol 1990; 191:691–706.

98. Chandler DE, Kazliek CJ. Calcium signals in neutrophils can be divided into three distinct phases. Biochim Biophys Acta 1987; 931:175–179.

99. Egan EA, Nelson RM, Beale EF. Lung solute permeability and lung liquid absorption in premature ventilated fetal goats. Pediatr Res 1980; 14:314–318.

100. Carlton DP. Surfactant alters lung liquid production and epithelial ion transport in fetal sheep. Pediatr Res 1996; 39:327A.

Dysfunction and Disease

15

The Physiological Significance of a Dysfunctional Lung Surfactant

TIMOTHY C. BAILEY and RUUD A. W. VELDHUIZEN

University of Western Ontario,
London, Ontario, Canada

I. Introduction

Pulmonary surfactant is essential for normal lung function (1). This physiological importance is obvious from the observed lung dysfunction in premature babies deficient in lung surfactant and the subsequent improvement in lung function following exogenous surfactant supplementation (2,3). In fact, the clinical term for lung impairment in premature neonates due to surfactant deficiency is neonatal respiratory distress syndrome (NRDS). The association of surfactant deficiency with this clinical syndrome has been the main rationale for the extensive studies on various aspects of the pulmonary surfactant system over the last 40 years (4,5). However, surfactant deficiency is not the only clinical situation in which the pulmonary surfactant contributes to physiological abnormalities. Several clinical conditions have been associated with alterations of the pulmonary surfactant system including acute lung injury (ALI) (6,7). In this chapter, we will focus on the role of surfactant in the development and treatment of ALI. First, we will briefly review the pulmonary surfactant system and ALI. This will be followed by a description of the alterations of surfactant in ALI. The rest of the chapters will then focus on the consequences of surfactant impairment in ALI, the mechanisms by which surfactant impairment occurs, and the potential of surfactant therapy for ALI. These discussions will be presented from a broad physiological–biochemical perspective. For further details on specific aspects, the reader will be referred to a number of recent review articles as well as other chapters in the current volume.

II. Physiological Function of Pulmonary Surfactant

The physiological importance of pulmonary surfactant can be explained by comparing the pressure–volume relationship (a PV curve) during inflation and deflation within lungs with a normal surfactant system and in lungs with an impaired or deficient surfactant system (Fig. 15.1). These pressure–volume curves are obtained by recording the volume during the stepwise inflation of lung by

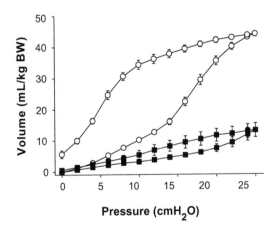

Figure 15.1 Pressure–volume curve from isolated rat lungs; nonventilated (open circles) with high volume at a pressure of 26 cmH$_2$O vs. mechanically ventilated (filled squared) with decreased volume at a pressure of 26 cmH$_2$O and decreased hysteresis.

2 cmH$_2$O pressure intervals. This is followed by a similar stepwise deflation of the lung. Figure 15.1 shows the pressure–volume curves of a normal rat lung (open circles) and a rat lung after impairment of the surfactant system through mechanical ventilation (filled squares) (8–10). It can be seen that, at every pressure >4 cmH$_2$O, the normal lung holds a higher volume of air than the injured lung such that at the highest pressure the normal lung contains only about three times the volume of air compared with that of the injured lung. This relation between the volume and the pressure in the lung is an indication of *lung compliance*. This difference between normal and injured lungs is also observed during deflation (the upper limb of each curve). In addition, it can be seen that the normal lung holds significantly more air during deflation than during inflation (this difference is called *hysteresis*), whereas only limited hysteresis is observed in the injured lung.

In this scenario of decreased compliance, less oxygen will be available inside the lung for gas exchange thus resulting in a lower level of partial pressure of oxygen in the arterial blood (PaO$_2$). Thus, the physiological role of surfactant can be defined as maintaining lung compliance, thereby allowing for adequate gas exchange.

The reason surfactant is needed to maintain lung compliance is related to the phenomenon of surface tension that arises at the air–liquid interface of the lung. Surface tension arises from an unequal distribution of attractive and repulsive forces that act on aqueous molecules at the interface in comparison to the equal distribution of forces acting on molecules in the bulk phase. This leads to the tendency for the aqueous bulk phase to shrink the surface area of the interface (this is the force that makes water form droplets). Within the confines of the lung, high surface tensions would lead to the spontaneous collapsing or flooding of alveoli, because a filled or collapsed alveolus would have the smallest air–liquid interface. This relationship between surface tension and pressure across a bubble is described more specifically by the law of Young and Laplace which states that the pressure across a bubble is equal to two times the surface tension divided by the radius. Within the lung, pulmonary surfactant reduces the surface tension at the air–liquid interface during exhalation. Within the context of the law of Young and Laplace, as the radius of the alveolus decreases, surfactant causes a parallel decrease in surface tension such that the pressure gradient across the bubble does not increase dramatically. The mechanism by which surfactant reduces the surface tension is through the formation of a phospholipid rich surface film at the air–liquid interface [reviewed in Refs. (11–13)]. The reduction of surface tension stabilizes each alveolus, which is important for maintaining the extremely high surface area for gas exchange; furthermore, patent alveoli promote balance of the Starling forces across the pulmonary capillaries. As will be discussed subsequently, pulmonary edema is one of the hallmarks of lung injury and a major contributor to surfactant dysfunction.

A second important role for the surfactant system in maintaining normal lung function is its contribution to the host defense of the lung. In order to facilitate gas exchange, the lung contains a large thin surface area that is constantly exposed to inhaled particles and infectious agents. To avoid chronic inflammation and to effectively clear the inhaled material, the lung requires a sophisticated host defense system which includes the pulmonary surfactant system (14). By lining the alveoli, surfactant is one of the first endogenous materials encountered by inhaled substances (15). Although both surfactant lipids and proteins may play a role in host defense, the crucial components for this function appear to be two of the surfactant proteins designated SP-A and SP-D. Numerous studies have provided evidence for this role for these proteins in the stimulation of alveolar macrophage phagocytosis, the alteration of chemotaxis of various inflammatory and immune cells, impacting reactive oxygen species production and regulation of cytokine release from various inflammatory cells [reviewed in Refs. (15–18)]. For example, mice deficient in SP-A are more susceptible to bacterial infections than the wild-type control mice (19–21).

In summary, pulmonary surfactant reduces the surface tension at the air–liquid interface of the alveoli of the lung. This reduces the amount of pressure that is needed to inflate the lung and reduces the tendency for lung collapse. Through this maintenance of lung compliance, surfactant allows for adequate gas exchange. In addition, components of the pulmonary surfactant system are also involved in the host defense mechanisms of the lung.

III. Surfactant Composition

As surfactant is present within the alveolar space of the lung it can easily be obtained by saline lavage of the lung. Surfactant is usually isolated from lavage by differential or sucrose gradient centrifugation. Although some methodological differences for obtaining and isolating lung surfactant exist, the reported composition in different studies and different mammalian species are remarkably consistent (22,23). Pulmonary surfactant is a mixture of ~85% phospholipids, 5% neutral lipids (mainly cholesterol), and ~10% surfactant-associated proteins (SPs) (24,25). Of the phospholipids ~60% are phosphatidylcholine (PC) of which 30–50% are the disaturated species dipalmitoylphosphatidylcholine (DPPC). Phosphatidylglycerol (PG) is the second most abundant phospholipid in surfactant, present at 7–15% of total phospholipid. Other phospholipids, such as phosphatidylinositol, phosphatidylserine, sphingomyelin, and phosphatidylethanolamine, make up the remainder of the surfactant phospholipids (26). The SPs can be divided into two general categories, the small hydrophobic proteins, SP-B and SP-C, and the two large multimeric, hydrophilic glycoproteins, SP-A and SP-D (27). The hydrophobic proteins are tightly associated with the surfactant lipids and play an important role in the surface tension reducing activity of surfactant [reviewed in Ref. (13)]. The other surfactant proteins, SP-A and SP-D, are members of the collectin family of proteins and are important in host defense mechanisms of the lung (16,17). SP-A may also play a relatively minor role in surface tension reduction and both SP-A and SP-D may influence surfactant metabolism (28–31).

IV. Surfactant Metabolism

Although it is ultimately the surface film of surfactant that accomplishes the main function of surface tension reduction, the generation and maintenance of this surface film is accomplished through a complex metabolic system involving synthesis, intracellular storage, secretion, surface film formation, and the generation of remnant particles for uptake and degradation or recycling (31–34). Briefly, the cell type responsible for surfactant synthesis is the alveolar type II cell. Substrates for surfactant synthesis, such as glucose and fatty acids, are taken up from the blood. Lipids and proteins are synthesized through the normal cellular processes and stored in lamellar bodies (32,35). Lamellar bodies contain all of the lipids and the hydrophobic proteins of surfactant as well as SP-A (36). A variety of signals, most notably lung stretch, can stimulate lamellar body secretion into the alveolar space (37). Subsequent to secretion, lamellar bodies unravel to form a unique lattice-like lipid–protein structure called tubular myelin as well as other organized lipid–protein structures (38–40). This freshly secreted surfactant can be isolated by differential centrifugation and is generally referred to as the surfactant large aggregate (LA) subfraction (41). It is believed that the LAs are the precursors of the surfactant film. Evidence for this stems from the observations that isolated LAs contain all surfactant lipid and protein components and are able to effectively reduce the surface tension *in vitro* and *in vivo* (42,43). During respiration, small unilamellar vesicles are formed for recycling by the type II cell or degradation through alveolar macrophages (44,45). This "spent" surfactant has been termed the small aggregate (SA) subfraction. Analyses of isolated SAs have shown that they contain mainly the lipid components of surfactant and are ineffective in reducing the surface tension (42,43). Overall, in a normal lung these metabolic pathways are responsible for maintaining a relatively constant amount of surfactant in the airspace. In humans, this alveolar surfactant is composed of $\sim$80–90% LAs and 10–20% SAs. It is not known how much of the surfactant obtained by lung lavage (either LA or SA) represents the material that was surface associated.

V. Acute Lung Injury

As mentioned earlier, there is strong evidence that pulmonary surfactant abnormalities play a role in the physiological lung dysfunction in patients with ALI (6,7). ALI has been defined by its acute onset and a number of physiological parameters developed by the American consensus conference (46). The two main physiological characteristics of ALI are decreased blood oxygenation and decreased lung compliance. It should also be noted that the consensus conference made a distinction between ALI and acute respiratory distress syndrome (ARDS), in which ARDS represent a more severe form of ALI (46). As all patients with ARDS also fall under the definition-criteria of ALI, we will utilize the term ALI throughout this review in reference to both conditions.

The overall mortality of ALI is 30–40% and, in addition, with many patients staying for prolonged periods in the intensive care unit this disease puts also a large financial burden on health care systems (47–50). As can be inferred from the physiologically based definition of ALI, there is no specific cause of ALI. Patients can develop ALI after one or more insults to the lung (51,52). Some of the most common causes of ALI are sepsis, pancreatitis, smoke inhalation, and acid aspiration. However, not all patients that have been exposed to one of these insults will develop ALI. It is thought that the initial host responses to an insult are protective, but if the patient is subsequently exposed to additional insults, the host inflammatory response becomes overwhelming and ALI ensues (52,53). One specific "secondary insult" that has been investigated is mechanical ventilation (9,54). Mechanical ventilation is often required in these patients but can also contribute to the progression of the disease (55,56). Regardless of the insult(s) that cause the initial injury to the lungs increased, permeability of the alveolar-capillary barrier, influx of serum proteins and accumulation of activated immune cells in the vasculature and airspace are characteristic of ALI (46) (Fig. 15.2). Alterations in the metabolism and functionality of pulmonary surfactant recovered from patients with ALI have also been consistently observed and are described below.

A Normal	B ALI
1. Capillaries Optimal gas exchange in capillaries	Impaired gas exchange, accumulation of inflammatory cells
2. Alveolar type II cell Regular phospholipid and surfactant associated protein metabolism	Decreased phospholipid and surfactant associated protein metabolism
3. Aqueous bulk phase Consistent ratio of LA (concentric circles and cross hatched) and SA (small vesicular forms)	Decreased LA and increased SA Increased inhibitory serum proteins (diagonally hatched form) Edema due to break down of alveolar-capillary barrier Infiltration of inflammatory cells and their secreted products
4. Air–liquid interface Surface film rich in DPPC (filled circles in Fig. 15.2) Favorable surface tension reduction	Decrease in DPPC in surface film replaced by less surface active phospholipids (open circles in Fig. 15.2) Insertion of inhibitory serum proteins Increased surface tension

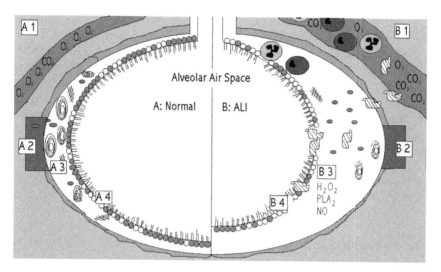

Figure 15.2 Schematic of normal alveolus compared with an alveolus of ALI.

VI. Alterations of Surfactant During ALI

The observation that the physiological impairments observed in ALI (decreased compliance and blood oxygenation) are similar to the effects of surfactant deficiency, led to the suggestion that surfactant may play a role in this condition. It was soon discovered that ALI injury was not associated with a surfactant deficiency but rather with an impairment of surfactant. Numerous studies have analyzed the pulmonary surfactant system from either patients with ALI (57–63) or from animal models of ALI (41,64–69). Interestingly, regardless of the underlying cause of ALI, the observations of the alterations of the surfactant system have been consistent, indicating that this represents a general mechanism of lung dysfunction in ALI.

Analysis of the phospholipid composition of surfactant from patients with ALI has demonstrated significant changes compared with controls [reviewed in Ref. (7)]. The relative amounts of the two most abundant lipids, PC and PG, are significantly reduced in patients with ALI with a concurrent increase in the other phospholipids of surfactant, as well as an increase in lyso-PC. In general, there also appears to be a significant decrease in the amount and/or activity of the SPs. In addition to these compositional changes, there are also changes in the relative amount of the LA and SA subfractions (58,62). In normal subjects, surfactant consists mostly of LA, whereas patients with ALI have a significant increase in the percentage of SA in the lavage material. Another consistent observation, although not directly related to surfactant, in the analysis of lavage material from patients with ALI is an increased concentration of nonsurfactant proteins. These proteins leak into the lung from the blood and are known to interfere with surfactant function (70–72).

The overall consequence of the altered composition, the shift in percentage of the surfactant subfractions, and the increase in nonsurfactant proteins is an impaired ability of the surfactant from patients with ALI to reduce the surface tension values required to maintain lung compliance (62). Thus, this impaired surface activity contributes to the physiological impairments observed in patients with ALI. The alterations of surfactant may also impact host defense functions of this material, although this has not yet been thoroughly investigated.

VII. Mechanisms by Which Alterations of Surfactant Occur

The observation that the alterations of pulmonary surfactant contribute to the lung dysfunction associated with ALI has initiated a large variety of studies investigating the mechanisms by which these changes occur. These studies have mostly relied on animal models of ALI as well as on a variety of *in vitro* studies. Although overlap exists, the proposed mechanisms can be categorized into three groups: (1) alterations of type II cell function, (2) inflammatory cells and their impact on the alveolar environment, and (3) contributions of therapeutic interventions.

Alterations of the synthetic pathways of the type II cell causing alteration of surfactant composition have been proposed. For example, it has been shown that tumor necrosis factor (TNF), a pro-inflammatory mediator associated with ALI, decreases the amount of choline incorporation into PC in type II cells (73–75). Similarly, decreased synthesis of SPs has been reported in response to TNF (76–78). The mechanisms by which TNF influences the metabolism of the type II cell have not been fully elucidated; however, p38 MAPK has been shown to play a role in the inhibition of SP-A *in vitro* (79). It has also been reported that TNF alters the morphology of type II alveolar cells (80). Other mediators may also affect type II cell function. Vivekananda et al. (81), reported that hepatocyte growth factor, which is increased in lung injury induced by hyperoxia, inhibits the synthesis and secretion of PC.

There are also several reported mechanisms by which the inflammatory cells, recruited to the lung during ALI, may contribute to alterations of surfactant. One proposed mechanism of inflammatory products directly causing alterations to surfactant is based on the observations of increased phospholipase A_2 activity in patients with ALI (82). Phospholipase A_2 can be secreted by inflammatory cells during inflammation in the lung and this enzyme can degrade PC (as well as PG) and generate lyso-PC and other lyso-phospholipids (83–86).

Another mechanism through which inflammatory cells affect surfactant is through the increased activity of inducible nitric oxide synthase (iNOS) (87). This increased activity of iNOS causes prolonged production of NO which reacts with reactive oxygen species, also produced by inflammatory cells, to nitrosylate various proteins including the SPs. The nitrosylation of SP-A has been reported in patients with ALI and *in vitro* studies have demonstrated that nitrosylated SP-A is less functionally active than normal SP-A (87–91).

Neutrophils can also secrete proteases such as elastase which could potentially degrade surfactant protein A (92,93). Increased protease activity in the airspace may also result in increased conversion of LA into SA, thereby contributing to the altered ratio of these subtypes (94–96).

Patients with ALI require mechanical ventilation to maintain blood oxygenation. Unfortunately, mechanical ventilation can also contribute to the surfactant alterations (8,97,98). Specifically, there is strong evidence that ventilation contributes to the conversion of LA into SA (99–101). It has been established by *in vitro* methods that a change in surface area is required for the conversion of LA into SA (96,102,103). Within the lung, this occurs due to ventilation as demonstrated by experiments with normal ventilated rabbits (101). This study demonstrated that when increased tidal volume was used (i.e., increased change in surface area), aggregate conversion increased as well. Furthermore, it was also shown that ventilated rabbits with ALI had increased conversion compared with noninjured control rabbits (100,101). Interestingly, spontaneously breathing injured animals did not show an increased conversion compared with controls, this has been attributed to the shallow breathing of these animals. These observations in animal models are consistent with clinical studies that mechanical ventilation plays an active role in the disease process. In a recent clinical trial low tidal volume ventilation was shown to be superior to higher tidal volumes (47). Although surfactant aggregates were not measured, it is possible that the lower tidal volumes limited the amount of conversion in this study.

Mechanical ventilation may also contribute to surfactant dysfunction due to some of the shear forces associated with the opening and closing of the lung with positive pressure (56,104). These forces may increase the leakage of serum proteins into the lung, which, as described earlier, can inhibit surfactant function. In addition to the mechanical-force aspect of ventilation, increased concentrations of oxygen are often part of this intervention. High levels of oxygen will increase the oxygenation of the blood but may also disturb the balance between oxidants and antioxidants. Thus, high levels of oxygen may cause oxidative damage to the surfactant (see chapter by Rodriquez-Capote et al., in the current volume for more details) (69). Thus mechanical ventilation can affect surfactant through altering the composition of the aggregates, increasing inhibition as well as through oxidative damage. Furthermore, these two contributing factors of mechanical ventilation will occur simultaneously. In a study in which mice were exposed to high oxygen for 48 h prior to mechanical ventilation, surfactant alterations induced by the stretch were more severe than mice exposed to room air prior to ventilation.

Taken as a whole, all of the earlier mechanisms contribute to the alterations of surfactant in ALI and all of the alterations combined result in the impaired activity. Thus, preserving surfactant function within the lung is difficult to achieve as multiple pathways are involved. It should also be noted that the numerous mechanisms of surfactant impairment overlap. For example, mechanical ventilation induced lung stretch may not only cause aggregate turnover but also cause the release of TNF-α into the alveolar space, which in turn can affect type II cell function.

VIII. Mechanisms by Which Alterations of Surfactant Lead to a Loss in Function

The functional consequences of the alterations of surfactant have been studied extensively. Particular focus has been on the role of serum proteins on surfactant's surface tension reducing activity (70–72,105–113). Addition of serum or purified serum proteins to surfactant will inhibit surfactant's ability to form a surface film and to effectively reduce surface tension values to ~0 mN/m. It is thought that one mechanism by which this inhibition by serum proteins occurs is by a direct physical interference at the air–liquid interface (105). Not all serum proteins inhibit surfactant to the same extent but fibrinogen appears to be one of the most potent inhibitory proteins that can leak into the lung (111). Interestingly, *in vitro* studies have demonstrated that SP-A can counteract serum protein inhibition of surfactant (110). However, as discussed earlier, SP-A levels during ALI are decreased and the SP-A itself could have decreased activity and/or altered function. The changes in phospholipids composition may also affect surfactant function. For example, the increased amount of lyso-PC may make the surfactant more susceptible to protein inhibition (109).

Many of the earlier studies on protein inhibition of surfactant have demonstrated that this inhibition is dependent on the concentration of surfactant. In this context, increased conversion of LA into SA within the airspace reduces the concentration of active (LA) surfactant subtype present, which may further enhance the sensitivity of the surfactant to inhibition. The influence of the increased SA fraction on the LA activity *in vivo* appears to be negligible, however, further studies are needed (43).

IX. Exogenous Surfactant Administration in ALI

To overcome the impairment of surfactant and thereby improve lung function, exogenous surfactant therapy has been investigated in animal studies and tested in clinical trials (114–121). As ALI has many different causes, a variety of animal models of ALI have been utilized to test the efficacy of surfactant therapy for ALI. In general, the reported studies have demonstrated that exogenous surfactant therapy can improve lung function and blood oxygenation in models of ALI (116,119,122). These promising results prompted several clinical studies varying from simple case reports to large multicenter clinical trials (114,115,117,118,120,121,123–125). The general outcome of all the clinical ALI studies combined, can be summarized as follows: exogenous surfactant treatment (1) is safe and feasible, (2) may improve oxygenation and lung function, and (3) has not significantly decreased the mortality of patients with ALI. These mortality results are obviously disappointing but, as will be discussed, do not necessarily imply a lack of clinical usefulness of surfactant therapy for ALI.

Numerous variables may have affected the outcomes in clinical trials, including the different types of exogenous surfactant utilized, the different methods of delivery and doses of material administered, the possible impact of ventilation strategy utilized prior, during and after surfactant treatment as well as the severity of the injury at the time of treatment (126). Although each of these variables has been investigated in preclinical animal studies, in the context of ALI, the jump from animal studies to clinical trials is very large. First, it should be noted that there is no ideal animal model of ALI and many investigators pick the model specifically to study one aspect of surfactant therapy which may not reflect all complications associated with ALI. For example, many investigation of surfactant therapy have been performed on adult animals with ALI induced by repetitive saline lavage. In this model, lung injury is induced by surfactant deficiency rather than impairment. Other studies have been performed on models that represent a specific cause of ALI such as sepsis or smoke inhalation but still these studies may not reflect the entire spectrum of patients tested in clinical trials. Other complications are the different timeframe and outcome parameters of animal studies vs. clinical trials. Whereas animal studies are usually performed over a period of hours and examine lung compliance, blood gas values and a number of other biochemical measurements, the clinical studies usually utilize 28 day mortality as one of the main outcome parameters. In fact, when examining the results from clinical trials, some of the short term benefits of surfactant therapy on compliance and/or blood gases are observed, in line with the animal studies. Unfortunately, the relationship short-term between the benefits observed after surfactant therapy and the potential long-term benefits are not known. The third issue that complicates the "translation" of animal studies into clinical practice is the fact that the reported results of animal studies will only reflect positive results as negative findings are not usually suitable for publication. Despite these limitations of animal studies, some insight into the variability of surfactant therapy in patients with ALI has been obtained.

The four factors that are thought to significantly influence the efficacy of surfactant therapy are: (1) the nature and severity of the lung injury, (2) the properties of the exogenous surfactant utilized, (3) the method and dose of surfactant delivery, and (4) the influence of supportive therapies such as mechanical ventilation. These four factors have been reviewed previously (126).

Briefly, the nature and severity of lung injury have been reported to be an important factor based on some trials that show trends for different outcomes in patients with direct lung injuries (i.e., acid aspiration, smoke inhalation, and pneumonia) vs. indirect causes of ALI (i.e., sepsis, pancreatitis). This concept of different initiating insults has not been tested in animal studies but intuitively it seems reasonable to assume that it can influence the efficacy (127). A few studies have studied the timing of surfactant treatment over the course of the development of ALI and showed that earlier treatment resulted in better outcomes than later treatments (128,129). The second factor, the properties of the exogenous surfactant, is also obviously important. Several natural based and a number of synthetic-based preparations are available. The most important property of the exogenous surfactant is having the biophysical activity needed to restore lung function (130). However, other issues also come in to play, such the host defense properties, the metabolic fate of the exogenous material once administered (including the resistance against potential inactivation by the same mechanisms as the endogenous material), the availability of the natural preparations and financial considerations. The goal of the dose and delivery method is to deliver sufficient amounts of surfactant to the alveolar space in a homogenous distribution pattern. Unfortunately, achieving this goal is not straightforward. For example, whereas tracheal instillation of surfactant may deliver a large dose of surfactant, its distribution may be heterogeneous and affected by the liquid volume and gravity (131–134). Aerosolization on the other hand may deliver surfactant in a most homogeneous fashion (at least in a homogeneous lung injury) but the dose delivered may be compromised (135). In general, the delivery of surfactant will be a compromise between dose delivered and distribution achieved, with feasibility and cost effectiveness being a secondary issue worth considering. Finally, the influence of therapeutic strategies should be considered. Specifically, the ventilation during and after surfactant administration may have significant effects on the efficacy of surfactant therapy in ALI (134,136,137). Animal studies have suggested that ventilation can affect the metabolism of exogenous surfactant similar to its effects on the endogenous material (134,136). The efficacy of the exogenous surfactant can also significantly be affected by the specific ventilation strategy.

The most relevant issue regarding these factors, however, is that they cannot easily be optimized in isolation, rather, surfactant therapy involves all of these issues which may need to be optimized for an individual patient. An example of this concept was observed in a study testing two different surfactants and two different delivery methods in a sheep model of ALI (116). It was found that one of the two surfactants, Survanta, improved the oxygenation of the saline lavaged sheep to a greater extent than the other surfactant, BLES, when delivered by aerosol. However, when these two surfactants were compared by tracheal instillation, BLES was superior to Survanta (116). In another study, the efficacy of aerosolized surfactant was compared between sheep with a homogeneous lung injury and a heterogeneous lung injury (138). Although physiologically, these animals had similar lung injury, aerosolized surfactant improved lung function in the homogeneous lung injury group but not in the heterogeneous group. This result was likely due to the distribution of the aerosol surfactant. In the heterogeneous group, more of the surfactant went to the "noninjured" areas (patent) of the lung rather than the injured areas (atelectatic) where surfactant was needed (135,138,139).

On the basis of these observations in clinical and animal studies, it is unlikely that one general surfactant treatment strategy will improve the outcome of patients with ALI. Rather, for surfactant treatment strategy to be effective it will need to be tailored to the individual patient. Initial studies examining patients with "direct" (i.e., smoke inhalation and acid aspiration) vs. "indirect" (i.e., sepsis, multiple trauma, etc.) lung injuries will provide a first indication of this concept. Further developments, such as the elucidation of biochemical markers of impending lung injury, would benefit tailored surfactant therapy IE: to allow for early or protective surfactant administration. Several strategies that may improve outcome are currently being developed and tested, most notably, combination therapies in which surfactant administration is combined with other therapeutic agents. For example, surfactant has been shown to enhance the delivery and expression of administered adenoviral vectors, and improve the peripheral distribution and activity of recombinant superoxide dismutases as well as antibiotics (140–144). Exogenous surfactant preparations have also been combined with urokinase and with polymers such as polyethyleneglycol (or dextran) in studies aimed at enhancing the effectiveness of the surfactant preparations (145–150).

X. Conclusions and Future Directions

This chapter focused on the role of surfactant in the development and treatment of ALI. Studies in animal models and data from lavage samples from patients have clearly demonstrated that a number of alterations of surfactant occur during ALI. Despite this knowledge, further studies are required to investigate in more detail how the compositional alterations cause surfactant impairment. Novel biophysical techniques are currently being employed to study the surface tension reducing activity of normal surfactant; similar approaches could be employed to understand how surfactant function is impaired in ALI. In addition to understanding the biophysical function of surfactant it is also imperative to consider its host defense role in the context of ALI. It is likely, for example, that reduced amounts or activity of SP-A in the injured lung may make the patient more susceptible to bacterial infection. Although this has not been studied experimentally, hospital-acquired pneumonia is frequently observed in patients with ALI. Further knowledge on the alterations of surfactant and the functional implication of these alterations will allow for improved therapeutic strategies for ALI.

In addition to the previous studies, further studies on the development of ALI are also required. ALI is a very heterogeneous disease with numerous causes and, consequently, diverse pathways leading to ALI. The endpoint of all these patients is similar, as defined by the physiological criteria. Surfactant treatment at this late stage of the disease has, to date, been unsuccessful. One approach to improve surfactant treatment would be an earlier administration. However, for early/protective treatments, a greater knowledge of the development of the disease is required. One interesting clinical scenario in which early surfactant treatment is possible in lung transplantation (151–153). It has been demonstrated in animal models of the ischemia-reperfusion injury associated with lung transplantation that physiological abnormalities and alterations of surfactant occur similarly to ALI (154,155). In follow-up studies, treatment of the donor lung prior to transplantation prevented the lung injury (151,152,156). The predictability of the lung insult in the setting of transplantation makes this protective treatment strategy very appealing. In the context of ALI, further research into biochemical markers of impending lung injury is warranted to allow for early treatments.

In summary, pulmonary surfactant is important for normal lung function. Alterations of surfactant contribute to lung dysfunction in patients with ALI. Surfactant treatment for patients with ALI holds promise but has been ineffective to date. It is believed that surfactant treatment needs to be tailored to the individual patients, possibly in combination with other therapies. We suggest that with a better knowledge of the functions of surfactant and with a greater understanding of the development of ALI, future successful therapies will be developed.

Acknowledgments

Work in the authors' laboratory is made possible through grants from the Canadian Institutes of Health Research and the Ontario Thoracic Society.

References

1. Van Golde LMG, Batenburg JJ, Robertson B. The pulmonary surfactant system. News Physiol Sci 1994; 9:13–20.
2. Robertson B, Halliday HL. Principles of surfactant replacement. Biochim Biophys Acta 1998; 1408:346–361.
3. Enhorning G, Shennan A, Possmayer F, Dunn M, Chen CP, Milligan J. Prevention of neonatal respiratory distress syndrome by tracheal instillation of surfactant: a randomized clinical trial. Pediatrics 1985; 76:145–153.
4. Avery ME, Mead J. Surface properties in relation to atelectasis and hyaline membrane disease. Am J Dis Child 1959; 97:517–523.
5. Avery ME. Surfactant deficiency in hyaline membrane disease: the story of discovery. Am J Respir Crit Care Med 2000; 161:1074–1075.

6. Lewis JF, Jobe AH. Surfactant and the adult respiratory distress syndrome. Am Rev Respir Dis 1993; 147:218–233.

7. Frerking I, Gunther A, Seeger W, Pison U. Pulmonary surfactant: functions, abnormalities and therapeutic options. Intensive Care Med 2001; 27:1699–1717.

8. Veldhuizen RA, Welk B, Harbottle R, Hearn S, Nag K, Petersen N, Possmayer F. Mechanical ventilation of isolated rat lungs changes the structure and biophysical properties of surfactant. J Appl Physiol 2002; 92:1169–1175.

9. Nakamura T, Malloy J, McCaig L, Yao LJ, Joseph M, Lewis J, Veldhuizen R. Mechanical ventilation of isolated septic rat lungs: effects on surfactant and inflammatory cytokines. J Appl Physiol 2001; 91:811–820.

10. Veldhuizen RA, Tremblay LN, Govindarajan A, van Rozendaal BA, Haagsman HP, Slutsky AS. Pulmonary surfactant is altered during mechanical ventilation of isolated rat lung. Crit Care Med 2000; 28:2545–2551.

11. Possmayer F, Nag K, Rodriguez K, Qanbar R, Schurch S. Surface activity *in vitro*: role of surfactant proteins. Comp Biochem Physiol A, (Mol. Integr. Physiol) 2001; 129:209–220.

12. Piknova B, Schram V, Hall SB. Pulmonary surfactant: phase behavior and function. Curr Opin Struct Biol 2002; 12:487–494.

13. Veldhuizen EJ, Haagsman HP. Role of pulmonary surfactant components in surface film formation and dynamics. Biochim Biophys Acta 2000; 1467:255–270.

14. Borron P, Veldhuizen RAW, Lewis JF, Possmayer F, Caveney A, Inchley K, McFadden RG, Fraher LJ. Surfactant associated protein-A inhibits human lymphocyte proliferation and IL-2 production. Am J Respir Cell Mol Biol 1996; 15:115–121.

15. Pison U, Max M, Neuendank A, Weissbach S, Pietschmann S. Host defence capacities of pulmonary surfactant: evidence for 'non-surfactant' functions of the surfactant system. Eur J Clin Invest 1994; 24:586–599.

16. Crouch E, Wright J. Surfactant proteins a and d and pulmonary host defense. Annu Rev Physiol 2001; 63:521–554.

17. McCormack FX, Whitsett JA. The pulmonary collectins, SP-A and SP-D, orchestrate innate immunity in the lung. J Clin Invest 2002; 109:707–712.

18. Haagsman HP. Interactions of surfactant protein A with pathogens. Biochim Biophys Acta 1998; 1408:264–277.

19. LeVine AM, Kurak KE, Wright JR, Watford WT, Bruno MD, Ross GF, Whitsett JA, Korfhagen TR. Surfactant protein-A binds group B *Streptococcus* enhancing phagocytosis and clearance from lungs of surfactant protein-A-deficient mice. Am J Respir Cell Mol Biol 1999; 20:279–286.

20. Korfhagen TR, LeVine AM, Whitsett JA. Surfactant protein A (*SP-A*) gene targeted mice. Biochim Biophys Acta 1998; 1408:296–302.

21. LeVine AM, Kurak KE, Bruno MD, Stark JM, Whitsett JA, Korfhagen TR. Surfactant protein-A-deficient mice are susceptible to *Pseudomonas aeruginosa* infection. Am J Respir Cell Mol Biol 1998; 19:700–708.

22. Postle AD, Heeley EL, Wilton DC. A comparison of the molecular species compositions of mammalian lung surfactant phospholipids. Comp Biochem Physiol A Mol Integr Physiol 2001; 129:65–73.

23. Shelley SA, Paciga JE, Balis JU. Lung surfactant phospholipids in different animal species. Lipids 1984; 19:857–862.

24. Yu S, Harding PG, Smith N, Possmayer F. Bovine pulmonary surfactant: chemical composition and physical properties. Lipids 1983; 18:522–529.

25. Goerke J. Pulmonary surfactant: functions and molecular composition. Biochim Biophys Acta 1998; 1408:79–89.

26. Veldhuizen RAW, Nag K, Orgeig S, Possmayer F. The role of lipids in pulmonary surfactant. Biochim Biophys Acta 1998; 1408:90–108.

27. Hawgood S, Poulain FR. Functions of the surfactant proteins: a perspective. Pediatr Pulmonol 1995; 19:99–104.

28. McCormack FX. Structure, processing and properties of surfactant protein A. Biochim Biophys Acta 1998; 1408:109–131.

29. Botas C, Poulain F, Akiyama J, Brown C, Allen L, Goerke J, Clements J, Carlson E, Gillespie AM, Epstein C, Hawgood S. Altered surfactant homeostasis and alveolar type ii cell morphology in mice lacking surfactant protein D. Proc Natl Acad Sci USA 1998; 95:11869–11874.

30. Ikegami M, Whitsett JA, Jobe A, Ross G, Fisher J, Korfhagen T. Surfactant metabolism in *SP-D* gene-targeted mice. Am J Physiol Lung Cell Mol Physiol 2000; 279:L468–L476.

31. Hawgood S, Poulain F. The pulmonary collectins and surfactant metabolism. Annu Rev Physiol 2001; 63:495–519.

32. Batenburg JJ, Haagsman HP. The lipids of pulmonary surfactant: dynamics and interactions with proteins. Prog Lipid Res 1998; 37:235–276.

33. Wright JR, Dobbs LG. Regulation of pulmonary surfactant secretion and clearance. Annu Rev Physiol 1991; 53:395–414.

34. Wright JR, Hawgood S. Pulmonary surfactant metabolism. Clin Chest Med 1989; 10:83–93.

35. Weaver TE, Na CL, Stahlman M. Biogenesis of lamellar bodies, lysosome-related organelles involved in storage and secretion of pulmonary surfactant. Semin Cell Dev Biol 2002; 13:263–270.

36. Oosterlaken Dijksterhuis MA, van Eijk M, van Buel BL, van Golde LM, Haagsman HP. Surfactant protein composition of lamellar bodies isolated from rat lung. Biochem J 1991; 274:115–119.

37. Rooney SA. Regulation of surfactant secretion. Comp Biochem Physiol A Mol Integr Physiol 2001; 129:233–243.

38. Poulain FR, Allen L, Williams MC, Hamilton RL, Hawgood S. Effects of surfactant apolipoproteins on liposome structure: implications for tubular myelin formation. Am J Physiol 1992; 262:L730–L739.

39. Voorhout WF, Veenendaal T, Haagsman HP, Verkleij AJ, Van Golde LM, Geuze HJ. Surfactant protein A is localized at the corners of the pulmonary tubular myelin lattice. J Histochem Cytochem 1991; 39:1331–1336.

40. Suzuki Y, Fujita Y, Kogishi K. Reconstitution of tubular myelin from synthetic lipids and proteins associated with pig pulmonary surfactant. Am Rev Respir Dis 1989; 140:75–81.

41. Lewis JF, Ikegami M, Jobe AH. Altered surfactant function and metabolism in rabbits with acute lung injury. J Appl Physiol 1990; 69:2303–2310.

42. Yamada T, Ikegami M, Jobe AH. Effects of surfactant subfractions on preterm rabbit lung function. Pediatr Res 1990; 27:592–598.

43. Brackenbury AM, Malloy JL, McCaig LA, Yao LJ, Veldhuizen RA, Lewis JF. Evaluation of alveolar surfactant aggregates *in vitro* and *in vivo*. Eur Respir J 2002; 19:41–46.

44. Baritussio A, Bellina L, Carraro R, Rossi A, Enzi G, Magoon MW, Mussini I. Heterogeneity of alveolar surfactant in the rabbit: composition, morphology, and labelling of subfractions isolated by centrifugation of lung lavage. Eur J Clin Invest 1984; 14:24–29.

45. Magoon MW, Wright JR, Baritussio A, Williams MC, Goerke J, Benson BJ, Hamilton RL, Clements JA. Subfractionation of lung surfactant. Implications for metabolism and surface activity. Biochim Biophys Acta 1983; 750:18–31.

46. Bernard GR, Artigas A, Brigham KL, Carlet J, Falke K, Hudson L, Lamy M, Legall JR, Morris A, Spragg R, the Consensus Committee. The American-European consensus conference on ARDS: definitions, mechanisms, relevant outcomes, and clinical trial coordination. Am J Respir Crit Care Med 1994; 149:818–824.

47. Brower RG, Matthay MA, Morris A, Schoenfeld D, Thompson BT, Wheeler A. Ventilation with lower tidal volumes as compared with traditional tidal volumes for acute lung injury and the acute respiratory distress syndrome. The Acute Respiratory Distress Syndrome Network. N Engl J Med 2000; 342:1301–1308.

48. Montgomery AB, Stager MA, Carrico CJ, Hudson ED. Causes of mortality in patients with the adult respiratory distress syndrome. Am Rev Respir Dis 1985; 132:485–489.

49. Abel SJ, Finney SJ, Brett SJ, Keogh BF, Morgan CJ, Evans TW. Reduced mortality in association with the acute respiratory distress syndrome (ards). Thorax 1998; 53:292–294.

50. Villar J, Slutsky AS. The incidence of the adult respiratory distress syndrome. Am Rev Respir Dis 1989; 140:814–816.

51. Hudson LD, Steinberg KP. Epidemiology of acute lung injury and ARDS. Chest 1999; 116:74S–82S.

52. Livingston DH, Mosenthal AC, Deitch EA. Sepsis and multiple organ dysfunction syndrome: a clinical- mechanistic overview. New Horiz 1995; 3:257–264.

53. Downey GP, Granton JT. Mechanisms of acute lung injury. Curr Opin Pulm Med 1997; 3:234–241.

54. Slutsky AS, Tremblay LN. Multi System Organ Failure: is mechanical ventilation a contributing factor? Am J Respir Crit Care Med 1998; 157:1721–1725.

55. Dreyfuss D, Soler P, Saumon G. Mechanical ventilation-induced pulmonary edema. Am J Respir Crit Care Med 1995; 151:1568–1575.

56. Dreyfuss D, Saumon G. Ventilator-induced lung injury: lessons from experimental studies. Am J Respir Crit Care Med 1998; 157:294–323.

57. Gregory TJ, Longmore WJ, Moxley MA, Whitsett JA, Reed CR, Fowler AA, Maunder RJ, Crim C, Hyers TM. Surfactant chemical composition and biophysical activity in acute respiratory distress syndrome. J Clin Invest 1991; 88:1976–1981.

58. Veldhuizen RA, McCaig LA, Akino T, Lewis JF. Pulmonary surfactant subfractions in patients with the acute respiratory distress syndrome. Am J Respir Crit Care Med 1995; 152:1867–1871.

59. Hallman M. Lung surfactant in respiratory distress syndrome. Acta Anaesthesiol Scand Suppl 1991; 95:15–20.

60. Pison U, Gono E, Joka T, Obertacke U. Phospholipid lung profile in adult respiratory distress syndrome–evidence for surfactant abnormality. Prog Clin Biol Res 1987; 236:517–523.

61. Schmidt R, Meier U, Yabut-Perez M, Walmrath D, Grimminger F, Seeger W, Gunther A. Alteration of fatty acid profiles in different pulmonary surfactant

phospholipids in acute respiratory distress syndrome and severe pneumonia. Am J Respir Crit Care Med 2001; 163:95–100.

62. Gunther A, Siebert C, Schmidt R, Ziegler S, Grimminger F, Yabut M, Temmesfeld B, Walmrath D, Morr H, Seeger W. Surfactant alterations in severe pneumonia, acute respiratory distress syndrome, and cardiogenic lung edema. Am J Respir Crit Care Med 1996; 153:176–184.

63. Pison U, Seeger W, Buchhorn R, Joka T, Brand M, Obertacke U, Neuhof H. Surfactant abnormalities in patients with respiratory failure after multiple trauma. Am Rev Respir Dis 1989; 140:1033–1039.

64. Lewis JF, Veldhuizen R, Possmayer F, Sibbald W, Whitsett J, Qanbar R, McCaig L. Altered alveolar surfactant is an early marker of acute lung injury in septic adult sheep. Am J Respir Crit Care Med 1994; 150:123–130.

65. Malloy JL, Veldhuizen RA, Lewis JF. Effects of ventilation on the surfactant system in sepsis-induced lung injury. J Appl Physiol 2000; 88:401–408.

66. Lachmann B, Hallman M, Bergmann KC. Respiratory failure following anti-lung serum: study on mechanisms associated with surfactant system damage. Exp Lung Res 1987; 12:163–180.

67. van Helden HP, Kuijpers WC, Steenvoorden D, Go C, Bruijnzeel PL, van Eijk M, Haagsman HP. Intratracheal aerosolization of endotoxin (LPS) in the rat: a comprehensive animal model to study adult (acute) respiratory distress syndrome. Exp Lung Res 1997; 23:297–316.

68. Davidson KG, Bersten AD, Barr HA, Dowling KD, Nicholas TE, Doyle IR. Lung function, permeability, and surfactant composition in oleic acid-induced acute lung injury in rats. Am J Physiol Lung Cell Mol Physiol 2000; 279:L1091–L1102.

69. Matalon S, Holm BA, Loewen GM, Baker RR, Notter RH. Sublethal hyperoxic injury to the alveolar epithelium and the pulmonary surfactant system. Exp Lung Res 1988; 14(suppl):1021–1033.

70. Seeger W, Grube C, Gunther A, Schmidt R. Surfactant inhibition by plasma proteins: differential sensitivity of various surfactant preparations. Eur Respir J 1993; 6:971–977.

71. Seeger W, Gunther A, Thede C. Differential sensitivity to fibrinogen inhibition of SP-C- vs. SP-B-based surfactants. Am J Physiol 1992; 261:L286–L291.

72. Nitta K, Kobayashi T. Impairment of surfactant activity and ventilation by proteins in lung edema fluid. Respir Physiol 1994; 95:43–51.

73. Vara E, Arias-Diaz J, Garcia C, Hernandez J, Balibrea JL. TNF-alpha-induced inhibition of PC synthesis by human type2 pneumocytes is sequentially mediated by PGE2 and NO. Am J Physiol 1996; 271:L359–L365.

74. Vara E, Arias-Diaz J, Garcia C, Hernandez J, Balibrea JL. Both prostaglandin E2 and nitric oxide sequentially mediate the tumor necrosis factor-alpha-induced inhibition of surfactant synthesis by human type2 pneumocytes. Arch Surg 1995; 130:1279–1286.

75. Arias-Diaz J, Vara E, Garcia C, Balibrea JL. Tumor necrosis factor-alpha-induced inhibition of phosphatidylcholine synthesis by human type 2 pneumocytes is partially mediated by prostaglandins. J Clin Invest 1994; 94:244–250.

76. Pryhuber GS, Bachurski C, Hirsh R, Bacon A, Whitsett JA. Tumor necrosis factor-a decreases surfactant protein B mRNA in murine lung. Am J Physiol 1998; 270:L714–L721.

77. Pryhuber GS, Khalak R, Zhao Q. Regulation of surfactant proteins a and b by tnf-alpha and phorbol ester independent of nf-kappa b. Am J Physiol 1998; 274:L289–L295.

78. Whitsett JA, Clark JC, Wispe JR, Pryhuber GS. Effects of TNF-alpha and phorbol ester on human surfactant protein and MnSOD gene transcription *in vitro*. Am J Physiol 1992; 262:L688–L693.

79. Miakotina OL, Snyder JM. TNF-alpha inhibits SP-A gene expression in lung epithelial cells via p38 MAPK. Am J Physiol Lung Cell Mol Physiol 2002; 283:L418–L427.

80. Sulkowska M. Effect of human recombinant tumour necrosis factor-alpha and pentoxifylline on the ultrastructure of type II alveolar epithelial cells in pregnant and nonpregnant rabbits. J Comp Pathol 1997; 117:227–236.

81. Vivekananda J, Awasthi V, Awasthi S, Smith DB, King RJ. Hepatocyte growth factor is elevated in chronic lung injury and inhibits surfactant metabolism. Am J Physiol Lung Cell Mol Physiol 2000; 278:L382–L392.

82. Kim DK, Fukuda T, Thompson BT, Cockrill B, Hales C, Bonventre JV. Bronchoalveolar lavage fluid phospholipase A2 activities are increased in human adult respiratory distress syndrome. Am J Physiol 1995; 269:L109–L118.

83. Hite RD, Seeds MC, Jacinto RB, Balasubramanian R, Waite M, Bass D. Hydrolysis of surfactant-associated phosphatidylcholine by mammalian secretory phospholipases A2. Am J Physiol 1998; 275:L740–L747.

84. Schrama AJ, de Beaufort AJ, Sukul YR, Jansen SM, Poorthuis BJ, Berger HM. Phospholipase A2 is present in meconium and inhibits the activity of pulmonary surfactant: an *in vitro* study. Acta Paediatr 2001; 90:412–416.

85. Flieger A, Gongab S, Faigle M, Mayer HA, Kehrer U, Mussotter J, Bartmann P, Neumeister B. Phospholipase A secreted by *Legionella pneumophila* destroys alveolar surfactant phospholipids. FEMS Microbiol Lett 2000; 188:129–133.

86. Touqui L, Arbibe L. A role for phospholipase A in ARDS pathogenesis. Mol Med Today 1999; 5:244–249.

87. Sittipunt C, Steinberg KP, Ruzinski JT, Myles C, Zhu S, Goodman RB, Hudson LD, Matalon S, Martin TR. Nitric oxide and nitrotyrosine in the lungs of patients with acute respiratory distress syndrome. Am J Respir Crit Care Med 2001; 163:503–510.

88. Haddad IY, Pataki G, Hu P, Galliani C, Beckman JS, Matalon S. Quantitation of nitrotyrosine levels in lung sections of patients and animals with acute lung injury. J Clin Invest 1994; 94:2407–2413.

89. Haddad IY, Zhu S, Ischiropoulos H, Matalon S. Nitration of surfactant protein A results in decreased ability to aggregate lipids. Am J Physiol 1996; 270:L281–L288.

90. Zhu S, Kachel DL, Martin WJ, Matalon S. Nitrated SP-A does not enhance adherence of pneumocystis carinii to alveolar macrophages. Am J Physiol 1998; 275:L1031–L1039.

91. Zhu S, Ware LB, Geiser T, Matthay MA, Matalon S. Increased levels of nitrate and surfactant protein a nitration in the pulmonary edema fluid of patients with acute lung injury. Am J Respir Crit Care Med 2001; 163:166–172.

92. Liau DF, Yin NX, Huang J, Ryan SF. Effects of human polymorphonuclear leukocyte elastase upon surfactant proteins *in vitro*. Biochim Biophys Acta 1996; 1302:117–128.

93. Lewis RW, Harwood JL, Tetley TD, Harris E, Richards RJ. Degradation of human and rat surfactant apoprotein by neutrophil elastase and cathepsin G. Biochem Soc Trans 1993; 21:206S.

94. Veldhuizen RA, Inchley K, Hearn SA, Lewis JF, Possmayer F. Degradation of surfactant-associated protein B (SP-B) during *in vitro* conversion of large to small surfactant aggregates. Biochem J 1993; 295:141–147.

95. Veldhuizen RAW, Hearn SA, Lewis JF, Possmayer F. Surface-area cycling of different surfactant preparations: SP-A and SP-B are essential for large-aggregate integrity. Biochem J 1994; 300:519–524.

96. Gross NJ. Extracellular metabolism of pulmonary surfactant: the role of a new serine protease. Annu Rev Physiol 1995; 57:135–150.

97. Veldhuizen RAW, Slutsky AS, Joseph M, McCaig L. Effects of mechanical ventilation of isolated mouse lungs on pulmonary surfactant and inflammatory cytokines. Eur Respir J 2001; 17:488–494.

98. Verbrugge SJ, Sorm V, Lachmann B. Mechanisms of acute respiratory distress syndrome: role of surfactant changes and mechanical ventilation. J Physiol Pharmacol 1997; 48:537–557.

99. Ito Y, Veldhuizen RAW, Yao L-J, McCaig LA, Bartlett AJ, Lewis JF. Ventilation strategies affect surfactant aggregate conversion in acute lung injury. Am J Respir Crit Care Med 1997; 155:493–499.

100. Veldhuizen RAW, Ito Y, Marcou J, Yao LJ, McCaig L, Lewis JF. Effects of lung injury on pulmonary surfactant aggregate conversion *in vivo* and *in vitro*. Am J Physiol 1997; 16:L872–L878.

101. Veldhuizen RAW, Marcou J, Yao L-J, McCaig L, Ito Y, Lewis JF. Alveolar surfactant aggregate conversion in ventilated normal and injured rabbits. Am J Physiol 1996; 270:L152–L158.

102. Gross NJ, Narine KR. Surfactant subtypes of mice: metabolic relationships and conversion *in vitro*. J Appl Physiol 1989; 67:414–421.

103. Veldhuizen RA, Yao L, Lewis JF. An examination of the different variables affecting surfactant aggregate conversion *in vitro*. Exp Lung Res 1999; 25:127–141.

104. Dreyfuss D, Saumon G. Role of tidal volume, FRC, and end-expiratory volume in the development of pulmonary edema following mechanical ventilation. Am Rev Respir Dis 1993; 148:1194–1203.

105. Holm BA, Enhorning G, Notter RH. A biophysical mechanism by which plasma proteins inhibit lung surfactant activity. Chem Phys Lipids 1988; 49:49–55.

106. Holm BA, Notter RH. Effects of hemoglobin and cell membrane lipids on pulmonary surfactant activity. J Appl Physiol 1987; 63:1434–1442.

107. Holm BA, Venkitaraman AR, Enhorning G, Notter RH. Biophysical inhibition of synthetic lung surfactants. Chem Phys Lipids 1990; 52:243–250.

108. Cockshutt AM, Absolom DR, Possmayer F. The role of palmitic acid in pulmonary surfactant: enhancement of surface activity and prevention of inhibition by blood proteins. Biochim Biophys Acta 1991; 1085:248–256.

109. Cockshutt AM, Possmayer F. Lysophosphatidylcholine sensitizes lipid extracts of pulmonary surfactant to inhibition by serum proteins. Biochim Biophys Acta 1991; 1086:63–71.

110. Cockshutt AM, Weitz J, Possmayer F. Pulmonary surfactant-associated protein A enhances the surface activity of lipid extract surfactant and reverses inhibition by blood proteins *in vitro*. Biochemistry 1990; 29:8424–8429.

111. Seeger W, Stohr G, Wolf HR, Neuhof H. Alteration of surfactant function due to protein leakage: special interaction with fibrin monomer. J Appl Physiol 1985; 58:326–338.

112. Kobayashi T, Nitta K, Ganzuka M, Inui S, Grossman G, Robertson B. Inactivation of exogenous surfactant by pulmonary edema fluid. Pediatr Res 1991; 29:353–356.

113. Venkitaraman AR, Baatz JE, Whitsett JA, Hall SB, Notter RH. Biophysical inhibition of synthetic phospholipid-lung surfactant apoprotein admixtures by plasma proteins. Chem Phys Lipids 1991; 57:49–57.

114. Walmrath D, Gunther A, Ardeschir H, Schermuly R, Schneider T, Grimminger F, Seeger W. Bronchoscopic surfactant administration in patients with severe adult respiratory distress syndrome and sepsis. Am J Respir Crit Care Med 1996; 154:57–62.

115. Wiswell TE, Smith RM, Katz LB, Mastroianni L, Wong DY, Willms D, Heard S, Wilson M, Hite RD, Anzueto A, Revak SD, Cochrane CG. Broncho-pulmonary segmental lavage with Surfaxin (KL(4)-surfactant) for acute respiratory distress syndrome. Am J Respir Crit Care Med 1999; 160:1188–1195.

116. Lewis JF, Goffin J, Yue P, McCaig LA, Bjarneson D, Veldhuizen RAW. Evaluation of exogenous surfactant treatment strategies in an adult model of acute lung injury. J Appl Physiol 1996; 80:1156–1164.

117. Anzueto A, Baughman RP, Guntupalli KK, Weg JG, Wiedemann HP, Artigas Raventos A, Lemaire F, Long W, Zaccardelli DS, Pattishall EN. Aerosolized surfactant in adults with sepsis-induced acute respiratory distress syndrome. N Engl J Med 1996; 334:1417–1421.

118. Lachmann B. Animal models and clinical pilot studies of surfactant replacement in adult respiratory distress syndrome. Eur Respir J Suppl 1989; 3:98s–103s.

119. So KL, de Buijzer E, Gommers D, Kaisers U, van Genderen PJ, Lachmann B. Surfactant therapy restores gas exchange in lung injury due to paraquat intoxication in rats. Eur Respir J 1998; 12:284–287.

120. Spragg R, Harris KW, Lewis J, Marsh JJ, Wurst W, Rathgeb F. Surfactant treatment of patients with ARDS may reduce acute lung inflammation. Am J Resp Crit Care Med 2001; 163:A23

121. Gregory TJ, Gadek JE, Weiland JE, Hyers TM, Crim C, Hudson LD, Steinberg KP, Maunder RA, Spragg RG, Smith RM, Tierney DF, Gipe B, Longmore WJ, Moxley MA. Survanta supplementation in patients with acute respiratory distress syndrome (ARDS). Am J Respir Crit Care Med 1994; 149(suppl 2):A567.

122. Brackenbury AM, Puligandla PS, McCaig LA, Nikore V, Yao LJ, Veldhuizen RA, Lewis JF. Evaluation of exogenous surfactant in HCL-induced lung injury. Am J Respir Crit Care Med 2001; 163:1135–1142.

123. Staudinger T, Bankier A, Strohmaier W, Weiss K, Locker GJ, Knapp S, Roggla M, Laczika K, Frass M. Exogenous surfactant therapy in a patient with adult respiratory distress syndrome after near drowning. Resuscitation 1997; 35:179–182.

124. Richman PS, Spragg RG, Robertson B, Merritt TA, Curstedt T. The adult respiratory distress syndrome: first trials with surfactant replacement. Eur Respir J Suppl 1989; 3:109s–111s.

125. Spragg RG, Gilliard N, Richman P, Smith RM, Hite RD, Pappert D, Robertson B, Curstedt T, Strayer D. Acute effects of a single dose of porcine surfactant on patients with the adult respiratory distress syndrome. Chest 1994; 105:195–202.

126. Lewis JF, Veldhuizen RAW. Factors influencing efficacy of exogenous surfactant in acute lung injury. Biol Neonate 1995; 67(suppl 1):48–60.

127. Puligandla PS, Gill T. The alveolar environment influences the metabolic and biophysical properties of exogenous surfactants. J Appl Physiol 2000; 88:1061–1071.

128. Ito Y, Goffin J, Veldhuizen R, Joseph M, Bjarneson D, McCaig L, Yao L-J, Marcou J, Lewis J. Timing of exogenous surfactant administration in a rabbit model of acute lung injury. J Appl Physiol 1996; 80:1357–1364.

129. Krause MF, Hoehn T. Timing of surfactant administration determines its physiologic response in a rabbit model of airway lavage. Biol Neonate 2000; 77:196–202.

130. Hafner D, Germann PG, Hauschke D. Effects of lung surfactant factor (LSF) treatment on gas exchange and histopathological changes in an animal model of adult respiratory distress syndrome (ARDS): comparison of recombinant LSF with bovine LSF. Pulm Pharmacol 1994; 7:319–332.

131. Lewis JF, Tabor B, Ikegami M, Jobe AH, Joseph M, Absolom D. Lung function and surfactant distribution in saline lavaged sheep given instilled vs. nebulized surfactant. J Appl Physiol 1993; 74:1256–1264.

132. Segerer H, VanGelder W, Angenent FWM, VanWoerkens LJPM, Curstedt T, Obladen M, Lachmann B. Pulmonary distribution and efficacy of exogenous surfactant in lung-lavaged rabbits are influenced by the instillation technique. Pediatr Res 1993; 34:490–494.

133. Gilliard N, Richman PM, Merritt TA, Spragg RG. Effect of volume and dose on the pulmonary distribution of exogenous surfactant administered to normal rabbits or to rabbits with oleic acid lung injury. Am Rev Respir Dis 1990; 141:743–747.

134. Kerr CL, Ito Y, Manwell SE, Veldhuizen RA, Yao LJ, McCaig LA, Lewis JF. Effects of surfactant distribution and ventilation strategies on efficacy of exogenous surfactant. J Appl Physiol 1998; 85:676–684.

135. Lewis J, Ikegami M, Higuchi R, Jobe A, Absolom D. Nebulized vs. instilled exogenous surfactant in an adult lung injury model. J Appl Physiol 1991; 71:1270–1276.

136. Ito Y, Manwell SEE, Kerr CL, Veldhuizen RAW, Yao L-J, McCaig LA, Bartlett AJ, Bjarneson D, Lewis JF. Effect of ventilation strategies on the efficacy of exogenous surfactant therapy in a rabbit model of acute lung injury. Am J Respir Crit Care Med 1998; 157:149–155.

137. Hartog A, Gommers D, Haitsma JJ, Lachmann B. Improvement of lung mechanics by exogenous surfactant: effect of prior application of high positive end-expiratory pressure. Br J Anaesth 2000; 85:752–756.

138. Lewis JF, Ikegami M, Jobe AH, Absolom D. Physiologic responses and distribution of aerosolized surfactant (Survanta) in a nonuniform pattern of lung injury. Am Rev Respir Dis 1993; 147:1364–1370.

139. Lewis JF, McCaig LA. Aerosolized versus instilled exogenous surfactant in a nonuniform pattern of lung injury. Am Rev Respir Dis 1993; 148:1187–1193.

140. Haitsma JJ, Lachmann U, Lachmann B. Exogenous surfactant as a drug delivery agent. Adv Drug Deliv Rev 2001; 47:197–207.

141. Jobe AH, Ikegami M, Yei S, Whitsett JA, Trapnell B. Surfactant effects on aerosolized and instilled adenoviral-mediated gene transfer. Hum Gene Ther 1996; 7:697–704.

142. van't Veen A, Mouton JW, Gommers D, Lachmann B. Pulmonary surfactant as vehicle for intratracheally instilled tobramycin in mice infected with *Klebsiella pneumoniae*. Br J Pharmacol 1996; 119:1145–1148.

143. Katkin JP, Husser RC, Langston C, Welty SE. Exogenous surfactant enhances the delivery of recombinant adenoviral vectors to the lung. Hum Gene Ther 1997; 8:171–176.

144. Davis JM, Rosenfeld WN, Koo HC, Gonenne A. Pharmacologic interactions of exogenous lung surfactant and recombinant human Cu/Zn superoxide dismutase. Pediatr Res 1994; 35:37–40.

145. Kobayashi T, Ohta K, Tashiro K, Nishizuka K, Chen WM, Ohmura S, Yamamoto K. Dextran restores albumin-inhibited surface activity of pulmonary surfactant extract. J Appl Physiol 1999; 86:1778–1784.

146. Tashiro K, Kobayashi T, Robertson B. Dextran reduces surfactant inhibition by meconium. Acta Paediatr 2000; 89:1439–1445.

147. Taeusch HW, Lu K, Goerke J, Clements J. Nonionic polymers revers inactivation of surfactant by meconium and other substances. Am J Respir Crit Care Med 1999; 159:1391–1395.

148. Sarin P, Taeusch HW, Lu K, Goerke J, Clements J. Polyethelene glycol results in concentration-dependent sedimentation of Survanta and improvement of its function. Pediatr Res 1999; 45:319A.

149. Lu KW, William TH, Robertson B, Goerke J, Clements JA. Polymer-surfactant treatment of meconium-induced acute lung injury. Am J Respir Crit Care Med 2000; 162:623–628.

150. Schermuly RT, Gunther A, Ermert M, Ermert L, Ghofrani HA, Weissmann N, Grimminger F, Seeger W, Walmrath D. Conebulization of surfactant and urokinase restores gas exchange in perfused lungs with alveolar fibrin formation. Am J Physiol Lung Cell Mol Physiol 2001; 280:L792–L800.

151. Erasmus ME, Petersen AH, Hofstede G, Haagsman HP, Bambang Oetomo S, Prop J. Surfactant treatment before reperfusion improves the immediate function of lung transplants in rats. Am J Respir Crit Care Med 1996; 153:665–670.

152. Novick R, MacDonald J, Veldhuizen R, Wan F, Duplan J, Denning L, Possmayer F, Gilpin A, Yao L-J, Bjarneson D, Lewis J. Evaluation of surfactant treatment strategies after prolonged graft storage in lung transplantation. Am J Respir Crit Care Med 1996; 154:98–104.

153. Hausen B, Rohde R, Hewitt CW, Schroeder F, Beuke M, Ramsamooj R, Schafers HJ, Borst HG. Exogenous surfactant treatment before and after sixteen hours of ischemia in experimental lung transplantation. J Thorac Cardiovasc Surg 1997; 113:1050–1058.

154. Veldhuizen RA, Lee J, Sandler D, Hull W, Whitsett JA, Lewis J, Possmayer F, Novick RJ. Alterations in pulmonary surfactant composition and activity after experimental lung transplantation. Am Rev Respir Dis 1993; 148:208–215.

155. Erasmus ME, Petersen AH, Oetomo SB, Prop J. The function of surfactant is impaired during the reimplantation response in rat lung transplants. J Heart Lung Transplant 1994; 13:791–802.

156. Novick RJ, Veldhuizen RAW, Possmayer F, Lee J, Sandler D, Lewis JF. Exogenous surfactant therapy in thirty-eight hour lung graft preservation for transplantation. J Thorac Cardiovasc Surg 1994; 108:259–268.

16

Pulmonary Surfactant in Asthma and Allergy

JENS M. HOHLFELD

Hannover Medical School and Fraunhofer Institute of Toxicology and
Experimental Medicine,
Hannover, Germany

I. Introduction

Pulmonary surfactant reduces the surface tension at the air–liquid interface in the entire lung. This surfactant lining layer, which is present in the alveoli and the airways, is composed of phospholipids, mainly dipalmitoylphosphatidylcholine (DPPC) and surfactant-specific proteins. Reduction of surface tension at the air–liquid interface prevents alveolar collapse at end expiration, contributes to airway stability and openness, and thus allows for cyclic ventilation of the lungs. This basic functional principle of pulmonary surfactant was invented more than 70 years ago. The pathogenetic relevance of surfactant was initially recognized in infant respiratory distress syndrome as a quantitative surfactant deficiency (1), but today biochemical and biophysical surfactant abnormalities have been reported in various lung diseases, such as acute respiratory distress syndrome, pneumonia, cardiogenic lung edema (2), following lung transplantation (3), as well as in patients with cystic fibrosis (4), and asthma (5).

The possible involvement of pulmonary surfactant in the pathophysiology of asthma has recently been addressed (6). There are two proposed mechanisms by which surfactant might alleviate airway obstruction in asthma. First, airway obstruction in asthma, which is commonly thought to be caused by smooth muscle constriction, mucosal edema, and secretion of fluid into the airway lumen, may be additionally due to a poor function of pulmonary surfactant. A dysfunction of surfactant has been demonstrated both in murine asthma models (7,8) and in patients with asthma (5,9). Poor-functioning surfactant looses the ability to stabilize airways and to prevent airway collapse (10). Therefore, surfactant dysfunction in asthma might contribute to airway obstruction. Accordingly, treatment strategies that act upon improving surfactant function might be of benefit in asthma. Secondly, airway obstruction in asthma occurs upon inhalation of a variety of stimuli due to bronchial hyperresponsiveness. This bronchial hyperresponsiveness is caused and sustained by a chronic inflammation of the airways (11). Surfactant components, such as the lung collectins SP-A and SP-D, have been found capable of modulating immune cells involved in the allergic inflammatory cascade in asthma (12–15). Moreover, SP-A and SP-D possess binding capacity for aeroallergens (16,17). Thus, surfactant components that down-regulate immune cell functions involved in this allergic inflammation might decrease bronchial hyperresponsiveness (18,19) and therefore protect against airway obstruction. Our current understanding of surfactant components acting on the cells involved in asthma will be reviewed in detail subsequently. Functional, morphological, and compositional aspects of surfactant with regard to asthma and the airway compartment will also be covered by this review.

II. General Aspects of Airway Surfactant

A. Functions

The best known function of surfactant according to its naming as "surface active agent" is surface activity. As in the alveoli, surfactant lowers surface tension at the air–liquid interface of conducting airways. According to the law of Laplace that applies for cylinders "$P = \gamma/r$", where P is the transmural pressure, γ the surface tension, and r the airway radius, it becomes obvious that the smaller the airways become, the higher the pressure would rise if surface active material would be absent, and therefore, γ would be constant. Accordingly, terminal airways would collapse. Fortunately, surfactant in the airways lowers surface tension and thereby minimizes the magnitude of negative pressure in the airway wall and its adjacent liquid layer which in turn reduces the tendency for airway wall collapse. Moreover, surfactant reduces the tendency of airway liquid to form bridges that occlude the airway lumen in the more narrow airways, because surface active material can stabilize the inner surface of the airways. Therefore, well-functioning surfactant secures airway stability and openness.

Surface tension in the conducting airways has been shown to range between 25 and 30 mN/m (20,21). Surface activity of airway surfactant is less when compared with alveolar surfactant, but the functional requirements of airway surfactant are also inferior because surface area changes during the respiratory cycle are much smaller in the airways when compared with the alveoli. A reduction of surface tension from water levels of 72 mN/m to values of 25–30 mN/m is obviously sufficient to keep airways open. The basic functional principle of surface active airway surfactant has been demonstrated experimentally by Liu et al. (22) who found that surfactant-containing fluid allowed a free airflow through glass capillaries, whereas saline lead to spontaneous refilling of the tubes. The ability of surfactant to maintain free airflow was lost with the addition of albumin or fibrinogen (two potent surfactant inhibitors). The principle findings of surfactant function and dysfunction in the rigid airway model using the glass capillaries and the capillary surfactometer have been confirmed in an elegant approach to study conducting airway function in excised isolated rat lungs (23). In a recent study with the capillary surfactometer, we have demonstrated that the surfactant dysfunction induced by proteins was further disturbed by cooling (24). This may, partly, explain the finding of increased airway resistance in patients with exercise-induced asthma. During exercise with hyperventilation of cold air, airway surfactant already affected by exuded proteins present in asthmatic airways (5) becomes further inactivated due to cooling. This in turn causes airway closure and might explain why exercise causes asthma attacks.

Besides the lowering of surface tension, surfactant also contributes to the regulation of airway fluid balance, improves bronchial clearance, and sets up a barrier to inhaled agents. First, the high surface pressure (low surface tension) of surfactant counteracts fluid influx into the airway lumen. Loss of surface activity would result in additional inward forces that cause fluid accumulation in the airway lumen. Secondly, surfactant improves bronchial clearance by optimizing transport of particles and bacteria from the peripheral to the more central airways. Moreover, surfactant has been shown to enhance mucociliary clearance (25), partly, by increasing ciliary beat frequency (26). Thirdly, several studies have suggested that surfactant sets up a barrier to the diffusion of inhaled agents including bacteria, allergens, and drugs (27,28). For example, depletion of the surfactant layer by lung lavage leads to augmented responses to drugs and allergens (29,30). Interestingly, exogenous surfactant treatment lessens the airway response to inhaled but not systemically given bronchoconstrictor stimuli in rats suggesting an airway barrier to drug diffusion (31). In addition, it has recently been shown that treatment of rats with exogenous phospholipids suppresses the neural activity of bronchial irritant receptors (32). This may support the view of a possible link between airway hyperresponsivenes and airway surfactant balance.

B. Morphology

Airway surfactant originates mainly from the alveoli where the majority of surfactant is synthesized and secreted by alveolar type II cells. During expiration, alveolar surfactant becomes extruded into adjacent conducting airways. In addition, local synthesis and release of phospholipids in tracheal epithelial cells have been demonstrated (33). Electron microscopy has revealed that surfactant material forming mono- and multilayers can be found at the air–liquid interface of the airway lumen. Additionally, multilamellar vesicles and lattice-like tubular myelin can be found within the hypophase of the epithelial lining fluid covering the airways (34).

As the surfactant phospholipids, surfactant proteins are mainly synthesized and secreted by alveolar type II cells. Surfactant-protein synthesis has also been shown in Clara cells (35,36), and SP-A and SP-D were found also in more proximal parts of the respiratory tract (37–39). In the adult human lung, SP-D was detected in type II cells, serous cells of tracheobronchial glands, and a subset of cells lining the peripheral airways (40). Whitsett and coworkers have shown that during lung development, the hydrophobic surfactant protein SP-B and SP-C mRNAs were first expressed in bronchi and bronchioles. Expression in epithelial cells of the bronchioloalveolar portals and in type II cells advanced with gestational age. In the fetal and adult human lung, SP-B and SP-C are expressed primarily in distal conducting and terminal airway epithelium (41). These data suggest that surfactant protein synthesis and secretion are not restricted to the alveolar compartment. Predominant expression of SP-B and SP-C in distal conducting and terminal airways might be related to local requirements with a major demand in optimizing biophysical surfactant properties. Presence of SP-A and SP-D in more proximal parts of the lung and even in extrapulmonary tissues indicates that they might be required for more ubiquitous functions, such as for innate and adaptive immune reactions, to protect against exogenous danger signals.

C. Composition

Data on the composition of airway surfactant are still limited by the fact that there is no method for selective sampling of surfactant from the conducting airways. Indirect evidence for airway surfactant to be mainly originated from the alveoli arises from analysis of airway secretions from tracheal aspirates that contain significant amounts of surfactant with a phospholipid composition similar to alveolar surfactant (9,21). In contrast, the concentrations of surfactant proteins have been found decreased in tracheal aspirates from porcine lungs (21).

An interesting approach to study airway surfactant function and composition arises from comparative biology. In contrast to the saccular or alveolar structure of mammalian lungs, the respiratory tract of birds has a completely different structure. Birds have tubular lungs that do not contain alveoli. Therefore, avian surfactant should predominantly function to maintain airflow through the lung tubules rather than preventing alveolar collapse. Therefore, we have recently investigated functional, structural, and biochemical parameters of avian surfactant. Although a uniform surfactant layer within the air tubules was demonstrable by electron microscopy, tubular myelin was absent in avian surfactant preparations. Although dynamic surface properties were impaired in bird surfactant, the ability to keep capillaries open was as good as with mammalian surfactant (42). When compared with mammalian surfactant, bird surfactant from duck and chicken was enriched in DPPC, but had less palmitoyl-myristoyl-phosphatidylcholine (PC16:0/14:0) and palmitoyl-pamitoleoyl-PC (PC16:0/16:1). For the latter two PC species, no defined role in mammalian surfactant has been established, but it has been shown that their concentrations increase during fetal development (43). This might indicate a specific function within the alveolus, such as promoting adsorption of DPPC which could serve to open or re-open collapsed alveoli. Although SP-B was detectable in avian surfactant, both SP-A and SP-C were absent. SP-B promotes film formation at the air–liquid interface (44). Accordingly, its presence in bird surfactant is consistent with good adsorption function demonstrated by studies with the pulsating bubble surfactometer (PBS) and the capillary surfactometer. The functional importance of SP-B for the airways is further supported by data from heterozygous SP-B $+/-$ mice that have a 50% decrease of SP-B mRNA and SP-B protein. These animals have increased residual volumes on pulmonary function testing, a variable that indicates an obstructive airway disease with air trapping (45). Further, in an animal model of asthma, it was demonstrated that the allergic inflammation resulted in a surfactant dysfunction, which was correlated with a reduction of SP-B in BALF (8). The assumption that SP-A and SP-C are less important for the biophysical function of surfactant in the airways is further supported by data from SP-A- and SP-C-deficient mice that have no apparent abnormalities in lung function or histopathology (46,47). In contrast, SP-D-deficient animals suffer from enlargement of terminal airways and emphysema (48). However, signs of obstructive airways disease in SP-D knock-out mice probably reflect the result of an imbalanced chronic lung inflammation with pathological airway remodeling rather than an impact of lacking SP-D on biophysical surfactant function in the airways.

III. Surfactant Alterations in Asthma

Data on surfactant composition and function in asthma have been derived both in asthmatic patients and from murine asthma models. In a murine model of asthma,

it has been reported that guinea pigs sensitized with ovalbumin, and then challenged with aerosolized antigen, reacted with a leakage of plasma proteins into
the airways, a markedly increased airway resistance, and an altered surfactant performance indicating a dysfunction (7). Recently, in mite allergen-induced airway
inflammation, decreased levels of SP-A and SP-D in BALF from sensitized mice
have been reported (49). In contrast, in various strains of sensitized mice allergen
challenge induced an increase of SP-A and SP-D immunostaining in nonciliated
airway epithelial cells, whereas SP-B immunostaining was unchanged (50).
This up-regulation of SP-A and SP-D was dependent on the presence of lymphocytes because gene-targeted mice lacking functional lymphocytes did not respond
with changes in their surfactant proteins. Furthermore, others have demonstrated
that allergen-induced airway inflammation is associated with down-regulation of
SP-C, whereas SP-A and SP-D were up-regulated (51). The down-regulation of
the hSP-C promoter in this animal model was found to be IL-5-dependent, high-
lighting the critical role for eosinophilic inflammation. Finally, in a murine asthma
model, it was shown that levels of SP-B and SP-C protein and mRNA decreased
and that SP-D levels increased, whereas SP-A was unchanged (52). These data on
changes of surfactant proteins upon allergen challenge in sensitized animals
suggest that the hydrophobic apoproteins SP-B and SP-C that are mainly responsible for surface activity probably become reduced, whereas the collectins SP-A
and SP-D are up-regulated upon allergen challenge. However, discrepancies in
the published results remain and might be explained because of differences in
animal models or differences in time points studied.

A further interesting finding on surfactant alterations in asthma results from
mice overexpressing IL-4 in the airways under the control of the Clara cell
secretory protein promotor. Although total SP-A and SP-B levels in bronchoalveolar fluids and lung homogenates were increased, SP-B positive cells were
decreased in bronchial and bronchiolar epithelial cells, but staining was
unchanged in alveolar type II cells (53). It might be speculated that in asthma,
the allergic inflammation with increased amounts of IL-4 in the airway environment leads to diminished local SP-B levels that can account for airway obstruction as seen in heterozygous SP-B deficient mice. This view is further supported
by data from Haczku et al. (8) who found decreased BAL levels of SP-B protein
and SP-B mRNA following intratracheal administration of IL-4 to aspergillus-
sensitized mice. The concept that the surfactant system is influenced during an
allergic inflammatory reaction is additionally strengthened by data from
Homer et al. (54) who showed alveolar type II cell hypertrophy with an increase
of BAL surfactant phospholipids and elevations of the SP-A, -B, -C, and -D in
mice overexpressing IL-13, an important TH2 cytokine in asthma. These data,
at least, suggest that cytokine changes with increases of IL-4 and IL-13 as they
occur in asthma are accompanied with alterations of surfactant proteins and
phospholipids.

In the last couple of years, data from patients with asthma are accumulating
but are still rare. Kurashima et al. (55) reported that sputum samples from patients

with asthma have a low surface activity. In addition, when asthma patients are compared with healthy controls, the percentage of DPPC decreased in sputum but not in BALF, SP-A levels were found unchanged (9). Interestingly, the percentage of DPPC in sputum correlated to the lung function variable FEV_1 (forced expiratory volume in 1 s). We have recently investigated the inflammatory changes of bronchoalveolar lavage fluid and the performance of BALF surfactant in healthy controls and patients with mild allergic asthma, before and after segmental allergen challenge. Allergen challenge of asthmatics, but not of healthy volunteers, significantly increased eosinophils, proteins, ratio of small to large surfactant aggregates (SA/LA), and decreased surface activity measured with the PBS and the capillary surfactometer (5). Analysis of phospholipid molecular species from BALF and plasma suggested that changes in PC composition in BALF in asthmatics subjects after allergen challenge were due to infiltration of plasma lipoproteins, but not due to phospholipid catabolism (56). Thus, the most likely reason for disturbed surfactant function was that proteins had invaded the airways as they reached a 10-fold increase in concentration. Proteins have extensively been proven to inhibit surfactant function (57,58). Interestingly, a washing procedure with saline that removed water-soluble inhibitors, such as the proteins, restored surfactant function. van de Graaf et al. (59) described that BALF levels of SP-A were lowered in patients with asthma. In contrast, Cheng et al. (60) found increased levels of SP-A and SP-D in bronchial and alveolar lavages in mild, stable asthmatics compared with controls. Taken together, data derived both in asthmatic patients and from murine asthma models undoubtedly suggest that surfactant alterations with disturbance of surfactant function, changes in surfactant protein expression and phospholipid levels occur following induction of an allergic inflammatory reaction.

IV. Modulation of Immune Cells in Allergic Inflammation

Besides the important biophysical properties of pulmonary surfactant, its role in immunomodulation has attracted increasing interest in asthma. The hydrophilic surfactant proteins SP-A and SP-D are important components of the innate immune response by modulating macrophage antimicrobial properties (61). The structural motifs of the lung collectins SP-A and SP-D suggest that these molecules in addition to microbial binding and interaction with cellular receptors of macrophages possess binding capacities for other environmentally derived invaders of the airways, such as allergens and particles, and might interact with cells of the adaptive immune response.

In asthma, the important immune cells in the allergic inflammatory response are dendritic cells, T-helper lymphocytes, IgE-producing B-lymphocytes (plasma cells), mast cells, and eosinophils. Of course, airway inflammation in asthma is a more complex scenario that also includes epithelial cells, smooth muscle cells, and parenchymal cells. However, available data on the effect of surfactant components on the latter cells are rare.

A. Allergen Binding

Inhaled allergens are initially dissolved into the airway lining fluid before they come into contact with immune cells. The airway lining fluid contains surfactant and therefore an initial contact between allergens and surfactant components will occur soon after inhalation and deposition into the airway lining fluid. Surfactant protein A has been shown to bind to water-extractable particles of pollen grains (16). Although pollen grains itself do not reach the lower airways because of their large diameter of 20–30 μm, they release starch granules that are readily inhalable and can reach the lower airways. It has been demonstrated that both SP-A and SP-D interact with inhalable mite allergens in a carbohydrate-specific and calcium-dependent manner (62). SP-A and SP-D were also found to inhibit allergen-specific IgE binding to mite allergens. Additionally, SP-A and SP-D bound to carbohydrate components on allergens from *Aspergillus fumigatus* (63). These data may suggest that lung collectins inhibit the induction of allergic reactions by direct allergen binding. This in turn would be beneficial both in preventing acute asthma attacks by inhibition of the allergen-specific IgE binding and possibly by inhibition of allergen uptake by dendritic cells. However, the fate of surfactant protein-bound allergen is unclear and needs future research.

B. Dendritic Cells

A very early step in the induction of the allergic inflammation is allergen uptake by dendritic cells (DCs), antigen processing, and subsequent antigen presentation to T lymphocytes. Antigens stimulate immature DCs in the lung to differentiate into mature DCs by changing their expression of surface markers, such as chemokine receptors or T cell regulatory molecules. Mature DCs migrate to the lymph nodes where they activate T cells. Endogenous and exogenous factors can modulate the immune responses of DCs. For example, lipopolysaccharide or microbial DNA binds to toll-like receptors on the DCs and thereby induce maturation. Recently, it has been shown that SP-A influenced the phenotypic and functional differentiation of immature DCs to become potent T cell stimulators. SP-A, but not SP-D, inhibited the maturation of DCs with decreased expression of MHC class II and CD86, resulting in a decreased T cell allostimulatory ability. Moreover, SP-A enhanced the endocytotic ability of DCs and enhanced chemotactic responses (15). These intriguing results demonstrate the potential role of surfactant proteins in regulating adaptive immune responses through interactions with DCs and suggest that the lung collectins are capable in determining the course of an immune response. In the allergen-induced inflammation, this might imply the potential of modulating Th1 vs. Th2 immune responses.

C. Lymphocytes

T lymphocyte proliferation or cytokine release is an important step in the further activation of the adaptive immune system in asthma. This T cell response can induce B lymphocyte differentiation into specific IgE antibody secreting plasma cells. In addition, IL-5 release by T lymphocytes attracts and activates eosinophils and prolongs eosinophil survival. Lymphocyte activity and proliferation can be down-regulated by the surfactant phospholipids and by the lung collectins SP-A and SP-D (12,13,64,65). Both SP-A and SP-D inhibited production and release of IL-2. The ability of lung collectins to regulate immune cells has been shown to be affected by the presence of lipids (66). Importantly, it has recently been demonstrated that surfactant proteins SP-A and SP-D inhibit allergen-induced proliferation of lymphocytes and inhibit histamine release from whole blood of atopic donors in response to the house dust mite allergen *Dermatophagoides pteronyssinus (Der p)* in a dose-dependent manner (14,62). These data suggest that lung collectins may be important molecules in asthma pathogenesis both during the acute asthma attack characterized by histamine release and in the chronic airway inflammation by modulating lymphocyte proliferation.

D. Eosinophils

Eosinophils play an important role in chronic airway inflammation in asthma. It has been shown by Cheng et al. (67) that SP-A suppresses the production and release of IL-8 by eosinophils stimulated by ionomycin. The SP-A effect was concentration dependent and reversed by addition of an SP-A antibody. We have recently demonstrated that the IL-5 stimulated expression of activation markers CD69 and HLA-DR on eosinophils was reduced in the presence of natural bovine lipid extract surfactant in a concentration-dependent fashion (68). This effect was presumably mediated by the lipid fraction of the surfactant preparation and definitely not mediated by SP-A as the lipid extracted surfactant contained no hydrophilic surfactant proteins. There is one recent report that zymosan-activated eosinophils stimulate phosphatidylcholine secretion in cultured type II pneumocytes (69). These findings may suggest a feedback-loop between surfactant release and eosinophil activation. However, much more research is needed to better understand the network between surfactant components, eosinophil activation, and their mediator release.

V. Therapeutic Potential and Clinical Aspects

Published data from the literature support the concept that a poor function of surfactant contributes to the pathophysiologic scenario in asthma. Thus, it seems justified to investigate the potential role of surfactant therapy in asthma. There are two different ways to improve the surfactant balance in the airways. First, various drugs that are commonly used in asthma therapy, such as corticosteroids, β-adrenergic agents, and theophylline, have been shown to stimulate surfactant synthesis or secretion (70–72). However, it remains to be determined whether pharmacological stimuli can augment surfactant secretion to an extent that could be clinically relevant. Secondly, treatment with exogenous surfactant has been shown to improve allergic airway obstruction in animal models of asthma. Prophylactic treatment of sensitized animals with intratracheal instillation of surfactant reduces the deteriorating lung function that otherwise would have developed (73). In studies from another laboratory, it was demonstrated that treatment of immunized guinea pigs with aerosolized surfactant alleviates an increase in airway resistance elicited by allergen challenge (74).

As the lung collectins SP-A and SP-D have various effects on immune cells involved in asthma, their therapeutic potential was tested in murine asthma models. Accordingly, treatment of aspergillus-sensitized mice with a recombinant fragment of human SP-D was effective in reducing the eosinophilic inflammation and specific IgE production in this asthma model. Furthermore, bronchial hyperresponsiveness in SP-D-treated animals compared with controls was inhibited and there was a shift from a TH2 cytokine pattern towards a TH1 response with increases of IL-12 and IFN-γ, but decreases of IL-4 and IL-5 (18,19). Our unpublished data revealed that this recombinant fragment of human SP-D also alleviates airway obstruction during the early phase reaction upon allergen challenge in aspergillus-sensitized mice. SP-A also decreased peripheral blood eosinophilia and reduced TH2 cytokine levels induced by allergen challenge in sensitized mice (18).

Human data are rare and are restricted to the use of commercially available natural or synthetic surfactant preparations. A small randomized controlled trial demonstrated a significant improvement of pulmonary function data after inhalation of surfactant in patients with acute asthma attacks (75). In addition, inhalation of a synthetic surfactant preparation artificial lung expanding compound (ALEC) reduced the degree of bronchoconstriction induced by allergen challenge in asthmatics compared with controls (76). In contrast, nebulized surfactant did not alter airway obstruction and bronchial responsiveness to histamine in asthmatic children with mild airflow limitation (77). A prospective randomized controlled trial of aerosolized synthetic surfactant (Exosurf) in 87 adult patients with stable chronic bronchitis revealed a significant improvement of forced expiratory volume in 1 s of 11%, a decrease of thoracic gas trapping by 6%, and an improvement of sputum transportability (78). Recently, it has been reported that exogenous surfactant improved disease course in infants with respiratory syncytial virus bronchiolitis (79), an obstructive airways disease where a surfactant dysfunction has been demonstrated (80). Taken together, these results demonstrate that exogenous surfactant therapy might have at least some beneficial effect in patients with asthma and obstructive airways disease. However, exogenous surfactant therapy is expensive and therefore still limited to research and case studies. Future investigations will help to unravel relevant surfactant components with the best antiobstructive effects and the most potent antiinflammatory capacity.

VI. Conclusions

Pulmonary surfactant with an optimal function in the airways is important because it stabilizes the conducting airways, prevents fluid accumulation within the airway lumen, improves bronchial clearance, acts as a barrier to the uptake of inhaled agents, and has important immunomodulatory properties. In asthma, it has been demonstrated that there is a surfactant dysfunction due to inhibition by proteins that have derived during the inflammatory process in the airways and due to diminished levels of SP-B, an apoprotein of evident importance for proper surfactant function. Besides the biophysical properties of airway surfactant, surfactant components, especially the lung collectins SP-A and SP-D have been shown to interact with immune cells that are involved in the allergic inflammation. Overall, the lung collectins seem to decrease the degree of allergic inflammation through a variety of interactions with DCs, lymphocytes, eosinophils, mast cells, and the allergens itself. Therefore, therapeutic interventions that improve airway surfactant function or modulate the allergic inflammation by exogenous surfactant supplementation or by stimulation of the endogenous surfactant system might prove beneficial in patients with asthma.

References

1. Avery ME, Mead J. Surface properties in relation to atelectasis and hyaline membrane disease. Am J Dis Child 1959; 97:517–523.
2. Günther A, Siebert C, Schmidt R, Ziegler S, Grimmiger F, Yabut M, Temmesfeld B, Walmrath D, Morr H, Seeger W. Surfactant alterations in severe pneumonia, acute respiratory distress syndrome, and cardiogenic lung edema. Am J Respir Crit Care Med 1996; 153:176–184.
3. Hohlfeld J, Tiryaki E, Hamm H, Hoymann HG, Krug N, Haverich A, Fabel H. Pulmonary surfactant activity is impaired in lung transplant recipients. Am J Respir Crit Care Med 1998; 158:706–712.
4. Griese M, Birrer P, Demirsoy A. Pulmonary surfactant in cystic fibrosis. Eur Respir J 1997; 10:1983–1988.
5. Hohlfeld JM, Ahlf K, Enhorning G, Balke K, Erpenbeck VJ, Petschallies J, Hoymann HG, Fabel H, Krug N. Dysfunction of pulmonary surfactant in asthmatics after segmental allergen challenge. Am J Respir Crit Care Med 1999; 159:1803–1809.
6. Hohlfeld JM. The role of pulmonary surfactant in asthma. Respir Res 2002; 3:4.
7. Liu M, Wang L, Enhorning G. Surfactant dysfunction develops when the immunized guinea-pig is challenged with ovalbumin aerosol. Clin Exp Allergy 1995; 25:1053–1060.
8. Haczku A, Atochina EN, Tomer Y, Cao Y, Campbell C, Scanlon ST, Russo SJ, Enhorning G, Beers M. The late asthmatic response is linked with increased surface tension and reduced surfactant protein B in mice. Am J Physiol Lung Cell Mol Physiol 2002; 283:L755–L765.
9. Wright SM, Hockey PM, Enhorning G, Strong P, Reid KBM, Holgate ST, Djukanovic R, Postle AD. Altered airway surfactant phospholipid composition and reduced lung function in asthma. J Appl Physiol 2000; 89:1283–1292.
10. Hohlfeld J, Fabel H, Hamm H. The role of pulmonary surfactant in obstructive airways disease. Eur Respir J 1997; 10:482–491.

11. Djukanovic R, Roche WR, Wilson JW, Beasley CR, Twentyman OP, Howarth RH, Holgate ST. Mucosal inflammation in asthma. Am Rev Respir Dis 1990; 142:434–457.

12. Borron P, Veldhuizen RAW, Lewis JF, Possmayer F, Caveney A, Inchley K, McFadden RG, Fraher LJ. Surfactant associated protein-A inhibits human lymphocyte proliferation and IL-2 production. Am J Respir Cell Mol Biol 1996; 15:115–121.

13. Borron PJ, Crouch EC, Lewis JF, Wright JR, Possmayer F, Fraher LJ. Recombinant rat surfactant-associated protein D inhibits human T lymphocyte proliferation and IL-2 production. J Immunol 1998; 161:4599–4603.

14. Wang JY, Shieh CC, You PF, Lei HY, Reid KBM. Inhibitory effect of pulmonary surfactant proteins A and D on allergen-induced lymphocyte proliferation and histamine release in children with asthma. Am J Respir Crit Care Med 1998; 158:510–518.

15. Brinker KG, Garner H, Wright JR. Surfactant protein A modulates the differentiation of murine bone marrow-derived dendritic cells. Am J Physiol Lung Cell Mol Physiol 2003; 284:L232–L241.

16. Malhotra R, Haurum J, Thiel S, Jensenius JC, Sims RB. Pollen grains bind to lung alveolar type II cells (A549) via lung surfactant protein A (SP-A). Biosci Rep 1993; 13:79–90.

17. Reid KB. Interactions of surfactant protein D with pathogens, allergens, and phagocytes. Biochim Biophys Acta 1998; 1408:290–295.

18. Madan T, Kishore U, Singh M, Strong P, Clark H, Hussain EM, Reid KB, Sarma PU. Surfactant proteins A and D protect mice against pulmonary hypersensitivity induced by *Aspergillus fumigatus* antigens and allergens. J Clin Invest 2001; 107:467–475.

19. Strong P, Reid KBM, Clark H. Intranasal delivery of a truncated recombinant human SP-D is effective at down-regulating allergic hypersensitivity in mice to allergens of *Aspergillus fumigatus*. Clin Exp Immunol 2002; 130:19–24.

20. Gehr P, Geiser M, Im Hof V, Schürch S, Waber U, Baumann M. Surfactant and inhaled particles in the conducting airways: structural, stereological, and biophysical aspects. Microsc Res Tech 1993; 26:423–436.

21. Bernhard W, Haagsman HP, Tschernig T, Poets CF, Postle AD, van Eijk ME, von der Hardt H. Conductive airway surfactant: surface-tension function, biochemical composition, and possible alveolar origin. Am J Respir Cell Mol Biol 1997; 17:4150.

22. Liu M, Wang L, Li E, Enhorning G. Pulmonary surfactant will secure free airflow through a narrow tube. J Appl Physiol 1991; 71:742–748.

23. Enhorning G, Duffy LC, Welliver RC. Pulmonary surfactant maintains patency of conducting airways in the rat. Am J Respir Crit Care Med 1995; 151:554–556.

24. Enhorning G, Hohlfeld J, Krug N, Lema G, Welliver RC. Surfactant function affected by airway inflammation and cooling: possible impact on exercise-induced asthma. Eur Respir J 2000; 15:532–538.

25. De Sanctis GT, Tomkiewicz RP, Rubin BK, Schürch S, King M. Exogenous surfactant enhances mucociliary clearance in the anaesthetized dog. Eur Respir J 1994; 7:1616–1621.

26. Kakuta Y, Sasaki H, Takishima T. Effect of artificial surfactant on ciliary beat frequency in guinea pig trachea. Respir Physiol 1991; 83:313–321.

27. Widdicombe JG. Airway liquid: a barrier to drug diffusion? Eur Respir J 1997; 10:2194–2197.

28. Hills BA. Asthma: is there an airway receptor barrier? Thorax 1996; 51:773–776.

29. So KL, Gommers D, Lachmann B. Bronchoalveolar surfactant and intratracheal adrenaline. Lancet 1993; 341:120–121.

30. Kiekhaefer CM, Kelly EAB, Jarjour NN. Enhanced antigen-induced eosinophilia with prior bronchoalveolar lavage. Am J Respir Crit Care Med 1999; 159:A99.

31. Hohlfeld J, Hoymann HG, Molthan J, Fabel H, Heinrich U. Aerosolized surfactant inhibits acetylcholine-induced airway obstruction in rats. Eur Respir J 1997; 10:2198–2203.

32. Hills BA, Chen Y. Suppression of neural activity of bronchial irritant receptors by surface-active phospholipid in comparison with topical drugs commonly prescribed for asthma. Clin Exp Allergy 2000; 30:1266–1274.

33. Barrow RE. Chemical structure of phospholipids in the lungs and airways of sheep. Respir Physiol 1990; 79:1–8.

34. Sims DE, Horne MM. Heterogeneity of the composition and thickness of tracheal mucus in rats. Am J Physiol (Lung Cell Mol Physiol) 1997; 273:L1036–L1041.

35. Auten RL, Watkins RH, Shapiro DL, Horowitz S. Surfactant apoprotein A (SP-A) is synthetized in airway cells. Am J Respir Cell Mol Biol 1990; 3:491–496.

36. Voorhout WF, Veenendaal T, Kuroki Y, Ogasawara Y, van Golde LM, Geuze HJ. Immunocytochemical localization of surfactant protein D (SP-D) in type II cells, Clara cells, and alveolar macrophages of rat lung. J Histochem Cytochem 1992; 40:1589–1597.

37. Khoor A, Gray ME, Hull WM, Whitsett JA, Stahlman MT. Developmental expression of SP-A and SP-A mRNA in the proximal and distal respiratory epithelium in the human fetus and newborn. J Histochem Cytochem 1993; 41:1311–1319.

38. Xu P, Hashimoto S, Miyazaki H, Asabe K, Shiraishi S, Sueishi K. Morphometric analysis of the immunohistochemical expression of Clara cell 10-kDa protein and surfactant apoproteins A and B in the developing bronchi and bronchioles of human fetuses and neonates. Virchows Arch 1998; 432:17–25.

39. Madsen J, Kliem A, Tornoe I, Skjodt K, Koch C, Holmskov U. Localization of lung surfactant protein D on mucosal surfaces in human tissues. J Immunol 2000; 164:5866–5870.

40. Stahlman MT, Gray ME, Hull WM, Whitsett JA. Immunolocalization of surfactant protein-D (SP-D) human fetal, newborn, and adult tissues. J Histochem Cytochem 2002; 50:651–660.

41. Khoor A, Stahlman MT, Gray ME, Whitsett JA. Temporal–spatial distribution of SP-B and SP-C proteins and mRNAs in developing respiratory epithelium of human lung. J Histochem Cytochem 1994; 42:1187–1199.

42. Bernhard W, Gebert A, Vieten G, Rau GA, Hohlfeld JM, Postle AD, Freihorst J. Pulmonary surfactant in birds: coping with surface tension in a tubular lung. Am J Physiol (Regul Integr Comp Physiol) 2001; 281:R327–R337.

43. Hunt AN, Kelly FJ, Postle AD. Developmental variation in whole human lung phosphatidylcholine molecular species: a comparison with guinea pig and rat. Early Hum Dev 1991; 25:157–171.

44. Possmayer F, Nag K, Rodriguez Capote K, Qanbar R, Schürch S. Role of surfactant apoproteins in surfactant function. Appl Cardiol 2000; 9:283–285.

45. Clark JC, Weaver TE, Iwamoto HS, Ikegami M, Jobe AH, Hull WM, Whitsett JA. Decreased lung compliance and air trapping in heterozygous SP-B-deficient mice. Am J Respir Cell Mol Biol 1997; 16:46–52.

46. Korfhagen TR, LeVine AM, Whitsett JA. Surfactant protein A (SP-A) gene targeted mice. Biochim Biophys Acta 1998; 1408:296–302.

47. Glasser SW, Burhans MS, Korfhagen TR, Na CL, Sly PD, Ross GF, Ikegami M, Whitsett JA. Altered stability of pulmonary surfactant in SP-C deficient mice. Proc Natl Acad Sci 2001; 98:6366–6371.

48. Wert SE, Yoshida M, LeVine AM, Ikegami M, Jones T, Ross GF, Fisher JH, Korfhagen TR, Whitsett JA. Increased metalloproteinase activity, oxidant production, and emphysema in surfactant protein D gene-inactivated mice. Proc Natl Acad Sci 2000; 97:5972–5977.

49. Wang JY, Shieh CC, Yu CK, Lei HY. Allergen-induced bronchial inflammation is associated with decreased levels of surfactant proteins A and D in a murine model of asthma. Clin Exp Allergy 2001; 31:652–662.

50. Haley KJ, Ciota A, Contreras JP, Boothby MR, Perkins DL, Finn PW. Alterations in lung collectins in an adaptive immune response. Am J Physiol Lung Cell Mol Physiol 2002; 282:L573–L584.

51. Mishra A, Weaver TE, Beck DC, Rothenberg ME. Interleukin-5-mediated allergic airway inflammation inhibits the human surfactant protein C promotor in transgenic mice. J Biol Chem 2001; 276:8453–8459.

52. Haczku A, Atochina EN, Tomer Y, Chen H, Scanlon ST, Russo S, Xu J, Panettieri RAJ, Beers M. *Aspergillus-fumigatus*-induced allergic airway inflammation alters surfactant homeostasis and lung function in BALB (c mice). Am J Respir Cell Mol Biol 2001; 25:45–50.

53. Jain-Vora S, Wert SE, Temann UA, Rankin JA, Whitsett JA. Interleukin-4 alters epithelial cell differentiation and surfactant homeostasis in the postnatal mouse lung. Am J Respir Cell Mol Biol 1997; 17:541–551.

54. Homer R, Zheng T, Chupp G, He S, Zhu Z, Chen Q, Ma B, Hite RD, Gobran LI, Rooney SA, Elias JA. Pulmonary type II cell hypertrophy and pulmonary lipoproteinosis are features of chronic IL-13 exposure. Am J Physiol Lung Cell Mol Physiol 2002; 283:L52–L59.

55. Kurashima K, Fujimura M, Matsuda T, Kobayashi T. Surface activity of sputum from acute asthmatic patients. Am J Respir Crit Care Med 1997; 155:1254–1259.

56. Heeley EL, Hohlfeld JM, Krug N, Postle AD. Phospholipid molecular species of bronchoalveolar lavage fluid after local allergen challenge in asthma. Am J Physiol (Lung Cell Mol Physiol) 2000; 278:L305–L311.

57. Fuchimukai T, Fujiwara T, Takahashi A, Enhorning G. Artificial pulmonary surfactant inhibited by proteins. J Appl Physiol 1987; 62:429–437.

58. Seeger W, Grube C, Günther A, Schmidt R. Surfactant inhibition by plasma proteins: differential sensitivity of various surfactant preparations. Eur Respir J 1993; 6:971–977.

59. van de Graaf EA, Jansen HM, Lutter R, Alberts C, Kobesen J, de Vries IJ, Out TA. Surfactant protein A in bronchoalveolar lavage fluid. J Lab Clin Med 1992; 120:252–263.

60. Cheng G, Ueda T, Numao T, Kuroki Y, Nakajima H, Fukushima Y, Motojima S, Fukuda T. Increased levels of surfactant protein A and D in bronchoalveolar lavage fluids in patients with bronchial asthma. Eur Respir J 2000; 16:831–835.

61. Crouch E, Wright JR. Surfactant proteins A and D and pulmonary host defence. Annu Rev Physiol 2001; 63:521–554.

62. Wang JY, Kishore U, Lim BL, Strong P, Reid KBM. Interaction of human lung surfactant proteins A and D with mite (*Dermatophagoides pteronyssinus*) allergens. Clin Exp Immunol 1996; 106:367–373.

63. Madan T, Kishore U, Shah A, Eggleton P, Strong P, Wang JY, Aggrawal SS, Sarma PU, Reid KB. Lung surfactant proteins A and D can inhibit specific IgE binding to the allergens of *Aspergillus fumigatus* and block allergen-induced histamine release from human basophils. Clin Exp Immunol 1997; 110:241–249.

64. Ansfield MJ, Kaltreider HB, Benson BJ, Caldwell JL. Immunosuppressive activity of canine pulmonary surface active material. J Immunol 1979; 122:1062–1066.

65. Sitrin RG, Ansfield MJ, Kaltreider HB. The effect of pulmonary surface-active material on the generation and expression of murine B- and T-lymphocyte effector functions *in vitro*. Exp Lung Res 1985; 9:85–97.

66. Kremlev SG, Umstead TM, Phelps DS. Effects of surfactant protein A and surfactant lipids on lymphocyte proliferation in vitro. Am J Physiol (Lung Cell Mol Physiol) 1994; 267:L357–L364.

67. Cheng G, Ueda T, Nakajima H, Kinjyo S, Motojima S, Fukuda T. Suppressive effects of SP-A on ionomycin-induced IL-8 production and release by eosinophils. Int Arch Allergy Immunol 1998; 117(suppl 1):59–62.

68. Hohlfeld JM, Knöß S, Schael M, Fabel H, Krug N. Pulmonary surfactant inhibits expression of HLA-DR and CD69 on human eosinophils (abstract). Am J Respir Crit Care Med 2000; 161(3 pt 2):A662.

69. Okumura M, Tsuruoka M, Isohama Y, Kai H, Takahama K, Miyata T. Activated eosinophils stimulate phosphatidylcholine secretion in primary culture of rat type II pneumocytes. Biochem Mol Biol Int 1996; 38:569–575.

70. Dobbs LG, Mason RJ. Pulmonary alveolar type II cells isolated from rats. Release of phosphatidylcholine in response to β-adrenergic stimulation. J Clin Invest 1979; 63:378–387.

71. Ekelund L, Burgoyne R, Brymer D, Enhorning G. Pulmonary surfactant release in fetal rabbits as affected by terbutaline and aminophyllin. Scand J Clin Lab Invest 1981; 41:237–245.

72. van Golde LMG. Synthesis of surfactant lipids in the adult lung. Annu Rev Physiol 1985; 47:765–774.

73. Liu M, Wang L, Li E, Enhorning G. Pulmonary surfactant given prophylactically alleviates an asthma attack in guinea-pigs. Clin Exp Allergy 1996; 26:270–275.

74. Kurashima K, Fujimura M, Tsujiura M, Matsuda T. Effect of surfactant inhalation on allergic bronchocontriction in guinea pigs. Clin Exp Allergy 1997; 27:337–342.

75. Kurashima K, Ogawa H, Ohka T, Fujimura M, Matsuda T, Kobayashi T. A pilot study of surfactant inhalation in the treatment of asthmatic attack. Aerugi (Jpn J Allergol) 1991; 40:160–163.

76. Babu KS, Woodcock DA, Smith SE, Staniforth JN, Holgate ST, Conway JH. Inhaled synthetic surfactant abolishes the early allergen-induced response in asthma. Eur Respir J 2003; 21:1046–1049.

77. Oetomo SB, Dorrepaal C, Bos H, Gerritsen J, van der Mark TW, Koeter GH, van Aalderen WMC. Surfactant nebulization does not alter airflow obstruction and bronchial responsiveness to histamine in asthmatic children. Am J Respir Crit Care Med 1996; 153:1148–1152.

78. Anzueto A, Jubran A, Ohar JA, Piquette CA, Rennard SI, Colice G, Pattishall EN, Barrett J, Engle M, Perret KA, Rubin BK. Effects of aerosolized surfactant in patients with stable chronic bronchitis. A prospective randomized controlled trial. J Am Med Assoc 1997; 278:1426–1431.

79. Tibby SM, Hatherill M, Wright SM, Wilson P, Postle AD, Murdoch IA. Exogenous surfactant supplementation in infants with respiratory syncytial virus bronchiolitis. Am J Respir Crit Care Med 2000; 162:1251–1256.

80. van Schaik SM, Vargas I, Welliver RC, Enhorning G. Surfactant dysfunction develops in BALB/c mice infected with respiratory syncytial virus. Pediatr Res 1997; 42:169–173.

17

Surfactant Treatment for Inflammatory Lung Disease

EGBERT HERTING

University of Lübeck,
Lübeck, Germany

BENGT ROBERTSON

Karolinska University Hospital,
Stockholm, Sweden

I. Introduction

During the last decade, surfactant administration has become standard for treatment of premature neonates with severe respiratory distress syndrome (RDS). Randomized controlled trials and meta-analyses clearly demonstrate improved gas exchange following surfactant instillation as well as significantly reduced neonatal morbidity and mortality (1).

More than 30 years ago, Ashbaugh et al. (2) described a form of severe respiratory failure in adults similar to neonatal RDS. However, in contrast to RDS caused by primary surfactant deficiency due to immaturity, the adult form of the disease, now called acute respiratory distress syndrome (ARDS), is caused by secondary surfactant dysfunction due to the liberation of surfactant inhibitors or leakage of plasma proteins into the bronchoalveolar space (3,4).

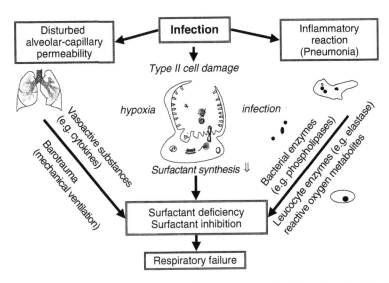

Figure 17.1 Pathophysiology of neonatal pneumonia and surfactant dysfunction (11).

Pulmonary or systemic infections are the major etiological factor for ARDS in all age groups including childhood (3). Proteins or enzymes and reactive oxygen metabolites released by leukocytes and/or bacteria inhibit surfactant function (Fig. 17.1) both *in vitro* and in animal studies (5–7). Recent clinical trials demonstrated improved gas exchange following surfactant treatment in newborn infants with bacterial pneumonia or meconium aspiration syndrome (8–10).

The large alveolar surface of the lung is constantly exposed to air polluted with microbial agents, dust, and other foreign particles. In the last decade, it was realized that surfactant and its major components, both the lipids and specific proteins, play an important role in the pulmonary host defense system [reviewed in Ref. (12)]. These "nonbiophysical" ("nonsurfactant") functions of the surfactant film seem to be of importance not only in directly limiting bacterial growth, but also in controlling the immune response and avoiding hypersensitivity reactions in the lung.

So far, exogenous surfactant has mostly been given to patients in acute respiratory failure, but future indications might include, for example, pneumonia, asthma, cystic fibrosis, bronchiolitis, and bronchopulmonary dysplasia, as inflammatory reactions are important features in the pathophysiology of these conditions as well. The role of surfactant in allergic lung disease is reviewed elsewhere in this book (Chapter 9).

II. *In Vitro* Studies

A. Influence of Surfactant on Bacterial Growth

Patients with severe respiratory failure due to bacterial pneumonia may receive exogenous surfactant. It has been speculated that surfactant given under such circumstances might serve as a nutrient for bacteria and thereby promote microbial growth (13). Only few reports, with diverging results, have been published concerning the direct influence of surfactant on bacterial growth (14–17). These studies evaluated the effects of low phospholipid concentrations (<1 mg/ mL). Also, the authors did not specify the phospholipid concentration of the surfactant material, as crude extracts of bronchoalveolar lavage fluid (BAL) from animal sources were used. Only two studies have analyzed bacterial growth in the presence of commercially available surfactant preparations currently used for replacement therapy in newborns. Sherman et al. (13) reported that complete natural surfactant derived from human amniotic fluid or natural sheep BAL fluid promoted growth of group B streptococci (GBS), whereas Exosurf®, a synthetic surfactant containing two alcohols as spreading agents, was bactericidal. Intermediate effects were observed for modified natural surfactants derived from bovine, porcine, or calf lungs. Neumeister et al. (18) observed that the modified bovine surfactant Survanta® significantly promoted the growth of *Escherichia coli*. However, these observations were either limited to one bacterial strain (13) and/or one phospholipid concentration (13,18).

We, therefore, examined the effects of different phospholipid concentrations of three modified natural (Curosurf®, Alveofact®, and Survanta) and two synthetic (Exosurf and Pumactant®) surfactant preparations on the *in vitro* proliferation of GBS, *Staphyloccocus aureus*, and *E. coli*, as these three bacteria are responsible for most cases of early onset infections in the neonatal period (19).

GBS, *S. aureus*, and *E. coli* were incubated in a nutrient-free medium (normal saline) for 5 h at 37°C together with different surfactants at concentrations of 0, 1, 10, and 20 mg/mL. With the exception of *E. coli*, incubation in saline alone led to a variable decrease in colony forming units (CFU). In the presence of Alveofact, Exosurf, and Pumactant, the decline in bacterial numbers was less marked than in saline alone (Fig. 17.2). Curosurf was bactericidal for GBS in a dose-dependent fashion and had a strong negative impact on the growth of a GBS subtype that lacked the polysaccharide capsule (GBS HD). In contrast, Survanta (10 and 20 mg/mL) significantly promoted the growth of *E. coli* indicating that surfactant components may actually serve as nutrients (Fig. 17.2). For *S. aureus*, incubation in saline alone had a bactericidal effect. When Curosurf was added, *S. aureus* were protected to some extent against the negative impact of the nutrient-free medium on microbial viability. In contrast, the viability of *E. coli* was unaffected by Curosurf as well as by Alveofact, Exosurf, and Pumactant. These results probably reflect variations in the metabolic demands of different bacteria. In our *in vitro* assay system, the bacteria were incubated in sterile saline, a nutrient-free medium. However, our own results of incubation of GBS and Curosurf in a culture medium containing glucose and protein as well as similar studies by Neumeister et al. (18) demonstrated that incubation of bacteria in nutrient-rich growth-promoting broth might mask the effects of surfactant that were observed when saline alone was used as a medium. Under normal physiological circumstances, the alveolar lining fluid may be considered to be relatively poor in nutrient content (20).

However, in the course of pneumonia and mechanical ventilation serum components including albumin and glucose may leak into the bronchoalveolar space and increase the amount of nutrients available for bacterial proliferation.

Both the nonencapsulated GBS HD and *S. aureus* showed a slight decline in CFU during 5 h incubation in sterile saline alone. GBS HD, the nonencapsulated phase variant, demonstrated a strong decline in viability when incubated with

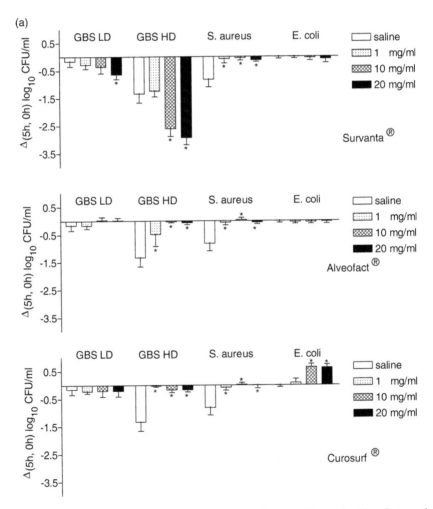

Figure 17.2 Effects of the natural modified surfactants Curosurf, Alveofact, and Survanta (a) and the synthetic surfactant preparations Exosurf and Pumactant (b) on *in vitro* growth of different bacterial strains. 7×10^7 CFU/mL of bacteria were incubated with different concentrations of surfactant (1, 10, and 20 mg/mL) and without surfactant (saline) for 5 h at 37°C. Values are mean Δ (5–0 h) $\log_{10}$ CFU/mL $\pm$ SD from six experiments. $^*p < 0.01$ vs. saline. [From Rauprich et al. (24).]

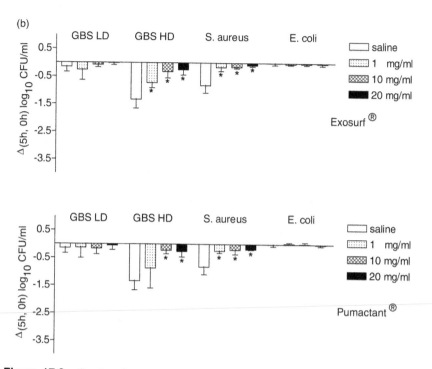

Figure 17.2 *Continued.*

Curosurf, whereas the GBS LD variant was clearly less susceptible under similar conditions, probably protected by the polysaccharide capsule. The capsule is an important virulence factor in GBS infections, and wild strains often contain a mixture of both encapsulated and nonencapsulated bacteria (21).

Connatal infections often trigger premature birth and may lead to respiratory failure within the first hours of life. Studies of surfactant treatment in infants with "idiopathic" RDS reveal that up to 20% of surfactant-treated neonates demonstrate signs of infection within the first days of life (19). All of the surfactant preparations investigated in this study have therefore been used in newborns with respiratory failure due to pneumonia.

Recommended doses for surfactant replacement therapy vary between 50 and 200 mg/kg body weight (bw) for the initial treatment of babies with RDS. It has been recognized that doses of 300 mg/kg bw of surfactant may be needed to overcome surfactant inhibition in pneumonia (22) or meconium aspiration syndrome (10). Such high doses would, even in babies devoid of endogenous surfactant, probably result in phospholipid concentrations well above 10 mg/mL in the alveolar lining layer, at least after resorption of fetal lung liquid (23). On the basis of these findings, the surfactant layer on the alveolar surface might be considered as an important part of the pulmonary defense system.

These findings underline that different subtypes of one bacterial species might differ in their interaction with surfactant. When we tested different clinical isolates from infants with GBS septicemia, the observed variation was small compared with the differences between different bacterial species. A similar observation was made by Neumeister et al. (18), who compared the influence of surfactant on different reference strains and several clinical isolates of GBS, *S. aureus*, and *E. coli*.

Several years ago, Coonrod and Yoneda (14) demonstrated that the surfactant fraction of rat alveolar lining material caused lysis of *Streptococcus pneumoniae* and several other Gram-positive bacteria (*Streptococcus viridans*, *Streptococcus pyogenes*, and *Streptoccoccus bovis*). The authors speculated that the observed bactericidal effect was due to free fatty acids contained in the lung lavage preparation (25). More recently, Brogden et al. (26) described an anionic bactericidal peptide in ovine pulmonary surfactant and one such peptide, prophenin-1, has also recently been isolated from porcine leukocytes (27). This antibacterial peptide has also been found to be associated to the lipids of Curosurf, a surfactant extracted from porcine lung homogenate (28). Part of the antibacterial effects of surfactant may thus be mediated by the binding of such microbicidal peptides to the bacterial cell wall and destabilization of the membranes by pore formation. The polarity of these peptides seems to be critical for their antibacterial activity (29). It has been shown that changes in, for example, sodium, zinc, calcium, or phosphorus content of the incubation medium can modify the *in vitro* bactericidal activity of the antimicrobial peptides. The bactericidal part of prophenin, a peptide rich in proline and phenylalanine, consists of 18 amino acids (PF-18). PF-18 can be added to surfactant (Curosurf) without negative effects on the biophysical function of the preparation (30), indirectly suggesting that surfactant could be used as a vehicle for the dispersion of the peptide on the alveolar surface.

We found that all the investigated surfactant preparations protected *S. aureus* from the negative effects of saline on bacterial growth. This might indicate that staphylococci can catabolize surfactant lipids to some extent, probably by the release of phospholipases (31). LaForce (32) reported increased growth of *S. aureus* after incubation with complete natural rabbit surfactant. Apparently, the bacteria can use surfactant components as nutrients. Natural surfactant isolated by lung lavage and subsequent sucrose gradient centrifugation contains a small proportion of carbohydrates (<1%) and ~10% proteins, including the specific surfactant-associated proteins (SP-A, SP-B, SP-C, and SP-D) (33). The hydrophilic proteins SP-A and SP-D are potent stimulators of macrophage function (34) and generally believed to serve as important components of the pulmonary host defense system against invading micro-organisms (35). SP-A and SP-D also have direct bacteriostatic effects (36). However, these proteins are removed by extraction with organic solvents and therefore absent in all the industrially produced modified natural surfactants examined in our study. SP-B, present in small amounts in all modified natural surfactants, may in itself have a bacteriostatic effect (discussed subsequently).

The relative resistance of Gram-negative *E. coli* to each of the investigated surfactants may reflect failure of the surfactant molecules to penetrate the lipopolysaccharide layer. In fact, incubation of *E. coli* with Survanta significantly promoted bacterial growth. This has also been reported by other investigators (18). Recently, it has been shown that proliferation of *E. coli* is inhibited by mature human pulmonary SP-B, or more specifically, by the residues 12–34 of SP-B (37). The reason for the observed proliferation of *E. coli* is unclear, but Survanta contains relatively little SP-B (38,39) and, in contrast to the other modified natural surfactants examined, it is enriched with artificial lipids. Increased growth of *E. coli* has also been reported after exposure to a crude surfactant preparation obtained from dog lungs (15). In the present study, synthetic surfactants containing lipids only (Pumactant) or lipids plus spreading agents (Exosurf) had no effect on the proliferation of *E. coli*. Although differences in surfactant composition might explain some of these seemingly conflicting results, species differences may also play a role. For example, the clearing rate of inhaled pneumococci varies between different animals (40).

Our finding that some surfactant preparations may enhance bacterial survival or even promote bacterial proliferation (as observed for Survanta and *E. coli*) is alarming and should be further studied in animal experiments. So far, most studies on surfactant for treatment of inflammatory lung disease have focused on gas exchange. Song et al. (41) demonstrated improved lung function in rats with *E. coli* pneumonia treated with Curosurf. Unfortunately, no attempts were made to quantify bacterial growth in this study. Interestingly, our *in vitro* data obtained with Curosurf and GBS are in keeping with observations in GBS-infected newborn rabbits (discussed subsequently), showing mitigation of bacterial proliferation in lung homogenate following treatment with this particular surfactant preparation (7,42).

Clinical and radiological signs do not differentiate with certainty between pneumonia and RDS in the first hours of life. As others and we observed that some surfactant preparations might promote bacterial growth, infants with severe respiratory failure treated with surfactant should receive antibiotic therapy until infection can be ruled out by culture and laboratory findings.

We conclude that bacterial growth in different surfactant preparations is influenced by microbial species and the composition and dose of surfactant. Further studies are necessary to elucidate the mechanisms involved and to evaluate the effects of surfactant on bacterial growth *in vivo*.

B. Influence of Surfactant on Leucocyte Function

Many studies have focused on the influence of BAL fluid, surfactant extracts, and isolated surfactant phospholipids, or proteins on the function of different inflammatory cells including granulocytes, lymphocytes, monocytes, and alveolar macrophages [reviewed in Ref. (12)].

We studied the influence of surfactant on oxygen metabolite release by polymorphonuclear neutrophilic granulocytes (PMN). Surfactant (Curosurf) at a concentration of 4 mg/mL suppressed the resting activity of unstimulated PMN significantly (Fig. 17.3). The nonencapsulated group B-streptococcal strain GBS HD stimulated PMN significantly in the absence of specific antiserum, whereas the encapsulated phase variant (GBS LD) needed opsonization by a specific antiserum. However, when the PMN were stimulated by GBS LD and a polyclonal anti-GBS antibody, the increase in oxygen metabolite release was not inhibited by surfactant (Fig. 17.3). These findings demonstrate that the polysaccharide capsule is an important virulence factor that protects GBS from phagocytosis in the absence of specific antibodies. Significant stimulation of oxygen metabolite release from PMN occurred only after the encapsulated bacteria had been opsonized with specific IgG.

In further studies using live bacteria, we found that the observed stimulation of nitroblue tetrazolium (NBT) reduction correlates to bacterial killing of GBS by isolated PMN. Again, Curosurf did not suppress the phagocytosis of opsonized GBS LD by PMN (43). The surfactant lipids seem to play a general immunoregulatory role and we demonstrated that large phospholipid doses decreased oxygen metabolite release (43,44), chemotaxis (44), and phagocytosis (45) of PMN. At lower concentrations, some stimulatory effects were

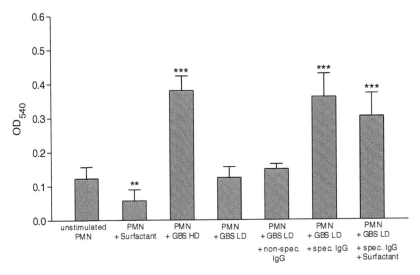

Figure 17.3 Oxygen metabolite release from PMN stimulated by encapsulated GBS LD or nonencapsulated GBS HD as measured spectrophotometrically (OD$_{540}$ = optical density at 540 nm) by NBT reduction test. GBS LD need opsonization by specific antibodies to elicit PMN stimulation. Surfactant does not suppress the antibody-mediated response. The bars represent mean and SD. $^{**}p < 0.01$; $^{***}p < 0.001$ vs. unstimulated PMN. [Modified from Herting et al. (43).]

noted, which might be related to biologically active substances like platelet activating factor (46) or antibacterial peptides (26,28) present in surfactants derived
from natural sources.

Reduced production of proinflammatory mediators like tumor necrosis factor
(TNFα) (47) and arachidonic acid metabolites (48) from monocytes and reduced
release of superoxide anions by stimulated monocytes and PMN (49,50) have
been demonstrated after incubation with surfactant phospholipids. In contrast,
stimulatory effects especially on alveolar macrophage function were triggered by
the surfactant proteins SP-A and SP-D (35). SP-A and SP-D (51) play a regulatory
role in surfactant homeostasis and have been shown to stimulate a variety of functions of alveolar macrophages. Mice deficient in SP-A or SP-D demonstrate
impaired immune function with increased susceptibility [e.g., to GBS (52)]. The
role of the surfactant proteins SP-A and SP-D in biophysical function, regulation
of surfactant metabolism, agglutination and presentation of bacterial, fungal, or
viral antigens, and in the control of the pulmonary immune defense system is
reviewed elsewhere in this book (Chapters 5 and 15).

III. Animal Studies

A variety of models have been used to study the effects of surfactant in animals
with inflammatory lung disease. Animals were infected either by direct needle
injection of bacteria into the trachea or by airway instillation of a bacterial suspension via a tracheotomy tube. Aerosol deposition, intraperitoneal injection, or
the cecal ligation/perforation model has been applied to spontaneously breathing
animals.

We designed a small animal model using ventilated newborn rabbits
infected with GBS via a tracheal cannula. This model allows evaluation of bacterial proliferation in lung homogenate, BAL fluid, or blood samples. In addition,
lung function can be monitored continuously and histological features can be
analyzed at the end of the experiments [Fig. 17.4(a)]. Surfactant (Curosurf) at
a dose of 200 mg/kg bw improved lung function (42) in immature rabbits (gestational age: 28 days) and mitigated bacterial growth (7,42) both in preterm and
near-term (gestational age: 29.5 days) animals as compared to littermate controls
receiving saline [Fig. 17.4(b)]. Similar findings were reported by Sherman et al.
(13). In the case of GBS infection, the impairment in surfactant function is
apparently mediated by the inflammatory cells and their products, as we could
demonstrate lipid peroxidation associated with impaired biophysical activity of
surfactant (6). Other bacterial strains seem to have a direct harmful effect on
pulmonary surfactant, for example, by the release of phopholipases (53) or the
cleavage of surfactant proteins by proteolytic enzymes (54).

In other studies, we evaluated the effects of different surfactant preparations
and different surfactant doses (55). *In vitro* and in animal models, SP-A improves
the resistance of surfactant against inhibition by plasma proteins or meconium

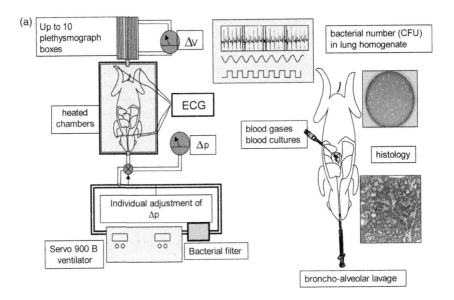

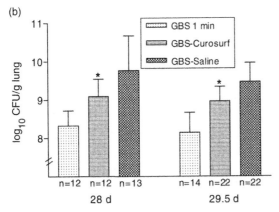

Figure 17.4 (a) Animal model of neonatal pneumonia (11). Rabbit fetuses are delivered by Cesarian section, anesthetized, tracheotomized, and ventilated in plethysmograph boxes that allow individual adjustment of the pressure (p) to reach a given tidal volume (V). In this way, dynamic compliance can be calculated. The animals are infected intratracheally with GBS and ventilated for 5 h. At the end of the experiments, blood is drawn from the right ventricle (e.g., for cultures or blood gas analysis), and the lung is used for bacterial counting or fixed for histological examination. Alternatively, airway lavage can be performed. Cardiovascular status is monitored by electrocardiogram (ECG); (b) Bacterial proliferation (CFU) in lung homogenates in preterm (28 days) and near-term (29.5 days) newborn rabbits (mean ± SD). Significant bacterial proliferation was observed in all GBS-infected ventilated rabbits as compared to the beginning of the experiments (GBS 1 min). Significantly less bacteria were found in lung homogenates of surfactant-treated animals (*$p < 0.05$ vs. GBS saline). [Modified from Herting et al. (7,42).]

(56–58). However, in the rabbit GBS pneumonia model, neither the intratracheal application of a monoclonal SP-A antibody (59) nor the addition of 2% SP-A to Curosurf had a significant influence on bacterial proliferation (55). These findings seem to contradict the increased bacterial proliferation in mice that are genetically deficient in SP-A (SP-A "knock outs"). However, the number of GBS instilled in our pneumonia model is more than 1000 times higher than in the mice experiments (52). Such a high inoculum apparently "overwhelms" the immune defense mechanisms. The newborn rabbit lung is relatively deficient in alveolar macrophages and under such circumstances the neutrophils present a "second line of defense" (60). It seems that SP-A controls the bacterial colonization of the lung mainly by stimulating alveolar macrophages and probably has a limited influence on the neutrophilic answer that is seen in severe bacterial pneumonia.

However, the inflammatory reaction has to be tightly controlled to avoid excessive lung damage by immune-competent cells and their products including cytokines, enzymes, or toxic oxygen metabolites. In additional experiments with the rabbit pneumonia model, we observed that surfactant caused a "downregulation" of the inflammatory response as regards both influx of neutrophils to the airspaces and release of elastase, a proteolytic enzyme, into BAL fluid or lung homogenate (61).

It seems tempting to use the unique spreading properties of surfactant to administer substances that can modulate the inflammatory response on the alveolar level. Using the neonatal GBS pneumonia model, we were able to demonstrate that surfactant can successfully be used as a carrier for specific immunoglobulins against pathogens like GBS (62) or pneumococci (63). Such antibodies can opsonize bacteria that are encapsulated by polysaccharides and evade phagocytosis in the absence of such "antigen presenting" IgG (43).

Using partial liquid ventilation in the same settings, we recently demonstrated that ventilation with perfluorocarbons resulted in a more homogeneous gas distribution in the lung and reduced bacterial proliferation as compared to mechanical ventilation with a tidal volume of ∼10 mL/kg bw (64,65). Conventional mechanical ventilation with large tidal volumes seems to promote translocation of bacteria from the alveolar compartment to the interstitial space and the blood stream (66).

In consequence, besides the direct effects of surfactant on bacterial growth that were demonstrated *in vitro*, improved mechanical properties of the lungs with a more homogeneous expansion, less epithelial damage, and reduced leak of plasma proteins into the airways probably contribute to the decrease in bacterial growth in animals undergoing surfactant therapy for bacterial pneumonia.

IV. Clinical Studies

Ablow et al. (67) were among the first to realize that surfactant deficiency was difficult to differentiate from severe pneumonia on clinical grounds, laboratory investigations, and X-ray findings. Pathologists had also noted the similarity to neonatal hyaline membrane disease in some patients dying from ARDS (2) or severe pneumonia. Case reports and smaller uncontrolled studies reported the use of surfactant in neonates with pulmonary and/or systemic infections (8,22,68,69). Studies on adults confirmed abnormalities of the surfactant system with decreased levels in surfactant proteins, increased protein and cytokine content in BAL fluid associated with altered phospholipid composition, and elevated minimum surface tension in a pulsating bubble surfactometer or increased conversion of large (surface active) to small surfactant aggregates (70–73).

In a European multicenter study (9), we were able to demonstrate that surfactant improved gas exchange both in term and preterm neonates with GBS infection. The study comprised 118 babies with respiratory failure, clinical and/or laboratory signs of acute inflammatory disease, and GBS infection proven by culture results. They were recruited retrospectively from a database of patients treated with surfactant at 28 neonatology units participating in European multicenter trials (1987–1993) and prospectively from the same units in the following years. A nonrandomized control group of 236 noninfected babies was selected from the same database. Main parameters evaluated were oxygen requirement, ventilator settings, and incidence of complications. Median birth weight in the GBS study group was 1468 g (25th–75th percentile: 1015–2170) and median gestational age was 30 weeks (27–33). Thirty-one percent of the infants weighed >2000 g. Median age at surfactant treatment was 6 h. The mean initial surfactant dose (SD) was 142 ± 53 mg/kg bw. Ninety of the infants were treated with Curosurf, 13 with Survanta, 12 with Alveofact, and 3 with Exosurf. Within 1 h of surfactant treatment, median FiO_2 (fraction of inspiratory oxygen) was reduced from 0.84 (25th–75th percentile: 0.63–1.0) to 0.50 (0.35–0.80) ($p < 0.01$). The response to surfactant was slower than in babies with RDS and repeated surfactant doses were often needed. Term infants and neonates with GBS septicemia demonstrated a slower response to surfactant treatment [Fig. 17.5(a)]. This might be due to a larger amount of surfactant inhibitors in the bronchoalveolar space. Probably, circulatory problems and a certain degree of pulmonary hypertension contributed to the disease severity in this subgroup of patients.

The mortality and morbidity were substantial considering the relatively high mean birth weight of the treated infants. In our study, mortality in the group of infants with GBS septicemia was as high as 49% and the overall incidence of intracerebaral hemorrhage was 42%, indicating that problems other than surfactant deficiency play a decisive role for the outcome of the disease. Even following adjustment for confounding variables by means of the propensity score technique, the relative risk for GBS infected infants to die or develop intracranial hemorrhage or chronic lung disease was more than doubled. Our results underline that the systemic inflammatory response is not only a pulmonary problem, but also equally affects the cerebral perfusion. Perinatal infections constitute an important risk factor for an adverse neurological outcome (74).

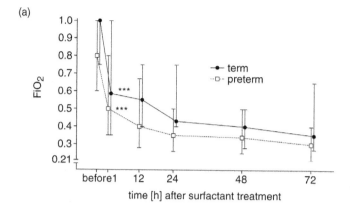

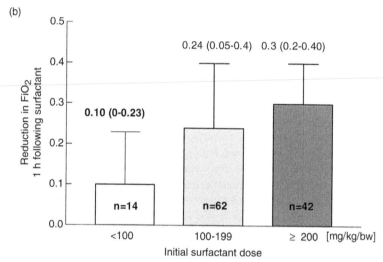

Figure 17.5 (a) Oxygen demand (FiO_2) in term ($n = 23$) and preterm ($n = 95$) neonates with respiratory failure and GBS infection following surfactant treatment (9). Values are median and 25th–75th percentile; (b) Reduction in oxygen demand (FiO_2) 1 h following surfactant treatment in neonates with respiratory failure and GBS infection in relation to initial surfactant dose. [From Herting et al. (9).]

Possibly, a higher dose of surfactant and/or earlier treatment could have improved these results. In a recent study on multiple-dose surfactant treatment for meconium aspiration syndrome initiated before the age of 6 h, a good effect on oxygenation was only observed after a cumulative surfactant dose of 300 mg/kg bw had been instilled into the airways (10). An initial surfactant dose of 300 mg/kg bw was also effective in adult patients with ARDS due to sepsis (22). Early treatment with large doses of surfactant may be required to counterbalance the presence of intra-alveolar surfactant inhibitors in this category of patients and to prevent ventilator-induced lung injury. A 100 mg/kg bw of surfactant is widely used as the standard initial dose to treat neonatal RDS. In infants with GBS infection, the improvement in oxygenation was more marked with a treatment dose of 200 mg/kg bw [Fig. 17.5(b)].

Infection is the most common cause of ARDS in children beyond the neonatal age. The lungs seem to be particularly vulnerable in the first year of life. Risk groups for development of ARDS include premature neonates with chronic lung disease developing viral (e.g., RSV) pneumonia and older children with immune deficiency syndromes and malignant neoplastic diseases that are especially prone to infections with *Pneumocystis carinii* [Fig. 17.6(a)]. It is not clear why pneumonia progresses to severe ARDS in certain children and not in others. Genetic predisposition may play a role, as some alleles of the SP-A and SP-B genes have been described more often in neonates with RDS and adults with ARDS (75).

Pneumonia in infancy and childhood may thus be associated with severe surfactant dysfunction and ARDS. We investigated the effects of surfactant treatment on oxygenation in eight infants (age: 1 month–13 years) with severe respiratory failure due to viral, bacterial, or *Pneumocystis carinii* pneumonia (76). Instillation of a modified porcine surfactant (Curosurf) improved gas exchange immediately. Median PaO_2/FiO_2 increased from 66 to 140 mmHg (8.8–18.7 kPa; $p < 0.01$) within 1 h of surfactant treatment. Seven of eight patients received multiple surfactant doses. Four patients (50%) died 3–62 days after surfactant treatment; six patients (75%) were immune deficient, and the observed mortality was mainly due to the underlying disease.

However, as the study population was nonuniform with a wide variation in age from 1 month to 13 years, the response to treatment was variable [Fig. 17.6(b)] and gas exchange was not normalized even following multiple-dose treatment. With the exception of infant 1, who was treated with 200 mg/kg bw of surfactant within 3 h after the onset of mechanical ventilation, all other patients demonstrated a response/relapse pattern and received multiple surfactant doses.

As mentioned, a subgroup analysis from our recent multicenter study of surfactant treatment for neonatal pneumonia (9) demonstrated that the decrease in FiO_2 within 1 h of surfactant treatment was most marked in patients receiving an initial treatment dose of ≥ 200 mg/kg bw [Fig. 17.5(b)]. Walmrath et al. (22) reported improved oxygenation after the use of 300 mg/kg bw of a bovine surfactant in 12 adults with ARDS and pneumonia. Obviously, high and repeated doses are necessary to antagonize the amount of surfactant inhibitors present in the bronchoalveolar space of patients with ARDS. In older patients, it might be possible to perform surfactant lavage by means of a bronchoscope to remove inhibitors of surfactant function from the airways (22). A modified lavage technique using catheters can be used in newborn infants as well (77). Although first reports of the lavage technique seem promising (e.g., in infants with meconium aspiration syndrome) (78,79), possible side effects have to be

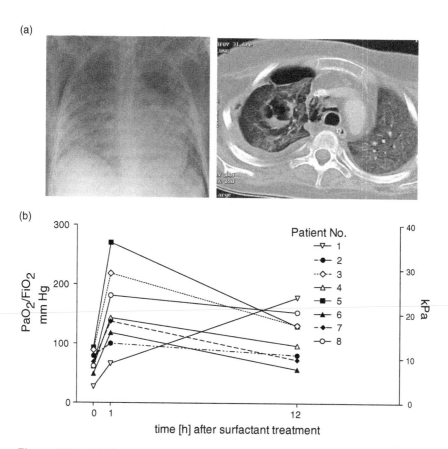

Figure 17.6 (a) Chest radiograph and CT-scan of a 13 year old immune deficient girl with ARDS due to *Pneumocystis carinii* pneumonia. Note the opaque appearance of the lungs resembling neonatal RDS. In addition, a lung abscess (isolated organism: *Nocardia* species), a pleural effusion, and a ventral small pneumothorax were present in the right upper lobe (see CT-scan); (b) PaO_2/FiO_2 ratio of infants and children ($n = 8$) with severe ARDS due to pneumonia prior to surfactant instillation (0 h) and at different time intervals (1 and 12 h) following the initial surfactant treatment. Retreatment was performed in seven of the eight infants. The median initial dose was 130 mg/kg bw and the median total dose was 245 mg/kg bw. [From Herting et al. (76).]

considered (80), and controlled randomized trials comparing lavage with early large dose bolus administration have to be performed before widespread clinical use can be recommended.

Apart from the case reports referred to earlier, little information is available on the effects of exogenous surfactant in patients with pediatric ARDS [reviewed in Ref. (3)]. Only one small controlled trial in infants and children with ARDS of different etiology has been published some years ago (81). A European controlled trial with a bovine surfactant has recently been reported (82). Both studies demonstrated improvement in oxygenation without improved survival. Larger controlled trials are therefore necessary before surfactant therapy can be recommended for pediatric ARDS.

The economic aspects of this therapy also must be considered. As the prices for surfactant are still based on the neonatal preparations, treatment costs for a child with a weight of ≥ 50 kg (e.g., patients 7 and 8 in our study) may amount to more than 50,000 Euros per case. Thus, identification of ARDS patients who would profit from surfactant treatment also in terms of survival seems mandatory. We speculate that early administration of surfactant should probably be superior to the late rescue therapy applied in our study at a stage when gas exchange was already critically impaired and the lungs had been exposed to the noxious effects of mechanical ventilation for several hours or even days.

In general, the incidence of pediatric ARDS has been decreasing over the last years (83), indicating that both better primary care and more gentle strategies of ventilation (e.g., "permissive hypercapnia") may help avoid the ventilator-induced lung injury involved in the pathophysiology of ARDS. A large randomized controlled trial in adults with ARDS (84) demonstrated reduced inflammatory response as measured by interleukin-6 levels in BAL fluid and decreased mortality in a group of patients ventilated with low tidal volumes (6–8 mL/kg bw) when compared with the previously advocated use of higher tidal volumes (10–12 mL/kg bw). As mentioned earlier, surfactant might also be of importance in this context by downregulating inflammatory responses in the lungs.

Future developments might lead to production of artificial surfactant preparations that are safe and hopefully less expensive, as they need not be extracted from animal lungs. In addition, it seems possible to design synthetic surfactants suitable for treatment of ARDS that are more resistant to inactivation (85). Clinical trials with synthetic surfactants containing either recombinant surfactant protein C [Venticute®, Altana (Byk Gulden), Konstanz, Germany] or the surfactant protein B-like peptide KL$_4$ (Surfaxin®, Discovery Laboratories, Doylestown, PA, USA) are in progress.

We conclude that surfactant improves gas exchange in patients with severe pediatric ARDS due to pneumonia. However, larger controlled trials are necessary to determine whether the improved oxygenation is associated with a better outcome.

V. Summary and Perspectives

Pulmonary inflammation is an important factor in the pathogenesis and pathophysiology of surfactant dysfunction. An inflammatory reaction may be the direct answer to the contact with bacterial antigens, allergens, and inhaled (e.g., smoke) or aspirated (e.g., blood, meconium) agents. Even in the absence of microbial antigens, an inflammatory reaction ("sterile pneumonia") is involved in the pathophysiology of numerous other diseases including asthma (Chapter 9), cystic fibrosis, or bronchopulmonary dysplasia (86). Contrary to what is seen for neonatal RDS based primarily on immaturity, for these ARDS-like conditions surfactant is just a symptomatic treatment. Although surfactant may improve gas exchange acutely under such circumstances, it is yet unclear whether surfactant treatment of ARDS actually reduces morbidity and mortality. Most of the studies reported so far used surfactant as a rescue treatment at a stage of the disease when the respiratory situation was already critical. We believe it would be wise to use surfactant at an earlier stage, perhaps even before the patient becomes ventilator dependent.

ARDS and sepsis-induced respiratory failure are different from the more uniform lung injury in neonatal RDS. The ARDS animal models (5) that demonstrated the effectiveness of surfactant treatment under such conditions used a "direct lung injury" (e.g., instillation of meconium, saline lavage). This situation may be quite different from the "indirect lung damage" that is observed in the clinical settings of a patient with ARDS and sepsis (5). The prognosis of many of the ARDS patients is not only influenced by the severity of the respiratory problems, but also by the degree of multiorgan dysfunction (3,4).

The obvious differences in the pathophysiology between neonatal and adult lung disease indicate that a surfactant that is suitable for the treatment of neonatal RDS may not be ideal for ARDS as well. Actually, it seems that new synthetic protein/peptide containing surfactants like KL_4 (Surfaxin) or recombinant SP-C surfactant (Venticute) are more resistant to inhibition than the currently available modified natural surfactants (85). Moreover, it seems possible to increase the resistance of surfactant to inhibition *in vitro* by adding dextran, polyethylene glycol (PEG), or hyaluronic acid (87–90). We recently reported the effects of polymyxin B (91), a cross-linking peptide that may mimic the function of SP-B (92) on the resistance of surfactant towards inhibition. As polymyxin B is an antibiotic as well, it could be of special value in the treatment of patients with ARDS due to pneumonia. Surfactant has also been proposed as a carrier for substances that reduce bacterial growth [e.g., antibiotics (93), lysozyme (94)] or modulate immune functions or oxygen metabolite toxicity [e.g., immunoglobulins (62,63), superoxide dismutase (95), phosphodiesterase inhibitors (96), or vitamins (6)].

Over the last decade, it has been realized that surfactants constitute "the frontline in lung host defense" (97). Both surfactant lipids and proteins exert antimicrobial and immune-regulatory effects. In addition to a direct antibacterial effect, the collectins SP-A and SP-D are involved in the regulation of the immune system and surfactant homeostasis. Recently, it has been demonstrated that SP-A and SP-D directly inhibit the growth of Gram-negative bacteria by increasing membrane permeability (36) without involving macrophages or aggregation of the micro-organisms. SP-A and SP-D are also expressed on other mucosal surfaces (97) (gastrointestinal tract, middle ear) suggesting a broader role of these proteins in host defense.

Bacterial growth in the presence of surfactant depends on the bacterial species and the origin and concentration of the applied surfactant preparation. Except for cultures of *E. coli* in Survanta, most surfactants do not promote bacterial growth. However, *E. coli* is nowadays rarely isolated from blood cultures or tracheal aspirate fluid in the neonatal period. Curosurf significantly diminished proliferation of GBS, the organism that accounts for most cases of neonatal early onset septicemia. First clinical observations give no reason to believe that treatment with surfactant should have adverse effects in neonates with connatal pneumonia but further *in vivo* studies are necessary to clarify this issue. Even if exogenous surfactant obtained from animal lungs influences bacterial growth *in vitro*, the effects of exogenous phospholipids on the microbiology of the human lung remain unclear. Careful follow-up of babies with bacterial infections treated with surfactant therefore seems mandatory. Recently, antibacterial peptides have been detected in a porcine surfactant. These peptides (e.g., defensins and cathelicidins) represent an ancient but effective part of the innate immune system (29).

Besides specific antimicrobial effects of surfactant components, part of the anti-inflammatory/antimicrobial activity is actually mediated by biophysical mechanisms. Surfactant prevents bacterial translocation from the alveolar compartment to the lung interstitium and to the blood stream. It probably serves as a "mechanical barrier" to bacterial invasion, improving mucociliary clearance and removal of inhaled particles from the airways. It also keeps the alveoli open, facilitating the recruitment of macrophages and granulocytes to the site of infection and preventing ventilation/perfusion mismatch and right to left shunting.

Surfactant also prevents intra-alveolar edema and protein leak into the airways. Ventilation with large tidal volumes in itself seems to induce an inflammatory reaction in the lungs. A large clinical study in patients with ARDS demonstrated significantly less cytokine release into BAL fluid and a decreased mortality in adults ventilated with a tidal volume of 6–8 mL/kg bw instead of 10–12 mL/kg bw (84).

Lung protective strategies [including "no ventilation"—by the use of CPAP and/or the early delivery of surfactant to spontaneously breathing patients by nebulization (98)] or the INSURE technique [INtubate SURfactant Extubate (99)] might of be of special benefit in patients with inflammatory lung disease and need to be studied in more detail.

VI. Conclusion

Surfactant treatment in inflammatory lung disease initially aimed at improving gas exchange and lung mechanics. We now begin to understand the important role of surfactant and its components in pulmonary host defense. Hopefully, this expanding knowledge will allow the design of new anti-inflammatory and antimicrobial treatment strategies in the future.

Acknowledgments

Our studies were supported by the German (DFG He 2072/2-2) and the Swedish Medical Research Council (Project No. 3351), Konung Oscar II's Jubileumsfond, and a collaborative project (313/S-PPP) of the German Academic Exchange Service (DAAD) and the Swedish Institute (SI).

References

1. Jobe AH. Pulmonary surfactant therapy. N Engl J Med 1993; 328:861.
2. Ashbaugh DG, Bigelow DB, Petty TL, Levine BE. Acute respiratory distress in adults. Lancet 1967; 2(7511):319–323.
3. Möller JC. Surfactant therapy for acute respiratory distress syndrome. In: Wauer R, ed. Surfactant Therapy. Basic Principles, Diagnosis. Stuttgart, New York: Georg Thieme Verlag, 1998:133–145.
4. Ware LB, Matthay MA. The acute respiratory distress syndrome. N Engl J Med 2000; 342:1334–1349.
5. Kobayashi T, Tashiro K, Cui X, Konzaki T, Xu Y, Kabata C, Yamamoto K. Experimental models of acute respiratory distress syndrome: clinical relevance and response to surfactant therapy. Biol Neonate 2001; 80(suppl 1):26–28.
6. Bouhafs RKL, Rauprich P, Herting E, Schröder A, Robertson B, Jarstrand C. Direct and phagocyte mediated lipid peroxidation of lung surfactant by group B streptococci. Lung 2000; 178:317–329.
7. Herting E, Jarstrand C, Rasool O, Curstedt T, Sun B, Robertson B. Experimental neonatal group B *Streptococcal pneumonia*. Effect of a modified porcine surfactant on bacterial proliferation in ventilated near-term rabbits. Pediatr Res 1994; 36:784–791.
8. Lotze A, Mitchell BR, Bulas DI, Zola EM, Shalwitz RA, Gunkel JH. Multicenter study of surfactant (beractant) use in the treatment of term infants with severe respiratory failure. Survanta in Term Infants Study Group. J Pediatr 1998; 132:40–47.
9. Herting E, Gefeller O, Land M, van Sonderen L, Harms K, Robertson B and members of the Collaborative European Multicenter Study Group. Surfactant treatment of neonates with respiratory failure and group B streptococcal infection. Pediatrics 2000; 106:957–964.
10. Findlay RD, Taeusch HW, Walther FJ. Surfactant replacement therapy for meconium aspiration syndrome. Pediatrics 1996; 97:48–52.
11. Herting E. Surfactant Treatment in Neonatal Group B Streptococcal Pneumonia. Ph.D. Thesis, Karolinska Institute Stockholm, Sweden, 1999; ISBN—91-628-3691-9, Available online at: http://diss.kib.ki.se.
12. Wright JR. Immunomodulatory functions of surfactant. Physiol Rev 1997; 77:931–962.
13. Sherman MP, Campbell LA, Merritt TA, Long WA, Gunkel JH, Curstedt T, Robertson B. Effect of different surfactants on pulmonary group B streptococcal infection in premature rabbits. J Pediatr 1994; 125:939–947.
14. Coonrod JD, Yoneda K. Detection and partial characterization of antibacterial factors in alveolar lining material of rats. J Clin Invest 1983; 71:129–141.

15. Jalowayski AA, Giammona ST. The interaction of bacteria with pulmonary surfactant. Am Rev Respir Dis 1972; 105:236–241.
16. Jonsson S, Musher DM, Goree A, Lawrence EC. Human alveolar lining material and antibacterial defenses. Am Rev Respir Dis 1986; 133:136–140.
17. LaForce FM, Boose DS. Sublethal damage of *Escherichia coli* by lung lavage. Am Rev Respir Dis 1981; 124:733–737.
18. Neumeister B, Woerndle S, Bartmann P. Effects of different surfactant preparations on bacterial growth *in vitro*. Biol Neonate 1996; 70:128–134.
19. Herting E. Surfactant therapy for neonatal pneumonia and for meconium aspiration syndrome. In: Wauer RR, ed. Surfactant Therapy: Basic Principles, Diagnosis, Therapy. Stuttgart, New York: Thieme, 1998:124–132.
20. Nielson DW. Electrolyte composition of pulmonary alveolar subphase in anesthetized rabbits. J Appl Physiol 1986; 60:972–979.
21. Håkansson S, Granlund-Edstedt M, Sellin M, Holm SE. Demonstration and characterization of buoyant-density subpopulations of group B *streptococcus* type III. J Infect Dis 1990; 161:741–746.
22. Walmrath D, Günther A, Ghofrani HA, Schermuly R, Schneider T, Grimminger F, Seeger W. Bronchoscopic surfactant administration in patients with severe adult respiratory distress syndrome and sepsis. Am J Respir Crit Care Med 1996; 154:57–62.
23. Kobayashi T, Shido A, Nitta K, Inui S, Ganzuka M, Robertson B. The critical concentration of surfactant in fetal lung liquid at birth. Respir Physiol 1990; 80:181–192.
24. Rauprich P, Möller O, Walter G, Herting E, Robertson B. Influence of modified natural or synthetic surfactant preparations on the growth of bacteria causing infections in the neonatal period. Clin Diag Lab Immunol 2000; 7:817–822.
25. Coonrod J, Lester RL, Hsu LC. Characterization of the extracellular bactericidal factors of rat alveolar lining material. J Clin Invest 1984; 74:1269–1279.
26. Brogden KA, De Lucca AJ, Bland J, Elliot S. Isolation of an ovine pulmonary surfactant-associated anionic peptide bactericidal for pasteurella haemolytica. Proc Natl Acad Sci USA 1996; 93:412–416.
27. Harwig SSL, Kokryakov VN, Swiderek KM, Aleshina GM, Zhao C, Lehrer RI. Prophenin-1, an exceptionally proline-rich antimicrobial peptide from porcine leukocytes. FEBS Letters 1995; 362:65–69.
28. Wang Y, Griffiths WJ, Curstedt T, Johansson J. Porcine pulmonary surfactant preparations contain the antibacterial peptide prophenin and a C-terminal 18-residue fragment thereof. FEBS Letters 1999; 460:257–262.
29. Zasloff M. Antimicrobial peptides of multicellular organisms. Nature 2002; 415:389–395.
30. Herting E, Wang Y, Agerbert B, Johansson J. Addition of the antimicrobial peptide prophenin (62–79) does not interfere with the biophysical activity of Curosurf [abstr]. Biol Neonate 2002; 81(suppl 1):34.
31. Matos JE, Harmon RJ, Langlois BE. Lecithinase reaction of staphylococcus aureus strains of different origin on Baird–Parker medium. Lett Appl Microbiol 1995; 21:334–335.
32. LaForce FM. Effect of alveolar lining material on phagocytic and bactericidal activity of lung macrophages against *Staphylococcus aureus*. J Lab Clin Med 1976; 88:691–699.

33. Johansson J. The proteins of the surfactant system. Eur Respir J 1994; 7:372–391.
34. Van Golde LMG. Potential role of surfactant proteins A and D in innate lung defense against pathogens. Biol Neonate 1995; 67(suppl 1):2–17.
35. McCormack FX, Whitsett JA. The pulmonary collectins, SP-A and SP-D, orchestrate innate immunity in the lung. J Clin Invest 2002; 109:707–712.
36. Wu H, Kuzmenko A, Wan S, Schaffer L, Weiss A, Fischer JH, Kim KS, McCormack FX. Surfactant proteins A and D inhibit the growth of Gram-negative bacteria by increasing membrane permeability. J Clin Invest 2003; 111:1589–1602.
37. Kaser MR, Skouteris GG. Inhibition of bacterial growth by synthetic SP-B1-78 peptides. Peptides 1997; 18:1441–1444.
38. Mizuno K, Ikegami M, Chen CM, Ueda T, Jobe AH. Surfactant protein-B supplementation improves *in vivo* function of a modified natural surfactant. Pediatr Res 1995; 37:271–276.
39. Seeger W, Grube C, Günther A, Schmidt R. Surfactant inhibition by plasma proteins: differential sensitivity of various surfactant preparations. Eur Respir J 1993; 6:971–977.
40. Coonrod JD, Varble R, Jarrells MC. Species variation in the mechanism of killing inhaled pneumococci. J Lab Clin Med 1990; 116:354–362.
41. Song GW, Robertson B, Curstedt T, Gan XZ, Huang WX. Surfactant treatment in experimental *Escherichia coli* pneumonia. Acta Anaesthesiol Scand 1996; 40:1152–1159.
42. Herting E, Sun B, Jarstrand C, Curstedt T, Robertson B. Surfactant improves lung function and mitigates bacterial growth in immature ventilated rabbits with experimentally induced neonatal group B streptococcal pneumonia. Arch Dis Child 1997; 76:F3–F8.
43. Herting E, Jarstrand C, Rasool O, Curstedt T, Håkansson S, Robertson B. Effect of surfactant on nitroblue tetrazolium (NBT) reduction of polymorphonuclear leucocytes stimulated with type Ia group B streptococci. Acta Paediatr 1995; 84:922–926.
44. Scholtes U, Wiegand N, Zwirner J, Herting E. Influence of porcine natural modified surfactant on chemotaxis and oxidative metabolism of polymorphonuclear leucocytes. Immun Biol 2002; 205:290–302.
45. Rauprich P, Möller O, Walter G, Herting E, Robertson B. Influence of modified porcine surfactant on *in vitro* growth and phagocytic killing of group B streptococci [abstr]. Biol Neonate 1997; 71(suppl 1):63.
46. Moya FR, Hoffman DR, Zhao B, Johnston JM. Platelet activating factor in surfactant preparations. Lancet 1993; 345:858–860.
47. Speer CP, Götze B, Curstedt T, Robertson B. Phagocytic functions and tumor necrosis factor secretion of human monocytes exposed to natural porcine surfactant (Curosurf). Pediatr Res 1991; 30:69–74.
48. Walti H, Polla BS, Bachelet M. Modified natural porcine surfactant inhibits superoxide anions and proinflammatory mediators released by resting and stimulated human monocytes. Pediatr Res 1997; 41:114–119.
49. Geertsma MF, Broos HR, van den Barselaar MT, Nibbering PH, van Furth R. Lung surfactant suppresses oxygen-dependent bactericidal functions of human blood monocytes by inhibiting the assembly of the NADPH oxidase. J Immunol 1993; 150:2391–2400.

50. Chao W, Spragg RG, Smith RM. Inhibitory effect of porcine surfactant on the respiratory burst oxidase in human neutrophils. Attenuation of p47phox and p67phox membrane translocation as the mechanism. J Clin Invest 1995; 96:2654–2660.

51. Botas C, Poulain F, Akiyama J, Brown C, Allen L, Goerke J, Clements J, Carlson E, Gillespie AM, Epstein C, Hawgood S. Altered surfactant homeostasis and alveolar type II cell morphology in mice lacking surfactant protein D. Proc Natl Acad Sci USA 1998; 95:11869–11874.

52. LeVine AM, Bruno MD, Huelsman KM, Ross GF, Whitsett JA, Korfhagen TR. Surfactant protein A-deficient mice are susceptible to group B streptococcal infection. J Immunol 1997; 158:4336–4340.

53. Holm BA, Keicher L, Liu M, Sokolowski J, Enhorning G. Inhibition of pulmonary surfactant function by phospholipases. J Appl Physiol 1991; 71:317–321.

54. Pison U, Tam EK, Caughey GH, Hawgood S. Proteolytic inactivation of dog lung surfactant-associated proteins by neutrophil elastase. Biochim Biophys Acta 1989; 992:251–257.

55. Herting E, Robertson B. Surfactant treatment in neonatal group streptococcal pneumonia. From experimental studies to clinical application. Appl Cardiopulm Pathophysiol 2000; 9:241–243.

56. Sun B, Curstedt T, Lindgren G, Franzén B, Alaiya AA, Calkovská A, Robertson B. Biophysical and physiological properties of a modified porcine surfactant enriched with surfactant protein A. Eur Respir J 1997; 10:1967–1974.

57. Strayer DS, Herting E, Sun B, Robertson B. Antibody to surfactant protein A increases sensitivity of pulmonary surfactant to inactivation by fibrinogen *in vivo*. Am J Respir Crit Care Med 1996; 153:1116–1122.

58. Sun B, Herting E, Curstedt T, Robertson B. Exogenous surfactant improves lung compliance and oxygenation in adult rats with meconium aspiration. J Appl Physiol 1994; 77:1961–1971.

59. Herting E, Strayer DS, Jarstrand C, Sun B, Robertson B. Lung function and bacterial proliferation in experimental neonatal pneumonia in ventilated rabbits exposed to monoclonal antibody to surfactant protein A. Lung 1998; 176:123–131.

60. Sherman MP, D'Ambola J, Aeberhard E, Barrett CT. Surfactant therapy of newborn rabbits impairs lung macrophage bactericidal activity. J Appl Physiol 1988; 65:137–145.

61. Herting E, Speer CP, Sun B, Jarstrand C, Curstedt T, Robertson B. Influence of surfactant on pulmonary inflammatory response and release of elastase in experimental neonatal group B *Streptococcal pneumonia*. Monatschr Kinderheilkd 1996; 144:1319–1325.

62. Herting E, Gan XZ, Rauprich P, Jarstrand C, Robertson B. Combined treatment with surfactant and specific immunoglobulin reduces bacterial proliferation in experimental neonatal group B-*Streptococcal pneumonia*. Am J Respir Crit Care Med 1999; 159:1862–1867.

63. Gan XZ, Jarstrand C, Herting E, Berggren P, Robertson B. Effect of surfactant and specific antibody on bacterial proliferation and lung function in experimental pneumococcal pneumonia. Int J Infect Dis 2001; 5:9–18.

64. Rüdiger M, Köpke U, Prösch S, Rauprich M, Wauer RR, Herting E. Effect of perfluorocarbons (PFC) and PFC/Surfactant-emulsions on growth and viability of group B streptococci and *Escherichia coli*. Crit Care Med 2001; 29:1786–1791.

65. Rüdiger M, Jarstrand C, Some M, Čalkovská A, Amato M, Robertson B, Herting E. Influence of partial liquid ventilation on bacterial growth and alveolar expansion in newborn rabbits with group B-*Streptococcal pneumonia*. Pediatr Res 2003; 54:803–813.

66. Van Kaam AHLC, Haitsma JJ, De Jaegere A, Lachmann R, Herting E, Kok JH, Lachmann B. Pulmonary surfactant reduces bacterial translocation and mortality in a piglet model of group B *Streptococcal pneumonia* [abstr]. Biol Neonate 2003; 84:34–35.

67. Ablow RC, Driscoll S, Effmann EL, Gross I, Jolles CJ, Uauy R, Washaw JB. A comparison of early onset group B streptococcal neonatal infection and the respiratory distress syndrome. N Engl J Med 1976; 294:65–70.

68. Harms K, Herting E. Successful surfactant replacement therapy in two infants with ARDS due to chlamydial pneumonia. Respiration 1994; 61:348–352.

69. Auten RL, Notter RH, Kendig JW et al. Surfactant treatment of full-term newborns with respiratory failure. Pediatrics 1991; 87:101–107.

70. Somerson NL, Kontras SB, Pollack JD, Weiss HS. Pulmonary compliance: alteration during infection. Science 1971; 171:66–68.

71. Günther A, Ruppert C, Schmidt R, Markart P, Grimminger F, Walmrath D, Seeger W. Surfactant alteration and replacement in acute respiratory distress syndrome. Respir Res 2001; 2:353–364.

72. Griese A. Pulmonary surfactant in health and human lung diseases: state of the art. Eur Respir J 1999; 13:1455–1476.

73. Walther FJ. Surfactant therapy for neonatal lung disorders other than respiratory distress syndrome. In: Robertson B, Taeusch WH, eds. Surfactant Therapy for Lung Disease. New York: Marcel Dekker, 1995:461–489.

74. Yoon BH, Romero R, Kim CJ et al. High expression of tumor necrosis factor-alpha and interleukin-6 in periventricular leukomalacia. Am J Obstet Gynecol 1997; 177:406–411.

75. Floros J, Ruzong F. Surfactant protein A and B genetic variants and respiratory distress syndrome: allele interactions. Biol Neonate 2001; 80(suppl 1):22–25.

76. Herting E, Möller O, Schiffmann JH, Robertson B. Surfactant improves oxygenation in infants and children with pneumonia and acute respiratory distress syndrome. Acta Paediatr 2002; 91:1174–1178.

77. Herting E, Schiffmann JH, Roth Ch, Zaltash S, Johansson J. Surfactant lavage demonstrates protein fibrils in a neonate with congenital surfactant protein B deficiency. Am J Respir Crit Care Med 2002; 166:1292–1294.

78. Lam BC, Yeung CY. Surfactant lavage for meconium aspiration syndrome: a pilot study. Pediatrics 1999; 103:1014–1018.

79. Wiswell TE, Knight GR, Finer NN, Donn SM, Desai H, Walsh WF, Sekar KC, Bernstein G, Keszler M, Visser VE, Merritt TA, Mannino FL, Mastrioianni L, Marcy B, Revak SD, Tsai H, Cochrane CG. A multicenter, randomized, controlled trial comparing Surfaxin (Lucinactant) lavage with standard care for treatment of meconium aspiration syndrome. Pediatrics 2002; 109:1081–1087.

80. Kattwinkel J. Surfactant lavage for meconium aspiration: a word of caution. Pediatrics 2002; 109:1167–1168.

81. Willson DF, Zaritsky A, Bauman LA, Dockery K, James RL, Conrad D, Craft H, Novotny WE, Egan EA, Dalton H. Instillation of calf lung surfactant extract (calfactant)

is beneficial in pediatric acute hypoxemic respiratory failure. Crit Care Med 1999; 27:188–195.

82. Möller JC, Schaible T, Roll C, Schiffmann JH, Bindl L, Schrod L, Reiss I, Kohl M, Demirakca S, Hentschel R, Paul T, Vierzig A, Groneck P, von Seefeld H, Schumacher H, Gortner L and the Surfactant ARDS Study Group. Treatment with bovine surfactant in severe acute respiratory distress syndrome in children: a randomized multicenter study. Intensive Care Med 2003; 29:437–446.

83. Martino Alba R, Pfenninger J, Bachmann DC, Minder C, Wagner BP. Changes in the epidemiology of the acute respiratory distress syndrome (ARDS) in children. An Esp Pediatr 1999; 50:566–570.

84. Brower RG, Matthay MA, Morris A, Schoenfeld D, Thompson BT, Wheeler A. Ventilation with lower tidal volumes as compared with traditional tidal volumes for acute lung injury and the acute respiratory distress syndrome. N Engl J Med 2000; 342:1301–1308.

85. Herting E, Rauprich P, Stichtenoth G, Walter G, Johansson J, Robertson B. Resistance of different surfactant preparations to inactivation by meconium. Pediatr Res 2001; 50:44–49.

86. Pandit PB, Dunn MS, Nelly KE, Pearlman M. Surfactant replacement in neonates with early chronic lung disease. Pediatrics 1995; 95:851–854.

87. Stichtenoth G, Curstedt T, Robertson B, Herting E. Increasing the resistance of Curosurf to meconium inactivation by adding lipids, phospholipids or dextran [abstr]. Biol Neonate 2001; 80(suppl 1):39.

88. Taeusch W, Lu KL, Goerke J, Clements J. Nonionic polymers reverse inactivation of surfactant by meconium and other substances. Am J Respir Crit Care Med 1999; 1590:1391–1395.

89. Kobayashi T, Ohta K, Tashiro K, Nishizuka K, Chen WM, Ohmura S, Yamamoto K. Dextran restores albumin-inhibited surface activity of pulmonary surfactant extract. J Appl Physiol 1999; 86:1778–1784.

90. Taeusch HW, Lu K. Are current surfactants good enough? Biol Neonate 2002; 82:277–278.

91. Stichtenoth G, Johansson J, Curstedt T, Robertson B, Herting E. Polymyxin B increases the resistance of Curosurf to inactivation by human meconium [abstr]. Biol Neonate 2003; 84:38.

92. Zaltash S, Palmblad M, Curstedt T, Johansson J, Persson B. Pulmonary surfactant protein B: a structural model and a functional analogue. Biochim Biophys Acta 2000; 1466:179–186.

93. van't Veen AJ, Mouton W, Gommers D, Lachmann B. Pulmonary surfactant as vehicle for intratracheally instilled tobramycin in mice infected with *Klebsiella pneumoniae*. Br J Pharmacol 1996; 119:1145–1148.

94. Sherman MP, Hall SL, Johanson JT, Aeberhard EE. Formulating a surfactant therapy for preterm infants who have bacterial pneumonia and respiratory distress syndrome. In: Bevilacqua G, Parmigiani S, Robertson B, eds. Surfactant in Clinical Practice. London: Harwood Academic Publishers, 1993:103–111.

95. Walther FJ, David CUR, Lopez SL. Antioxidant surfactant liposomes mitigate hyperoxic lung injury in premature rabbits. Am J Physiol 1995; 269:L613–L617.

96. Häfner D, Germann PG. Additive effects of phosphodiesterase-4 inhibition on effects of rSP-C surfactant. Am J Respir Crit Care Med 2000; 161:1495–1500.

97. Wright JR. Pulmonary surfactant: a front line of lung host defense. J Clin Invest 2003; 111:1453–1455.

98. Berggren E, Liljedahl M, Winbladh B, Andreasson B, Curstedt T, Robertson B, Schollin J. Pilot study of nebulized surfactant therapy for neonatal respiratory distress syndrome. Acta Paediatr 2000; 89:460–464.

99. Stevens TP, Blennow M, Soll RF. Early surfactant administration with brief ventilation vs. selective surfactant and continued mechanical ventilation for preterm infants with or at risk for RDS. Cochrane Database Syst Rev 2002; (2):CD003063.

18

Alteration of Alveolar Surfactant Function by Reactive Oxygen Species

KARINA RODRIGUEZ-CAPOTE, JONATHAN R. FAULKNER, and FRED POSSMAYER

University of Western Ontario,
London, Ontario, Canada

KAUSHIK NAG

Memorial University of Newfoundland,
St. John's, Newfoundland and Labrador, Canada

I. Introduction

The toxicity of oxygen originates from its property to dismutate into oxygen radicals known as reactive oxygen species (ROS). These radicals can react with biomolecules, thus changing and inactivating these molecules. ROS are produced continuously in the body as byproducts of normal aerobic respiration and other biochemical processes. However, when an organ or tissue is placed under oxidative stress, ROS production can overwhelm the body's endogenous antioxidant defense systems and lead to tissue damage. The lung is the first to encounter inspired oxygen. Its cells are exposed to higher oxygen concentrations than cells in other organs, and owing to its large surface area, the lung is a primary target of oxidant injury.

   Pulmonary surfactant is essential for normal lung function. It forms a lipid film at the alveolar air–water interface which reduces the surface tension (ST). By lowering ST during inspiration, surfactant reduces the work of breathing. The low STs generated with adequate surfactant minimize the differences in surface forces among alveoli. The high spreadability of surfactant also limits differences between adjacent alveolar regions. By lowering ST far below the 70 mN/m of saline at 37°C, surfactant also tends to reduce transudation of fluid from interstitial spaces (1). In addition to its surface-active properties, surfactant acts in the lung's host defense system and as an inflammatory reducing agent (2).

   Surfactant chemical composition is highly conserved among different species. Surfactant is composed of ~85% phospholipids (PLs), 5% neutral lipids, and 10% surfactant associated proteins (SPs) (Fig. 18.1). The SPs consist of SP-A and SP-D, which are hydrophilic glycoproteins, and SP-B and SP-C, which are low molecular weight hydrophobic proteins (1,3).

   Surfactant dysfunction is an important factor contributing to the pathophysiology of several diseases (4,5). Different mechanisms have been proposed to explain the alterations in interfacial properties occurring in such lung diseases. These include biophysical interactions with serum proteins in edema fluid (6), decreases in surfactant apoprotein content as a result of degradation mediated

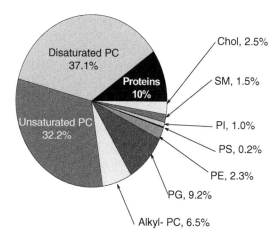

Figure 18.1 Bovine pulmonary surfactant composition [from Possmayer (1)].

by leukocyte proteases (7) or down regulation of their synthesis, and altered surfactant lipid and protein composition as a result of chemical modifications caused by ROS (4,8,9).

Considerable evidence suggests that oxidative stress, defined as an increased exposure to oxidants and/or decreased antioxidant capacities, can be implicated in airway diseases. ROS, produced both intracellularly by lung parenchymal cells and extracellularly by lung macrophages and infiltrating neutrophils, can play a central role in the pathogenesis of various lung diseases such as adult respiratory distress syndrome (ARDS) (4,5,10), asthma (11), chronic obstructive pulmonary disease (COPD) (8), and infection (10).

Oxidative stress has been a topic of research for many years. This chapter will focus on the effects of oxidant damage, caused by ROS, on the pulmonary surfactant and its function. See Eberhardt (12) for a review of the chemistry of ROS and their medical relevance. For more detailed information on the surfactant system itself, the reader is referred to recent reviews (1,9).

II. Reactive Oxygen Species

A free radical is any molecule or atom that contains one or more unpaired electrons in its outer orbit (12,13). The unpaired electron makes the species highly reactive. These compounds can be formed by the loss of a single electron from a nonradical, by the gain of a single electron from a nonradical, or by homolytic fission. The most important radicals in biological systems are the superoxide anion ($^{\pm}O_2$), hydroxyl radical ($^{\uparrow}OH$), nitric oxide (NO), and the lipid-derived peroxyl (ROO$^{\bullet}$) and alkoxyl (RO$^{\bullet}$) radicals (12,14,15).

The primary ROS are $^{\pm}O_2$ and H_2O_2. All other oxygen-related reactive compounds such as singlet oxygen ($^1O_2$), alkoxyl radicals (RO$^{\bullet}$), and peroxyl radicals (ROO•) are generated via secondary reactions of these primary oxygen metabolites (13,14,16). All of these atoms and compounds have the potential to cause free radical reactions (12,15).

The initial reaction in ROS chemistry is the reduction of molecular oxygen and the formation of $^{\bullet}O_2$ (12,14,15). Although the reactivity of $^{\bullet}O_2$ is quite low, it is capable of initiating free-radical chain reactions. Superoxide undergoes either spontaneous or enzymatic dismutation to form H_2O_2. This dismutation reaction, catalyzed by superoxide dismutases (SODs), is 10^4 times faster than the spontaneous reaction (Fig. 18.2) (13,14,17). Hydrogen peroxide is more stable than $^{\bullet}O_2$. It can diffuse through the plasma membrane and be transformed to $^{\bullet}OH$, $^1O_2$, or HOCl, thus promoting radical reactions far from its origin if not scavenged locally by catalase or glutathione peroxidase (GPX, 12).

Hypochlorous acid (HOCl), synthesized by a myeloperoxidase-mediated reaction from H_2O_2 and chloride ions, is the main product of activated neutrophils and is much more reactive than H_2O_2 (Fig. 18.2) (18,19). HOCl is a relatively long-lived oxidant and both unsaturated aliphatic groups of PLs and protein amino acids are targets of this reactive species (12).

The $^{\bullet}OH$ is considered the most reactive and potentially harmful radical. The hydroxyl radical is generated from H_2O_2 through the Fenton reaction catalyzed by the transition metals, iron or copper, or from $^{\bullet}O_2$ and H_2O_2 through the Haber–Weiss reaction again catalyzed by transition metals, iron or copper. Owing to its short lifetime, $^{\bullet}OH$ can be expected to react at or close to its site of formation (12,17,20).

Another possible source of $^{\bullet}OH$, which has been the focus of considerable attention during the last decade, is the reaction of superoxide with NO to form

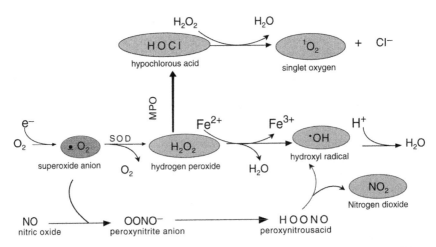

Figure 18.2 Formation of ROS. SOD, superoxide dismutase; MPO, myeloperoxidase; e−, electron. (Modified from *Reactive Oxygen Species*. R&D systems 1997 catalog.)

peroxynitrite (ONOO⁻). At physiological pH (7.4), this anion can be protonated to peroxynitrous acid, which then decomposes to generate $\cdot$OH (21,22). An alternative pathway for $\cdot$OH formation, which does not require the presence of transition metals, is the reaction of $^{\cdot}O_2$ with hypochlorous acid. When a free-radical reacts with a nonradical molecule, the target molecule can be converted to a radical, which may then initiate a chain reaction (12).

A. Sources of ROS in the Lung

Lung cells are exposed to higher oxygen concentrations than cells in other organs. Production of ROS is increased upon exposure to high oxygen concentrations, to exogenous oxidants like ozone, asbestos fibers, cigarette smoke, radiation, and to certain drugs (9,23). Not only can environmental pollutants react directly with vital targets, but also they can stimulate leukocytes and thereby increase the production of ROS.

Mitochondria are an important source of superoxide, ROS and H_2O_2. Superoxide generation is associated with NADH dehydrogenase and the ubiquinone cytochrome b complex, and exposure to hyperoxia increases mitochondrial ROS generation in the lung (23). Mitochondrial H_2O_2 is mainly derived from the dismutation of $^{\cdot}O_2$ with $\sim 1-2\%$ of the oxygen consumed by the mitochondria being converted to $^{\cdot}O_2$ and H_2O_2.

In addition, ROS are formed by intracellular enzymes. Xanthine dehydrogenase/xanthine oxidase (XDH/XO) is a cytoplasmic enzyme that under normal conditions is in its dehydrogenated form with no detectable ROS generation. In ischemic tissues, it is converted to the oxidase form leading to the production of $^{\cdot}O_2$ and H_2O_2 during reoxygenation (24). Sources of XDH/XO that mediate lung injury include resident pulmonary cells, both important sources of this enzyme in some species (25). In addition, diverse pathologic processes can result in circulating XDH/XO (26). XDH/XO released from tissues into the plasma can bind to sulfated glycosoaminoglycans on vascular endothelial cells producing site-specific oxidant injury to organs remote from the site of release (27). For example, XDH/XO from reperfused ischemic liver has been shown to accumulate in the lung in its enzymatically active form (24,28). Importantly, patients with ARDS, infections, or ischemia–reperfusion injury have markedly increased levels of XDH/XO in plasma (26,27). These observations provide a possible explanation for lung injury due to oxidative damage following a peripheral insult.

A nonenzymatic source of ROS is the generation of $\cdot$OH by iron-catalyzed reactions [Fenton and Haber–Weiss reactions, (17)]. The "catalysis" by Fe^{2+} of the formation of ROS (Fig. 18.2) through redox cycling has been well documented in biological systems, tissue injuries, and many pathological conditions (16). Pro-oxidant iron is present in normal human pulmonary epithelial lining fluid (ELF) and is greatly increased in ARDS patients (29,30).

In vivo, surfactant may be exposed not only to ongoing Fenton chemistry but also to local high concentrations of HOCl/⁻OCL, ⁻OONO, and $^{\cdot}O_2$

generated by phagocytic cells recruited to the alveolar space during the inflammation process. Activated neutrophils can produce large amounts of $HOCl/^-OCl$. For example, it has been reported that 5×10^6 activated neutrophils generate 44.2 ± 12.8 nmol of $HOCl/^-OCl$ per h (18,31).

It has been shown recently that overproduction of endogenous NO by alveolar macrophages, epithelial, interstitial, and endothelial cells, as well as by inhalation of NO, contributes to the alveolar epithelium's oxidant burden by the production of reactive oxygen–nitrogen intermediates (32). It has been proposed that inhaled NO could be used for the treatment of a number of pulmonary diseases such as acute lung injury, severe RDS, asthma, lung transplantation, and congenital heart diseases (33). The rationale for such therapy is that inhaled NO produces relaxation in pulmonary capillaries, thereby leading to increased blood flow specifically in regions adjacent to aerated alveoli. Owing to the short half-life of NO in blood, NO therapy selectively enhances pulmonary circulation without lowering systemic blood pressure and avoiding the induction of hypotensive shock. However, NO therapy can have a dark side as it has become evident that NO inhalation can lead to the generation of reactive oxygen–nitrogen species, thus contributing to the alveolar epithelium's oxidative burden (32).

Cigarette smoking is a major risk factor for the development of pulmonary disease, including emphysema, chronic bronchitis, and lung cancer. Free radicals in both gas and particulate/tar phases are among the many toxic components of cigarette smoke. These include superoxide and NO, which may combine to produce peroxynitrites, the highly damaging hydroxyl radical, tar semiquinone-free radicals, and various xenobiotic electrophiles (34). Pulmonary inflammatory cells which are a secondary source of free-radical production are increased in cigarette smokers (35,36). These cells can significantly contribute to oxidative damage in the airways. Furthermore, smoking is associated with increased lipid peroxidation products in plasma, exhaled breath, and lung tissue (37,38).

III. Antioxidant Defense Mechanisms

Antioxidant, as defined by Halliwell and Gutteridge (20), refers to "any substance that, when present in low concentration compared with those of an oxidable substrate, significantly delays or inhibits oxidation of that substrate." Lung cells differ profoundly in their resistance to oxidative stress, which may be due to differences in their antioxidant capacity or in the balance between oxidants and antioxidants in these cells. These enzymatic and nonenzymatic antioxidant defenses are discussed subsequently. The ELF and bronchial epithelium are among the first tissue elements to come into contact with gaseous pollutants. Therefore, the antioxidant defenses of ELF and lung tissues are important for protection of the respiratory system from oxidant damage. If these antioxidants are depleted, the lung epithelium will undergo oxidative injury. These biochemical changes can result in a wide variety of pathophysiological responses including airway inflammation, alterations in airway permeability, and increased airway reactivity to bronchoconstrictor agents (5).

A. Antioxidant Enzymes in the Lung

Superoxide Dismutases

SODs, mentioned earlier, are metalloenzymes which catalyze the dismutation of $^{\cdot}O_2$ to H_2O_2 and O_2 at a rate 10^4 times faster than spontaneous dismutation at neutral pH (13,16,20). Three different classes of SODs have been characterized; a copper/zinc-containing form (Cu/ZnSOD) localized in the cytosol, a manganese-containing form (MnSOD) in the mitochondria, and a copper/zinc-containing form in the extracellular matrix (ECSOD) (14,39).

Cu/ZnSOD, mainly localized in the cytosol, is also found in the nucleus and peroxisomes of human cells. Cu/ZnSOD contains both Cu(II) and Zn(II) at its active sites. Manganese SOD, which constitutes $\sim 10–15\%$ of total cellular SOD activity, is localized in the matrix of the mitochondria. This location is optimal for removal of $^{\cdot}O_2$ produced by the respiratory chain (40).

The overall expression of MnSOD in healthy lung is low. *In situ* hybridization of normal rat lung showed a consistent pattern of MnSOD mRNA distribution in the lung. The most prominent labeling occurred in the septal tips of alveolar ducts, around arterioles near airways, alveolar type II pneumocytes, and mesothelial cells (41). Immunohistochemical studies indicated that MnSOD protein is present in the mitochondria of all lung cells in the rat, with the highest staining in type II epithelial cells and bronchial epithelium (42). Both MnSOD and ECSOD are expressed at low levels in human bronchial epithelium, alveolar type II pneumocytes, and alveolar macrophages (43,44).

Extracellular SOD is a secretory tetrameric Cu/Zn-containing glycoprotein. ECSOD is the rarest of the SODs in tissues, but it is the major SOD in extracellular fluids such as plasma and extracellular matrix (45). Most animals have relatively high ECSOD activity in their lungs when compared with other tissues, however, ECSOD accounts for only $5–10\%$ of total lung SOD activity. ECSOD mRNA is found in airway epithelial cells, type II pneumocytes, and fibroblasts of human lung (45). Furthermore, rat macrophages and neutrophils invading the lung during inflammation have shown intensive staining for ECSOD protein (46).

Catalase

Catalase is a tetrameric hemoprotein that decomposes H_2O_2 to water and oxygen. Catalase is mainly localized in the peroxisomes, but is also localized in the cytosol of human neutrophils (44,47). The Michaelis–Menten constant (K_m) of catalase is higher than the K_m of GPx, suggesting that catalase scavenges H_2O_2 efficiently at high H_2O_2 concentrations (12). In healthy human lung, catalase is primarily expressed in alveolar type II pneumocytes, with lower levels in the bronchial epithelium and alveolar macrophages (48).

Glutathione Peroxidase and Glutathione Reductase

In contrast to catalase, the glutathione redox cycle is a mechanism for scavenging lipid peroxides and H_2O_2. The enzymes in the cycle include GPx and glutathione reductase (GR). GPx is a tetrameric selenoprotein, which uses reduced glutathione as a co-substrate. The glutathione cycle is complementary to catalase in scavenging H_2O_2 with the K_m value of GPx for H_2O_2 being lower than that for catalase. GPx mRNA and protein are expressed in both the alveolar and the bronchial lung epithelia, but the most prominent labeling of GPx protein is seen in the extracellular connective tissue of the lung (49).

B. Nonenzymatic Antioxidants

A number of low molecular weight compounds act as nonenzymatic antioxidants. The major ELF antioxidants in the upper and lower respiratory tract are ascorbate and urate. However, GSH is present at significant concentrations in bronchoalveolar ELF (50).

Vitamin C and Vitamin E

Vitamin C (ascorbic acid) and vitamin E (various tocopherols, of which α-tocopherol is the most active radical scavenger) co-operate in cellular defense against ROS. Vitamin C, a hydrophilic scavenger of ROS, is considered the most important antioxidant in extracellular fluids (50), whereas α-tocopherol is lipophilic and acts to block the chain reaction of lipid peroxidation (12). Ascorbic acid reduces the oxidized α-tocopherol radical back to α-tocopherol (12).

Glutathione

Other important low molecular weight antioxidant is reduced glutathione. In addition to being essential in the glutathione redox cycle, glutathione can scavenge ROS nonenzymatically (51), and detoxify xenobiotics via the glutathione S-transferase reaction. Glutathione protects SH-groups of proteins from oxidation and maintains vitamin C levels (52). Finally, the precursor of glutathione, N-acetyl-cysteine, scavenges ROS and has been studied in a number of clinical trials (28).

Uric Acid

Uric acid is formed together with the superoxide radical anion during the oxidation of xanthine by XDH/XO. Uric acid is an effective scavenger of hydroxyl radicals, peroxyl radicals, peroxynitrites, and singlet oxygen (12).

IV. Biophysical and Biochemical Alterations of the Surfactant System by ROS

A. Effects of ROS on Pulmonary Surfactant

ROS are harmful because they interact with each other and modify critical biomolecules. Lipid peroxidation is a complex process that occurs in the presence of oxygen and transition metal ions or enzymes. It is a radical-mediated chain reaction initiated by abstraction of a hydrogen atom from a polyunsaturated lipid and terminated by chain-breaking antioxidants such as α-tocopherol (13,53). Hydroxyl radical, ROO$^\bullet$, RO$^\bullet$, and some iron complexes, but not $^\pm O_2$ or H_2O_2, are reactive enough to initiate lipid peroxidation. Excessive peroxidation of membrane lipids disrupts the bilayer arrangement, decreases membrane fluidity, increases membrane permeability, and modifies the activity of membrane-bound proteins (12).

The major ST reducing component of pulmonary surfactant is DPPC. Depending on the species, unsaturated PLs represent 50–65% of the weight of mammalian surfactants, and 10–15% of surfactant PLs contain two or more double bonds (3,54). Mixing DPPC with unsaturated PLs lowers its transition temperature, facilitating adsorption to the air–water interface at physiological temperatures. It has been proposed that during compression of the surfactant film, part of the unsaturated components is squeezed out of the monolayer, leading to an increase in the relative proportion of DPPC, thereby enabling the film to achieve a ST near $0 \, mN/m$. The availability of unsaturated lipids to act as liquefiers is thought essential for efficient surfactant adsorption and the reincorporation of material during expansion of the film during the breathing cycle (1).

In the alveolus, the fatty acids of unsaturated surfactant lipids are exposed to strong oxidizing conditions, including direct exposure to oxidative air pollutants and, in the subphase, ROS produced by activated neutrophils and macrophages (9). Oxidation leads to degradation of the unsaturated fatty acids and modification of proteins, thus changing the composition of alveolar surfactant (55,56). This will alter the physicochemical properties, providing a mechanism for loss of surfactant function without a decrease in the concentration of DPPC. The decrease in these unsaturated species, as well as accumulation of lipoperoxidation subproducts such as aldehydes and lysophospholipids, can lead to surfactant dysfunction (9,57). Previous reports from our laboratory and others have shown that LysoPC inhibits surfactant activity (58–62). In addition, lipid peroxidation products can inhibit the synthesis and secretion of new surfactant (63) and reduce the viability of alveolar macrophages and type II pneumocytes (64).

Proteins are also susceptible to oxidative modification (65). It has been reported that the oxidation of SP-A is associated with alterations in its biological activity (66,67). The ability of SP-A to aggregate PLs and to act synergistically with SP-B to lower ST was impaired after *in vitro* exposure to peroxynitrite (56). Exposure of SP-A to NO and superoxide separately did not decrease SP-A-mediated lipid aggregation as observed during concurrent exposure. The concurrent exposure resulted in nitrotyrosine formation, which can only be generated by peroxynitrite (66). Furthermore, *in vivo* oxidative modifications of SP-A have been detected in bronchoalveolar lavage of ARDS patients (68,69), and nitrotyrosine residues were observed in human lung tissue obtained from patients suffering acute lung injury (68,69), indicating that peroxynitrite plays a role in acute lung injury.

Specific structural changes in the hydrophobic proteins exposed to oxidative stress have not yet been reported. When lipid peroxidation occurs in the presence of proteins or peptides, the reactive lipid products such as malondialdehyde (MDA) can form stable adducts with these molecules. Furthermore, SP-B and SP-C exposed to peroxynitrite became less effective in lowering the ST of PL (56).

Biochemical Modifications of Surfactant by ROS

Studies by a number of groups, including our own, have shown that oxidizing either natural or therapeutic lipid extract surfactants results in an increase in the levels of conjugated dienes and the appearance of secondary lipoperoxidation products such as MDA and HNE (55,70). Because of the relatively low levels of polyunsaturated fatty acids, relatively low levels of these primary and secondary oxidative products are observed during surfactant oxidation when compared with those observed with studies on serum lipoproteins (12,62,71,72). In addition, surfactant oxidation occurs rapidly when compared with oxidation of serum lipoproteins where prolonged lag phases are normally encountered (12,62,71,72). The lack of a delay with isolated pulmonary surfactants can be attributed to the low levels of the usual endogenous antioxidants such as ascorbic acid, urate, and reduced glutathione. Rapid reaction times are particularly evident with a number of modified therapeutic surfactants such as bovine lipid extract surfactant (BLES, Fig. 18.3), Curosurf, and Survanta, where the endogenous lipid-soluble α-tocopherol is removed during processing (55,62,72).

Relatively little is known about the individual events occurring during peroxidation of complex mixtures such as pulmonary surfactant. Not surprisingly oxidation of surfactant, for example, either by the hypochlorous acid or by the Fenton reaction leads to a reduction in the levels of unsaturated PLs and increase in the levels of PLs containing peroxide and hydroperoxide modifications. These changes tend to be less evident with oxidation using hypochlorous acid than with the Fenton reaction (72). Alkyl-PC species, which have been suggested as PL protectors (73,74), are not altered significantly during oxidation (72).

The generation of conjugated dienes, MDA and HNE, which indicates reactions of PLs containing unsaturated fatty acids with two or more double bonds, has been studied with serum lipoproteins as well as surfactant (55,62,72). Initial events in the formation of conjugated dienes may involve removal of *bis*-allylic hydrogen atoms, which are prone to abstraction and bond rearrangement. Molecular oxygen could then react to produce alkoxy radicals. Shortened sn-2 residues would then be generated through beta-scission at the site of the former double bond (75).

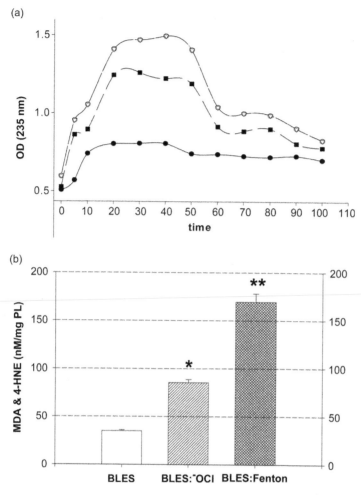

Figure 18.3 (a) The formation of conjugated dienes was monitored, by reading the absorbance at 235 nm. BLES alter the exposure of BLES at 0.25 mg/mL to oxidation. BLES in the absence of oxidants (filled circles), reacted with HOCL/$^-$OCL 0.5 mM (filled squares), and BLES reacted with the Fenton reagents (FeCl$_2$/EDTA/H$_2$O$_2$, 0.65/ 0.65/30 mM, open triangles). (b) The secondary peroxidation products formed during oxidation were measured after 24 h of incubation as the content of MDA and 4-HNE in the surfactant sample. The Fenton reaction, which acts through generation of reactive hydroxyl radical, caused 4.5 times more MDA and HNE than the reaction with HOCL/$^-$OCL, 2.01 (BLES vs. BLES: HOCL/$^-$OCL $p < 0.005$, BLES vs. BLES:Fenton $p < 0.001$).

The resulting lipid hydroperoxides can decompose to aldehydes (76). Uhlson et al. (64) have recently reported that exposure of calf lung surfactant to high concentrations of ozone led to the formation of significant amounts of the oxidation byproducts of 1-palmitoyl-2-oleoyl-PC, a major surfactant PL (64). This suggests that monoenoic fatty acids, thought to be relatively inert, can also be degraded through oxidative reactions.

Studies have reported that oxidative reactions of unsaturated PLs can generate lyso-derivatives (18,31). It appears likely that these compounds arise as a result of two sequential events: oxidation and fragmentation of the sn-2 residues of phosphatidylcholine, followed by the hydrolysis of the shortened fatty acyl residues (75,77). Oxidation of surfactant leads to the liberation of both saturated and unsaturated fatty acids (62,72). Thus oxidation can result in phospholipase A_1- and A_2-like reactions, resulting in the liberation of free fatty acids and loss of the parent PLs (18,31,72).

B. Effects of Oxidation on the Interfacial Properties of Pulmonary Surfactant

A large number of studies by various groups, including our own, have reported that subjecting natural, modified natural (therapeutic), or artificial surfactants to oxidative conditions results in decreased surface activity (55,78). Such investigations include studies on a number of therapeutic modified surfactants such as BLES, Curosurf, Survanta, and artificial therapeutic surfactants such as Exosurf and KL4. In general, it appears that natural surfactants are much less susceptible to the effects of oxidation than the modified natural therapeutic preparations or the artificial surfactants (55,78). Studies on oxidized surfactant using a variety of techniques including the Langmuir–Wilhelmy surface balance, the pulsating bubble surfactometer, and more recently the captive bubble tensiometer (CBT) have revealed that oxidative stress results in a marked decrease in adsorption to equilibrium ST, higher minimal surface tension (ST_{min}) during surface area reduction and higher maximal surface tensions (ST_{max}) during film expansion (62,78).

Recent studies with the CBT have noted that exposure of the bovine surfactant extract, BLES, to HOCl leads to film instability so that oxidized preparations lose the ability to attain ST near 0 mN/m (62,72). In addition, treatment with HOCl resulted in a decrease in surfactant respreadability during film expansion. In contrast, exposing BLES to the Fenton reaction led to a marked increase in compressibility during surface area reduction (62,72).

As discussed earlier, it has long been thought that certain low molecular weight compounds including ascorbate, urate, and reduced glutathione play important roles in contravening surfactant oxidation. In addition, the critical roles of certain antioxidant enzymes, in particular catalase and SOD, are well recognized (79). Recent studies have revealed that other nonenzymatic proteins may also function in contravening the effects of oxidative stress. Studies with serum lipoproteins have shown that apoE and apoAIV can function to limit lipid peroxidation and may be important in the prevention of atherosclerosis (80). It has also been observed that a number of serum proteins including albumin possess the ability to inhibit lipid peroxidation (70,71). Recently, it has been reported that SP-A and SP-D counteract lipid peroxidation (71,81). Although the precise mechanism remains unclear, these surfactant apoproteins block accumulation of conjugated dienes and thiobarbituric acid-reactive substances in oxidant-exposed surfactant and in low density lipoproteins (LDL). The available information suggests that the carbohydrate recognition domains of these C-type lectins are important for the antioxidant properties. Interestingly, neither the closely related, acute-phase, mannose-binding protein nor the structurally similar complement component, C1Q, has the ability to block lipid peroxidation (71).

SP-A and SP-D appear to have a number of important roles in lung homeostasis and function. SP-A has been implicated in the formation of tubular myelin, enhancing ST reduction by surfactant, retarding surfactant secretion, and promoting surfactant uptake by type II cells (1,2). SP-D does not appear to have a major role in ST reduction but can influence surfactant structure (1,2). SP-D has important roles in regulating surfactant homeostasis and in regulating alveolar oxidative capacity. In addition, both SP-A and SP-D play similar but independent critical roles in the innate host defense system, where they promote the host's response to alveolar microbes and particulates (82). Furthermore, it appears that in addition to the ability of SP-A to counteract surfactant inhibition by serum proteins (83,84), SP-A can block the inhibitory effects of oxidation of surfactant function (62,72). Addition of 5% SP-A by weight was able to reverse the debilitating effects of HOCl or Fenton reaction on surfactant adsorption. It is important to mention that in these studies, SP-A was added long after the surfactant oxidation was complete. Furthermore, SP-A restored the ability of the oxidized surfactants to achieve ST_{min} near zero and to maintain ST_{max} near equilibrium (62,72).

It would also be important to determine whether the effects observed here derive from direct interactions between SP-A and surfactant lipids, particularly DPPC, or involve co-operative interactions with other surfactant proteins. Previous investigations have demonstrated that SP-A can interact directly with DPPC (85–87). However, SP-A has only slight effects in enhancing DPPC adsorption by itself, where it interacts with DPPC monolayers to improve compressibility (86,87). SP-A also improves compressibility with DPPC:cholesterol spread films, possibly by reducing SP-A:cholesterol interactions and generating aggregated DPPC domains. SP-A binds DPPC ripple phase and, in the presence of DPPC, can form long strands which could contribute to the formation of tubular myelin (88,89). Recent studies indicate that SP-A binds to liquid condensed phase of spread surfactant monolayers (90). As SP-B and SP-C preferentially locate in liquid expanded phases, this would suggest SP-A and SP-B could occupy different regions of the surfactant monolayers. These observations indicate that SP-A has independent effects on oxidized surfactant films.

In contrast, there is considerable evidence which shows that SP-A can have co-operative effects with SP-B. SP-A can enhance surfactant adsorption, reduce film compressibility, increase respreadability, and limit the surface area

reductions required to attain low STs with surfactant extracts and model surfactant systems containing SP-B but not with systems containing only SP-C
(83,84,91–94). SP-A and SP-B, but not SP-C, are required for reconstitution
of tubular myelin and SP-A can contribute to the formation and maintenance
of the highly surface active large aggregate form of surfactant (95). Whether
SP-A reversal of the effects of surfactant oxidation requires SP-B or SP-C
must be determined through reconstitution studies.

As indicated earlier, it appears that surfactant oxidation by hypochlorous
acid or the Fenton reaction can have distinct effects on surfactant biophysical
function. Hypochlorous acid treatment did not have an apparent effect on film
compressibility but induced film stability as ST was reduced. HOCl also resulted
in poor film respreadability above equilibrium ST. The Fenton reaction greatly
increased film compressibility and appeared to have an effect on respreadability
above equilibrium ST (62,72). The mechanisms responsible for these distinct
effects of oxidation must still be clarified.

Studies on the oxidation of LDL and HDL have shown $HOCl/^-OCl$ is
effective in oxidizing proteins, whereas the Fenton reaction more specifically oxi-
dizes lipids containing unsaturated fatty acyl groups (19,96). Further studies are
required to determine the contribution of oxidation to the SP-B and/or SP-C as
opposed to PL oxidation in surfactant function and the salutary effects of SP-A.

Future studies will be necessary to determine the manner in which SP-A
reverses the effects of oxidation of surfactant biophysical function. As these
effects occur long after oxidation is complete, it is thought that the mechanisms
are separate from those involved in the prevention of lipid peroxidation by SP-A
and SP-D (71,81). That separate mechanisms that are involved also appears likely
from the observation that SP-D has very limited effects on surfactant surface
chemistry (97). It would be important to establish whether the ability of SP-A
to reverse oxidative inhibition is related to selective interactions of SP-A with
DPPC (86–90) or the ability of SP-A to promote co-operative effects with
SP-B (83,84,91–94). Crossover studies with purified surfactant lipids and apoproteins from control and oxidized surfactants are required to address these
issues. In addition, studies using recombinant SP-As and perhaps SP-A:SP-D
and SP-A:mannose binding protein chimeras could also provide considerable
insight into the mechanisms responsible for the dramatic reversal of surfactant
inhibition by oxidative processes.

C. Pathological Processes Involving ROS in the Lung

The upper airways of the normal lung are lined by pseudostratified ciliated cells,
goblet and basal cells. Further down the airways, the epithelium becomes progressively thinner and simplifies. The alveolar epithelium consists of type I pneumocytes,
covering ~90% of the surface area. Type II pneumocytes, present in equal number
to type I cells, cover only ~10% of the alveolar surface. Type II cells produce
surfactant and also act as progenitor cells of the alveolar epithelium (1).

Hyperoxia

The lung is the organ most severely damaged by exposure to hyperoxia. Different animal species show similar morphological changes in response to high oxygen tension (98). Exposure of rats to a lethal dose of hyperoxia (e.g., 100%) shows an initiation phase (first 24–72 h) with no morphological changes, but increased production of ROS (23). Changes in endothelial cell structure leading to increased capillary permeability are the earliest morphological changes in the hyperoxic rat lung, followed by accumulation of inflammatory blood cells (platelets and neutrophils) into intravascular and interstitial spaces and release of inflammatory mediators. The final stage of lethal oxygen toxicity is characterized by endothelial cell damage after 80 h of hyperoxic exposure (98). In rats exposed to high oxygen, the numbers of type I and II pneumocytes remain constant. In contrast, 4 days of hyperoxia exposure to monkeys can result in almost complete destruction of type I pneumocytes leading to hyperplasia of type II pneumocytes (99).

Adult Respiratory Distress Syndrome

ARDS is characterized by severe hypoxemia, pulmonary infiltration, pulmonary edema, and decreased respiratory compliance, occurring in a variety of clinical settings and with uniformly poor prognosis. Massive infiltration of the lungs by neutrophils occurs with consequent oxidant injury. It has been suggested that increased production of ROS by activated neutrophils combined with decreased antioxidant capacity plays a central role in the pathogenesis of ARDS (5,100). Several factors may magnify the production of ROS in acute and chronic lung diseases: (i) during the course of these diseases, oxygenotherapy is commonly necessary to ameliorate the hypoxemia (4,5,100), (ii) in response to proinflammatory cytokines, activated neutrophils and macrophages are recruited into the lung and release ROS (18,100), and (iii) under ischemia, decreased perfusion, low oxygen tension, or trauma, the enzyme xanthine dehydrogenase is converted to xanthine oxidase, which can serve as a locus for the intense production of ROS (24,101). It has been shown recently that overproduction of endogenous NO by alveolar macrophages, epithelial, interstitial, and endothelial cells, as well as by inhalation of NO, contributes to the alveolar epithelium's oxidant burden by the production of reactive oxygen–nitrogen intermediates (102). As it has been proposed that therapy with inhaled NO could be used to treat pulmonary diseases such as lung injury, severe RDS, asthma, lung transplantation, and congenital heart diseases, it is clearly important to consider the potential negative effects of NO on lung oxidant status (13).

Numerous studies have confirmed that patients with ARDS show clear evidence of increased oxidative damage to lipids, proteins, and DNA. There are multiple biophysical and biochemical alterations of lung surfactant associated with ARDS. First, the minimum ST achieved during the film compression increases to $>15–20 \, mN/m$ when compared with near zero in healthy controls (5,10).

The PL profile is also altered with reduction of the relative percentages of PC and phosphatidylglycerol and an increase in the relative percentages of phosphatidylinositol, phosphatidylethanolamine, and sphingomyelin (5). Alterations to the fatty acid composition include a marked reduction of the relative content of the saturated PL fraction, especially palmitic acid (103). Surfactant apoproteins are also affected with decreased levels of SP-A (5,104) and SP-B (10). The content of large aggregates, the active surfactant subfraction, is reduced in patients with ARDS (5).

Asthma

Asthma is a major health problem worldwide, with a prevalence of $\sim 10\%$ among children and 5% among adults in western countries. It is defined by reversible airflow obstruction, bronchial hyper-responsiveness, and chronic inflammation characterized by the influx and activation of inflammatory cells and epithelial cell damage (11,105). Allergic disorders, such as asthma and rhinitis, may be mediated by oxidative stress. Oxidative stress occurs from environmental exposure to air pollution and cigarette smoke as well as a result of inflammation (53,106). In addition, it has recently been shown that in the airway epithelium of asthmatic patients, CuZnSOD, but not catalase or GPx, is decreased (107). Decreased antioxidant defense in the airways of asthmatic patients may be associated not only with the increased oxidant burden, but also with the epithelial injury of these patients. Whatever the underlying factors precipitating asthma, airway inflammation is a key feature (53) characterized by the presence of eosinophils, T lymphocytes, and masts cells in the airways, which can produce free radicals.

Enhörning et al. (108) reported that lavage fluid from antigen-challenged human asthmatics contains agents inhibiting surface activity, particularly at reduced temperatures. Surfactant function was inhibited by segmental allergen challenge in asthmatics (11), whereas the reduced concentration of DPPC in BAL fluid correlated with an increase in protein content (106,108). A complementary study in stable asthmatics revealed decreased DPPC only in sputum but not in BAL fluid, without any change in protein concentration (109).

SP-A levels in the BAL fluid of asthmatic patients are decreased when compared with healthy controls (110), possibly reflecting an impaired resistance against pulmonary inflammation, with further disturbance of the surfactant system. SP-A binds to allergenic glycoproteins from pollen grains, whereas both SP-A and SP-D inhibit binding of allergen-specific IgE to house dust mite extracts. Furthermore, SP-A and SP-D inhibit histamine release in the early phase of allergen provocation and suppress lymphocyte proliferation in the late phase of bronchial inflammation (111). These effects on the two essential steps in the development of asthmatic symptoms point to a possible important protective role for these two proteins.

COPD and Emphysema

COPD is an obstructive airway disorder characterized by a gradually progressive and irreversible decrease in forced expiratory volume (112). This decrease is due to narrowing of the airway lumen and occurs as a direct result of disturbances in airway and interstitial lung tissue. A strong relationship exists between smoking and COPD, with nearly 90% of the patients being smokers.

Considerable evidence links COPD with oxidative stress (112,113), with iron playing a key role. Iron concentrations of smokers are known to be increased in alveolar macrophages, ELF, and upper lobes (30). This is due to a combination of iron present in the cigarette and to the increased release of iron from its binding proteins. As superoxide and hydrogen peroxide will react in the presence of iron to produce the most potent oxidizing agent, the hydroxyl radical, the resultant increase in oxidative stress is obvious (12,30). Cigarette smoke is estimated to contain 500 mg/kg NO and 10^{15} free radicals per puff and so will provide a rich source of oxidants which will again contribute to the increase in oxidative stress (34,114).

In the pathogenesis of COPD, generation of ROS by activated inflammatory cells plays a central role. Cigarette smoke also contributes to the recruitment of inflammatory cells to the airways. Furthermore, this inflammation is stimulated by other inhaled pollutants and by cytokines. A protease–antiprotease imbalance plays an important role in the progression of COPD, but an imbalance between oxidants and antioxidants has also been proposed as playing a role in the pathogenesis of this disease (115).

Damage of Surfactant by Cigarette Smoke

As stressed throughout this chapter, cigarette smoke is a major contributor to oxidative lung damage. Well-established biochemical and biophysical studies support this smoke induced impairment of lung function. Cigarette smoke itself contains ROS. One puff of cigarette smoke has been estimated to contain 10^{15} radicals (34). Cigarette smoke alters the surface activity of pulmonary surfactant as endobronchial washings from long-term cigarette smokers show a significant rise in minimum ST when compared with nonsmokers (116). The data on the contents of PLs are less clear, even though they are the main ST-reducing constituent of surfactant. In the BAL fluid of smokers, reports vary from lower total PL content to no difference and significantly higher levels in smokers compared with nonsmokers (117).

V. Summary

Pulmonary surfactant is essential for normal lung function. The low STs generated with adequate surfactant minimize the differences in surface forces amongst alveoli. Surfactant chemical composition is highly conserved among different species, composed of 85% PL, 5% neutral lipids, and 10% SPs. ROS can damage pulmonary surfactant, altering both biophysical and biochemical properties.

Considerable evidence suggests that oxidative stress, defined as an increased exposure to oxidants and/or decreased antioxidant capacities, is implicated in airway diseases. ROS, produced both intracellularly by lung parenchymal cells and extracellularly by lung macrophages and infiltrating neutrophils, play a central role in the pathogenesis of various lung diseases such as ARDS, asthma, COPD, and infections.

Exposing surfactant to ROS can have several significant effects. There was a marked inhibition in its surface-active properties, including prolonged adsorption times, and elevated ST_{min} and ST_{max}. Recent studies have shown that SP-A can play an important role in the functioning of oxidized BLES. This is accomplished by decreasing compressibility of surfactant films during compression at low STs, stabilizing surface films at low STs, and enhancing respreadability of surfactant lipids during film expansion, thereby maintaining ST_{max} near equilibrium.

Although the negative effects of ROS on surfactant composition and function are obvious, some key areas remain unclear. Further studies are required to determine the relative contributions of oxidized SP-B and/or SP-C, and that of the oxidized PLs, to the observed surfactant function impairment and the mechanisms behind SP-A's "rescue" of surfactant function. Of clinical interest are new methods for preventing pulmonary surfactant oxidation and ultimately inactivation in the course of lung diseases.

References

1. Possmayer F. Physicochemical aspects of pulmonary surfactant. In: Polin RA, Fox WW, eds. Fetal and Neonatal Physiology, 3rd ed. Philadelphia: W.B. Saunders Company, 2004:1014–1034.
2. McCormack FX, Whitsett JA. The pulmonary collectins, SP-A and SP-D, orchestrate innate immunity in the lung. J Clin Invest 2002; 109(6):707–712.
3. Postle AD, Heeley EL, Wilton DC. A comparison of the molecular species compositions of mammalian lung surfactant phospholipids. Comp Biochem Physiol A Mol Integr Physiol 2001; 129(1):65–73.
4. Creuwels LA, van Golde LM, Haagsman HP. The pulmonary surfactant system: biochemical and clinical aspects. Lung 1997; 175(1):1–39.
5. Lewis JF, Veldhuizen R. The role of exogenous surfactant in the treatment of acute lung injury. Annu Rev Physiol 2003; 65:613–642.
6. Seeger W et al. Alteration of surfactant function due to protein leakage: special interaction with fibrin monomer. J Appl Physiol 1985; 58(2):326–338.
7. Pison U et al. Proteolytic inactivation of dog lung surfactant-associated proteins by neutrophil elastase. Biochim Biophys Acta 1989; 992(3):251–257.
8. Saugstad OD. Chronic lung disease: oxygen dogma revisited. Acta Paediatr 2001; 90(2):113–115.

9. Putman E, van Golde LM, Haagsman HP. Toxic oxidant species and their impact on the pulmonary surfactant system. Lung 1997; 175(2):75–103.
10. Gunther A et al. Surfactant alterations in severe pneumonia, acute respiratory distress syndrome, and cardiogenic lung edema. Am J Respir Crit Care Med 1996; 153(1):176–184.
11. Hohlfeld JM. The role of surfactant in asthma. Respir Res 2002; 3(1):4.
12. Eberhardt MK. Reactive Oxygen Metabolites: Chemistry and Medical Consequences. Boca Raton: CRC Press, 2000.
13. Gutteridge JM, Halliwell B. Free radicals and antioxidants in the year 2000. A historical look to the future. Ann N Y Acad Sci 2000; 899:136–147.
14. Fridovich I. Fundamental aspects of reactive oxygen species, or what's the matter with oxygen? Ann N Y Acad Sci 1999; 893:13–18.
15. Pryor WA. Oxy-radicals and related species: their formation, lifetimes, and reactions. Annu Rev Physiol 1986; 48:657–667.
16. Halliwell B, Gutteridge JM. Role of free radicals and catalytic metal ions in human disease: an overview. Methods Enzymol 1990; 186:1–85.
17. Liochev SI, Fridovich I. The Haber–Weiss cycle—70 years later: an alternative view. Redox Rep 2002; 7(1):55–57; discussion 59–60.
18. Downey GP et al. Regulation of neutrophil activation in acute lung injury. Chest 1999; 116(suppl 1):46S–54S.
19. Hawkins CL, Davies MJ. Hypochlorite-induced oxidation of proteins in plasma: formation of chloramines and nitrogen-centred radicals and their role in protein fragmentation. Biochem J 1999; 340(Pt 2):539–548.
20. Halliwell B, Gutteridge JM. The antioxidants of human extracellular fluids. Arch Biochem Biophys 1990; 280(1):1–8.
21. Pryor WA, Squadrito GL. The chemistry of peroxynitrite: a product from the reaction of nitric oxide with superoxide. Am J Physiol 1995; 268(5 Pt 1):L699–L722.
22. Squadrito GL, Pryor WA. Oxidative chemistry of nitric oxide: the roles of superoxide, peroxynitrite, and carbon dioxide. Free Radic Biol Med 1998; 25(4–5):392–403.
23. Freeman BA, Crapo JD. Hyperoxia increases oxygen radical production in rat lungs and lung mitochondria. J Biol Chem 1981; 256(21):10986–10992.
24. Weinbroum A et al. Liver ischemia–reperfusion increases pulmonary permeability in rat: role of circulating xanthine oxidase. Am J Physiol 1995; 268(6 Pt 1):G988–G996.
25. Linder N, Rapola J, Raivio KO. Cellular expression of xanthine oxidoreductase protein in normal human tissues. Lab Invest 1999; 79(8):967–974.
26. Hoidal JR et al. Lung injury and oxidoreductases. Environ Health Perspect 1998; 106(suppl 5):1235–1239.
27. Kishi M et al. Role of neutrophils in xanthine/xanthine oxidase-induced oxidant injury in isolated rabbit lungs. J Appl Physiol 1999; 87(6):2319–2325.
28. Weinbroum AA et al. N-Acetyl-L-cysteine for preventing lung reperfusion injury after liver ischemia–reperfusion: a possible dual protective mechanism in a dose-response study. Transplantation 2000; 69(5):853–859.
29. Gutteridge JM et al. Pro-oxidant iron is present in human pulmonary epithelial lining fluid: implications for oxidative stress in the lung. Biochem Biophys Res Commun 1996; 220(3):1024–1027.
30. Quinlan GJ, Evans TW, Gutteridge JM. Iron and the redox status of the lungs. Free Radic Biol Med 2002; 33(10):1306–1313.

31. Saran M et al. Phagocytic killing of microorganisms by radical processes: consequences of the reaction of hydroxyl radicals with chloride yielding chlorine atoms. Free Radic Biol Med 1999; 26(3–4):482–490.

32. Eiserich JP et al. Formation of nitric oxide-derived inflammatory oxidants by myeloperoxidase in neutrophils. Nature 1998; 391(6665):393–397.

33. Kinsella JP, Abman SH. Recent developments in inhaled nitric oxide therapy of the newborn. Curr Opin Pediatr 1999; 11(2):121–125.

34. Pryor WA, Stone K. Oxidants in cigarette smoke. Radicals, hydrogen peroxide, peroxynitrate, and peroxynitrite. Ann N Y Acad Sci 1993; 686:12–27; discussion 27–28.

35. Ludwig PW et al. Cigarette smoking causes accumulation of polymorphonuclear leukocytes in alveolar septum. Am Rev Respir Dis 1985; 131(6):828–830.

36. MacNee W et al. Cigarette smoke and ozone-induced epithelial perturbation *in vivo* and *in vitro*. The role of glutathione. Chest 1996; 109(suppl 3):39S.

37. Morrow JD et al. Increase in circulating products of lipid peroxidation (F2-isoprostanes) in smokers. Smoking as a cause of oxidative damage. N Engl J Med 1995; 332(18):1198–1203.

38. Petruzzelli S et al. Pulmonary lipid peroxidation in cigarette smokers and lung cancer patients. Chest 1990; 98(4):930–935.

39. Fridovich I. The trail to superoxide dismutase. Protein Sci 1998; 7(12):2688–2690.

40. Crapo JD et al. Copper, zinc superoxide dismutase is primarily a cytosolic protein in human cells. Proc Natl Acad Sci USA 1992; 89(21):10405–10409.

41. Clyde BL et al. Distribution of manganese superoxide dismutase mRNA in normal and hyperoxic rat lung. Am J Respir Cell Mol Biol 1993; 8(5):530–537.

42. Chang LY et al. Immunocytochemical localization of the sites of superoxide dismutase induction by hyperoxia in rat lungs. Lab Invest 1995; 73(1):29–39.

43. Kinnula VL et al. Primary and immortalized (BEAS 2B) human bronchial epithelial cells have significant antioxidative capacity *in vitro*. Am J Respir Cell Mol Biol 1994; 11(5):568–576.

44. Lakari E et al. Manganese superoxide dismutase and catalase are coordinately expressed in the alveolar region in chronic interstitial pneumonias and granulomatous diseases of the lung. Am J Respir Crit Care Med 2000; 161(2 Pt 1):615–621.

45. Marklund SL. Extracellular superoxide dismutase. Methods Enzymol 2002; 349:74–80.

46. Loenders B et al. Localization of extracellular superoxide dismutase in rat lung: neutrophils and macrophages as carriers of the enzyme. Free Radic Biol Med 1998; 24(7–8):1097–1106.

47. Asikainen TM et al. Expression and developmental profile of antioxidant enzymes in human lung and liver. Am J Respir Cell Mol Biol 1998; 19(6):942–949.

48. Erzurum SC et al. *In vivo* antioxidant gene expression in human airway epithelium of normal individuals exposed to 100% O2. J Appl Physiol 1993; 75(3):1256–1262.

49. Coursin DB et al. Immunolocalization of antioxidant enzymes and isozymes of glutathione S-transferase in normal rat lung. Am J Physiol 1992; 263(6 Pt 1): L679–L691.

50. van der Vliet A et al. Determination of low-molecular-mass antioxidant concentrations in human respiratory tract lining fluids. Am J Physiol 1999; 276(2 Pt 1):L289–L296.

51. Morris PE, Bernard GR. Significance of glutathione in lung disease and implications for therapy. Am J Med Sci 1994; 307(2):119–127.
52. Barrios R et al. Oxygen-induced pulmonary injury in gamma-glutamyl transpeptidase-deficient mice. Lung 2001; 179(5):319–330.
53. Bowler RP, Crapo JD. Oxidative stress in allergic respiratory diseases. J Allergy Clin Immunol 2002; 110(3):349–356.
54. Yu S et al. Bovine pulmonary surfactant: chemical composition and physical properties. Lipids 1983; 18(8):522–529.
55. Andersson S, Kheiter A, Merritt TA. Oxidative inactivation of surfactants. Lung 1999; 177(3):179–189.
56. Haddad IY et al. Mechanisms of peroxynitrite-induced injury to pulmonary surfactants. Am J Physiol 1993; 265(6 Pt 1):L555–L564.
57. Zhu S et al. Contribution of reactive oxygen and nitrogen species to particulate-induced lung injury. Environ Health Perspect 1998; 106(suppl 5):1157–1163.
58. Cockshutt AM, Possmayer F. Lysophosphatidylcholine sensitizes lipid extracts of pulmonary surfactant to inhibition by serum proteins. Biochim Biophys Acta 1991; 1086(1):63–71.
59. Enhorning G et al. Phospholipases introduced into the hypophase affect the surfactant film outlining a bubble. J Appl Physiol 1992; 73(3):941–945.
60. Holm BA et al. Biophysical inhibition of synthetic lung surfactants. Chem Phys Lipids 1990; 52(3–4):243–250.
61. Holm BA et al. Inhibition of pulmonary surfactant function by phospholipases. J Appl Physiol 1991; 71(1):317–321.
62. Rodriguez Capote K, Possmayer F. SP-A restores the surface activity of oxidized pulmonary surfactant. Biopys J 2002; 82:2554-Pos.
63. Warburton D et al. Sublethal oxidant injury inhibits signal transduction in rat type II pneumocytes. Am J Physiol 1989; 257(4 Pt 1):L217–L220.
64. Uhlson C et al. Oxidized phospholipids derived from ozone-treated lung surfactant extract reduce macrophage and epithelial cell viability. Chem Res Toxicol 2002; 15(7):896–906.
65. Stadtman ER, Levine RL. Protein oxidation. Ann N Y Acad Sci 2000; 899:191–208.
66. Haddad IY et al. Nitration of surfactant protein A results in decreased ability to aggregate lipids. Am J Physiol 1996; 270(2 Pt 1):L281–L288.
67. Zhu S et al. Nitrated SP-A does not enhance adherence of *Pneumocystis carinii* to alveolar macrophages. Am J Physiol 1998; 275(6 Pt 1):L1031–L1039.
68. Sittipunt C et al. Nitric oxide and nitrotyrosine in the lungs of patients with acute respiratory distress syndrome. Am J Respir Crit Care Med 2001; 163(2):503–510.
69. Zhu S et al. Increased levels of nitrate and surfactant protein A nitration in the pulmonary edema fluid of patients with acute lung injury. Am J Respir Crit Care Med 2001; 163(1):166–172.
70. Marzan Y et al. Effects of simultaneous exposure of surfactant to serum proteins and free radicals. Exp Lung Res 2002; 28(2):99–121.
71. Bridges JP et al. Pulmonary surfactant proteins A and D are potent endogenous inhibitors of lipid peroxidation and oxidative cellular injury. J Biol Chem 2000; 275(49):38848–38855.
72. Rodriguez-Capote K, McCormack FX, Possmayer F. Pulmonary surfactant protein-A (SP-A) restores the surface properties of surfactant after oxidation by a

mechanism that requires the Cys6 interchain disulfide bond and the phospholipid binding domain. J Biol Chem 2003; 278(23):20461–20474.

73. Rustow B et al. Synthesis and secretion of plasmalogens by type-II pneumocytes. Biochem J 1994; 302(Pt 3):665–668.

74. Smiley PL et al. Oxidatively fragmented phosphatidylcholines activate human neutrophils through the receptor for platelet-activating factor. J Biol Chem 1991; 266(17):11104–11110.

75. Porter NA, Caldwell SE, Mills KA. Mechanisms of free radical oxidation of unsaturated lipids. Lipids 1995; 30(4):277–290.

76. Kanazawa K, Ashida H. Dietary hydroperoxides of linoleic acid decompose to aldehydes in stomach before being absorbed into the body. Biochim Biophys Acta 1998; 1393(2–3):349–361.

77. Kanazawa K, Ashida H. Catabolic fate of dietary trilinoleoylglycerol hydroperoxides in rat gastrointestines. Biochim Biophys Acta 1998; 1393(2–3):336–348.

78. Seeger W et al. Alteration of alveolar surfactant function after exposure to oxidative stress and to oxygenated and native arachidonic acid *in vitro*. Biochim Biophys Acta 1985; 835(1):58–67.

79. Macnee W, Rahman I. Oxidants and antioxidants as therapeutic targets in chronic obstructive pulmonary disease. Am J Respir Crit Care Med 1999; 160(5 Pt 2): S58–S65.

80. Qin X et al. Apolipoprotein AIV: a potent endogenous inhibitor of lipid oxidation. Am J Physiol 1998; 274(5 Pt 2):H1836–H1840.

81. Blanco O, Catala A. Surfactant protein A inhibits the non-enzymatic lipid peroxidation of porcine lung surfactant. Prostaglandins Leukot Essent Fatty Acids 2001; 65(4):185–190.

82. Hickman-Davis JM et al. Lung surfactant and reactive oxygen–nitrogen species: antimicrobial activity and host-pathogen interactions. Am J Physiol Lung Cell Mol Physiol 2001; 281(3):L517–L523.

83. Cockshutt AM, Weitz J, Possmayer F. Pulmonary surfactant-associated protein A enhances the surface activity of lipid extract surfactant and reverses inhibition by blood proteins *in vitro*. Biochemistry 1990; 29(36):8424–8429.

84. Venkitaraman AR et al. Enhancement of biophysical activity of lung surfactant extracts and phospholipid-apoprotein mixtures by surfactant protein A. Chem Phys Lipids 1990; 56(2–3):185–194.

85. King RJ et al. Interaction between the 35 kDa apolipoprotein of pulmonary surfactant and saturated phosphatidylcholines. Effects of temperature. Biochim Biophys Acta 1986; 879(1):1–13.

86. Yu SH, Possmayer F. Interaction of pulmonary surfactant protein A with dipalmitoylphosphatidylcholine and cholesterol at the air/water interface. J Lipid Res 1998; 39(3):555–568.

87. Yu SH et al. Interactions of pulmonary surfactant protein SP-A with monolayers of dipalmitoylphosphatidylcholine and cholesterol: roles of SP-A domains. J Lipid Res 1999; 40(5):920–929.

88. Palaniyar N et al. Domains of surfactant protein A that affect protein oligomerization, lipid structure and surface tension. Comp Biochem Physiol A Mol Integr Physiol 2001; 129(1):109–127.

89. Palaniyar N et al. Formation of membrane lattice structures and their specific interactions with surfactant protein A. Am J Physiol 1999; 276(4 Pt 1):L642–L649.

90. Taneva SG, Keough KM. Differential effects of surfactant protein A on regional organization of phospholipid monolayers containing surfactant protein B or C. Biophys J 2000; 79(4):2010–2023.

91. Hawgood S et al. Nucleotide and amino acid sequences of pulmonary surfactant protein SP 18 and evidence for cooperation between SP 18 and SP 28–36 in surfactant lipid adsorption. Proc Natl Acad Sci USA 1987; 84(1):66–70.

92. Rodriguez-Capote K et al. Surfactant protein interactions with neutral and acidic phospholipid films. Am J Physiol Lung Cell Mol Physiol 2001; 281(1):L231–L242.

93. Yu SH, Possmayer F. Effect of pulmonary surfactant protein A (SP-A) and calcium on the adsorption of cholesterol and film stability. Biochim Biophys Acta 1994; 1211(3):350–358.

94. Yu SH, Possmayer F. Role of bovine pulmonary surfactant-associated proteins in the surface-active property of phospholipid mixtures. Biochim Biophys Acta 1990; 1046(3):233–241.

95. Veldhuizen RA et al. Surfactant-associated protein A is important for maintaining surfactant large-aggregate forms during surface-area cycling. Biochem J 1996; 313(Pt 3):835–840.

96. McIntyre TM, Zimmerman GA, Prescott SM. Biologically active oxidized phospholipids. J Biol Chem 1999; 274(36):25189–25192.

97. Poulain FR et al. Ultrastructure of phospholipid mixtures reconstituted with surfactant proteins B and D. Am J Respir Cell Mol Biol 1999; 20(5):1049–1058.

98. Crapo JD. Morphologic changes in pulmonary oxygen toxicity. Annu Rev Physiol 1986; 48:721–731.

99. Kinnula VL et al. Oxidants and antioxidants in alveolar epithelial type II cells: *in situ*, freshly isolated, and cultured cells. Am J Physiol 1992; 262(1 Pt 1):L69–L77.

100. Chabot F et al. Reactive oxygen species in acute lung injury. Eur Respir J 1998; 11(3):745–757.

101. Weinbroum AA et al. Multiple organ dysfunction after remote circulatory arrest: common pathway of radical oxygen species? J Trauma 1999; 47(4):691–698.

102. Matthay MA et al. Oxidant-mediated lung injury in the acute respiratory distress syndrome. Crit Care Med 1999; 27(9):2028–2030.

103. Hall SB et al. Altered function of pulmonary surfactant in fatty acid lung injury. J Appl Physiol 1990; 69(3):1143–1149.

104. Greene KE et al. Serial changes in surfactant-associated proteins in lung and serum before and after onset of ARDS. Am J Respir Crit Care Med 1999; 160(6):1843–1850.

105. Maddox L, Schwartz DA. The pathophysiology of asthma. Annu Rev Med 2002; 53:477–498.

106. Heeley EL et al. Phospholipid molecular species of bronchoalveolar lavage fluid after local allergen challenge in asthma. Am J Physiol Lung Cell Mol Physiol 2000; 278(2):L305–L311.

107. Smith LJ et al. Reduced superoxide dismutase in lung cells of patients with asthma. Free Radic Biol Med 1997; 22(7):1301–1307.

108. Enhorning G et al. Surfactant function affected by airway inflammation and cooling: possible impact on exercise-induced asthma. Eur Respir J 2000; 15(3):532–538.

109. Wright SM et al. Altered airway surfactant phospholipid composition and reduced lung function in asthma. J Appl Physiol 2000; 89(4):1283–1292.

110. van de Graaf EA et al. Surfactant protein A in bronchoalveolar lavage fluid. J Lab Clin Med 1992; 120(2):252–263.

111. Wang JY et al. Inhibitory effect of pulmonary surfactant proteins A and D on allergen-induced lymphocyte proliferation and histamine release in children with asthma. Am J Respir Crit Care Med 1998; 158(2):510–518.

112. MacNee W. Oxidative stress and lung inflammation in airways disease. Eur J Pharmacol 2001; 429(1–3):195–207.

113. Rahman I et al. 4-Hydroxy-2-nonenal, a specific lipid peroxidation product, is elevated in lungs of patients with chronic obstructive pulmonary disease. Am J Respir Crit Care Med 2002; 166(4):490–495.

114. Eiserich JP et al. Molecular mechanisms of damage by excess nitrogen oxides: nitration of tyrosine by gas-phase cigarette smoke. FEBS Lett 1994; 353(1):53–56.

115. Rahman I et al. Is there any relationship between plasma antioxidant capacity and lung function in smokers and in patients with chronic obstructive pulmonary disease? Thorax 2000; 55(3):189–193.

116. Honda Y et al. Decreased contents of surfactant proteins A and D in BAL fluids of healthy smokers. Chest 1996; 109(4):1006–1009.

117. Subramaniam S et al. Alteration of pulmonary surfactant proteins in rats chronically exposed to cigarette smoke. Toxicol Appl Pharmacol 1996; 140(2):274–280.

19

Novel Surfactant Therapy for Developing Countries: Current Status and Future Directions

RINTI BANERJEE

School of Biosciences and Bioengineering, Indian Institute of Technology, Mumbai, India

I. Introduction

Pulmonary surfactant lines the alveoli and is composed of saturated and unsaturated phospholipids, neutral lipids, and surfactant specific proteins SP-A, -B, -C, and -D. It prevents the alveoli from collapsing during expiration and decreases our work of breathing. Surfactant may be quantitatively and/or qualitatively dysfunctional in various respiratory diseases. A replacement surfactant would be beneficial for the therapy of such diseases. In this chapter, I will describe the potential of herbal oil based surfactants for neonatal and adult respiratory distress syndromes. I will also explore some less documented areas of respiratory diseases where surfactants might be altered and there may be a scope for future surfactant applications.

II. Surfactant Therapy in Neonatal Respiratory Distress Syndrome

Neonatal respiratory distress syndrome (NRDS) occurs in newborn infants, especially in those who are born prematurely. In such babies, development of the alveolar type II cells has not yet arrived at a stage sufficient to generate the necessary surfactant material. This lack of surfactant interferes with the ability of the lungs to properly inflate during respiration. Avery and Mead were the first to demonstrate that a deficiency in lung surfactant is a major cause of NRDS and that such a deficiency leads to a high surface tension in the alveoli. Our knowledge of the lung surfactant system has grown vastly over the decades, and exogenous surfactants have been used with a high success rate in NRDS, all over the world.

Meta-analysis of surfactant therapy in NRDS has evaluated the efficacy of surfactant therapy, as well as compared the effects of high doses vs. low doses, prophylactic therapy vs. rescue therapy, single dose vs. multiple doses, and natural surfactants vs. synthetic surfactants. While comparing the natural and synthetic surfactants, meta-analysis has revealed a reduced risk of pneumothorax and a borderline reduced risk of neonatal mortality in those treated with natural surfactants than those treated with synthetic surfactants (1). However, the differences were not very large, and the choice of the type of surfactant is to be determined keeping the entire situation in mind such as the speed of action required, cost, and availability.

III. Status of Surfactant Therapy for NRDS in Developing Countries

In spite of the tremendous success of surfactant therapy across the world, the progress in surfactant therapy in developing countries has been limited.

However, in developing countries like India, the animal-derived surfactants, such as Curosurf and Survanta and the synthetic products ALEC and

Exosurf, are neither affordable nor readily available. Thousands of babies are dying every day due to lack of adequate intensive care, delay in transfer to the elite intensive care units, and more specifically, due to the lack of an affordable and effective surfactant replacement therapy. NRDS affects 7–12% of newborns in India and is associated with a high mortality rate (2,3). It is only in the last 5–6 years that surfactant therapy is being used sparingly to treat infants with NRDS. Similarly, in Malaysia also the advent of surfactant therapy in NRDS has been recent, and the high costs are hindering in its widespread use.

For India and many other developing countries, there is an urgent need for the development of new, effective, and affordable surfactants for NRDS. In this chapter, I will highlight some of the initial promising findings with respect to the development of an affordable herbal oil based surfactant. In the next section, I will briefly enumerate the methods that are used for the *in vitro* evaluation of replacement surfactants for therapy.

IV. *In Vitro* Evaluation of Surfactants

The models that are the most widely used to evaluate the efficacy of surfactants are the Langmuir balance (4), the pulsating bubble surfactometer (5), and the captive bubble surfactometer (6). All these instruments model the air–aqueous interface of the alveoli and study the dynamic surface activity of the surfactants at this interface. Details regarding the assumptions, advantages, and disadvantages of these techniques have been discussed in earlier reviews (7).

V. Parameters of Physiological Relevance

Using the *in vitro* models mentioned in the last section, the dynamic surface activity of surfactants are compared and their possible physiological effects *in vivo* are inferred. The surface properties that are of physiological relevance for an effective therapeutic surfactants are (1) minimum surface tension on dynamic compression, (2) adsorption rate, (3) film compressibility, (4) stability of monolayer, (5) phase transitions of the monolayer, and (6) re-spreading ability from hypophase to interface on repeated compressions.

The criteria for an ideal replacement surfactant are (1) ability to reduce the surface tension to <5 mN/m on dynamic compression at the respiratory rate as the *in vivo* surface tension of lung surfactant has been documented to reach near zero values of surface tension by fluorescent droplet studies. This property will allow the surfactant to prevent alveolar collapse during expiration. (2) An adsorption time of the order of few milliseconds. The lung surfactant needs to form a surface-active monolayer at the air–aqueous interface of the alveoli within the time frame of a single breath and hence a quick adsorption is a prerequisite for a substitute surfactant. (3) A low compressibility of the monolayer of the order of 0.005–0.01 mN/m of the first compression monolayer. The compressibility will be calculated as a measure of the inverse of the slope of the surface tension area isotherm of the surfactant. A low value is observed in the case of lung surfactant and is beneficial as it implies that the surface tension is reduced with minimal film compression leaving a large area behind in the lungs for gas exchange. (4) High stability given by a low desorption coefficient of the monolayer that is held constant at its minimum surface tension. This would ensure that an active functional surfactant remains at the alveolar interface for maintaining alveolar patency.

Two other characteristics of relevance are the phase transition of the monolayer from liquid expanded to condensed and solid phase and as the re-spreading of the surfactant. Dipalmitoyl phosphatidylcholine (DPPC), the main constituent of lung surfactant, was found to be effective owing to a high transition temperature, above body temperature enabling close packing of the monolayer to near "solid" phases capable of maintaining high surface pressures required for lung function. The re-spreading ratio is a parameter that is evaluated from the length of the collapse plateaus of the surfactant monolayers during successive cycles. It evaluates the ability of the lung surfactant to re-enter the interface from the hypophase during successive respiratory cycles causing replenishment and effective functioning. A higher re-spreading is considered effective to prevent depletion of the surfactant from the interface.

All these criteria are to be fulfilled ideally at 37°C and a pH of 7.4 to simulate body conditions. In the absence of an ideal performance, surfactants are compared on their relative performance in these criteria.

VI. *In Vitro* Results for Herbal Oil Surfactants for NRDS

We have evaluated the surface activity of phospholipids in combination with herbal oils as surfactants that may act as promising alternatives to the existing products and may be of particular importance to developing countries. The herbal oil surfactants have been evaluated in a modified Langmuir balance and a pulsating bubble surfactometer. Figures 19.1 and 19.2 show the performance of some of the promising novel herbal oil based surfactants in comparison with those of the commercial surfactants with respect to surface parameters of physiologic relevance. We evaluated the surfactants in a pulsating bubble surfactometer. We cycled the bubble in automatic mode between R_{min} and R_{max} at 40 cycles/min (cpm) for 10 cycles. Cycling was stopped at R_{min} and the bubble was expanded manually to R_{max} and held static for 10 s. The static surface tension was measured. This gives an indication of the adsorption of the surfactant. Stability index (SI) was calculated as $SI = 2(\gamma_{max} - \gamma_{min})/(\gamma_{max} + \gamma_{min})$ at 40 cpm. A 40 cpm was chosen as the frequency of oscillation because it corresponds to the neonatal respiratory rate and is the frequency which is used clinically in ventilator settings for a neonate with respiratory distress syndrome.

For evaluation of the re-spreading, we studied surface excess films of the surfactants in a Langmuir trough. Surfactants were dissolved in chloroform to

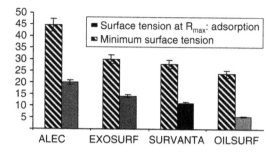

Figure 19.1 Surface tension achieved by oil based surfactant and therapeutic surfactants in a pulsating bubble surfactometer. *Y*-axis shows the surface tension (mN/m). Lower values of surface tension are beneficial. The study was conducted in a pulsating bubble surfactometer at a temperature of 37°C, and the surface tension on adsorption to a bubble of radius R_{max} 0.5 mm and the minimum surface tension on pulsation for 30 s at the rate of 40 cpm were compared. [Figure is based on data from Banerjee and Bellare (8,9).]

a concentration of 1 mg/mL, and the solution was spread drop-wise from a syringe at the air–water interface under surface excess conditions. This refers to a high initial surface concentration of monolayer coverage (15 Å^2 per molecule). All experiments were carried out at a body temperature of 37°C ± 0.5°C

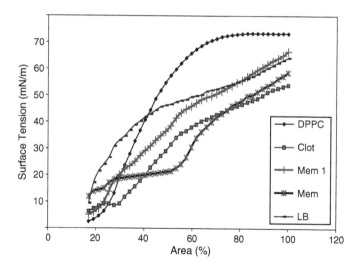

Figure 19.2 Comparison of stability index and re-spreading ratio of therapeutic surfactants and herbal oil based surfactants. The quantities are unitless ratios. Higher values of stability index and re-spreading ratio are beneficial physiologically. Stability index was calculated from the experiments in a pulsating bubble surfactometer, whereas the re-spreading ratio was calculated from the surface pressure-area isotherms in a Wilhelmy balance. Due to the aqueous nature of Survanta, re-spreading was not studied. [Figure is based on data from Banerjee and Bellare (8,9).]

using Ringer's lactate as the subphase adjusted to a pH of 7.4 and a calcium concentration of 2.5 mM. A time span of 10 min was allowed for solvent evaporation before commencing cycling. Seven successive cycles of compression/expansion at the interface were recorded between maximum and minimum areas with a compression ratio of 4:1 at a constant speed of 1.2 cpm. The compression ratio of 4:1 is much higher than that found in normal respiratory cycles. However, this ratio was used in order to obtain information regarding the re-spreading capability of the surfactants. This was done by comparison of collapse–plateau ratios which could be obtained on maximum compression of the films past collapse.

The figures indicate that at a concentration of 1 mg/mL of phospholipid, the herbal oil added surfactant denoted as OILSURF achieved lower values of minimum surface tension and adsorption surface tension when compared with ALEC and Exosurf, two commercially available therapeutic surfactants, in the state of art *in vitro* models such as the pulsating bubble surfactometer. Further, OILSURF had a higher stability, a higher re-spreading, and a higher hysteresis area (data not shown) when compared with the commercial surfactants. These properties in turn determine the ability of the surfactant to form a film at the air–aqueous interface in the alveoli, prevent alveolar collapse, reduce the work of breathing, and re-enter the interface on successive breaths.

VII. Proposed Mechanism of Action of Herbal Oil Surfactants

The herbal oil surfactants have superior properties with respect to adsorption and re-spreading when compared with some of the existing surfactants. We propose that this is due to the possible effects of the herbal oils in shifting the phase transition temperature of the surfactant mixture as explained subsequently.

DPPC alone is unable to be an effective surfactant replacement therapy due to its poor adsorption to the air–liquid interface. This is due to its gel to liquid crystalline transition temperature being higher than that of body temperature. The herbal oils studied have various short chain alcohols as their main components. It is proposed that the alcohols in the herbal oils allow the fluidization of the surfactant to allow the adequate adsorption of the surfactant. The transition temperature of the lamellar aggregates of lung surfactant or any of its replacements should be close to body temperature as the rate of fusion of vesicles at an air–water interface are highest at the transition temperature of the substance. This then promotes rapid monolayer formation at the alveolar interface. This is achieved by reducing the phase transition temperature of the phospholipid–herbal oil mixture. Herbal oils can either directly adsorb to the interface along with the phospholipids and then get selectively squeezed out from the surfactant monolayers on compression or they could aid the selective enrichment of DPPC to the interface. The mechanism by which this occurs is as yet unknown. Whether the oils remain in a surface associated reservoir and aid in re-spreading of the film during expansion remains to be seen. The surfactant specific proteins are known to cause an improved functioning of the lung surfactant *in vivo* by similar mechanisms.

VIII. Surfactant Therapy in Adult Respiratory Distress Syndrome

Apart from NRDS, surfactant is also dysfunctional in adult respiratory distress syndrome (ARDS). ARDS is a condition of secondary dysfunction of lung surfactant due to inactivation by the presence of plasma proteins and edema fluid in the lungs. However, most replacement surfactants have been designed for the NRDS, which is caused by a primary deficiency of pulmonary surfactant. The properties essential for a surfactant to be effective in ARDS will differ from those required for the neonatal condition as the pathophysiology of the two diseases differ markedly. Inhibition of the function of pulmonary surfactant in the alveolar space is an important element of the pathophysiology of ARDS.

The known mechanisms by which surfactant dysfunction occurs are (a) competitive inhibition of phospholipid entry into the surface monolayer (e.g., by plasma proteins) and (b) infiltration and destabilization of the surface film by extraneous lipids (e.g., meconium-derived free fatty acids). Surfactant secreted in ARDS is qualitatively different from normal surfactant and is further responsible for the stimulation of macrophages which release phospholipase A_2 causing oxidation of the phospholipids in lung surfactant. In addition the leakage of protein-rich edema fluid into the lungs in ARDS may be a major factor contributing to abnormal surface activity due to the inhibition of surfactant caused by blood, plasma, serum proteins, fibrin, fibrin degradation products, oxygen radicals, and a number of enzymes.

Although some impairment of production and secretion of surfactant constituents may be present in ARDS, surfactant inactivation is probably a more important factor in this disease. Until recently, surfactants available for human use have been easily susceptible to inactivation and this may explain why they have been less successful for treatment of ARDS than for NRDS.

Studies have indicated that the present day protein-free surfactants are more susceptible to inhibition than the animal-derived surfactants containing surfactant-specific proteins. We are trying to fill this gap by developing more effective protein-free herbal oil based surfactants that will have an improved ability to withstand inhibition.

Research is actively being carried out internationally for the development of a surfactant that can withstand inactivation and hence will be suitable for therapy in ARDS. The research is directed both toward development of synthetic protein analogs and other agents which when added to the surfactants available for NRDS will withstand inactivation by plasma proteins, meconium, and other inhibitory agents. Recent data suggest that addition of nonionic polymers, such as dextran and polyethylene glycol, to surfactant mixtures may significantly improve resistance to inhibition (10,11). Polymers have been found to neutralize the effects of several different inhibitors and can produce near-complete restoration of surfactant function. The anti-inhibitory properties of polymers, and their possible role as an adjunct to surfactant therapy deserve further exploration. Tashiro et al. (12) have shown that an addition of dextran to surfactant increases resistance to inactivation by albumin and meconium.

Most of the *in vitro* studies using inhibitory models for ARDS use various plasma proteins as models for the inactivating fluid flooding the alveoli (13–15). However, the interaction of pure plasma proteins with the surfactant system may not be suitable in predicting the inhibition caused by more complex systems, such as whole blood, lysed blood, serum, and so on, that may reach the alveoli during ARDS and alter the lung surfactant function.

IX. Surfactant Inhibition Studies *In Vitro*

We have been evaluating the relative inhibitory capacities of different blood components on the lung surfactant system. In our initial studies, we have used DPPC monolayers as simple models of lung surfactant and have studied the interaction of blood components with this monolayer using a Langmuir trough. Our preliminary results show that complex physiological fluids, such as whole blood, serum, platelet rich plasma, lysed erythrocytes, differ in their abilities to inhibit the surface activity of the DPPC monolayers. The inhibitory capacity of these systems is not predicted by the behavior of the individual proteins. We have used whole blood and its components as inhibitors in our surface activity studies. The inhibitors are mixed in the subphase of physiological saline prior to spreading the DPPC monolayers. DPPC was spread on the surface at a concentration of 100 Å^2 permolecule. After allowing time for solvent evaporation, the monolayers were compressed to one-fifth the original area at 37°C and a speed of 1.2 cpm. Figure 19.3 shows the preliminary results of the surface tension isotherms of DPPC in the absence and presence of the blood components. The ratio of lipid to inhibitor was 10 parts of DPPC per million parts of inhibitor. Most of the pure plasma proteins were not inhibitory to the surface activity of DPPC (data not shown) and even in mixtures of albumin, fibrinogen, and hemoglobin were unable to achieve the same inhibition as serum, clot, lysed blood, and erythrocyte membranes. Serum, lysed blood, and red cell membranes caused an increase in the minimum surface tension reached as well as the percentage area change required to reach a surface tension <10 mN/m. Both of these would have deleterious effects on pulmonary physiology. We are presently evaluating the relative effects of blood components in the form of platelet rich and poor plasma, combinations of pure proteins, serum, and so on, on the minimum surface tension, compressibility, percentage area change, and adsorption of more complex models of lung surfactant mixtures.

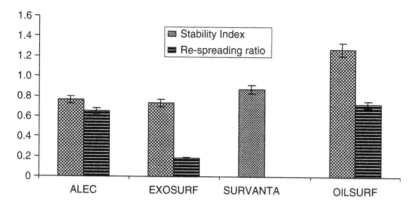

Figure 19.3 Surface activity of DPPC in presence of hematological inhibitors. RBC membranes (Mem), clot (Clot), and lysed blood (LB) were used as inhibitors in a ratio of 10 parts of DPPC per million parts of inhibitor (w/v). For RBC membranes, a lower concentration of inhibitor in the ratio of 50 parts DPPC per million parts of inhibitor is also depicted (Mem 1).

The surface activity of DPPC with eucalyptus oil was also tested in the presence of erythrocyte membranes. Some preliminary isotherms of herbal oil added surfactants have been depicted in Fig. 19.4. The inhibitors used were the same as in the previous experiment, only eucalyptus oil was added to DPPC as a model surfactant monolayer. The results were promising and further studies

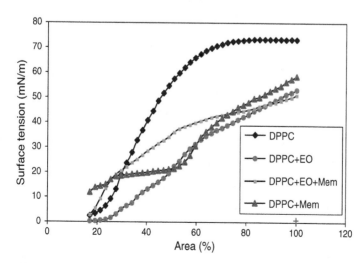

Figure 19.4 Surface activity of DPPC and herbal oils in the presence of red cell membranes RBC membranes are added in a concentration of 10 parts of surfactant to 1 million parts of the inhibitor. Eucalyptus oil was added to DPPC as a model herbal oil surfactant.

need to be done to evaluate the effects of herbal oil surfactants to overcome inhibition of increasing concentrations of hematological inhibitors. It would be interesting to explore the effects of other known protective agents, such as polymers, in combination with the herbal oil surfactants.

X. Tropical Causes of ARDS

Apart from the well-recognized causes of lung injury and sepsis leading to ARDS, there are certain infective causes that are common in the tropical countries. Specifically, malaria, typhoid, sepsis, and strongyloides infections account for major causes of ARDS in the tropics. Interesting among these is the widely occurring number of cases of malaria and typhoid that lead to ARDS (16).

Malaria is one of the major world public health problems resulting in more than 1 million deaths worldwide. It is a protozoan disease transmitted by the bite of infected Anopheles mosquitoes. Four species of the genus *Plasmodium* cause all infections in humans, that is, *Plasmodium vivax, P. ovale, P. malariae*, and *P. falciparum*. Clinically significant pulmonary involvement is seen in up to 5% of infected patients, ranging from mild cough to respiratory failure due to ARDS. Fulminant respiratory failure is an often-fatal manifestation of *P. falciparum* malaria in adults and is usually associated with cerebral malaria, acute renal failure, high levels of parasitemia, or delayed treatment (17,18). The central pathologic feature of severe falciparum malaria is the sequestration of parasitized erythrocytes in the microvasculature of organs including the lung (19).

Strongyloides stercoralis is a free-living parasite that is endemic throughout the tropics. The larvae of *S. stercoralis* penetrate the skin and enter the patient's blood, traveling to the lung *en route* to the small intestine to complete their life cycle. It develops when larvae, which have hatched from eggs laid by adult worms in the duodenum develop into the infective stage, re-penetrate the bowel and develop into adult forms and spread throughout the body, particularly into the lungs. The patients suffering from this infestation develop spiking fever, anemia, weight loss, diffuse alveolar infiltrates, and hypoxic respiratory failure resembling ARDS (20).

It would be interesting to evaluate whether the alterations in surface activity of bronchoalveolar lavage fluid in these cases are different from that of the other well-known causes. Further, there may be subtle changes in the inhibition seen in ARDS depending on the causative factor. These may be manifested by the different degrees to which the different surface activity parameters are affected. Further, it will be a challenge to try and tailor make surfactants for specific causes of ARDS. The effect of antimalarial drugs or antiparasitic drugs, as the case may be, encapsulated in surfactant formulations needs to be explored.

So far, the discussion has been restricted to the presence and alteration of surfactant in the alveoli in NRDS and ARDS. The next section describes the roles assigned to airway surfactants and their effects on mucociliary clearance and mucus biophysical properties.

XI. Role of Airway Surfactant in Chronic Obstructive Pulmonary Diseases

Effective mucociliary clearance requires the transmission of the kinetic energy from the beating cilia to the respiratory mucus layer. The mucociliary apparatus consists of the cilia surrounded by periciliary fluid and the airway surfactant and respiratory mucus gel at the tips of the cilia. The beating cilia are surrounded by a periciliary fluid layer that appears to be regulated in depth and composition by transepithelial and pericellular ion and water transport. There is strong evidence that this periciliary fluid layer is separated from the mucus layer by surfactant phospholipids. Surfactant is functionally beneficial to the airways for mainten-ance of airway patency and reduction of airway resistance (21–23) Hence, the layer of surface-active material in the airways by its ability to reduce surface tension causes a decrease in the pressure required to keep small airways dis-tended. Surfactant in the airways can decrease the mucus adhesivity to the airway epithelium and thus help to facilitate clearance (24). A high adhesivity inhibits the changes in surface architecture required to produce waves on the surface of the mucus. This in turn prevents adequate mucus propagation and clearance.

In many airway diseases, such as bronchial asthma and chronic bronchitis, there is an alteration in the airway surfactant composition and function as well as a change in the rheological parameters of the mucus that affect the mucociliary and airflow or cough clearance. A surfactant that can favorably alter the biophysi-cal properties of mucus aiding in clearance of secretions either by the mucociliary apparatus or by the cough clearance would be promising in such conditions. Exogenous surfactants can have therapeutic benefits in airway diseases if they favorably alter the rheological properties of mucus.

XII. Rheological Properties of Airway Mucus

Airway mucus is a non-Newtonian fluid and behaves as a viscoelastic gel having both viscous and elastic responses. It is important to evaluate the frequency dependence of the rheological parameters as low frequency deformations are rel-evant to mucus transport by ciliary beating and high frequency deformations are relevant to the cough clearance of mucus. Several studies of dynamic rheology of mucus have indicated that the parameters associated with mucus clearance are the overall mucus impedance and the ratio of viscosity to elasticity. These par-ameters are evaluated by analyzing the response of mucus after subjecting it to a sinusoidal oscillatory stress. G^* is the vectorial sum of the elastic and viscous moduli and represents the overall impedance or rigidity of the mucus.

During sinusoidal deformations, the elastic component of the mucus viscoelasticity (G') is in phase with the applied stress, whereas the viscous component (G'') lags 90° out of phase. The ratio of G''- to -G' is tan δ, also called loss tangent, where δ is the phase shift.

Mucociliary clearance and cough clearance are negatively correlated with log G^* at low and high frequencies, respectively. Mucociliary clearance also correlates negatively with tan δ at low frequencies. However, cough clearance is positively correlated with tan δ at high frequencies. Thus, an increase in the ratio of viscosity and elasticity of the mucus usually leads to a decrease in its mucociliary clearance and an increase in its cough clearance (25–27). For optimal mucociliary clearance, the rheological characteristics of respiratory mucus must lie within certain limits. The requirement for mucus with specific rheological characteristics may be due to the need for efficient transfer of energy from the cilia to the mucus for effective transport. Table 19.1 enumerates some rheological properties of respiratory mucus that are favorable for mucociliary clearance.

Changes in either the mucus viscosity or the mucus elasticity lead to impaired mucus clearance and syndromes of mucus hypersecretion as in chronic bronchitis, cystic fibrosis, and chronic asthma. King et al. (28) have found a negative correlation between surface tension and mucus clearance. This has been confirmed by Rubin et al. (29) in their study of interfacial tension and rheology of respiratory mucus. In this study, sputum from patients of chronic bronchitis had a high surface tension and was associated with an increased mucus viscoelasticity.

Though the role of surfactants in lowering surface tension is well documented, very few studies have considered the effect of surfactants on the rheology of respiratory mucus. Rubin et al. (30) have described the efficacy of Exosurf in reducing the viscoelasticity of mucus in respiratory distress syndrome. de Sanctis et al. (31) studied the effect of Curosurf on mucus viscosity and mucociliary clearance in dogs suffering from respiratory distress syndrome. The tracheal mucus velocity was found to increase significantly, but no changes were observed in viscoelastic parameters. Our group is interested in studying the effects of herbal oil surfactants on rheology of mucus. Our preliminary studies with mucus gel simulants have shown that various phospholipid mixtures as

Table 19.1 Properties of Respiratory Mucus Favoring Mucociliary Clearance

Mucus properties	Values
Elastic modulus	$1-2 \text{ N/m}^2$
Concentration of macromolecules	$1.5-2\%$
Dynamic viscosity	$5-20 \text{ Pa s}$
Spinnability	$>70 \text{ mm}$

well as herbal oil based surfactants decrease the viscosity of these simulants. We are presently exploring the effects of these surfactants on the rheological profile of mucus from asthmatic patients.

Before ending this chapter, I will introduce two other promising areas of surfactant research that are gaining increasing importance in recent times: pollution and pulmonary tuberculosis. First, the effects of environmental pollutants on the lung surfactant system is presented.

XIII. Interaction of Surfactants with Environmental Pollutants

There is an overwhelming increase in the levels of air pollution worldwide due to the increased emissions from manufacturing industries and transportation exhausts. Our lungs are particularly vulnerable to damage by extrinsic inhalation agents. The large alveolar surface area is ventilated by $\sim 10 \times 10^3$ L of air daily that may be contaminated by a diverse range of gaseous, particulate, or liquid aerosol pollutant. Pulmonary surfactant lines the air–liquid interface of the alveoli and, thus, is in direct contact with this potentially harmful environment of pollutants. An alteration of lung surfactant would make our lungs prone to collapse and increase the respiratory distress. Identification of the specific functions of lung surfactant that are altered due to specific pollutants is of extreme importance today.

Pollutants of particular interest worldwide are ozone, particulates, and nitrogen dioxide. Ozone is a strong oxidizing agent formed in the troposphere through a series of reactions involving the action of sunlight on nitrogen dioxide and hydrocarbons. Ozone has been shown to have a powerful oxidant activity and activates stress-signaling pathways of epithelial cells and alveolar inflammatory cells (32). Currie et al. (33) have demonstrated that the bronchoalveolar lavage fluid from rats exposed to 2 ppm ozone for a period of 2–8 h had a significantly decreased ability to maintain airway patency as evaluated by a capillary surfactometer. Ozone exposure was found to alter the structural characteristics of lamellar bodies in type II alveolar cells. There was a decrease in the lysozyme levels associated with these lamellar bodies and these changes preceded an increase in the alveolar levels of plasma protein due to ozone exposure (34). This evidence implies the ability of ozone to adversely affect the lung surfactant system.

"Particulate air pollutants" is a term used to describe a complex mixture of anthropogenic and naturally occurring airborne particles. The site of attack or reaction of a particulate air pollutant within the respiratory system is dependent on the solubility of the reactant chemicals in aqueous media and on the diameter of the particle or aerosol. A distinction is made between PM 10 which are particles smaller than 10 μm in diameter that can penetrate into the lower respiratory system, PM 2.5 or respirable particles smaller than 2.5 μm that can penetrate into

the gas-exchange region of the lungs, and ultra-fine particles smaller than 100 nm
that can contribute little to particle mass but which are most abundant in terms of
numbers and offer a very large surface area and are able to reach the alveoli.
Although it is not clear from epidemiology whether it is the nature, mass,
number, or surface area of particles that is the most important determinant of
health impact, some toxicological studies show that ultra-fine particles exert a
much larger physiological effect than the same mass of larger particles.
Johnston et al. (35) showed that inhalation exposure to ultra-fine particles
of ∼16 nm of polytetrafluorethylene, a low toxicity material in the particle
form of diameter >0.5 μm, caused acute pulmonary toxicity and mortality in
rats. Fine and ultra-fine particles are mainly found in emissions from combustion
processes and are mostly composed of carbonaceous material, metals, sulfate,
nitrate, and ammonium ions. Recent studies have shown that road traffic and
stationary combustion sources generate a significant number of nanoparticles
of diameter <10 nm (36). It has been documented that an increase in the concentration of respirable and particulate matter is associated with an increase in the
overall mortality rates (37).

Exposure to silica is an especially effective stimulus that causes massive
increases in surfactant concentrations both within the type II pneumocytes and
in the alveolar lining fluid. The condition induced in the lungs of rats by
inhaled and/or intratracheally instilled silica closely resembles the human lung
disease known as pulmonary alveolar proteinosis (38). Pulmonary surfactant
floods the alveoli on exposure to numerous other toxic agents, either particulate
or chemical. Particulates other than silica known to induce surfactant flooding in
the lungs include asbestos, aluminum, titanium dioxide, nickel, and diesel
exhaust. The increased lung surfactant could be the result of an attempt to try
and protect the alveoli from cytotoxic effects of the pollutants. For mineral
dust induced surfactant accumulation, there was little or no change in the composition of extracellular surfactant phospholipid and fatty acid composition of phosphatidyl choline (39). In contrast, diesel particles given intratracheally to rats
produced an increased level of lavage phospholipids with elevated phosphatidyl
choline content (40). Further details of the ratio of the various saturates and surfactant proteins, their surface activity, and structural changes induced in the accu-
mulated surfactant will help to improve our understanding of the interactions due
to specific pollutants.

Nitrogen dioxide is mainly found in the atmosphere due to the combustion
of fossil fuels and from motor vehicles. In ambient conditions, the atmospheric
nitric oxide is rapidly transformed into nitrogen dioxide by oxidants such as
ozone. Not much is known about the respiratory effects of nitrogen dioxide. It
has an oxidant action and is responsible for impairing the function of alveolar
macrophages and epithelial cells. Both short (3–16 ppm for 1 h and 15 ppm
for 28 h) and chronic (3 ppm, 24 h daily, 5 days a week for 9 months) exposures
to nitrogen dioxide caused an increase in the minimal surface tension of alveolar
surfactant (41,42). Surfactant protein-A gets functionally impaired on exposure

to nitrogen dioxide and ozone as certain amino acids, such as methionine and tryptophan get oxidized (43,44).

For millions of people living in rural areas in developing countries, indoor pollution from the use of biomass fuels occurs at concentrations that are several orders of magnitude higher than currently seen in the developed world (45). This exposure has been shown to be associated with an increased incidence of respiratory infections. Table 19.2 enumerates some of the ways by which air pollutants can adversely affect the pulmonary surfactant system. We are evaluating the effects of the ambient atmospheric pollutants in the form of PM 2.5 fractions, diesel exhausts and the indoor pollutants in the form of biofuel combustion sources for their effects on the lung surfactant system.

There is a need for further evaluation of the effects of air pollutants on different components of the lung surfactant system. Research should be directed at the relative importance of various characteristics of the pollutants on their adverse effects, their mechanisms of action and at identifying specific surfactant components that minimize the adverse interactions between the pollutants and the respiratory function.

XIV. Surfactant System in Pulmonary Tuberculosis

The other disease that is regaining importance, not only in developing countries but also worldwide, is tuberculosis (TB). TB continues to plague us even today with rising morbidity and mortality. The respiratory system is the first site of entry of the TB bacilli and they will primarily interact with molecules in their immediate environment. There is a close proximity between the bacilli and the lung surfactant suggesting close interactions between them. The cell wall of the mycobacterium has many components, such as glycopeptidolipids (GPLs), mycolic acid, and phosphatidyl inositol, that may interfere with the surface activity of pulmonary surfactant. Further, the phospholipids of lung surfactant

Table 19.2 Possible Adverse Effects of Air Pollutants on the Lung Surfactant System

Damage to Clara cells
Altered number of alveolar macrophages and epithelial cells
Replacement of type I cells by type II cells
Impaired antibacterial defense mechanism of the alveoli
Oxidation and decreased biological activity of SP-A
Impaired tubular myelin formation
Abnormal structure of lamellar bodies
Increased accumulation of extracellular phospholipids in the alveoli
Flooding of serum proteins in the alveoli

may be responsible for the resuscitation of the dormant tubercular bacilli. The interactions between the bacilli and the lung surfactant could determine the extent of spread of the disease as well as the ventilation/perfusion mismatch due to localized collapse of the alveoli. There is a need to explore these interactions. The biophysical interactions between lung surfactant and tubercular cell wall components could lead to a better understanding of the role of surfactants in pathogenesis and progress of active pulmonary TB. The ability of lung surfactant to alter progression of the disease should be evaluated and can lead to new therapeutic options in TB. Given the universal nature of the problem of pulmonary TB, any research that helps in understanding the disease and in alleviating its harmful effects will have a tremendous impact on health globally.

A study by Vergne and Desbat (46) using GPLs from opportunistic tubercular pathogens, such as *Mycobacterium avium*, *M. intracellulare*, and *M. scrofulaceum*, evaluated the surface activity of these GPLs with a Langmuir trough individually and on insertion beneath a preformed DPPC monolayer. The isotherms depict that these molecules by themselves have the ability to adsorb to the air–aqueous interface. GPLs are also present in tubercular cell wall. When tested individually, GPLs reached a surface pressure of 30 mN/m; whereas for an effective lung surfactant, we require a surface pressure of the order of ~70 mN/m. The presence of GPLs could, thus, lower the surface pressure of the lung surfactant monolayer. GPLs could get inserted in the pure DPPC films and have a fluidizing effect which would then increase the tendency of the lungs to collapse.

Cord factor consisting of mycolic acids are found in mycobacterium TB and is believed to be one of the virulence factors. Such cord factors have also been isolated from norcardia asteroids. It strongly inhibits fusion between the unilamellar vesicles containing acidic phospholipids (47). It is seen that cord factor increases molecular area of preformed phospholipid monolayer as measured by isothermal compression of the monolayer. The cord factor can then actually cause a similar effect on lung surfactant hindering the ability to reach low surface pressures.

Unlike most bacteria, which are killed by macrophages, pathogenic mycobacteria are able to survive and even multiply in the cytoplasm of macrophages. The survival of the mycobacteria depends on their ability to overcome the microbicidal power of the macrophages. It is likely that their entry path may provide mycobacteria with a survival advantage (48). Indeed, studies have demonstrated that the attachment of mycobacteria to the phagocytes varies according to the mycobacterial strain and the activation state of the phagocyte. It has been demonstrated that two key elements of innate immunity against airborne pathogens, pulmonary SP-A and SP-D, interact with *M. tuberculosis*. Although the interaction of *M. tuberculosis* with SP-D reduces the uptake of the bacilli by macrophages (49), it has been shown that the interaction with SP-A promotes this uptake (50). This suggests that SP-A may provide mycobacteria with an important target-cell entry pathway. The carbohydrate recognition domain (CRD) of

SP-A is believed to interact with a glycoprotein on the surface of the tubercle bacilli because binding was inhibited either by deglycosylated SP-A or by competition with mannosyl bovine serum albumin.

In summary, tubercular cell wall lipids have the capability to get detached from the cell wall and get inserted and adsorbed to the air–aqueous interface. They may thereby alter the surface-active properties of lung surfactant making the patient prone to increased work of breathing and alveolar collapse. Though there is some evidence in the literature of the potential harmful effects of these tubercular components on the lung surfactant system, the number of studies is few. The immunological aspects of lung surfactant in TB has been studied to some extent, but there is a dearth of studies that evaluate various biophysical surface properties of lung surfactant in the presence of tubercular bacteria and their physiological consequences. The evaluation of the surface activity of bronchoalveolar lavage and sputum of cases of pulmonary TB as well as the detailed evaluation of the surface activity of components of lung surfactant in the presence of the tubercle bacilli and their components will help us to gain further insight into this condition.

XV. Improved Delivery Forms of Lung Surfactant

Our increasing knowledge of the importance of lung surfactant in various diseases will have an increased impact if the surfactant can be delivered in a non-invasive manner. Lung surfactant is mostly administered in the form of intratracheal instillations. This method allows delivery of a known amount of the surfactant directly into the lungs and avoids losses in the upper airways. However, tracheal instillation causes a heterogenous distribution of the surfactant in the alveoli. Intratracheal inhalation has been shown to overcome this problem and ensure that a large amount of the dispensed substance reaches the lungs as well as ensuring a more uniform distribution in the alveoli (51). Figure 19.5 schematically shows the relative distributions of particles using intratracheal instillation and inhalation. This method needs to be explored further, and improvements in this technique could be applied to surfactant delivery to ensure a more uniform distribution in the alveoli.

A further improvement from the intratracheal inhalation technique would be effective use of nebulizers such that the losses of drug are minimized and the alveolar deposition is improved. The respiratory tract has become an increasingly attractive route for drug delivery not only to the alveoli but also for the systemic effects. The challenge in pulmonary application of drugs is in atomization of the drug or surfactant formulation in a form suitable for inhalation. It is generally accepted that aerosol particles of $1–5$ μm are required for deposition in the alveoli. Nanoparticle formulations having particles of diameter < 1 μm are more easily incorporated in the respirable percentage of aerosolized droplets (droplets exhibiting a mass median aerodynamic diameter of $1–5$ μm). Recent studies

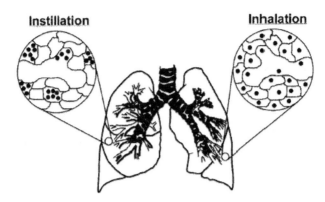

Figure 19.5 Comparison of the alveolar particle distribution using intratracheal instillation and intratracheal inhalation. [Reproduced with permission from Osier and Oberdörster (51).]

have generated respirable aerosols with jet nebulizers using colloidal dispersions of beclomethasone diproprionate with mean particle diameter <400 nm (52). In addition, small battery operated ultrasonic nebulizers have been developed, and Ostrander et al. (53) have demonstrated an increased respirable fraction by using a concentrated nanocrystalline dispersion of beclomethasone diproprionate. The use of nanocrystalline material enhances the probability that each vehicle droplet will possess a drug population for a given homogenous suspension. Improved nebulization techniques that improve the postinhalation alveolar deposition will greatly improve the widespread application of surfactants. However, it should be kept in mind that this should not be at the cost of surfactant efficacy. Wagner et al. (54) found that the ultrasonic nebulization of surfactant suspensions at frequencies >1.8 MHz resulted in a decreased phospholipid content. A challenging direction for future research will be the development of more effective alveolar deposition of surfactant using less invasive routes without sacrificing the surface activity of the formulation.

XVI. Issues of Toxicity of Herbal Oil Surfactants

For the future application of these herbal oil surfactants, their safety must be unequivocally established. There have been concerns regarding the safety of these oils. The literature has evidence of both its safety and incidents regarding its toxic effects (55–58). Although the purity of the pharmaceutical grade of herbal oils ensures >98% of the main constituent, it is of importance to evaluate the exact composition of the herbal oils being evaluated. Even trace amounts of a secondary component could be responsible for toxic effects and a purer component would overcome any toxic effects. We are evaluating the detailed effects of these herbal oils and their components to ensure the safety of the substance without losing out on its therapeutic potential. Our preliminary results have shown their safety in certain *in vitro* cell models, but further evaluation is underway.

XVII. Summary

Surfactant therapy has come a long way from the initial discovery of surface-active material in the lungs and its deficiency in NRDS several decades ago. Researchers all over the world have gained an insight into the working of pulmonary surfactant and have developed improved surfactants for therapy of NRDS. Apart from the recent advances made in the field of recombinant surfactant proteins, herbal oil based surfactants are one promising angle and need to be further explored. Surfactant research has broadened into its applications in many respiratory conditions and identifying the exact dysfunctions of the surfactant systems in these conditions is an interesting field of research. Further, this could lead to the development of tailor-made surfactants that would be effective in various respiratory conditions depending on the underlying pathogenesis of the condition. Side-by-side, the delivery forms of surfactant also need to be improved to be able to make a significant impact on many respiratory diseases.

Acknowledgments

I would like to thank Dr. Neil Morton for allowing me to use the Pulsating Bubble Surfactometer at the Royal Hospital for Sick Children, Glasgow, United Kingdom. I acknowledge the contributions made by my doctoral students Ms. Rachana Rastogi and Dr. Geetanjali Chimote on ARDS and tuberculosis.

References

1. Robertson B, Halliday HL. Principles of surfactant replacement. Biochim Biophys Acta 1998; 1408:346–361.
2. Neonatal Morbidity and Mortality: Report of the National Neonatal Perinatal Database. Indian Pediatr 1997; 34:1089–1092.
3. Narang A, Kumar P, Dutta S, Kumar R. Surfactant therapy for hyaline membrane disease: the Chandigarh experience. Indian Pediatr 2001; 38:640–646.
4. Clements J. Surface tension of lung extracts. Proc Soc Exp Biol Med 1957; 95:170–172.
5. Enhorning G. Pulsating bubble technique for evaluating pulmonary surfactant. J Appl Physiol 1977; 43:198–203.
6. Schurch S, Bachofen H, Goerke J, Possmayer F. A captive bubble method reproduces the *in situ* behavior of lung surfactant monolayers. J Appl Physiol 1989; 67:2389–2396.
7. Banerjee R. Surface chemistry of the lung surfactant system: techniques for *in vitro* evaluation. Curr Sci 2002; 82:420–428.

8. Banerjee R, Bellare JR. Comparison of *in vitro* surface properties of clove oil–phospholipid suspensions with those of ALEC, Exosurf and Survanta. Pulm Pharmacol Ther 2001; 14:85–91.

9. Banerjee R, Bellare JR. *In vitro* evaluation of surfactants with eucalyptus oil for respiratory distress syndrome. Respir Physiol 2001; 126:141–151.

10. Dargaville PA, Morley CJ. Overcoming surfactant inhibition with polymers. Acta Paediatr 2000; 89:1397–1400.

11. Lu KW, Taeusch WH, Robertson B, Goerke J, Clements JA. Polymer-surfactant treatment of meconium-induced acute lung injury. Am J Respir Crit Care Med 2000; 162:623–628.

12. Tashiro K, Kobayashi T, Robertson B. Dextran reduces surfactant inhibition by meconium. Acta Paediatr 2000; 89:1439–1445.

13. Notter RH, Wang Z, Holm B. Function and dysfunction of endogenous and exogenous lung surfactants. Res Adv Lipids 2000; 1:73–105.

14. Kuo R, Chang C, Yang Y, Maa J. Induced removal of DPPC by exclusion of fibrinogen from compressed monolayers at air/liquid interfaces. J Colloid Interf Sci 2003; 257:108–115.

15. Wen X, Franses EI. Adsorption of bovine serum albumin at the air–water interface and its effects on the formation of DPPC surface film. Colloid Surf 2001; 190:319–322.

16. Jindal SK, Aggarwal AN. and Gupta D. Adult respiratory distress syndrome in the tropics. Clin Chest Med 2002; 23:445–455.

17. Lichtman AR, Mohrcken S, Engelbrecht M et al. Pathophysiology of severe forms of falciparum malaria. Crit Care Med 1990; 18:666–668.

18. Aursudkij B, Wilairatana P, Vannaphan S et al. Pulmonary edema in cerebral malaria patients in Thailand. Southeast Asian J Trop Med Public Health 1998; 29:541–545.

19. Urquhart AD. Putative pathophysiological interactions of cytokines and phagocytic cells in severe human falciparum malaria. Clin Infect Dis 1994; 19:117–131.

20. Cook GA, Rodriguez ZH, Silva H et al. Adult respiratory distress secondary to strongyloidiasis. Chest 1987; 92:1115–1116.

21. Enhorning G, Holm BA. Disruption of pulmonary surfactant's ability to maintain openness of a narrow tube. J Appl Physiol 1993; 74:2922–2927.

22. Yager D, Butler JB, Bastacky J et al. Amplification of airway constriction due to filling of airway interstices. J Appl Physiol 1989; 66:2873–2884.

23. Kamm RD, Scrofer RC. Is airway closure caused by a liquid film instability? Respir Physiol 1989; 75:141–156.

24. Reifenrath R. Open airways—an engineering achievement of nature. Bull Eur Physiopath Respir 1978;14:79–81.

25. King M. Mucus and mucociliary clearance. Respir Care 1983; 28:335–344.

26. Lethem MI. The role of tracheobronchial mucus in drug administration to the airways. Adv Drug Delivery Rev 1993; 11:271–298.

27. Griese M, App EM, Derouix A, Burkert A, Schams A. Recombinant human DNase (rhDNase) influences phospholipid composition, surface activity, rheology and consecutively clearance indices of cystic fibrosis sputum. Pulm Pharmacol Ther 1997; 10:21–27.

28. King M, Zahm JM, Pierrot D, Vaquez-Girod S, Puchelle E. The role of mucus gel viscosity, spinnability and adhesive properties in clearance by simulated cough. Biorheology 1978; 26:737–745.

29. Rubin BK, Tomkiewicz RP, Ramirez OE, King M. Surface properties of respiratory secretions: relationship with mucus transport. Biorheology 1990; 32:213–217.
30. Rubin BK, Ramirez O, King M. Mucus rheology and transport in neonatal respiratory distress syndrome and the effect of surfactant therapy. Chest 1992; 101:1080–1085.
31. de Sanctis, GT, Tomkiewicz RP, Rubin BK, Schurch S, King M. Exogenous surfactant enhances mucociliary clearance in the anaesthetised dog. Eur Respir J 1994; 7:1616–1621.
32. Brunekreef B, Holgate ST. Air pollution and health. Lancet 2002; 360:1234–1242.
33. Currie WD, van Schaik SM, Vargas I, Enhorning G. Ozone affects breathing and pulmonary surfactant function in mice. Toxicology 1998; 125:21–30.
34. Shelley SA, Paciga JE, Balis JU. Lysozyme is an ozone-sensitive component of alveolar type II cell lamellar bodies. Biochim Biophys Acta 1991; 1096:338–344.
35. Johnston CJ, Finkelstein JN, Mercer P et al. Pulmonary effects induced by ultrafine PTFE particles. Toxicol Appl Pharmacol 2000; 168:208–215.
36. Ping SJ, Evans DE, Khan AA, Harrison RM. Sources and concentration of nanoparticles <10 nm diameter in the urban atmosphere. Atmos Environ 2001; 35:1193–1202.
37. Pope CA III, Thun MJ, Namboodiri MM et al. Particulate air pollution as a predictor of mortality in a prospective study of US adults. Am J Respir Crit Care Med 1995; 151:669–674.
38. Hepplestone AG. Pulmonary toxicology of silica, coal and asbestos. Environ Health Perspect 1984; 55:111–127.
39. Kornbrust DJ, Hatch GR. Effect of silica and volcanic ash on the contents of lung alveolar and tissue phospholipids. Environ Res 1984; 35:140–153.
40. Eskelson CD, Chvapil M, Strom KA, Vostal JJ. Pulmonary phospholipidosis in rats respiring air containing diesel particulates. Environ Res 1984; 44:260–271.
41. Williams RA, Rhoades RA, Adams WS. The response of lung tissue and surfactant to nitrogen dioxide exposure. Arch Intern Med 1971; 128:101–108.
42. Arner EC, Rhoades RA. Long-term nitrogen dioxide exposure. Arch Environ Health 1973; 26:156–160.
43. Muller B, Seifart C, Barth PJ. Effect of air pollutants on the pulmonary surfactant system. Eur J Clin Invest 1998; 28:762–777.
44. Oosting RS, van Greevenbroek MMJ, Verhoef J, van Golde LMG, Haagsman HP. Structural and functional impairment of surfactant protein A induced by ozone. Am J Physiol 1991; 261:L77–L83.
45. Smith KR, Samet JM, Romieu I, Bruce N. Indoor air pollution in developing countries and acute lower respiratory infections in children. Thorax 2000; 55:518–532.
46. Vergne I, Desbat B. Influence of the glycopeptidic moiety of mycobacterial glycopeptidolipids on their lateral organization in phospholipid monolayers. Biochim Biophys Acta Biomembr 2000; 1467:113–123.
47. Crowe L, Spargo J, Ioneda T, Beaman L, Crowe H. Interaction of cord factor with phospholipids. Biochim Biophys Acta 1994; 1194:53–60.

48. Sidobre S, Puzo G, Rivieare M. Lipid-restricted recognition of mycobacterial lipoglycans by human pulmonary surfactant protein A: a surface-plasmon-resonance study. Biochem J 2002; 365:89–97.

49. Ferguson JS, Voelker DR, McCormack FX, Schlesinger LS. Surfactant protein D binds to *Mycobacterium tuberculosis* bacilli and lipoarabinomannan via carbohydrate lectin interactions resulting in reduced phagocytosis of the bacteria by macrophages. J Immunol 1999; 163:312–321.

50. Downing JF, Pasula R, Wright JR, Twigg HLD, Martin WJD. Surfactant protein A promotes attachment of *Mycobacterium tuberculosis* to alveolar macrophages during infection with human immunodeficiency virus. Proc Natl Acad Sci USA 1995; 92:4848–4852.

51. Osier M, Oberdörster G. Intratracheal inhalation vs. intratracheal instillation: differences in particle effects. Fundam Appl Toxicol 1997; 40:220–227.

52. Wiedman TS, DeCastro L, Wood RW. Nebulization of nanocrystals: production of a respirable solid-in-liquid-in-air colloidal dispersion. Pharm Res 1997; 14:112–116.

53. Ostrander KD, Bosch HW, Bondanza DM. An *in vitro* assessment of a Nano-Crystal[TM] beclomethasone dipropionate colloidal dispersion via ultrasonic nebulization. Eur J Pharm Biopharm 1999; 48:207–215.

54. Wagner MH, Wiethoff S, Friedrich W et al. Ultrasonic surfactant nebulization with different exciting frequencies. Biophys Chem 2000; 24:35–43.

55. Gerosa R, Borin M, Menegazzi G, Puttini M, Cavalleri G. *In vitro* evaluation of the cytotoxicity of pure eugenol. J Endod 1996; 22:532–534.

56. Rompelberg CJ, Vogels JT, de Vogel N et al. Effect of short-term dietary administration of eugenol in humans. Hum Exp Toxicol 1996; 15:129–135.

57. Shapiro S, Meier A, Guggenheim B. The antimicrobial activity of essential oils and essential oil components towards oral bacteria. Oral Microbiol Immunol 1994; 9:202–208.

58. Tibballs J. Clinical effects and management of eucalyptus oil ingestion in infants and young children. Med J Aust 1995; 163:177–180.

Index